VOLUME II

ACLS
COMPREHENSIVE REVIEW

Volume II
ACLS
COMPREHENSIVE REVIEW
Third Edition

Ken Grauer, M.D., F.A.A.F.P.

Professor
Department of Community Health and Family Medicine
Assistant Director, Family Practice Residency Program
College of Medicine, University of Florida, Gainesville
ACLS National Affiliate Faculty

Daniel Cavallaro, REMT-P

Research Director
The Center for Cardiopulmonary Research
Children's Research Institute
   at All Children's Hospital, St. Petersburg, Florida
Past ACLS National Affiliate Faculty

with 286 illustrations

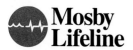

St. Louis Baltimore Boston Chicago London Philadelphia Sydney Toronto

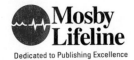
Dedicated to Publishing Excellence

Publisher: David T. Culverwell
Executive Editor: Richard A. Weimer
Assistant Editor: Julie Scardiglia

Printed in the United States of America

Mosby–Year Book, Inc.
11830 Westline Industrial Drive
St. Louis, Missouri 63146

Library of Congress Cataloging in Publication Data
Grauer, Ken.
    ACLS / Ken Grauer, Daniel L. Cavallaro.—3rd ed.
      p.   cm.
    Includes bibliographical references and index.
    Contents: v. 1. Certification preparation—v. 2. Comprehensive review.
    ISBN 0-8016-7069-1 (v. 1) : $19.95.—ISBN 0-8016-7070-5 (v.2) : $34.95
    1. Cardiovascular emergencies—Problems, exercises, etc.
2. Cardiac arrest—Treatment—Problems, exercises, etc. 3. CPR (First aid)—Problems, exercises, etc. I. Cavallaro, Daniel L.
II. Title.
    [DNLM: 1. Heart Arrest—problems. 2. Life Support Care—problems.
3. Resuscitation—problems. WG 18 6774a]
RC675.G73   1993
616.1′025′076—dc20
DNLM/DLC
for Library of Congress   92-48248
                               CIP

93 94 95 96 97 GW/VH 9 8 7 6 5 4 3 2

Authors' Commentary
As This Book Goes to Press
The New Guidelines: *How We Compare*

Revised and updated Guidelines for Cardiopulmonary Resuscitation and Emergency Cardiac Care (put forth by the Emergency Cardiac Care Committee/Subcommittees and American Heart Association) have now been published in the Journal of the American Medical Association (JAMA 268:2171-2295, 1992). The contents of this work reflect proceedings of the 1992 National Conference on Cardiopulmonary Resuscitation (CPR) and Emergency Cardiac Care (ECC)—and forms the basis of the soon-to-be published revised American Heart Association Textbook on ACLS.

As emphasized in its introduction, the new guidelines "do not represent broad changes, nor do they suggest that care provided under past guidelines is either unsafe or ineffective" (ECC/AHA Committee—JAMA, 1992). Note is made in the document of how the term "standards" is conspicuous by its absence from the title of the new recommendations, underscoring a definite lack of "legalistic or prohibitory function" (Paraskos—1992). The authors then go on to openly acknowledge that "deviations from (the new) recommendations and guidelines *may* be warranted when a trained physician (or medical care provider) proficient in CPR and ECC recognizes that such is in the best interest of the patient" (ECC/AHA Committee—JAMA, 1992). Thus the new guidelines are in no way put forth as the sole acceptable approach to cardiopulmonary resuscitation.

For the most part, suggestions and recommendations in our ACLS materials are in close conformance with those presented in the new ECC/AHA guidelines. Nevertheless, *minor differences do exist.* In cases where this occurs, our preferences and opinions are clearly stated as such—based on our approach to clinical integration of existing literature. For purposes of successfully completing the ACLS Provider Course we therefore suggest checking *beforehand* with ACLS faculty of the particular course you are taking *to clarify the range of responses that will be acceptable for the various clinical code simulations of that particular course.*

We summarize below the principle areas where differences arise between our approach and that recommended in the new guidelines:

Use of Magnesium—The new ECC/AHA guidelines primarily favor use of magnesium sulfate for treatment of ventricular arrhythmias (including ventricular fibrillation/tachycardia) in patients with *documented* hypomagnesemia.

In addition to this indication, we favor consideration of magnesium administration for treatment of these arrhythmias in patients with normal (or unknown) serum magnesium levels—especially in lifethreatening situations—when standard antiarrhythmic therapy has been ineffective—and in patients who are *likely to be* intracellularly depleted of this cation.

Use of Epinephrine—The new ECC/AHA guidelines favor administration of **S**tandard-**D**ose **E**pinephrine **(SDE)** in a dose of 1 mg IV as the first agent to be used in cardiac arrest, with repetition of this dose at 3 to 5 minute intervals. Use of **H**igh-**D**ose **E**pinephrine **(HDE)** "is acceptable (after the 1 mg dose has been tried and failed)—but can be neither recommended nor discouraged." Higher doses of epinephrine (of at least 2 to 2.5 times the peripheral IV dose) are likely to be needed when the drug is administered by the *endotracheal route.*

While acknowledging the lack of data demonstrating improved survival from the use of HDE, we nevertheless favor strong consideration for rapidly escalating the dose of epinephrine administered to HDE (i.e., up to a dose of 0.1 to 0.2 mg/kg) for cases of ventricular fibrillation, asystole, and EMD if one (or *at most two*) doses of SDE fail to produce the desired response. We especially favor the use of HDE for treatment of cardiac arrest that occurs outside of the hospital and/or in patients known (or suspected) of having been unresponsive for an extended period of time. Use of HDE should also translate to the use of higher epinephrine doses for *endotracheal route* administration—with increases to 2 mg to 3 mg— *or more*—if the patient fails to respond to the initial 1 mg ET dose.

Use of Atropine—The new ECC/AHA guidelines allow for an increase in atropine dosing to a total of 0.04 mg/kg (or about 3 mg).

While acknowledging 0.04 mg/kg as the full vagolytic dose, we feel the key concepts are the cautions and reduced indications for the use of this drug—and appreciation of the fact that patients who fail to respond to the previously recommended 2 mg total dose are not very likely to respond to higher atropine doses.

Use of Verapamil/Adenosine—The new ECC/AHA guidelines favor use of adenosine as the antiarrhythmic agent of first choice for pharmacologic treatment of PSVT.

While fully acknowledging the beneficial features of adenosine and the clear need for caution when administering verapamil, we favor consideration of both drugs as *alternative* first-line agents of comparable efficacy for treatment of PSVT. Because each drug has advantages and drawbacks, we base distinction in our selection between these two agents on clinical parameters of the particular case.

Energy Requirements for Defibrillation—Recommendations in the new ECC/AHA guidelines are similar to those put forth in the 1986 Guidelines. Thus, 200 joules are recommended for the *initial* defibrillation attempt—200 to 300 joules are *acceptable* for the second attempt—360 joules are recommended for the third and subsequent attempts—and the recommendation for ventricular fibrillation recurrence is for treatment with countershock at the same energy level that last resulted in successful defibrillation.

We differ slightly from these recommendations by regularly favoring an increase in energy selection for the second defibrillation attempt from 200 to 300 joules (to *ensure* greater current flow)—and in favoring a drop back to 200 joules for the initial countershock delivery if (and when) ventricular fibrillation recurs at a later point in the code.

Approach to Management of a Regular Wide Complex Tachycardia of Uncertain Etiology—Emphasis must always be on "treating the patient and not the monitor." Thus *all* wide complex tachycardias must be assumed ventricular in etiology until proven otherwise. The new ECC/AHA Guidelines downplay the potential role of the 12-lead ECG in the diagnostic process. They recommend treatment initially with lidocaine—to be followed with adenosine if there is no response.

While fully agreeing that the overwhelming majority of wide complex tachycardias of uncertain etiology are ventricular tachycardia (and that they need to be *treated accordingly* until *proven* otherwise), we firmly believe that attention to selected morphologic features on the 12-lead tracing will often be of invaluable assistance for increasing the certainty of one's preliminary diagnosis. As a result, we strongly favor obtaining a 12-lead ECG on all hemodynamically stable patients who present with a wide complex tachycardia *whenever* this is feasible. We also favor stronger consideration of procainamide as a first-line agent for medical treatment of wide complex tachyarrhythmias of uncertain etiology.

Use of the Term Pulseless Electrical Activity (PEA)—The new ECC/AHA guidelines introduce the term **PEA** to encompass EMD (i.e., electromechanical dissociation) *and* a heterogeneous group of rhythms that includes "pseudo-EMD", ventricular escape rhythms, post-defibrillation IVR (idioventricular rhythm), and other bradyasystolic rhythms.

While acknowledging the overlap in definition and management of these entities, we favor continued use of traditional terminology with distinction between EMD, asystole, and other bradyarrhythmias (including slow IVR).

KEN GRAUER
DAN CAVALLARO

References

Emergency Cardiac Care Committee and Subcommittees, American Heart Association: Guidelines for Cardiopulmonary Resuscitation and Emergency Cardiac Care, *JAMA* 268:2171-2295, 1992.

Paraskos JA: Emergency Cardiac Care: The Science Behind the Art, *JAMA* 268:2295-2297, 1992.

PREFACE to the Third Edition: Why This Book Now Consists of Two Volumes

(and How to Find What You're Looking For)

Since publication of the second edition of this book six years ago, numerous advances have been made in the field of cardiopulmonary resuscitation and emergency cardiac care. In response to these advances, to recent revision by the American Heart Association of their guidelines for cardiopulmonary resuscitation, and to feedback received from readers of our second edition, the need was felt to revise this book.

Medical knowledge continues to expand at an exponential rate. Thus, our second edition published in 1987 was double the size of our first edition. This third edition again *doubles* the size of its predecessor. Yet despite the ever increasing size of this book, our dual motivation for writing it remains the same:

i) To provide a practical, easy-to-read *study guide* that facilitates preparation for the ACLS course and *complements* American Heart Association guidelines (and their textbook).

ii) To provide a state-of-the-art, clinically relevant reference source for *comprehensive review* on key topics of interest that relate to cardiopulmonary resuscitation and emergency cardiac care.

Practical space constraints have made these two goals mutually exclusive. There simply was no way to retain the convenient size required of a study guide with the amount of expansion needed to accommodate all of the new material. Fortunately, a solution soon became obvious: *Expand the book into two separate volumes.*

In an attempt to preserve the style and format of our second edition, we have kept the structural organization from that book largely intact. Thus with one exception,* chapter numbers and contents are the same in the third edition as they were in the second edition. **Volume I** of this third edition is therefore now entitled, ***"ACLS: Cer-***

*In the second edition, Chapter 13 was devoted to detailed discussion on the "Use of Lidocaine." To create a place in the third edition for our new chapter on "Special Resuscitation Situations," we have incorporated the information on lidocaine into our greatly expanded chapter on *Acute Myocardial Infarction.*

tification Preparation." Its principal aim is to serve as an easy-to-read *study guide* for preparing to take the ACLS course. It also serves as a targeted review of the key components of cardiopulmonary resuscitation. Volume I contains what were the first three parts of our second edition: Part I on the *Essentials of Running a Code* (Chapters 1 through 6), Part II on the *Essentials of Airway and IV Access* (Chapters 7 and 8), and Part III on *Pearls and Pitfalls in Management of Cardiac Arrest* (Chapter 9).

The remaining chapters from our second edition now comprise **Volume II,** which is entitled, ***"ACLS: A Comprehensive Review."*** It includes Part IV on *Topics of General Interest in Emergency Cardiac Care* (Chapters 10 through 13), Part V on *Beyond the Basics* (Chapters 14 through 16), Part VI on *Pediatric Resuscitation* (Chapter 17), and Part VII on *Medicolegal Aspects* (Chapter 18).

How To Use This Book

The entire contents of these two volumes have been rewritten and updated to reflect the *most recent* developments in the field.* *Each volume stands completely on its own.* How each volume may best be used will depend primarily on the needs of the reader:

If the Principal Need is to Review/Prepare for the ACLS Course— *Volume I is the key.* When the time available for review/preparation is exceeding limited (i.e., 3 days or *less*), the primary focus might best be concentrated on Chapter 1. The essence of the ACLS course is now contained in this chapter, which includes an overall perspective for running a code and detailed algorithms with a suggested step-by-step approach for the management of ventricular fibrillation, ventricular tachycardia, bradycardia/asystole/EMD, supraventricular tachyarrhythmias, and use of the AED. Explanatory commentary highlighting key points of interest accompanies each of the treatments recommended. Following each algorithm, concepts are crystallized in a section entitled, *"Questions To Further Understanding."* Thorough review of Chapter 1 may be the most

*Numerous references are cited throughout to support our discussion. The sense of currency is conveyed by the fact that many of the sources cited relate to work just recently published (i.e., in 1991 or 1992).

time-effective manner of preparing for the ACLS course (as well as for quickly reviewing the essentials of cardiopulmonary resuscitation).

If after completing Chapter 1 time still remains before the course, preparation (particularly for the MEGA CODE station) might best be facilitated by going through a number of the simulated code scenarios presented in Chapter 4 *(Putting It All Together)*. Additional practice for MEGA CODE is provided in the code vignettes presented in Chapter 5 *(Finding the Error)*. Preparation for the written test is best afforded by working through the *Self-Assessment Section* (Chapter 6), which features 100 multiple choice and true-false questions on various aspects of ACLS. Explained answers provide immediate feedback, and indicate where in the text to refer for additional information.

Readers with the luxury of more time to prepare/review will be rewarded by the wealth of material contained within the remaining chapters of this volume. Essential drugs and treatment modalities are extensively covered in Chapter 2, with suggested recommendations for dosing and a detailed commentary on the use of each agent. Special features included in this chapter are brief overview of the actions of the various alpha- and beta-adrenergic receptors in the autonomic nervous system, full discussion on the pros and cons of using high vs standard dose epinephrine, the "hows and whys" of energy selection for defibrillation, discussion of newer essential drugs expected to have an impact in emergency cardiac care (such as adenosine, magnesium, and amiodarone), explanation of a simplified method for remembering how to calculate IV infusions, and discussion of the role of modalities such as pacing, synchronized cardioversion, the precordial thump, and cough version.

The gamut of cardiac arrhythmias encountered in emergency cardiac care follows in Chapter 3. More than 150 illustrative tracings rapidly advance the reader from basic rhythm interpretation to a fairly high level of sophistication. Clinical relevance and a problem-solving approach aimed to stimulate and actively recruit reader participation is stressed throughout. Numerous practice tracings (with explained answers) have been included to reinforce concepts discussed.

Finishing touches to Volume I are applied in the last three chapters: *Management of the Airway and Ventilation* (Chapter 7), *IV Access* (Chapter 8), and *Pearls and Pitfalls in the Management of Cardiac Arrest* (Chapter 9).

If the Principal Need/Desire is to Explore *Beyond the Basics* in Cardiopulmonary Resuscitation and Emergency Cardiac Care—*Volume II is the key.* This volume begins with Part IV on *Topics of General Interest in Emergency Cardiac Care,* and includes *New Developments in CPR* (Chapter 10), *Sudden Cardiac Death* (Chapter 11), *Acute Myocardial Infarction* (Chapter 12), and *Special Resuscitation Situations* (Chapter 13). This last chapter is completely new and consists of a practical approach to evaluation and management of patients who present with unusual code situations including drowning or near drowning, hypothermia, heat stroke, lightning and electrical injuries, overdose from cocaine or tricyclic antidepressant agents, cardiopulmonary arrest in pregnancy, airplane emergencies, and traumatic cardiac arrest.

Chapters 10 through 12 illustrate the extent to which this third edition has been expanded compared to our previous edition. Thus, our chapter on *Acute Myocardial Infarction* now encompasses six subsections and over 80 pages. Issues that are thoroughly explored include clinical evaluation of the patient with acute ischemic chest pain, standard medical treatments, newer treatments (such as potential use of magnesium for prophylaxis and/or treatment of ventricular arrhythmias), use of thrombolytic therapy, anticoagulation, and antiplatelet agents, when to consider invasive intervention, and an illustra-

tive case study that challenges the reader to clinically apply the material covered. Chapter 11 on *Sudden Cardiac Death* has been similarly expanded, and now includes subsections on out-of-hospital cardiac arrest, the role of electrolytes (potassium and magnesium) in cardiac arrest, in-hospital cardiac arrest, options for management of sudden death survivors, and a special section entitled, *"What To Do If the Patient Dies . . . "* Features contained in our chapter on *New Developments in CPR* (Chapter 10) include discussion of the mechanisms, efficacy, and potential complications of CPR, clinical application of End-Tidal CO_2 monitoring, a historical review tracing the development of CPR, the rationale for current BLS recommendations, and frank discussion of potential problems that may be encountered in trying to implement CPR. This latter subsection directly confronts controversial issues such as administration of mouth-to-mouth ventilation when you know (or suspect) that the patient may have AIDS.

The additions we have made to Part V of Volume II (on *Beyond the Basics*) should delight the most sophisticated of our readers. Among the new drugs added to Chapter 14 are labetalol, esmolol, IV diltiazem, and discussion on the use of digoxin antibody fragments (for acute treatment of life-threatening digitalis intoxication). Chapters 15 *(Differentiation of PVCs from Aberrancy)* and 16 *(More Advanced Concepts in Arrhythmia Interpretation)* have each nearly doubled in size, and explore their respective topic from every facet imaginable. Numerous clinical examples constantly challenge the reader and illustrate important points that are made.

Chapters 17 *(Pediatric Resuscitation)* and 18 *(Medicolegal Aspects of ACLS)* complete Volume II. Each has been updated and suitably expanded to reflect new developments and advances accomplished since publication of our second edition.

Regardless of one's clinical background and training, there should be more than enough material in these two volumes to satisfy the most demanding of needs. *We emphasize that Volume II is not essential reading for those whose primary concern is successful completion of the ACLS course.* However, the contents of this volume should prove invaluable for those with an interest in delving beyond the core of the ACLS course and/or expanding their horizons in emergency cardiac care.

For the Reader Who Wants More . . . .

IN 1988 we published a series of approximately 350 flash cards in conjunction with the second edition of this book (*ACLS: Mega Code Review/Study Cards*—Mosby–Year Book, St. Louis). The aim of these cards was twofold:

i) To provide another type of *study aid* that might supplement the second edition of our book.

ii) To provide an additional method of preparing for the challenging MEGA CODE station that would simulate testing conditions, but at the same time allow the student to individualize their preparation, *and proceed at their own pace.*

The first goal was easily accomplished by posing a clinical question or simply listing a drug or arrhythmia on the front of a card, and providing explanatory discussion on the back. The latter goal was attained by incorporating a portion of the cards into simulated code scenarios in which the front of a card presented the patient's rhythm and clinical status, and the back of that card indicated our suggested approach to treatment.

We have completely revised the cards in this study aid (*ACLS: MEGA CODE Review/Study Cards—Second Edition*, Mosby–Year Book, 1993). In addition to updating the cards and greatly expanding the extent of their content, the new set of cards features a much more "user-friendly" format that reinforces *without* duplicating the material we cover in the third edition of our book. Utilization of these *Study Cards* therefore provides an additional, time-effective way of reviewing the essentials of cardiopulmonary resuscitation and preparing for the ACLS course.

We hope you enjoy reading our ACLS material, and find it clinically useful. It was written with YOU—the reader—in mind.

Author's Note

Our recommendations for management in the key algorithms of cardiopulmonary resuscitation are generally very consistent with those put forth by the American Heart Association. However, we do not always adhere strictly to their guidelines. In cases where we differ, we clearly state the rationale for our views, and appropriately reference any points of contention.

We do *not* feel such differences of opinion represent a departure from the objectives of the American Heart Association, since this agency freely acknowledges that their algorithms for treatment are not all inclusive. On the contrary, we firmly believe that acknowledging areas of controversy and presenting potential alternative approaches for selected situations is beneficial and may lead to improved emergency care. Our book is therefore aimed to *complement* the American Heart Association ACLS Textbook. We hope combined use will not only prove insightful, but also add an extra dimension to the learning experience of the reader.

Foreword

The tremendous success of the American Heart Association program on advanced cardiac life support (ACLS) has been evident from the continued demand for this course among the health care professionals. Clearly the course provides the most time-efficient method for improving one's skills in the area of cardiopulmonary resuscitation.

The principal difficulty posed by the ACLS course lies with the large amount of material that the participant is expected to assimilate in a short period of time. Even though the American Heart Association ACLS textbook will ideally be distributed well in advance of the course, this text has not solved the problem of preparing the student for the intensive program to follow. Despite its extensive scope, much of the material in the ACLS textbook is not conveniently organized into a decision-making format for patient care. In addition, practice exercises in arrhythmia interpretation and management of cardiac arrest are entirely lacking.

ACLS: Certification Preparation and a Comprehensive Review by Grauer and Cavallaro was developed in an attempt to meet the educational needs of the reader. Now in its third edition, this book should keenly interest *anyone* who is either taking the ACLS course or involved in emergency cardiac care. Written in a style that transcends medical specialties, the two volumes of this third edition masterfully succeed in accomplishing the authors' goals of producing a practical, easy-to-read study guide that facilitates preparation for the ACLS course, as well as a comprehensive, state-of-the-art review in the field of cardiopulmonary resuscitation.

I find each of the two volumes in this third edition to be stimulating, informative, and invaluable as a *complement* to the American Heart Association ACLS Textbook.

Richard J. Melker, M.D., Ph. D.
Emergency Cardiac Care Committee,
    American Heart Association
Associate Professor
Surgery, Anesthesiology, Pediatrics
University of Florida
College of Medicine
Gainesville, Florida

To my father,

Samuel Grauer

*without whom this book
would not have been possible.*

About the Authors

KEN GRAUER, M.D., F.A.A.F.P., is a professor in the Department of Community Health and Family Medicine, College of Medicine, University of Florida, and assistant director of the Family Practice Residency Program in Gainesville. He is board certified in family practice, and is a National ACLS Affiliate Faculty member and former contributor to the American Heart Association ACLS Textbook who served on the Task Force for ACLS Post-Testing. In addition to this book, Dr. Grauer is the principal or sole author of the following books and teaching resources: *ACLS: Mega Code Review/Study Cards* (Second edition—Mosby–Year Book, 1993), *A Practical Guide to ECG Interpretation* (Mosby–Year Book, 1992), *ECG Interpretation Pocket Reference* (Mosby–Year Book, 1992), *Clinical Electrocardiography: A Primary Care Approach* (Second edition—Blackwell Scientific Publications, 1992), and *ACLS Teaching Kit: An Instructor's Resource* (Mosby–Year Book, 1990). He has lectured widely and is primary author of numerous articles on cardiology for family physicians, including several "ECG of the Month" columns that have been published for a period of more than seven years in various primary care journals. He also serves on the Editorial Board of the following journals: ACLS Alert, Family Practice Recertification, Procedural Skills and Office Technology, and Internal Medicine Alert.

Dr. Grauer has become well known throughout Florida and nationally for teaching ACLS courses and ECG/arrhythmia workshops to diverse medical audiences including nurses, paramedics, medical students, physicians in training, and physicians in practice. His trademark has always been the ability to simplify otherwise complicated topics into a concise, practical, and easy-to-remember format.

DAN CAVALLARO, REMT-P, is research director of the Center for Cardiopulmonary Research at All Children's Hospital in St. Petersburg, Florida. He is a former ACLS National Affiliate Faculty member, and a former contributor to the American Heart Association ACLS Textbook who served on the Task Force for ACLS Post-Testing. In addition to co-authoring this book, he has co-authored the following teaching resources: *ACLS: Mega Code Review/Study Cards* (Second edition—Mosby–Year Book, 1993), and *ACLS Teaching Kit: An Instructor's Resource* (Mosby–Year Book, 1990). Clinically, he has worked in the critical care and emergency medical fields for the past 15 years. During that time, he has also been extremely active developing and participating in courses on prehospital care and emergency medicine, and has taught in well over 150 ACLS courses.

Acknowledgments

I am indebted to the following people whose contributions were instrumental to the preparation of this book:

Dan Cavallaro, whose expertise has continued to enrich my knowledge over the years, and whose friendship and enthusiasm helped keep me going during the seemingly "endless" three years it took to complete the writing (and constant rewriting) of this book. His contributions to each of the two volumes in this third edition have truly been *invaluable* to me.

Jorge Giroud, MD, and **Al Saltiel,** MD, for their assistance in helping to write the chapters on intravenous access and pediatrics.

John Gums, Pharm D, for his assistance in helping me write the chapters relating to cardiovascular pharmacology. Nowhere could there possibly be another Pharm D the equal of John, whose encyclopedic, photographic memory and unfathomable clinical insight become the instant envy of all who are lucky enough to work with him.

Fred Langer, RN, for his ingenuity in conceiving our ACLS poetry addendum: *"The Night Before Morning."* The birth of this poem is the result of Fred's labor.

Ellie Green, RN, for her help with the finishing touches of our poem. I'm eternally grateful to Ellie for her assistance in targeting (and retargeting) selected portions of this text to the audience we wanted to reach—as well as for her valued friendship. *Has there ever been a better teacher to bless the nursing profession?*

Arlene Marrin, RN, **Marvin A. Dewar,** MD, JD, and **Ray Moseley,** PhD, for their assistance in helping me write the chapter on medicolegal aspects of ACLS—and for their assistance in the numerous rewritings of this chapter that marked our attempt to keep up with this everchanging field. *What better combination of coauthors could one ask for to write this chapter than a nurse/claims examiner, a doctor/lawyer who happens to be your director, and the best medical ethicist there is?*

Janet Silverstein, MD, Des Schatz, MD, and John Hellrung, MD, for their input in the chapter on pediatrics. To Richard Bucciarelli, MD, Greg Gaar, MD, John Santamaria, MD, and Bonnie Sklaren, for their assistance in helping with the original version of the chapter on pediatrics that appeared in the second edition of our book.

Geno Romano, MD, Brent Leytem, MD, Mike Ware, MD, Karen Hall, MD, Lou Kuritzky, MD, R. Whitney Curry, Jr., MD, René Lee-Pack, MD, Doug Coran, MD, Frank Foster, MD, Boyd Kellet, MD, for their assistance in writing selected portions of the special resuscitation situations chapter.

Larry Kravitz, MD, Harry Sernaker, MD, Jerry Diehr, MD, and Paul Augereau, MD, for their assistance in helping with the original version of the chapter on intravenous access that appeared in the second edition of our book.

Geno Romano, MD, Holly Jensen, RN, Karen Hall, MD, Brent Leytem, MD, Aixa Rey, Pharm D, for reviewing significant portions of the manuscript, and "keeping me honest."

Sherry Wingate, Virginia Hungerford, Steve Roark, MD, Anne Curtis, MD, and Betty Arnette, REMT-P, for their assistance and expertise in reviewing selected portions of this text—and to Jim Nimocks, MD and Garth Vaz, MD for the "fascinoma" tracings they contributed.

J. Daniel Robinson, Pharm D, for contributing the SIMKIN figures which I modified in the chapter on lidocaine.

Robyn Lyemance for her kindness and wonderful patience in the endless photographic sessions needed to prepare the chapters on airway management and IV access.

Kinsey Judkins-Waldron, RN, for her invaluable insight, unfailing support, and tremendously welcome 100%-biased positive feedback during the "middle ages" period of the writing of this book.

Anita Wofford (my career counselor), for dancing into my life during the "final ages" period of this book—and for sustaining me when I needed a friendly attentive "ear" and a caring lifelong friend.

R. Whit Curry, Jr., MD, for allowing me to "pump his brain" on numerous occasions throughout the years on primary care questions about cardiology issues—and for his unwavering support of me in his capacity as Director-Chairman of our Family Practice program.

Rick Weimer of Mosby–Year Book—for his encouragement, enthusiasm, and motivation, out of which this book was born—and out of which came the rebirth of this third edition. **Julie Scardiglia** of Mosby–Year Book, for helping to make the rebirth possible. *Nowhere could there be another pair more deserving of credit (as well as a raise) than Rick and Julie for their positive influence and total involvement in the development and fruition of this project.*

Diana Laulainen of Mosby–Year Book—for jumping in during the "final" stages. *This book would NOT be without Diana!*

Jan and **Jackie Katz** of *Resource Applications,* for making it possible for me to teach (and learn from) nurses across the country.

Mikel Rothenberg, MD—*my favorite pen pal*—for "alerting" me monthly to *What's New in ACLS.*

Pat and **"Tree"** (and the rest of the crew at Sonny's)—and **Phil Heflin** (and the crew at Chaucer's), for their great food and ever EXCELLENT service, and for providing me with a peaceful, pleasant, and inspiring environment for writing (and forever rewriting), and reviewing much of the text. And ditto for Ruby Tuesday.

Maria Alvarez—the BEST dance teacher I know—as well as my other "best" dance teacher, Ray Parris, for their inspiration toward excellence in ballroom dancing, and who together with all my friends at the *Maria Alvarez Imperial Dance Studio,* were instrumental in helping me to maintain my sanity (and still have fun by dancing) for much of the time I was working on this book.

Barney Marriott, MD, and **William P. Nelson,** MD, *for teaching me more about ECGs than I can ever say.*

Brian Kennedy, MD and **Andres Ticzon,** MD, for teaching and inspiring a family physician (= me!) to better appreciate the magic of cardiology.

The Cardiology staff at Alachua General Hospital (Burt Silverstein, MD; Steve Roark, MD; Mike Dillon, MD; Gary Cooper, MD, and Fraser Richards, MD), for their tremendous support of me, and for teaching cardiology to our residents.

ALL of the other excellent cardiologists who have inspired me, and from whom I have learned.

ALL those who have knowingly (and unknowingly) provided me with tracings through the years.

ALL the nurses, medical students, residents, and other paramedical personnel who have allowed me to learn by teaching them.

Ken Grauer, MD

Contents

PART VI Pediatric Resuscitation

VOLUME I
Brief Contents

VOLUME II

ACLS

COMPREHENSIVE REVIEW

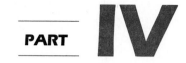

Topics of General Interest in Emergency Cardiac Care

CHAPTER 10

NEW DEVELOPMENTS IN CPR:
Optimizing Ventilation-Perfusion in the Arrested Heart

SECTION A

BASIC LIFE SUPPORT ASPECTS OF CPR

CPR: Definition/Semantic Problems

CPR is one of the most important treatment modalities for the victim of cardiopulmonary arrest. Its impact is immense. In addition to being the first line of therapy for cardiopulmonary arrest, CPR plays a major role in educating the public about primary prevention (risk factor modification) and recognition of coronary artery disease, acute myocardial infarction, and sudden cardiac death.

It is well known that the letters **"CPR"** stand for **C**ardio**P**ulmonary **R**esuscitation. Unfortunately, a semantic problem has developed with the use of this designation because many emergency care providers have come to equate the abbreviation "CPR" with **BLS.** BLS (= **B**asic **L**ife **S**upport) measures entail external chest compression and mouth-to-mouth (or mouth-to-mask) ventilation. More advanced life support measures (i.e., defibrillation, definitive airway control, establishment of IV access, and administration of medications) are covered under the umbrella terms of **ACLS** (= **A**dvanced **C**ardiac **L**ife **S**upport). In truth, the term *"cardiopulmonary resuscitation"* really encompasses *all* aspects of *both* basic *as well as* advanced life support.

Thus technically speaking,

CPR = BLS + ACLS

. . . . *whereas according to common usage, it may be that:*

CPR = BLS *or* **BLS + ACLS** (depending on the clinical context and semantic perception of the user)

Although admittedly the meaning of the term CPR will usually be clear from the context of use, it may be necessary at times to clarify the issue by specifying whether advanced cardiac life support measures are also meant to be involved.

Awareness of CPR in this country has mushroomed; almost 90% of adult Americans have heard of the technique, and well over 40 million individuals have already received formal training. The technique does save lives, although there is not universal agreement on the manner in which it accomplishes this goal (Valenzuela, 1989).

Our goal for this chapter is to review current recommendations for performance of basic life support in adults (Section A). We take a historical look at the development of CPR (Section B). In Section C, we focus on recent developments that have improved our understanding of cardiopulmonary resuscitation, and attempt to relate the clinical impact of these developments to practical aspects of basic *and* advanced cardiac life support. Among the questions we'll examine in this section are:

1. *How effective is CPR?*
2. How can we optimize the fundamental parameters of basic life support (i.e., ventilation and perfusion of the arrested heart)?
3. Are changes likely to be forthcoming in the techniques utilized to perform basic life support? (If so, what is the rationale prompting consideration of these changes?)
4. How has our relatively new understanding of the mechanism for blood flow with CPR influenced our utilization of basic life support? How has it affected recommendations for advanced cardiac life support? What may be anticipated for the future?

We conclude the chapter in Section D by addressing some of the difficulties involved in implementing BLS training among the lay public including the increasing reluctance of health care providers to perform mouth-to-mouth ventilation on victims of cardiopulmonary arrest.

Basic Life Support: Recommendations for One-Rescuer CPR

Performance of basic life support (BLS) is predicated on patient assessment and management of the ABCs (**A**irway, **B**reathing, and **C**irculation). In addition to **A**irway, the **A** should also help recall that **A**ssessment is the *initial* step of each phase. Current recommendations for the sequence of one- and two-rescuer CPR in adults follow:

Recommendations for One-Rescuer CPR

Airway:
1. **Assessment**—Determine unresponsiveness. (*"Are you OK?"*)
2. Call for help.
3. Position the victim (so he/she is supine on a flat firm surface).
4. Open the airway. (Use the head-tilt/chin-lift or jaw-thrust maneuver.)

Breathing:
1. **Assessment**—Determine breathlessness. (*Look, listen,* and *feel* for air movement.)
2. If the victim is not breathing, *begin rescue breathing.* Give two *slow,* full breaths (over a total inspiratory time of 3 to 4 seconds).

Circulation:
1. **Assessment**—Determine pulselessness. (Spend a good 5 to 10 seconds feeling for a carotid pulse.)
2. If there is no pulse, *begin external chest compressions.* Compress at a rate of 80 to 100 per minute.
3. Perform 15 chest compressions and then stop to deliver two *slow,* full breaths (with an inspiratory time of 1.5 to 2 seconds per breath). Perform four complete cycles of this 15:2 compression/ventilation ratio, and then reassess the patient. If the patient is still breathless and pulseless, resume CPR and continue until help arrives.

SELECTED COMMENTS

After attending to (and securing) the **A**irway of an unconscious victim, **B**reathing must be *assessed* and the rescuer must ensure that there is adequate ventilation. Three possible situations may be encountered:

1. *The victim is breathing adequately.* In this case, maintain an open airway while waiting for help to arrive.
2. *The victim is not breathing adequately (or is not breathing at all).* In this case, deliver two *slow,* full breaths to initiate CPR.

   "Staircase" breathing is no longer recommended. This phenomenon is an artifact of Resusci Annie that was produced only because of the mannikin's exhalation valve. Staircase breaths are impossible to achieve in human subjects because practically speaking, air is expired as rapidly as it is taken in (Melker et al, 1981). Even if one could staircase breaths in humans, this would not be desirable. The gastroesophageal sphincter of most patients opens as soon as pressure in the unprotected airway exceeds 25 cm H_2O. Were one to deliver 2 L of air within 1 second as required by the staircase effect, pressures much higher than this would have to be generated. Gastric insufflation would certainly result leading to ineffective CPR and potential regurgitation of gastric contents with aspiration (Melker and Banner, 1985).

3. *The victim is not breathing and you are unable to ventilate.* Instead, there is resistance to your attempts at delivering rescue breaths and the chest does not rise. If you are still unable to ventilate after repositioning the victim, suspect *airway obstruction* (i.e., by a foreign body) until proved otherwise!

   To treat the patient for suspected foreign body airway obstruction, apply the Heimlich maneuver (subdiaphragmatic abdominal thrusts or chest thrusts). Follow this with a finger sweep to dislodge and/or remove the foreign body obstruction. Reposition the victim's head and attempt to ventilate again. If unsuccessful, repeat this sequence.

THE RATE OF COMPRESSION

After ensuring adequate ventilation, assess the victim for the presence of a pulse (i.e., **C**irculation). If a pulse is present, maintain an open airway and continue rescue breathing (at a rate of 12 per minute) while waiting for help to arrive. If there is no pulse, begin external chest compressions, and compress at a rate of between 80 to 100 per minute.

A major change that was incorporated into the 1986 guidelines for CPR was an increase in the recommended *rate* of compressions to 80 to 100 per minute for both one- and two-rescuer CPR. There were two reasons for this change. First, insertion of the 1- to 1.5-second pause for each ventilation reduced the total time allotted for chest compressions. A faster rate of compressions was needed to make up for this.

Equally important is the fact that an increased rate improves the *efficacy* of chest compression. Traditionally, a rate of 60 compressions per minute had been recommended for two-rescuer CPR, with each compression ideally lasting 50% of the compression-relaxation cycle. In practice, more attention was usually directed to complying with the rate criterion. Rescuers tended to meticulously count off one per second cardiac compressions while paying little attention to whether each compression was maintained for the proper amount of time.

Actually, *force* and *duration* of chest compression appear to be more important determinants of blood flow than *rate* per se (Taylor et al, 1977; Luce et al, 1980; Maier et al, 1984). Carotid blood flow increases in direct relation to increases in compression duration, and maximal antegrade flow is achieved when compression duration is extended to occupy 60% to 70% of the compression-relaxation cycle (Luce et al, 1980; Parmley et al, 1982).

The problem is that sustaining each compression for at least 50% of the cycle is hard to accomplish at slow compression rates. With faster rates of compression, however, the total time for each cycle is less. As a result, the *percentage* of time devoted to compression becomes proportionately greater. In addition, rescuers tend to apply greater *force* with each compression when working at a faster rate *(high-impulse CPR)*. Thus the end result of increasing the recommended rate for chest compressions is improved efficiency of CPR because the faster rate proportionately lengthens the period of compression duration as it increases the amount of force applied with each compression (Swenson et al, 1988; Kern and Ewy, 1990). As we suggest in Section C of this chapter, aiming for the *upper end* of the rate range for compressions (i.e., compressing as close to a rate of 100 per minute as possible) is likely to optimize potential blood flow during CPR.

Recommendations for Two-Rescuer CPR

Performance of CPR by two rescuers has never been shown to improve survival compared to performance of CPR by a single rescuer. Nevertheless, one might intuitively expect this to be the case. Data supportive of this concept appear in Figure 10A-1, which illustrates the effect of one- and two-rescuer CPR on key hemodynamic parameters during cardiac arrest. Note how dramatically cerebral and systemic perfusion drop off during the ventilatory phase of one-rescuer CPR (when compressions are stopped). In contrast, cerebral and systemic perfusion are maintained at a consistent level throughout performance of two-rescuer CPR. Mean aortic and pulmonary artery pressures, as well as mean flow in the common carotid artery are all significantly higher with two-rescuer CPR. It would therefore seem that the best possible results from cardiopulmonary resuscitation are obtained when two-rescuer CPR is initiated as early as possible during resuscitation.

Despite the improved hemodynamics that are possible with two-rescuer CPR, this technique is no longer recommended by the American Heart Association for lay individuals. Incorporating a second rescuer to the CPR sequence adds complexity to the task, especially when lay person rescuers are unfamiliar with each other's CPR technique. Failure to coordinate their efforts could sufficiently detract from overall performance enough to counteract the benefit of the second rescuer. Practically speaking, out-of-hospital cardiac arrest

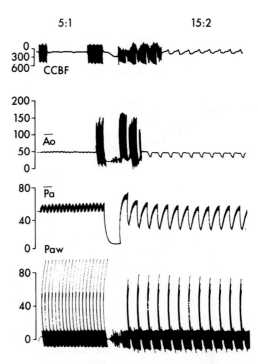

Figure 10A-1. Comparison of key hemodynamic parameters during one- and two-rescuer CPR. Mean common carotid blood flow (CCBF), mean aortic pressure (Ao), and mean pulmonary artery pressure (Pa) all drop off markedly during the ventilatory phase of one-rescuer CPR. Peak airway pressure (Paw) remains relatively constant throughout both one- and two-rescuer CPR. (Cavallaro D: Personal correspondence and ongoing research.)

only rarely occurs in the presence of more than one lay individual who is proficient in CPR. Even when this happens, a much more vital role for the second rescuer than assisting in CPR is to contact the EMS system—since realistic chances for survival of a victim of out-of-hospital cardiac arrest who does not respond to initial attempts at rescue breathing depend on early defibrillation.

In contrast, in a hospital setting, performance of CPR by *two* rescuers (who are trained health care providers) is essential for optimizing hemodynamics during resuscitation while ACLS measures are being carried out.

Recommendations for Two-Rescuer CPR

Airway:
Same as for One-Rescuer CPR

Breathing:
1. **Assessment**—Determine breathlessness. (*Look, listen,* and *feel* for air movement.)
2. If the victim is not breathing, *begin rescue breathing.* (Give two *slow* full breaths over 3 to 4 seconds.)

Circulation:

Same as for One-Rescuer CPR, except that one rescuer ventilates the patient while the other performs chest compressions. After completing 5 compressions (given at a rate of 80 to 100 per minute), the first rescuer *pauses* for 1.5 to 2 seconds while the second rescuer delivers a *slow*, full ventilation. The first rescuer then resumes compressions. The 5:1 compression/ventilation ratio is continued.

Comments

In the past, the recommendation was to *interpose* ventilations between the upstroke of the fifth compression and the downstroke of the first compression of the subsequent cycle. The time allotted to complete each ventilation by this method was necessarily short. As a result, there was a tendency to prematurely terminate ventilations so as to be sure to finish before the first compression of the next cycle. Because of our improved understanding of the mechanism of blood flow with CPR, we now know that interposing ventilations is not essential for optimal ventilation and perfusion during resuscitation (Melker and Cavallaro, 1983). Moreover, the limited time allotted for respiration when ventilations are interposed may result in excessive generation of airway pressures (and lead to gastric insufflation and regurgitation) without necessarily providing sufficient time for adequate lung expansion.

Instead, the key to effective ventilation appears to be delivery of *slow* and full breaths (over 1.5 to 2 seconds). In the victim with an unprotected airway, ventilation is delivered during a pause after each fifth compression. The purpose of the pause is that it reduces intrathoracic pressure. This makes it much more likely that air (which follows the path of least resistance) will enter the trachea rather than the esophagus.

> In an attempt to further reduce the chance of producing gastric insufflation in patients with an unprotected airway, the recommendation has recently been made to slow delivery of rescue breathing to an even greater degree. Thus, each rescue breath should be delivered over a period of 1.5 to 2 seconds (compared to the 1 to 1.5 second inspiratory time recommended previously).

Once the patient has been intubated, delivery of air into the trachea is ensured. As a result, there is no longer any need to coordinate the timing of ventilation and compression. The theoretical concern that chance occurrence of simultaneous ventilation and compression might excessively increase intrathoracic pressure and impede blood flow with CPR has not been borne out in practice. On the contrary, the occurrence of simultaneous ventilation and compression if anything *increases* blood flow (Chandra et al, 1990). Once the airway is protected, it no longer matters when ventilation is delivered with respect to compression. Performance of *asynchronous* (totally independent) ventila-

tion and compression maximizes efficiency by allowing each rescuer to concentrate on a particular task.

Recommendations for Two-Rescuer CPR in the Intubated Patient

Airway:
Same as for Two-Rescuer CPR

Breathing:
1. **Assessment**—Determine breathlessness. (*Look, listen,* and *feel* for air movement.)
2. If the victim is not breathing, *begin rescue breathing.* (Give two *slow* full breaths over 3 to 4 seconds.)
3. In the intubated patient, the ventilatory pause is no longer needed so that ventilation and compression are now *asynchronous.*

Circulation:
One rescuer performs 80 to 100 compressions per minute, while the other independently (i.e., *asynchronously*) delivers 12 to 15 ventilations per minute.

MAXIMIZING PERFORMANCE OF CPR

Performance of CPR *is* important. Without it, blood will not flow in the arrested heart. With properly performed two-rescuer CPR, cardiac output may approach 25% of normal values (although admittedly blood flow to essential organs may be significantly less than this—unless medications such as epinephrine are used). Key points we have emphasized in this section for maximizing blood flow with CPR in adults are to:

1. Deliver ventilations *slowly* and completely (over an inspiratory time of *no less* than 1.5 to 2 seconds per breath).
2. *Be sure ventilations are effective.* The chest should rise as breaths are delivered, and the rescuer should *feel* the sensation of air entering and expanding the lungs. If this does not occur, the airway is not patent—either due to inadequate airway control (which should resolve with repositioning of the victim) or a mechanical cause (such as a foreign body).
3. Compress *rapidly* (at a rate of *at least* 80, and up to 100 times per minute). Err on the side of *faster* rather than slower rates (i.e., closer to 100 per minute).

4. Compress with *adequate* (but not excessive) *force.*

> After locating the xiphoid process and placing the heel of the compressing hand two fingerbreaths above this point,

pressure is then delivered over the midline (lower half of the sternum) with sufficient force to depress the sternum 1 to 1½ inches. The fingers may be either extended or interlaced while compressing (as long as they are kept *off* the chest wall). Leaning forward (so that the compressor's shoulders are directly over the patient's sternum), keeping the arms straight (to minimize fatigue) and at a 90-degree angle to the victim's chest further helps to optimize the mechanics of compression delivery.

5. Get help.

All too often, cardiopulmonary resuscitation at the bedside of a hospitalized patient becomes an overcrowded event. An important function that extra health care providers may serve at the bedside is to monitor the quality of CPR being performed and constructively provide ongoing feedback to rescuers on parameters of CPR that they may not be aware of (such as the rate of compression or adequacy of ventilation).

References

Chandra NC, Tsitlik JE, Halperin HR, Guerci AD, Weisfeldt ML: Observations of hemodynamics during human cardiopulmonary resuscitation, *Crit Care Med* 18:929-934, 1990.

Kern KB, Ewy GA: Future directions in cardiopulmonary resuscitation, Discussion at the Learning Center, University of Arizona, June 11-13, 1990.

Luce JM, Cary JM, Ross BK, Culver BH, Butler J: New developments in cardiopulmonary resuscitation, *JAMA* 244:1366-1370, 1980.

Maier GW, Tyson GI, Olsen CO, Kernstein KJ, Davis JW, Cohn EH, Sabiston DC, Rankin JS: The physiology of external cardiac massage: high-impulse cardiopulmonary resuscitation, *Circulation* 70:86-101, 1984.

Melker R, Cavallaro D, Krischer J: One-rescuer CPR: a reappraisal of present recommendation for ventilation, *Crit Care Med* 9:423, 1981.

Melker RJ, Cavallaro DL: Cardiopulmonary resuscitation during synchronous and asynchronous ventilation, *Ann Emerg Med* 12:142, 1983 (abstract).

Melker RJ, Banner MJ: Ventilation during CPR: two-rescuer standards reappraised, *Ann Emerg Med* 14:397-402, 1985.

Parmley WW, Hatcher CR, Ewy GA, Furman S, Redding J, Weisfeldt ML: Task force V: physical interventions and adjunctive therapy, Thirteenth Bethesda Conference on Emergency Cardiac Care, *Am J Cardiol* 50:409-420, 1982.

Swenson RD, Weaver WD, Niskanen RA, Martin J, Dahlberg S: Hemodynamics in humans during conventional and experimental methods of cardiopulmonary resuscitation, *Circulation* 78:630-639, 1988.

Taylor GJ, Tucker WM, Greene HL, Rudikoff MT, Weisfeldt ML: Importance of prolonged compression during cardiopulmonary resuscitation in man, *N Engl J Med* 296:1515-1518, 1977.

Valenzuela TD: Bystander CPR—discouragement or reaffirmation? *Ann Emerg Med* 18:324-325, 1989.

SECTION B

THE HISTORY OF CPR

The history of CPR is fascinating. Brief review of development of the art is extremely insightful to our current understanding and clinical practice.

The first reference to artificial respiration dates back to the biblical prophet Elisha, who revived an apparently dead child. As recorded in the Book of Kings:

> Elisha then went to the house, and there on his bed lay the child, dead . . . he climbed onto the bed and stretched himself on top of the child, putting his mouth on his mouth, his eyes to his eyes, and his hands on his hands, and as he lowered himself onto him, the child's flesh grew warm . . . he lowered himself onto the child seven times in all; then the child sneezed and opened his eyes.

It should always be so easy. . . .

Development of Methods for Ventilation

In 177 AD, Galen used a bellows to inflate a dead animal's lungs. Although other techniques were periodically tried over the ensuing centuries, little real progress was made in the art of resuscitation until the 18th century. Perhaps the first "Policy Statement" was made in 1740 when the Paris Academy of Sciences officially recommended mouth-to-mouth resuscitation for drowning victims. There followed a series of newer, "more advanced" techniques for artificial respiration (*JAMA* Suppl, 1974; DeBard, 1980; Criley et al, 1984; Liss, 1986). These included:

- The *Inversion Method* (1770),* in which the victim was suspended upside down (by the feet) in an attempt to force air entry into and out of the lungs.
- The *Barrel Method* (1773), in which a rolling barrel literally compressed the chest to produce expiration and inspiration. In a variation of this method, the victim was placed *inside* the barrel as it was rolled.
- The *Trotting Horse Method* (1812), in which the victim was mounted face down on top of a cantering horse (with the up and down motion from the canter aimed at producing air movement).
- The *Le Roy Method* (1829), *Marshall Hall Method* (1856), *Sylvester Method* (1861), and *Howard Method* (1871) — in which the anterior chest or back was compressed in various ways with the patient either supine or rolled over to effect rhythmic inflation and deflation of the lungs.
- Additional unnamed methods aimed at "waking up" the nonresponding individual included yelling, crying, star-

tling (with loud noises), hitting, slapping, or whipping the victim.* . . . . and many other methods . . . .

In the early 1900s, the *Schafer Method* became a popular means for administering artificial respiration. The technique was based on intermittent delivery of pressure on the *back* of the prone victim. It was felt to be advantageous because it maintained an open airway, allowed drainage of aspirated water by gravity, posed no risk to internal organs, was easy to learn, could be performed without fatigue, and was thought to provide an efficient method of gas exchange (Liss, 1986). The Schafer Method was recommended as the standard for resuscitation in the United States until the late 1940s when it finally became apparent that ventilation was inadequate with this technique. Definitive proof of the clear superiority of mouth-to-mouth ventilation compared to manual methods of ventilation was provided a decade later by Safar et al (1958). It is ironic that it took more than 200 years after the Paris Academy's 1740 Policy Statement before the superiority of mouth-to-mouth ventilation was finally realized.

Development of Electrical Defibrillation and Cardiac Compression

The first recorded use of electricity in cardiopulmonary resuscitation dates back to 1775 when Squires described successful defibrillation of a 3-year-old child who had fallen out of a window (Julian, 1975). Some 30 years later Burns combined lung inflation with electric countershock in attempted resuscitation.

At about the same time, other investigators were exploring the use of chest compression. The technique was initially tried in animals, and then in humans (Kouwenhoven et al, 1960). Surprisingly, use of *external chest compression (ECC)* was quickly replaced by a "more advanced" technique — *open chest cardiac massage (OCCM)*. Interest in the use of closed-chest cardiac massage (i.e., ECC) wasn't revived until more than a half century later. Then, in 1903, Crile reported the first successful use of ECC in human resuscitation.† Despite Crile's successful report with the use of ECC, the belief that opening the chest

---

*A similar type of inversion had been used in Egypt 3,500 years earlier on victims of drowning (Liss, 1986).

---

*In a sense, the *precordial thump* may be our last remaining "vestige" of *beating on the victim* in an attempt to restore spontaneous respiration and circulation (Liss, 1986).

†It is of historical interest that Crile was probably also the first investigator to recognize the key role of epinephrine in increasing aortic diastolic pressure and coronary perfusion in the arrested heart (Crile, 1904).

(to perform OCCM) was necessary for successful resuscitation of the arrested heart generally persisted until the mid-1950s.

Impetus for development of the modern defibrillator was provided by the Consolidated Electric Company of New York in 1926 (Sladen, 1984). Research on the use of electricity in industry was funded by the company out of concern for the excessive number of electric shock accidents to their linesmen. The goal was to develop a technique for defibrillation of electrocuted victims that did not require opening the chest (i.e., closed-chest or external defibrillation). Research led to a series of advancements including successful use of external defibrillation in dogs (Gurvich and Yuniev, 1939), successful use of internal (open-chest) defibrillation of man (in conjunction with OCCM) by Beck in 1947 (Jude et al, 1961), and successful use of external defibrillation in man by Zoll (Zoll et al, 1956).

Modern success with ECC was reported by both Bahnson and Jude in 1958 (Sladen, 1984). Two years later, Kouwenhoven, Jude, and Knickerbocker (1960) achieved the momentous milestone of successfully integrating all three components (ECC, mouth-to-mouth ventilation, and external defibrillation) in a resuscitation effort. *The modern era of cardiopulmonary resuscitation had begun!*

As with so many other discoveries in science and medicine, verification of the efficacy of closed-chest cardiac massage was the result of a *chance observation*. Thus in 1958, while preparing to defibrillate a dog in ventricular fibrillation, Kouwenhoven and Knickerbocker noted that the pressure exerted by defibrillator paddles (which were relatively heavy) on the chest wall of the dog produced a marked rise in femoral arterial pressure. They then postulated that intentional application of manual pressure in a rhythmic fashion to the chest wall of the animal might produce a corresponding rhythmic increase in arterial pressure—and were rewarded by generation of blood flow in the arrested heart.

The Modern Era of CPR

Application of cardiopulmonary resuscitation techniques have continuously expanded in the modern era. Use in the prehospital setting was advanced by Pantridge and Gedders in Belfast (1967) with initiation of a program for delivering ambulances (called "mobile coronary care units"), medical equipment, and health care providers to victims at the scene of out-of-hospital cardiac arrest. Subsequent work by Leonard Cobb resulted in development of an exceedingly effective EMS (emergency medical services) system in Seattle, Washington, that has since become the prototype for the rest of the country (Cobb et al, 1980). Interestingly, initial statements by the American Red Cross and American Heart Association restricted application of ECC and mouth-to-mouth ventilation to *trained* medical personnel. It has since become apparent that the cornerstone of any effective resuscitation program must be the active involvement of the community. Although ultimate survival from out-of-hospital cardiac arrest is determined by early defibrillation, extension of teaching basic life support skills to the lay public (with emphasis on early recognition of cardiac arrest and impending arrest) is the essential first step for implementing successful EMS programs.

References

American Heart Association Subcommittee on Emergency Cardiac Care: Standards and guidelines for cardiopulmonary resuscitation (CPR) and emergency cardiac care (ECC), *JAMA* 227 (suppl): 833-868, 1974.

Cobb LA, Hallstrom AP, Thompson RG, Mandell MA, Copass MK: Community cardiopulmonary resuscitation, *Ann Rev Med* 31:453-462, 1980.

Crile WG: Surgical anemia and resuscitation, New York, 1904, D Appleton and Co.

Criley JM, Niemann JT, Rosborough JP: Cardiopulmonary resuscitation research 1960-1984: discoveries and advances, *Ann Emerg Med* 13:756-758, 1984.

DeBard ML: The history of cardiopulmonary resuscitation, *Ann Emerg Med* 9:273-275, 1980.

Gurvich HL, Yuniev GS: Restoration of heart rhythm during fibrillation by condenser discharge, *Am Rev Soviet Med* 4:252-256, 1947.

Jude JR, Kouwenhoven WB, Knickerbocker GG: Cardiac arrest, *JAMA* 178:1063-1070, 1961.

Julian DG: Cardiac resuscitation in the eighteenth century, *Heart Lung* 4:46-48, 1975.

Kings II, 4:34-35 (KJV).

Kouwenhoven WB, Jude JR, Knickerbocker GG: Closed-chest cardiac massage, *JAMA* 173:1064-1067, 1960.

Liss HP: A history of resuscitation, *Ann Emerg Med* 15:65-72, 1986.

Pantridge JF, Gedders JS: A mobile intensive care unit in the management of myocardial infarction, *Lancet* 2:271-273, 1967.

Safar P, Escarraga LA, Elam JO: A comparison of the mouth-to-mouth and mouth-to-airway methods of artificial respiration with the chest-pressure arm-lift methods, *N Engl J Med* 258:671-677, 1958.

Sladen A: Closed-chest massage, Kouwenhoven, Jude, Knickerbocker, *JAMA* 251:3137-3140, 1984.

Zoll PM, Linenthal AJ, Gibson W, Paul MH, Norman LR: Termination of ventricular fibrillation in man by externally placed electric countershock, *N Engl J Med* 254:727-732, 1956.

SECTION C

MECHANISMS, EFFICACY, AND COMPLICATIONS OF CPR

The Cardiac Pump Theory

Despite more than 30 years of experience with modern CPR techniques, much remains to be learned regarding the mechanism for blood flow during cardiac arrest. As we indicated in the previous section, the initial discovery of modern CPR was serendipitous, resulting from the chance observation that downward pressure from the weight of defibrillator paddles placed on the chest wall of a fibrillating animal produced an increase in femoral artery pressure. From this observation came the theory that rhythmic application of manual pressure on the chest wall might produce meaningful blood flow in the arrested state, and that the mechanism for such blood flow was direct compression of the heart between the sternum and vertebral column *(cardiac pump theory)*.

Recent evidence suggests that other mechanisms are operative with CPR. While the cardiac pump theory may explain blood flow during cardiac arrest in infants, young children, and other individuals with thin and/or compliant chest walls, direct cardiac compression is probably *not* the major mechanism for generating blood flow in many

(most?) adults (Niemann et al, 1981; Weisfeldt et al, 1981; Rogers, 1983).

A number of observations have led researchers to believe in the importance of other mechanisms. If blood flow were simply the result of direct cardiac compression, one would expect pressure in the left ventricle to dramatically increase as blood was "squeezed" out of this chamber. The mitral valve would then close in response to the high pressure gradient produced between the left ventricle and the left atrium, and heart size would decrease as blood was ejected from the aorta. Similar events should occur on the right side of the heart as blood was ejected into the pulmonary bed (Fig. 10C-1).

Evidence against the cardiac pump theory derives from studies suggesting that cardiac chamber size does not change significantly during CPR, pressures remain equal in all cardiac chambers and intrathoracic vessels, and heart valves remain open throughout the entire cardiac cycle (Luce et al, 1980; Bircher, 1982). This evidence suggests that rather than acting as a pump, the heart serves more as a *passive conduit* for blood flow during CPR. No pressure gradient is produced anywhere within the thorax,

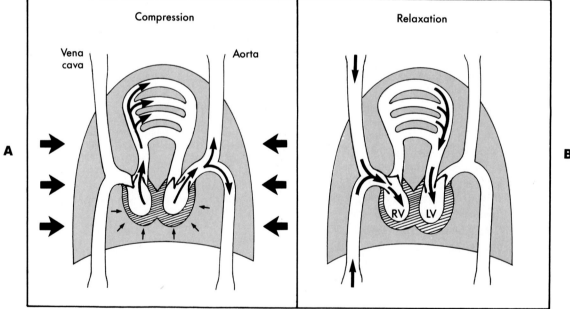

Figure 10C-1.   Sequence of events that should occur during the compression and relaxation-phases of CPR *if the* **cardiac pump theory** *was operative.* **A,** External chest *compression* would produce an increase in intraventricular pressure. This would generate a pressure gradient, causing the mitral and tricuspid valves to close while blood is simultaneously ejected from the aorta and pulmonary artery. **B,** During the *relaxation* phase, pressure in the ventricles drops significantly, and blood is returned to the thorax. Opening of the tricuspid valve allows the right ventricle to fill, while opening of the mitral valve allows blood from the pulmonary bed to return to the left side of the heart. The drop in intraventricular pressures (in the right and left ventricle) explains the closure of the pulmonary and aortic valves during the relaxation phase.

and the increase in intrathoracic pressure that occurs with external chest compression is generalized.

Additional evidence against the cardiac pump theory is provided by observations of blood flow during CPR performed on patients with emphysema and flail sternum. If the heart did function as a pump, one would expect blood flow during CPR to be minimal in emphysematous patients since direct cardiac compression should be much more difficult to accomplish in "barrel-chested" individuals. In contrast, one would expect blood flow to be maximal in traumatized patients with flail sternum. What better opportunity for direct cardiac compression could there be than when the sternum is unrestricted by its costal attachments?

In fact, neither of these expectations is realized. Blood flow in emphysematous individuals is comparable to blood flow in individuals with normal chest wall configurations. Traumatized victims with flail sternum demonstrate minimal blood flow with CPR *unless* the thorax is bound and stabilized to allow for a generalized increase in intrathoracic pressure.

Final evidence against the cardiac pump theory was provided by Criley et al (1976) with the introduction in the 1970s of the technique known as *cough CPR*. With this self-administered form of CPR, a number of subjects were able to sustain consciousness during ventricular fibrillation for periods of up to 90 seconds simply by forceful repetitive coughing. Such coughing generated high intrathoracic pressures (of up to 140 mm Hg!) that somehow resulted in adequate blood flow despite the presence of a nonperfusing rhythm (ventricular fibrillation or asystole). *How could the cardiac pump theory be the only mechanism operative when coughing alone* (without any chest compression) *was enough to maintain consciousness?*

The Thoracic Pump Theory

To try and answer the question of how cough CPR could sustain consciousness despite the presence of a nonperfusing rhythm, the *thoracic pump theory* was proposed. Rather than saying that a pressure gradient is generated between cardiac and vascular structures *within* the thorax, this theory suggests that the pressure gradient develops *outside* the thorax. The intrathoracic-extrathoracic pressure differential produced provides the impetus for forward (antegrade) flow of blood out of the aorta (Fig. 10C-2).

Three factors allow unidirectional flow of blood to occur with sternal compression. They are:

1. Functional venous closure at the thoracic inlet
2. Preserved patency of the carotid artery
3. Greater *capacitance* of the extrathoracic venous bed*

Researchers have postulated that a valve exists in the jugular vein at the thoracic inlet. Competence of this valve would explain why retrograde flow does not occur out of the thoracic cavity with chest compression. That valves exist elsewhere in the jugular vein is evidenced by the fact that blood does not flow up the neck during a Valsalva

---

*Because veins have greater capacitance than arteries, lower pressures are generated in the venous system for an equal volume of blood.

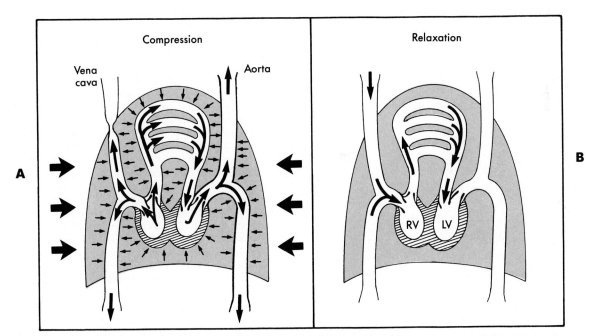

Figure 10C-2.   Sequence of events that should occur during the compression and relaxation-phases of CPR if the **thoracic pump theory** was operative. **A,** The impetus for blood flow with the thoracic pump theory results from generation of an **intra***thoracic*-**extra***thoracic* pressure gradient. However, *the increase in intrathoracic pressure with compression is generalized.* Undirectional forward flow is made possible by functional venous closure at the thoracic inlet, preserved patency of the thick-walled carotid artery, and greater capacitance of the extrathoracic venous bed. The heart merely serves as a *passive conduit* for blood flow. **B,** The drop in intrathoracic pressure with *relaxation* allows blood return to the thorax. Blood flow below the diaphragm is minimal due to the lack of valves in the inferior vena cava.

maneuver. However, whether or not a valve is present precisely at the thoracic inlet is still the subject of controversy. In any event the lack of retrograde flow out of the thoracic cavity can at least be explained by a *functional* closure that occurs when the thin-walled jugular vein is collapsed by the increase in intrathoracic pressure generated by external chest compression.

In contrast, the thick-walled carotid artery resists compression and remains patent throughout CPR. By doing so it allows transmission of intrathoracic pressure to the extrathoracic arterial bed. This increase in pressure is also transmitted to the extrathoracic venous bed, but because of the greater *capacitance* of venous structures, pressures do not rise to nearly the same degree as they do on the arterial side. An *intrathoracic-extrathoracic* pressure gradient is thus established, and blood flows out of the thorax (Luce et al, 1980; Niemann et al, 1981).

Blood returns during the relaxation phase of CPR. With release of chest compression, pressure within the thorax drops to virtually zero. The residual pressure in the extrathoracic venous bed now exceeds pressure within the thorax, and blood flows back into the chest (see Fig. 10C-2). Cardiac valves remain open throughout the process, and the heart merely serves as a "passive conduit" for blood flow.

> The presence of venous valves is essential for producing and maintaining a pressure difference between the carotid artery and the internal jugular vein. Without this valving mechanism, blood would not flow during CPR. In contrast, no such valving mechanism is present in the inferior vena cava. As a result, pressures in the arteries and veins of the abdomen and lower extremities are nearly equal during external chest compression, and circulation to the lower extremities is significantly less than that to the thorax and head (Niemann et al, 1981). Clinically this is important in explaining why the femoral vein is no longer a favored route for drug administration during CPR.

Additional Means for Improving Blood Flow with CPR

Researchers reasoned that if the thoracic pump mechanism was operative, a number of modifications in CPR technique might enhance blood flow during cardiac arrest. These included:

- SCV-CPR (simultaneous compression-ventilation CPR)
- Abdominal binding
- Increase in the ventilatory rate to 40 per minute (with a corresponding reduction in the rate of compression to the same rate of 40 per minute)
- Prolongation of compression duration to 60% of the compression-relaxation cycle

Taken together, these modifications formed the *"New CPR,"* a research technique that received much attention in the early 1980s (Bircher, 1982). Understanding the rationale for suggesting these modifications provides insight to the mechanism for blood flow during CPR in the arrested heart. If blood flow during CPR is dependent on generation of an intrathoracic-extrathoracic pressure gradient (as postulated by the thoracic pump theory), then maximizing intrathoracic pressure should maximize blood flow during CPR. Coordinating external chest compression so that it occurs *simultaneously* with ventilation (i.e., **S**imultaneous **C**ompression-**V**entilation or **SCV**-CPR) maximizes intrathoracic pressure. When this is done experimentally, peripheral and common carotid blood flow increase dramatically (Chandra et al, 1980; 1990).

Abdominal binding is another way of increasing intrathoracic pressure during CPR. Abdominal binding limits passive movement of the diaphragm during CPR (Niemann et al, 1982). This results in an increase in common carotid blood flow. Aortic afterload also increases, and presumably leads to preferential redistribution of blood to the coronary and cerebral vascular beds. Other investigators have suggested that *application of military anti-shock trousers* (MAST suit) or *interposed abdominal compressions* (IAC)* might result in a similar favorable redistribution of carotid blood flow during CPR (Ohomoto et al, 1976; Lilja et al, 1981; Ward et al, 1989; Sack et al, 1992).

> It should be emphasized that the New CPR is a research tool that has *never* been recommended for clinical application by either the lay public or trained health care personnel (Krischer et al, 1989). For a number of reasons, this technique simply would not work in practice. First, the high pressure ventilation of the New CPR requires endotracheal intubation. This alone prevents its use by the lay public. With the New CPR, one ventilation is delivered for each chest compression (SCV-CPR). At a rate of 40 compressions per minute, this means that 40 ventilations would have to be delivered each minute—a rate far too rapid for use in the field. Finally, coordinating ventilation so that it occurs simultaneously with compression, and extending compression duration to occupy at least 60% of the cardiac cycle are both difficult objectives to achieve consistently by human endeavor. Laboratory use of a mechanical compression device (thumper) is needed.
>
> Despite these limitations, the New CPR has been instrumental in providing us with a wealth of information about the mechanism of blood flow during cardiopulmonary resuscitation. Application of this knowledge has led to our realization that *duration of compression* is at least equally important as rate as a determinant of cardiac output during CPR. Awareness that an *increase* in intrathoracic pressure is a major mechanism for blood flow has resulted in elimination of the previous recommendation to interpose ventilations with compression, and has led to adoption of the asynchronous mode of CPR for the intubated patient.

---

*Application of IAC-CPR requires the addition of a third rescuer whose task is to *interpose* an abdominal compression (performed with approximated open hands centered over the umbilicus) between each chest compression. Thus, the rate of abdominal compressions equals the rate of chest compressions—and the goal is to increase intra-abdominal (and abdominal aortic) pressure in the hope of increasing aortic diastolic pressure *(see Addendum at the end of this section)*.

Clinical Implications of CPR Mechanisms

It should be realized that the thoracic pump model has not been unquestionably accepted by all investigators in the field as the principal mechanism for blood flow in adults during CPR. Advocates of another theory known as *high-impulse CPR* assert that direct cardiac compression *is* an important mechanism in many adults, and that maximal cardiac output will only be obtained when manual massage is performed at a rapid rate with brief compression of moderate force (Maier et al, 1984). Compressing more rapidly naturally increases the *force* of each compression. It may be that force rather than (or in conjunction with) faster rates and a longer relative duration of compression is the key. Advocates of this theory question the validity of the thoracic pump theory in view of more recent echocardiographic studies demonstrating mitral valve closure with high-impulse chest compression and the occurrence of antegrade transmitral blood flow *only* during compression diastole (Deshmukh et al, 1985; Feneley et al, 1987).

Although the full story is not yet known, the "true" explanation for blood flow during CPR is likely to be part of a spectrum. Direct cardiac compression appears to play a major role in infants, young children, and individuals with thin and compliant chest walls.* At the other end of the spectrum (i.e., in many adults—especially those with emphysema), the thoracic pump model appears to provide a more rational explanation for blood flow. In between these two extremes, a combination of cardiac and thoracic pump models (and perhaps high-impulse CPR) is probably operative.

> Recent results from echocardiographic studies performed during CPR suggest that the mechanism for blood flow may actually *change* during resuscitation (Deshmukh et al, 1989; Higano et al, 1990). During the early minutes (? first 10 minutes) of the code, the mechanism for blood flow may be direct cardiac compression (i.e., cardiac pump theory) with increased force (i.e., high-impulse) compressions providing the major impetus for blood flow. Later on in the process, cardiac valves no longer appear to actively close and open during compression systole and diastole, at which point the thoracic pump theory (in which the heart acts more as a *passive conduit* for blood flow) may become the predominant model.

Clinical implications of determining the mechanism for blood flow with CPR are that this knowledge might shed light on the optimal rate for chest compression. Assuming force and compression duration time remain relatively constant, faster rates (up to 120 beats per minute) should optimize blood flow according to the cardiac pump theory. This is because the relatively constant stroke volume associated with the cardiac pump theory should produce a greater cardiac output if the rate of compression is increased* (Maier et al, 1984; Swenson et al, 1988; Kern and Ewy, 1990).

> In the laboratory, the "ideal" compression rate appears to be between 100 and 120 times per minute. Faster rates (i.e., greater than 120 per minute) are not recommended because they would excessively abbreviate diastolic filling time and thus compromise cardiac perfusion (Feneley et al, 1988). Practically speaking, compression rate is limited by the human factor of fatigue. It is extremely difficult (tiring) to continue to perform chest compressions at a rate of 120 times per minute for any length of time (Kern and Ewy, 1990).

In contrast, compression *duration* (rather than rate) appears to be the primary determinant of cardiac output with the thoracic pump theory. Slower rates (performed so as to maintain compression duration) should produce optimal blood flow according to this theory. However, faster rates could also be beneficial because they might make it easier to achieve the desired 50% compression-relaxation ratio believed to be optimal by advocates of the thoracic pump theory. This was the reasoning for changing the recommended compression rate from 60 per minute to a rate of between 80 to 100 per minute for both one- and two-rescuer CPR (AHA ACLS Text, 1986). *Increasing the rate represented a compromise* that should lead to increased blood flow regardless of whether the cardiac pump theory, thoracic pump theory, or high-impulse CPR was the predominant mechanism for blood flow in a particular individual. If anything, *we would favor erring on the higher side of this range* (i.e., compressing as close to a rate of 100 per minute as possible), especially during the early minutes of the resuscitation process—as this may be the most effective noninvasive way to optimize blood flow during CPR.

> Although the AHA recommendation to perform chest compressions at a rate of *at least* 80 per minute has been generally well accepted, many emergency care providers just don't maintain rates within this range in practice. Instead (and despite the best of intentions), when left to their own, emergency care providers tend to slow down the rate of compression as the code progresses (Kern et al, 1992). Moreover, many emergency care providers appear to be *unaware* of the rate at which they are compressing (Ewy, 1990; Kern et al, 1992).
>
> To remedy this situation (and help optimize cardiac output during CPR), consideration might be given to the use of some objective method for timing (and pacing the rate of) cardiac compressions. This may be done with a *metronome* (as is used to keep time in music) or an *audiorecording*. Use of an audio-prompted, rate-directing signal in this manner is a simple, practical way to ensure awareness of the correct rate of compressions. Doing so not only facilitates maintenance of the rate of compressions within the correct range throughout the resuscitation effort, but it also leads to objective improvement (as demonstrated by increased ET CO_2 readings) in compression efficacy (Kern et al, 1992).

---

*As discussed in Section A of Chapter 2, **Cardiac output = stroke volume × heart rate.** Assuming stroke volume is kept relatively constant, cardiac output should become greater as heart rate is increased.

---

*See Addendum at the end of this section.

Efficacy of CPR: Are the Vital Organs Perfused?

Two final questions remain:
1. *Does the increase in common carotid blood flow produced by the New CPR result in improved cerebral perfusion?*
2. *Does it improve coronary blood flow?*

Under the best of circumstances, cardiac output generated by performance of basic life support during cardiac arrest is no more than 20% to 30% of cardiac output during spontaneous circulation (Del Guercio et al, 1963; Falk et al, 1988). Without the use of medication, however, no more than a fraction of this output is delivered to the two key organs: the heart and the brain. Although one might logically assume that increases in common carotid blood flow as produced by the New CPR should result in improved cerebral perfusion, this is not necessarily the case (Luce et al, 1980; Rogers, 1983; Sanders et al, 1984). The common carotid artery divides into two branches: the external and the internal carotid arteries. The tongue, face, scalp, and neck are supplied by the former, while the internal branch supplies the brain. *When CPR is performed in the absence of pharmacologic therapy, blood is preferentially shunted to the external carotid artery.* Thus, even though common carotid blood flow may more than double with SCV-CPR, cerebral perfusion remains minimal.

Use of adjuncts such as abdominal binding has been advocated in the hope of improving coronary and cerebral blood flow. However, such measures are of unproven benefit and may even be deleterious. Blood flow to the brain is determined by cerebral perfusion pressure. This is equal to mean arterial pressure minus resting intracranial pressure (ICP):

```
Cerebral Perfusion  =  Mean Arterial  -  ICP
    Pressure               Pressure
```

Abdominal binding increases intrathoracic pressure. Because of free communication between veins in the intrathoracic and intracerebral compartments, increases in intrathoracic pressure lead to increases in resting ICP. But as can be seen from the above equation, an increase in ICP will *reduce* blood flow to the brain (Rogers, 1983; Ewy 1984; Michael et al, 1984).

> Potential benefits from application of procedures such as IAC-CPR are exciting but remain controversial. Although this technique may produce more favorable hemodynamics than standard CPR, improvement in cerebral blood flow is uncertain, and it remains to be proved whether neurologically intact survival rates can be consistently increased (Berryman and Phillips, 1984; Howard et al, 1987; Ward et al, 1989). Nevertheless, initial results by Sack et al (1992) are encouraging

and hold promise in the interim awaiting results from further clinical trials.

What about coronary perfusion? Although external chest compression may generate *systolic* blood pressure peaks of more than 100 mm Hg, *diastolic blood pressure is extremely low in the absence of pharmacologic therapy.* It is essential to remember that **the coronary arteries are perfused during diastole.** Increasing systolic blood pressure by external chest compression without also increasing diastolic blood pressure will therefore have little (if any) beneficial effect on coronary blood flow (Luce et al, 1980; Niemann et al, 1982; Sanders et al, 1984; Martin et al, 1986).

Once again, abdominal binding, application of the MAST suit, and IAC (interposed abdominal compression)-CPR have all been advocated in the hope of favorably redistributing blood flow to the coronary circulation during CPR. However, these techniques are cumbersome to employ during cardiopulmonary resuscitation, their benefit is unproven, and their use cannot be recommended at the present time. Moreover, to encourage application of a MAST suit or abdominal binding while CPR is being performed on patients in ventricular fibrillation might divert attention and delay treatment (defibrillation) of the primary disorder.

Another intervention that had been recommended in the past for increasing common carotid blood flow is *volume loading.* Utilization of the MAST suit hoped to take advantage of this concept by *autotransfusion* of lower extremity circulating volume to the intravascular compartment above the diaphragm. Although volume loading does increase common carotid flow, overall perfusion of vital organs (the heart and brain) is paradoxically decreased by this technique (Ditchey and Lindenfeld, 1984). Volume loading cannot be recommended for the normovolemic victim in cardiac arrest.

Open-Chest CPR

The problem of perfusing vital organs by closed-chest cardiac massage (CCCM) can be resolved by thoracotomy, cross-clamping the aorta, and direct manual cardiac compression *(open-chest CPR)*. This technique was first described in the 1800s and remained the most commonly accepted method of cardiac resuscitation until after introduction of CCCM in 1960. Survival with open-chest CPR varied greatly, but success rates of up to 50% were reported in selected cases when open-chest CPR was performed in the operating room. Unlike CCCM, the limitations of blood flow to vital organs imposed by the heart being contained within the intrathoracic cavity (compartment) are obviated by opening the chest (thoracotomy). Direct cardiac compression more than *triples* cardiac output, and blood flow to the heart and brain is favored (Bircher and Safar, 1984; Sanders et al, 1984; Sanders et al, 1985). The technique may be lifesaving when patients fail to respond to CCCM. However, if it is to be effective, it appears that open-chest CPR must be started early (Sanders et al, 1985; Kern et al, 1987). Even though hemodynamics may be temporarily improved, delay of open-chest CPR beyond 10 to 12 minutes will usually negate any beneficial effect of the procedure on survival (Kern and Ewy, 1990). Because of the risks of the procedure, its restriction to centers with readily accessible trained personnel comfortable in performing the procedure, and a lack of convincing evidence of its superiority in improving ultimate survival compared to CCCM, the impact of open-chest CPR has not been (and is not likely to be) appreciable.

Epinephrine

Short of opening the chest, *how can one increase blood flow to vital organs (the heart and brain) during CPR?*

The answer lies with pharmacologic therapy—and specifically with epinephrine. As discussed in detail in Chapter 2, epinephrine exerts both α-adrenergic and β-adrenergic effects. In the setting of cardiopulmonary arrest, the α-adrenergic (or vasoconstrictor) effect is by far the most important action of this drug (Michael et al, 1984; Koehler et al, 1985).

Epinephrine works by:

1. Increasing aortic *diastolic* pressure—which increases the gradient for blood flow to the coronary arteries.
2. Preserving carotid artery tone—which allows intrathoracic pressure to be transmitted intact to the extrathoracic arterial bed (which is a prerequisite for circulation of blood according to the thoracic pump theory).
3. Increasing extracranial arterial resistance—which results in shunting of blood from the external to the internal carotid artery, thus increasing cerebral perfusion (Rogers, 1983; Michael et al, 1984; Koehler et al, 1985).

As already emphasized, the coronary arteries are perfused during diastole. As a result, the gradient for blood flow to the coronary arteries (i.e., *coronary perfusion pressure*) is determined by the difference in pressure between the aorta and the right atrium at the onset of diastole (Fig. 10C-3):

Coronary Perfusion Pressure	=	Aortic Diastolic Pressure	−	Right Atrial Diastolic Pressure

Performance of basic life support during cardiac arrest does little to favor coronary blood flow because the pressure generated by external chest compressions is primarily *systolic* in nature. Instead, it is the α-adrenergic (vasoconstrictor) effect of epinephrine that holds the key for assuring adequate blood flow during cardiac arrest. Vasoconstriction increases aortic diastolic pressure. As can be seen from the above equation, increasing aortic diastolic pressure produces a corresponding increase in coronary perfusion pressure.

Paradis et al suggest that achieving an adequate aortic diastolic pressure during cardiopulmonary resuscitation may be

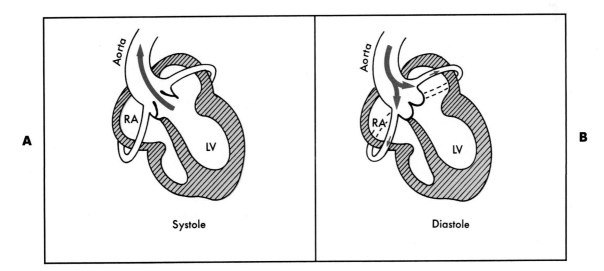

Figure 10C-3. Blood flow to the coronary arteries. **A,** During *systole*, blood is ejected from the left ventricle. The aortic valve opens, allowing entry to the systemic circulation. **B,** Soon after the onset of *diastole*, the aortic valve closes. Returning blood now perfuses the coronary arteries (which terminate in the coronary sinus that drains into the right atrium). The gradient for blood flow to the coronary arteries (i.e., *coronary perfusion pressure*) is determined by the difference in pressure between the aorta and the right atrium at the onset of diastole.

the single most important determinant of survival. Return of spontaneous circulation (ROSC) is improbable when maximal coronary perfusion pressure during resuscitation is less than 15 mm Hg. ROSC only becomes likely if coronary perfusion pressure exceeds 20 mm Hg (Paradis et al 1990).

The optimal dose of epinephrine during cardiac arrest is still unknown. Despite an absence of data demonstrating improved long-term survival, it appears that *high-dose epinephrine* (i.e., administration of more than 1 mg of epinephrine every 5 minutes) is needed to ensure achievement of adequate coronary perfusion pressure during cardiopulmonary resuscitation of adults (Paradis et al, 1991).

Assessment of the Efficacy of Resuscitative Efforts

Up until recently there had been no practical way to monitor the efficacy of resuscitative efforts. Despite the predictive value of coronary perfusion pressure as an indicator of ultimate survival, this technique is invasive and requires rapid insertion of a catheter into the right atrium at the onset of cardiac arrest. It is often neither practical nor feasible to perform this procedure in the acute setting.

As discussed in Chapter 2, arterial blood gas (ABG) analysis is not the reliable indicator of acid-base status during cardiac arrest that it was previously thought to be. This is because a significant discrepancy (of up to several pH units) develops between arterial and mixed venous blood within seconds of the onset of cardiac arrest (Grundler et al, 1985; Weil et al, 1986). Thus, the pH measured by ABGs may differ substantially from the true pH at the cellular level (which is more closely reflected by the pH of mixed venous blood). In addition, the low flow state associated with cardiac arrest dramatically reduces pulmonary flow. This significantly prolongs the time available for gas exchange in the lungs. As a result, arterial oxygen concentrations may be deceptively normal, or even increased despite the absence of an effective cardiac output.

Palpation of arterial pulses cannot be depended upon to accurately reflect hemodynamic status during external chest compression either. Although it is reasonable to assume that arterial pressure (and coronary flow) during CPR will not be adequate if chest compression fails to produce a palpable pulse, the converse is *not* necessarily true. That is, *the presence of a palpable pulse during CPR does not assure that coronary flow will be adequate* (Paradis et al, 1990; Kern and Ewy, 1990).

Detection of a palpable pulse (during CPR or with spontaneous circulation) depends on *pulse pressure* (i.e., the *difference* between systolic and diastolic pressure readings). **Pulse pressure is not an indicator of coronary perfusion pressure.** Consider the following example in which pressure recordings from the aorta and right atrium are given for two patients (A and B) during compression systole and diastole:

	Patient A	Patient B
Aortic systolic pressure	80 mm Hg	80 mm Hg
Aortic diastolic pressure	25 mm Hg	25 mm Hg
Right atrial diastolic pressure	5 mm Hg	20 mm Hg

PROBLEM   **1. For which patient (A and/or B) should you feel a pulse in the carotid artery during CPR?**
2. For which patient (A and/or B) will coronary perfusion pressure during CPR be adequate (i.e., ≥20 mm Hg)?

ANSWER   As noted, detection of palpable pulse depends on achieving an appreciable pulse pressure. In this example, the pulse pressure (i.e., the difference between aortic systolic and diastolic pressure) for *both* patients A and B is 55 mm Hg (80 − 25), a value which should be sufficient to produce a palpable pulse. However, coronary perfusion pressure will *not* be the same for the two patients. Coronary perfusion pressure (i.e., the difference between aortic and right atrial *diastolic* pressure) is 20 mm Hg for patient A (25 − 5), a value which should be sufficient to ensure adequate coronary flow. In contrast, coronary perfusion pressure for patient B is only 5 mm Hg (25 − 20), a value which is clearly too low to provide adequate coronary flow, *despite the fact that a carotid pulse will be palpable.* **Thus, the presence of a palpable pulse during CPR in no way ensures that coronary perfusion will be adequate!**

Emergency care providers frequently palpate for the femoral artery when attempting to determine the presence of a pulse during CPR. It is important to realize that detection of an impulse in the femoral area in association with chest compression does *not* necessarily indicate the presence of an *arterial* pulse.

Lower extremity veins lack valves. As a result, retrograde *venous* transmission of the impulse from chest compression may occasionally be felt as a pulsation in the femoral area (and be mistakenly perceived as an arterial pulsation).

Because of these shortcomings with standard monitoring methods, efforts have been directed at developing a noninvasive, easy-to-perform technique for predicting survival and assessing the efficacy of ongoing resuscitation. Measurement of end-tidal CO_2 (carbon dioxide) by capnography seems to satisfy these needs (Grauer, Cavallaro, and Gums, 1991).

End-Tidal CO_2 Monitoring

End-tidal CO_2 (ET CO_2) is the amount of carbon dioxide present in expired air.* This amount depends on three factors (Garnett et al, 1987; Falk et al, 1988):

1. CO_2 production
2. Pulmonary perfusion
3. Minute ventilation

---

*The initial part of an expired breath contains no CO_2 because it comes from the "dead space" (i.e., residual air in the airway space). It is the last ("end-tidal") portion of expired air that reflects the CO_2 content of alveolar equilibration.

CO_2 is produced in cells of the body as an end product of metabolism **(1).** It is then transported in the systemic circulation to the heart, and ultimately to the lungs (pulmonary perfusion) where it is eliminated in expired air **(2).** Under normal circumstances (i.e., with spontaneous circulation and adequate peripheral perfusion), the amount of CO_2 eliminated by the lungs will depend on the minute ventilation (i.e., the product of tidal volume and the number of respirations per minute—**3).** Under normal circumstances, hyperventilation would therefore be expected to increase ET CO_2 values.

In contrast, with a low flow state (such as cardiac arrest), the *limiting factor* for determining CO_2 content in expired air becomes *pulmonary perfusion.* If CO_2 is inadequately delivered to the lungs, it cannot be eliminated, regardless of the efficacy of ventilation (Garnett et al, 1987; Falk et al, 1988). Thus one would expect ET CO_2 values to remain relatively low with cardiac arrest even when the patient is being hyperventilated.

Pulmonary perfusion depends on cardiac output (Falk et al, 1988). In cardiac arrest, cardiac output and pulmonary perfusion are both negligible. With return of spontaneous circulation (ROSC), cardiac output dramatically improves. As a result, pulmonary perfusion improves, more CO_2 is delivered to and eliminated from the lungs, and ET CO_2 increases. Support for this concept is provided from the excellent correlation that has been shown to exist between coronary perfusion pressure and ET CO_2 values (Sanders et al, 1985).

However, in contrast to measurement of coronary perfusion pressure, ET CO_2 monitoring is an entirely noninvasive procedure that is extremely easy to perform during cardiac arrest. All it requires is attachment of a device to the endotracheal tube that measures the content of CO_2 in expired air. Studies on human subjects demonstrate lowest ET CO_2 values with cardiopulmonary arrest, higher values with performance of cardiopulmonary resuscitation (which may generate 20% to 30% of baseline cardiac output), and a dramatic increase with ROSC.

In a study by Sanders et al (1989) of 35 patients with cardiac arrest, each of the 9 survivors had an average ET CO_2 partial pressure ($P_{ET}CO_2$) of ≥10 mm Hg. (average value = 15 mm Hg).* Only 6 of the 26 nonresuscitated patients had a $P_{ET}CO_2$ ≥10 mm Hg, and the average $P_{ET}CO_2$ value among nonsurvivors was 7 mm Hg (P < 0.001). Of even more clinical significance than the absolute $P_{ET}CO_2$ reading, however, may be the *trend* of this value during resuscitation (Brown and Hendee, 1990; Weil et al, 1990). Thus, a patient whose value remains low is unlikely to be resuscitated unless the therapeutic approach is changed. In contrast, the chance for successful re-

suscitation becomes much greater for patients who respond to therapeutic measures with an increase in $P_{ET}CO_2$. Continued resuscitative efforts should be strongly encouraged in such cases. In fact, *an abrupt rise in ET CO_2 will often be the first clinical indicator that ROSC has occurred* (Garnett et al, 1987; Callaham and Barton, 1990).

PITFALLS IN THE USE OF ET CO_2 MONITORING

A few words of caution are in order. Although $P_{ET}CO_2$ values ≥10 mm Hg are highly correlated with survival, *not* all patients with such values survive. Clearly other factors (e.g., underlying disease, patient age, the mechanism of the arrest, time until defibrillation) are equally important parameters for determining the likelihood of survival. What can be said is that *survival is extremely unlikely in patients with $P_{ET}CO_2$ values that are consistently below 10 mm Hg.*

Emergency care providers should also be aware of the fact that administration of sodium bicarbonate increases $P_{ET}CO_2$ because it liberates CO_2 which must then be excreted through the lungs. The effect is transient, of a much lesser degree than occurs with ROSC, and $P_{ET}CO_2$ usually returns to its baseline value within 5 minutes (Garnett et al, 1987; Sanders et al, 1989; Brown and Hendee, 1990). In contrast, epinephrine administration may slightly decrease $P_{ET}CO_2$ values despite the fact that this drug increases the chance of successful resuscitation (Weil et al, 1990). Epinephrine-induced vasoconstriction may increase afterload and thus reduce overall cardiac output, leading to decreased pulmonary perfusion. The beneficial effect of epinephrine on coronary and cerebral perfusion probably outweighs this drawback.

USE OF ET CO_2 MONITORING IN CLINICAL DECISION MAKING

The potential of ET CO_2 monitoring for predicting outcome from cardiopulmonary resuscitation is extremely promising, especially when sophisticated capnometer sensors are used with in-line connections to the endotracheal tube and continuous $P_{ET}CO_2$ recordings are made. In a prospective study of 55 adult, nontraumatic prehospital cardiac arrest patients, the **initial $P_{ET}CO_2$ reading** (obtained as soon as intubation was accomplished) was highly predictive of whether ROSC would occur at any point during resuscitation (Callaham and Barton, 1990). In this study, an initial $P_{ET}CO_2$ reading of ≥15 mm Hg had a 71% sensitivity and 98% specificity for correctly predicting ROSC. In contrast, patients who never developed a spontaneous pulse had a mean initial $P_{ET}CO_2$ reading of 5 mm Hg.

Although each case must be individualized and considered on its own merit, awareness of the predictive and prognostic value of the initial $P_{ET}CO_2$ reading (immediately after intubation) may greatly assist in clinical decision making (Weil and Gazmuri, 1990).

---

*ET CO_2 readings are typically reported *either* in units of pressure (i.e., mm Hg) or as a percentage figure that indicates the content (i.e., %) of CO_2 in expired air. Normally, the CO_2 content of expired air is approximately 4%. This corresponds to a partial pressure of CO_2 ($P_{ET}CO_2$) of approximately 30 mm Hg. As noted above, partial pressures of ≥10 mm Hg (i.e., a 1% to 2% expired air CO_2 content) appear to be necessary for there to be a reasonable chance for ultimate survival.

1. Since the chance for ultimate survival in patients with low initial values is so small, prolonged resuscitation (beyond 20 to 30 minutes) would seem futile (and may not be warranted) unless values begin to rise.
2. Low initial $P_{ET}CO_2$ values (or values that decrease as the code progresses) may indicate a need for alteration in CPR technique or methodology (a need for open-chest CPR?) if there is to be a realistic chance for survival.
3. In patients with asystole, relatively high initial values with CPR at least suggest that closed-chest compression is successfully perfusing the pulmonary circuit (Callaham and Barton, 1990).
4. Relatively high initial values make it unlikely that a clinical diagnosis of EMD is correct. A surprisingly high percentage of patients are mistakenly diagnosed as having "EMD" when in fact they have measurable systolic blood pressures (between 40 to 100 mm Hg) by transducer (Berryman, 1986). Thus, despite the absence of a palpable pulse, a greater than expected initial $P_{ET}CO_2$ reading is evidence against a clinically presumptive diagnosis of EMD and strongly favors the presence of a perfusing rhythm. Direct arterial pressure monitoring, continued intensive therapy (i.e., high-dose epinephrine), and search for a potentially correctable underlying cause of hypotension (i.e., hypovolemia) is indicated in such cases. In contrast, prolonged resuscitation is probably not warranted for patients with true EMD, low initial $P_{ET}CO_2$ readings, and no potentially correctable cause of their nonperfusing rhythm.

USE OF ET CO₂ MONITORING TO VERIFY ET TUBE PLACEMENT

A final important use of ET CO_2 monitoring is to verify correct placement of the endotracheal tube after intubation. Surprisingly, unrecognized esophageal placement occurs *even in the hands of experienced anesthesiologists* in the controlled setting of the operating room (MacLeod et al, 1991). It is much more likely to occur when intubation is performed by less experienced personnel under the stressful conditions of cardiopulmonary arrest (Anton et al, 1991). Although direct observation of endotracheal tube passage through the vocal cords and auscultation for equal, bilateral breath sounds are commonly used as clinical (bedside) standards for verification of correct tube placement, these procedures are *not* infallible (Brunel et al, 1989). Moreover, emergency care providers often assume care of patients who are already intubated, and thus have no knowledge of whether the intubator was able to view the tube pass directly through the cords. Considering the potentially disastrous consequences of unrecognized esophageal intubation (cerebral hypoxia, brain damage, and death), the importance of having a quick, reliable method for verifying correct endotracheal tube placement is obvious (Anton et al, 1991). Realistically, radiographic confirmation of endotracheal tube placement takes too much time. However, ET CO_2 monitoring appears to satisfy the requirements of being a rapid, reliable method for confirming correct ET tube placement.

Disposable CO_2 detection devices are color-coded for ease of use. A change in the indicator from a CO_2 content of less than 0.5% to the 2.5% to 5% range confirms correct endotracheal tube placement. In contrast, failure of the ET CO_2 reading to rise after intubation suggests either incorrect (i.e., esophageal) placement or inadequate perfusion with CPR. The latter is likely when other clinical evidence (equal bilateral breath sounds, direct visualization of endotracheal tube passage through the vocal cords) suggests proper endotracheal tube placement. In such cases, persistent low ET CO_2 readings are an extremely poor prognostic sign (MacLeod et al, 1991; Anton et al, 1991).

Does Lay Bystander CPR Improve Survival?

Much controversy has centered around the question of whether CPR initiated by a lay bystander is important in saving lives of patients with out-of-hospital cardiac arrest. This is understandable considering our previous discussion of how blood flow to the heart and brain is minimal when CPR is performed without pharmacologic therapy. Determining the true value of CPR is made all the more difficult because of the problem in separating out bystander-initiated CPR from the host of other variables that influence survival from cardiac arrest. Response time from patient collapse until arrival of EMS units capable of providing ACLS is especially hard to control for. Lay person perception of time under the stress of witnessing a cardiac arrest (especially if it is on a loved one) is notoriously inaccurate (Hoekstra, 1990). Although one may clock in the time that a witness notifies EMS and accurately calculate response time from that moment, *there is no way to verify how long it really took the witness to recognize the arrest in the first place.* Nor is there any way to determine how long it actually took the witness to make the emergency phone call after recognizing the arrest.

Many of the studies performed to examine this issue suffer from these problems (Hoekstra, 1990). For example, the comprehensive review of the literature by Cummins and Eisenberg (1985) suggests that performance of lay bystander CPR improves survival from prehospital cardiac arrest. Unfortunately, the studies quoted by these authors do not control for the variables of witnessed arrest or paramedic response time, and only a few of them controlled for the variable of presenting rhythm. Uncontrolled studies that demonstrate improved survival with bystander-initiated CPR can be misleading because they are more likely to select cases in which the arrest was witnessed, where the initial rhythm was ventricular tachycardia/fibrillation, and for whom the call for help was put in sooner.

Stueven et al (1986) reached a different conclusion about the efficacy of CPR in a retrospective review of 1,500 prehospital cardiac arrests that occurred in the Milwaukee area over a 10-year period. Their results suggest that when the variables of witnessed arrest, paramedic response times, and presenting rhythm are controlled for, performance of CPR by lay bystanders is *not* of benefit in improving ultimate survival from ventricular fibrillation, ventricular tachycardia, or asystole. Both BLS and ALS response times in the Milwaukee system were extremely rapid (2 and 5 minutes, respectively), and it could be that prompt provision of prehospital care "overpowered" the effect of bystander-initiated CPR in this study

(Spaite et al, 1990). A subsequent retrospective study conducted by Spaite et al (1990) suggested that even in EMS systems with very short response times, performance of bystander CPR prior to the arrival of paramedic units improved long-term outcome.

In view of such conflicting conclusions, how should the data on the effect of lay bystander CPR be interpreted? In other words, *what is the true value of CPR?*

Because of the difficulty in standardizing study protocols and assessing hard-to-control-for variables, it is likely that the controversy will continue. Nevertheless, the conclusion reached in a recent review by Hoekstra (1990) suggests that most studies on the subject do support the premise that early initiation of lay bystander CPR improves outcome.

> We feel it more important to emphasize the concept that the most effective treatment of out-of-hospital cardiac arrest is defibrillation. The sooner patients with ventricular fibrillation or pulseless ventricular tachycardia can be countershocked, the better the chances for survival. CPR, in and of itself, is no substitute for definitive therapy, although it may "buy time" (i.e., prolong the period of potential viability) until the defibrillator arrives (Niemann, 1985; Spaite et al, 1990). It is true that in cases of pure respiratory arrest (as may occur with victims of near-drowning, lightning strikes, or drug overdoses), the *rescue breathing* component of CPR alone may be curative. However, in the overall perspective, it is likely that the greatest impact of CPR on survival from cardiopulmonary arrest derives from teaching the lay public to recognize cardiac arrest sooner and mobilize EMS systems and personnel in a more timely fashion (Eisenberg et al, 1979; Thompson et al, 1985).

Complications from CPR

CPR is not benign. In addition to the almost universal subjective complaint of sore chest reported by CPR survivors, serious complications may occur in up to 25% of all recipients (Nagel et al, 1984; Kern et al, 1986; Bedell and Fulton, 1986). Rib and sternal fractures are exceedingly common, occurring in more than 40% of cases (Krischer et al, 1987). These may lead to pneumothorax, pericardial tamponade, and flail chest. As discussed in Chapter 7, pulmonary contusions and parenchymal damage are also surprisingly common, and may significantly impair the efficacy of CPR. Other complications that may directly result from CPR include aspiration, aortic laceration, myocardial contusion, esophageal or gastric mucosal tears with hemorrhage, gastric rupture, liver lacer-

ation, pulmonary edema, and lung herniation (Bjork et al, 1982; McDonnel et al, 1984; Nagel et al, 1984; Batra, 1986).

> *This is **not** to say that CPR should not be promptly initiated by witnesses at the scene of a cardiac arrest.* Instead it merely emphasizes how common complications from CPR apparently are. Fortunately, the overwhelming majority of such injuries are not life-threatening (Krischer et al, 1987). Thus, it is clear that prompt initiation of CPR is indicated at the onset of cardiopulmonary arrest, and that this potentially life-saving procedure should *never* be withheld for fear of causing a complication. Nevertheless, awareness of the frequency and nature of such complications may be instrumental in assisting with management decisions during resuscitation (i.e., in suggesting a potentially reversible iatrogenic cause of EMD), as well as in post-resuscitation managment of survivors.

Because of the high incidence of CPR-associated injury, it is important to verify that true cardiopulmonary arrest has occurred *before* beginning external chest compression. For this reason, stressing the *recognition* of clinical signs of cardiopulmonary arrest at lay-person CPR courses should assume *equal importance* as teaching the mechanical skills of CPR itself.

Practically speaking, many of the injuries that occur in association with CPR are virtually unavoidable. As such, they should not be considered as "unanticipated" consequences of CPR (Krischer et al, 1987). Such unavoidable injuries include fractures of ribs 3 through 5, and/or sternal fractures at the 3rd and 4th intercostal spaces. On the other hand, *up to 20% of resuscitation victims suffer potentially avoidable injury.* Fractures of the lateral portion of a rib, of higher ribs (i.e., ribs 1 or 2), of lower ribs (ribs 6 through 8), or of ribs 8 through 11 at the sternochondral junction suggest injuries that could possibly have been avoided if CPR technique were more proficient (Krischer et al, 1987). Other injuries such as liver or spleen rupture, anterior mediastinal hemorrhage, and cardiac contusions are also potentially avoidable. Thus, attention to aspects of proper technique (i.e., correct hand placement position, avoidance of overzealous application of force) *must* receive high priority from *all* who undergo training in CPR—lay individuals and skilled health care professionals alike! Only by doing so can CPR performance be optimized while keeping the incidence of complications at a minimum (Bedell and Fulton, 1986; Krischer et al, 1987).

Addendum

Much remains to be learned regarding the actual mechanism of CPR in human subjects. In infants and young children, current theory still attributes a major role to *direct cardiac compression* as the explanation for blood flow during CPR. However, preliminary data from an echocardiographic study performed by Giroud, Cavallaro et al (1992) suggest that direct cardiac compression does not necessarily take place in subjects of this age group. Instead, an increase in intrathoracic pressure may be needed to generate blood flow not only for adults, but also for infants and children.

> In practice, resuscitation techniques that produce a *generalized* increase in intrathoracic pressure are unlikely to generate effective coronary flow. This is because of their tendency to elevate intrathoracic pressure during chest compression to a similar degree in all vascular structures within the thorax. For coronary flow to occur, a *pressure differential* is needed between aortic pressure in diastole and right atrial pressure in diastole (Halperin and Weisfeldt, 1992). Maximizing this perfusion gradient for coronary flow with each compression cycle appears to hold the key for optimizing the efficacy of CPR.

We have already emphasized the importance of epinephrine as a pharmacologic means for augmenting coronary perfusion pressure. Recent research in the field of CPR has focused on development of mechanical ways to accomplish the same goal. Halperin et al have worked on a *vest technique* that employs rapid cyclical inflation and deflation of a garment around the chest, intermittently generating pressure levels of 200 mm Hg or more (Halperin et al, 1986; Halperin and Weisfeldt, 1992). The key to the experimental success of this technique appears to reside in the *cyclical* application of inflation and deflation of the vest, which results in production of the pressure differential needed for coronary flow.

Another mechanical technique for augmenting coronary perfusion pressure employs an *active compression-decompression (ACD) device* (Cohen et al, 1992). The device was initially inspired by the anecdotal account of a successful resuscitation effort by a layperson who performed external chest compressions for 10 minutes with a simple household toilet plunger (Lurie et al, 1990). Presumably, the seal formed by application of the rubber suction cup of the plunger to the victim's chest produced enough negative pressure after each compression to ventilate the patient. Cyclical application of negative pressure by the plunger after each chest compression may have also favored coronary flow by increasing chest expansion and enhancing the pressure differential between intrathoracic and extrathoracic compartments.

> The ACD device described by Cohen et al (1992) consists of a rubber suction header, a bellows, and a circular disk with a cushioned upper surface for compression and an undercut grip for decompression. Advantages of the device are that it is easy to use, it only requires a single rescuer, and it does not produce excessive operator fatigue. The principle of the ACD technique is that the passive decompression phase of CPR is converted to an active process, in the hope that doing so will increase the pressure differential between intrathoracic vascular structures.

Performance of CPR with interposed abdominal compressions (i.e., IAC-CPR) is the final technique discussed in this section. Theoretically, IAC-CPR augments coronary perfusion by a mechanism similar to that invoked with use of the intra-aortic balloon pump (Halperin and Weisfeldt, 1992). Application of this technique requires active coordination of two sets of "trained hands" that alternately compress the chest and abdomen 80 times each minute. Interposition of abdominal compression in this manner is thought to increase intrathoracic pressure by one or more of a variety of mechanisms. These include: (1) transmission of increased subdiaphragmatic pressure to the intrathoracic compartment; (2) prolongation of the duration of compression; (3) an increase in the absolute number of compressions (since there will be 80 chest + 80 abdominal compressions/min with the IAC-CPR technique); and (4) upward displacement of abdominal contents and the diaphragm so as to impinge on the contents of the thoracic cavity (Sack et al, 1992). In addition, manual compression of the abdomen during IAC-CPR may at least indirectly compress the abdominal aorta, thus raising aortic diastolic pressure and further favoring the gradient for coronary flow.

> At the present time, each of the mechanical techniques described above remain investigational. Additional clinical trials demonstrating improved long-term survival are clearly needed. Nevertheless, these exciting advances have enhanced our understanding of the mechanism of blood flow during CPR, and place us on the threshold of optimizing meaningful survival from cardiopulmonary resuscitation.

References

American Heart Association Subcommittee on Emergency Cardiac Care: Standards and guidelines for cardiopulmonary resuscitation (CPR) and emergency cardiac care (ECC), *JAMA* 255:2905-2992, 1986.

Anton WR, Gordon RW, Jordan TM, Posner KL, Cheney FW: A disposable end-tidal CO_2 detector to verify endotracheal intubation, *Ann Emerg Med* 20:271-275, 1991.

Batra AK: Lung herniation after CPR, *Crit Care Med* 14:595-596, 1986.

Bedell SE, Fulton EJ: Unexpected findings and complications at autopsy after cardiopulmonary resuscitation (CPR), *Ann Int Med* 146:1725-1728, 1986.

Berryman R, Phillips GM: Interposed abdominal compression-CPR in human subjects, *Ann Emerg Med* 13:226-229, 1984.

Berryman CR: Electromechanical dissociation with directly measurable arterial blood pressures, *Ann Emerg Med* 15:625, 1986 (abstract).

Bircher N: New concepts in cardiopulmonary resuscitation, *ER Reports* 3:45-48, 1982.

Bircher N, Safar P: Manual open-chest cardiopulmonary resuscitation, *Ann Emerg Med* 13:770-773, 1984.

Bjork RJ, Snyder BD, Campion BC, Loewenson RB: Medical complications of cardiopulmonary arrest, *Arch Intern Med* 142:500-503, 1982.

Brown E, Hendee WR: End-tidal PCO_2 during cardiopulmonary resuscitation, *JAMA* 263:814-815, 1990.

Brunel W, Coleman DL, Schwartz DE, Peper E, Cohen NH: Assessment of routine chest roentgenograms and the physical examination to confirm endotracheal tube position, *Chest* 96:1043-1045, 1989.

Callaham M, Barton C: Prediction of outcome of cardiopulmonary resuscitation from end-tidal carbon dioxide concentration, *Crit Care Med* 18:358-362, 1990.

Chandra N, Rudikoff M, Weisfeldt ML: Simultaneous chest compression and ventilation at high airway pressure during cardiopulmonary resuscitation, *Lancet* 1:175-178, 1980.

Chandra NC, Tsitlik JE, Halperin HR, Guerci AD, Weisfeldt ML: Observations of hemodynamics during human cardiopulmonary resuscitation, *Crit Care Med* 18:929-934, 1990.

Cohen TJ, Tucker KJ, Lurie KG, Redberg RF, Dutton JP, Dwyer KA, Schwab TM, Chin MC, Gelb AM, Scheinman MM, Schiller NB, Callaham ML: Active compression-decompression: a new method of cardiopulmonary resuscitation, *JAMA* 267:2916–2923, 1992.

Criley JM, Blaufuss AH, Kissel GL: Cough-induced cardiac compression: self-administered form of cardiopulmonary resuscitation, *JAMA* 236:1246-1250, 1976.

Cummins RO, Eisenberg MS: Prehospital cardiopulmonary resuscitation: is it effective? *JAMA* 253:2408-2412, 1985.

Del Guercio LRM, Coomaraswamy RP, State D: Cardiac output and other hemodynamic variables during external cardiac massage in man, *N Eng J Med* 269:1398-1404, 1963.

Deshmukh HG, Weil MH, Rackow EC, Trevino RP, Bisera J: Echocardiographic observations during cardiopulmonary resuscitation with a preliminary report. *Crit Care Med* 13:904-906, 1985.

Deshmukh HG, Weil MH, Gudipati CV, Trevino RP, Bisera J, Rackow EC: Mechanism of blood flow generated by precordial compression during CPR: studies on closed chest compression, *Chest* 95:1092-1099, 1989.

Ditchey RV, Lindenfeld J: Potential adverse effects of volume loading on perfusion of vital organs during closed chest resuscitation, *Circulation* 69:181-189, 1984.

Eisenberg MS, Bergner L, Hallstrom A: Cardiac resuscitation in the community: importance of rapid provision and implications for program planning, *JAMA* 241:1905-1907, 1979.

Ewy GA: Current status of cardiopulmonary resuscitation, *Mod Conc Cardiovasc Dis* 53:43-45, 1984.

Ewy GA: Personal communication, 1990.

Falk JL, Rackow EC, Weil MH: End-tidal carbon dioxide concentration during cardiopulmonary resuscitation, *N Engl J Med* 318:607-611, 1988.

Feneley MP, Maier GW, Gaynor JW, Gall SA, Kisslo JA, Davis JW, Rankin JS: Sequence of mitral valve motion and transmitral blood flow during manual cardiopulmonary resuscitation in dogs, *Circulation* 76:363-375, 1987.

Feneley MP, Maier GW, Kern KB, Gaynor JW, Gall SA, Sanders AB, Raissler K: Influence of compression rate on initial success of resuscitation and 24 hour survival after prolonged manual cardiopulmonary resuscitation in dogs, *Circulation* 77:240-250, 1988.

Garnett AR, Ornato JP, Ganzalez ER, Johnson EB: End-tidal carbon dioxide monitoring during cardiopulmonary resuscitation, *JAMA* 257:512-515, 1987.

Giroud JM, Cavallaro DL, Satiel AM, Nichter MA, Quintessenza JA: Echocardiographic evaluation of CPR in infants, The American Pediatric Society/The Society for Pediatric Research, Jan 1992 (abstract).

Goldberg RJ, Gore JM, Love DG, Ockene JK, Dalen JE: Layperson CPR—are we training the right people? *Ann Emerg Med* 13:701-704, 1984.

Grauer K, Cavallaro D, Gums J: New developments in cardiopulmonary resuscitation, *Am Fam Phys* 43:832–844, 1991.

Grundler W, Weil MH, Rackow EC, Falk JL, Bisera J, Miller JM, Michaels S: Selective acidosis in venous blood during human cardiopulmonary resuscitation: a preliminary report, *Crit Care Med* 13:886-887, 1985.

Halperin HR, Guerci AD, Chandra N, Herskowitz A, Tsitlik JE, Niskanen RA, Wurmb E, Wesfeldt ML: Vest inflation without simultaneous ventilation during cardiac arrest in dogs: improved survival from prolonged cardiopulmonary resuscitation, *Circulation* 74:1407–1415, 1986.

Halperin HR, Weisfeldt ML: New approaches to CPR: four hands, a plunger, or a vest, *JAMA* 267:2940–2941, 1992 (editorial).

Higano ST, Oh JK, Ewy GA, Seward JB: The mechanism of blood flow during closed chest cardiac massage in humans: transesophageal echocardiographic observations, *Mayo Clin Proc* 65:1432-1440, 1990.

Hoekstra J: Bystander CPR: a review, *Resuscitation* 20:97-113, 1990.

Howard M, Carrubba C, Foss F, Janiak B, Hogan B, Guinness M: Interposed abdominal compression-CPR: its effects on parameters of coronary perfusion in human subjects, *Ann Emerg Med* 16:253-259, 1987.

Kern KB, Carter AB, Showen RL, Voorhees WD, Babbs CF, Tacker WA, Ewy GA: CPR-induced trauma: comparison of three manual methods in an experimental model, *Ann Emerg Med* 15:674-679, 1986.

Kern KB, Sanders AB, Badylak SF, Janas W, Carter AB, Tacker WA, Ewy GA: Long-term survival with open-chest cardiac massage after ineffective closed-chest compression in a canine preparation, *Circulation* 75:498-503, 1987.

Kern KB, Ewy GA: Future directions in cardiopulmonary resuscitation, Discussion at the Learning Center, University of Arizona, pp 1-15, June 11-13, 1990.

Kern KB, Sanders AB, Raife J, Milander MM, Otto CW, Ewy GA: A study of chest compression rate during cardiopulmonary resuscitation in humans: the importance of rate-directed chest compressions, *Arch Int Med* 152:145-149, 1992.

Koehler RC, Michael RJ, Guerci, AD, Chandra N, Schleien CL, Dean JM, Rogers MC, Weisfelt ML, Traystman RJ: Beneficial effect of epinephrine infusion on cerebral and myocardial blood flows during CPR, *Ann Emerg Med* 14:744-749, 1985.

Krischer JP, Fine EG, Davis JH, Nagel EL: Complications of cardiac resuscitation, *Chest* 92:287-291, 1987.

Krischer JP, Fine EG, Weisfeldt ML, Guerci AD, Nagel E, Chandra N: Comparison of prehospital conventional and simultaneous compression-ventilation cardiopulmonary resuscitation, *Crit Care Med* 17:1263-1269, 1989.

Lilja GP, Long RS, Ruiz E: Augmentation of systolic blood pressure during external cardiac compression by use of the MAST suit, *Ann Emerg Med* 10:182-184, 1981.

Luce JM, Cary JM, Ross BK, Culver BH, Butler J: New developments in cardiopulmonary resuscitation, *JAMA* 244:1366-1370, 1980.

Lurie KG, Lindo C, Chin J: The p stands for plumber's helper, *JAMA* 264:1661, 1990.

MacLeod BA, Heller MB, Gerard J, Yealy DM, Menegazzi JJ: Verification of endotracheal tube placement with colorimetric end-tidal CO_2 detection, *Ann Emerg Med* 20:267-270, 1991.

Maier GW, Tyson GS, Olsen CO, Kernstein KJ, Davis JW, Conn EH, Sabiston DC, Rankin JS: The physiology of external cardiac massage: high-impulse cardiopulmonary resuscitation, *Circulation* 70:86-101, 1984.

Martin GB, Carden DL, Nowak RM, Lewinter JR, Johnston W, Tomlanovich MC: Aortic and right atrial pressures during standard and simultaneous compression and ventilation CPR in human beings, *Ann Emerg Med* 15:125-130, 1986.

McDonnell PJ, Hutchins GM, Hruban RH, Brown CG: Hemorrhage from gastric mucosal tears complicating cardiopulmonary resuscitation, *Ann Emerg Med* 13:230-233, 1984.

Michael JR, Guerci AD, Koehler RC, Shi AY, Tsitlik J, Chandra N, Niedermeyer E, Rogers MC, Traystman RJ, Weisfeldt ML: Mechanisms by which epinephrine augments cerebral and myocardial perfusion during cardiopulmonary resuscitation in dogs, *Circulation* 69:822-835, 1984.

Nagel EL, Fine EG, Krischer JP, Davis JH: Complications of CPR, *Crit Care Med* 9:424, 1984.

Niemann JT, Rosborough J, Ung S, Criley JM: Blood flow without cardiac compression during closed chest CPR, *Crit Care Med* 9:380-381, 1981.

Niemann JT, Rosborough J, Hausknecht M, Ung S, Criley JM: Coronary perfusion pressure during experimental cardiopulmonary resuscitation, *Ann Emerg Med* 11:127-131, 1982.

Niemann JT: Artificial perfusion techniques during cardiac arrest: questions of experimental focus versus clinical need, *Ann Emerg Med* 14:761-768, 1985.

Ohomoto T, Miura I, Konno S: A new method of external cardiac massage to improve diastolic augmentation and prolong survival times, *Ann Thorac Surg* 21:284-290, 1976.

Paradis NA, Martin GB, Rivers EP, Goetting MG, Appleton TJ, Feingold M, Nowak RM: Coronary perfusion pressure and the return of spontaneous circulation in human cardiopulmonary resuscitation, *JAMA* 263:1106-1113, 1990.

Paradis NA, Martin GB, Rosenberg J, Rivers EP, Goetting MG, Appleton TJ, Feingold M, Cryer PE, Wortsman J, Nowak RM: The effect of standard- and high-dose epinephrine on coronary perfusion pressure during prolonged cardiopulmonary resuscitation, *JAMA* 265:1139-1144, 1991.

Rogers MC: New development in cardiopulmonary resuscitation, *Pediatrics* 71:655-658, 1983.

Sack JB, Kesselbrenner MB, Bregman D: Survival from in-hospital cardiac arrest with interposed abdominal counterpulsation during cardiopulmonary resuscitation, *JAMA* 267:379-385, 1992.

Sanders AB, Kern KB, Ewy GA, Atlas M, Bailey L: Improved resuscitation from cardiac arrest with open-chest massage, *Ann Emerg Med* 13:672-675, 1984.

Sanders AB, Kern KB, Ewy GA: Time limitations for open-chest cardiopulmonary resuscitation from cardiac arrest, *Crit Care Med* 13:897-898, 1985.

Sanders AB, Ewy GA, Bragg S, Atlas M, Kern KB: Expired PCO_2 as a prognostic indicator of successful resuscitation from cardiac arrest, *Ann Emerg Med* 14:948-952, 1985.

Sanders AB, Kern KB, Otto CW, Milander MM, Ewy GA: End-tidal carbon dioxide monitoring during cardiopulmonary resuscitation: a prognostic indicator for survival, *JAMA* 262:1347-1351, 1989.

Spaite DW, Hanlon T, Criss EA, Valenzuela TD, Wright AL, Keeley KT, Meislen HW: Prehospital cardiac arrest: the impact of witnessed collapse and bystander CPR in a metropolitan EMS system with short response times, *Ann Emerg Med* 19:1264-1269, 1990.

Stueven H, Troiano P, Thompson B, Mateer JR, Kastenson EH, Tonsfeldt D, Hargarten K, Kowalski R, Aprahamian C, Darlin J: Bystander/first responder CPR: ten years experience in a paramedic system, *Ann Emerg Med* 15:707-710, 1986.

Swenson RD, Weaver WD, Niskanen RA, Martin J, Dahlberg S: Hemodynamics in humans during conventional and experimental methods of cardiopulmonary resuscitation, *Circulation* 78:630-639, 1988.

Thompson BM, Stueven HA, Mateer JR, Aprahamian CC, Tucker JF, Darin JC: Comparison of clinical CPR studies in Milwaukee and elsewhere in the United States, *Ann Emerg Med* 14:750-754, 1985.

Ward KR, Sullivan RJ, Zelenak RR, Summer WR: A comparison of interposed abdominal compression CPR and standard CPR by monitoring end-tidal PCO_2, *Ann Emerg Med* 18:831-837, 1989.

Weil MH, Rackow EC, Trevino R, Grundler W, Falk JL, Griffel MI: Difference in acid-base state between venous and arterial blood during cardiopulmonary resuscitation, *N Engl J Med* 315:153-156, 1986.

Weil MH, Gazmuri RJ: Immediate resuscitation, *Crit Care Med* 18:455, 1990 (editorial).

Weil MH, Gazmuri RJ, Kette F, Bisera J: End-tidal PCO_2 during cardiopulmonary resuscitation, *JAMA* 263:814-815, 1990 (letter).

Weisfeldt ML, Chandra N, Tsitlik J: Increased intrathoracic pressure—not direct heart compression—causes the rise in intrathoracic vascular pressures during CPR in dogs and pigs, *Crit Care Med* 9:377-378, 1981.

SECTION D

PROBLEMS IN IMPLEMENTING CPR

Layperson CPR: Are We Training the Right People?

CPR is our link with the community in the treatment and prevention of cardiopulmonary arrest. However, people in the community cannot become involved with CPR unless they receive training in this area. *Are we training the right people?* A study by Goldbert et al (1984) of family members of patients with coronary artery disease suggests that we may not be. Despite the fact that CPR training was felt to be important by the overwhelming majority of family members in this study, only 22% of these family members had ever taken a CPR course, and only 9% had done so within the past 3 years!

One might expect doctors to feel at least equally positive about the importance of CPR as the lay public. Yet a large Massachusetts survey revealed only 6% of physicians in that area routinely provided information about CPR training to family members of their patients with coronary artery disease (Goldberg et al, 1984). Considering the current emphasis in primary care on health maintenance procedures such as mammography, testing for occult blood, and sigmoidoscopy, education about the signs and symptoms of a heart attack and instruction in CPR should probably command at least equal priority.

The Usual Scenario

What is the usual scenario of out-of-hospital cardiac arrest? Most such arrests occur in the home. Frequently, only one other person (most often the spouse) is around. Since the most common victims are men over 40, women over 40 (spouses) form the most likely group to witness a cardiac arrest, and are therefore the most logical focus group to receive CPR training (Dracup et al, 1989). Yet those people who seek instruction in CPR tend to be younger (in their 20s and 30s), and men seek training more commonly than do women (Goldberg et al, 1984; Mandel and Cobb, 1985). Even after the episode, most spouses of surviving victims still do not learn CPR. *Are we training the right people?*

One of the most commonly cited reasons for the reluctance (failure) of health care professionals to recommend CPR training for family members of patients at high risk of cardiac arrest is concern for the psychologic stress such family members might experience in the event that their attempt at resuscitating a loved one was unsuccessful. This concern does not appear to be well founded. A majority of family members *can* be taught to perform CPR effectively on a loved one (Dracup et al, 1989). Patients and their families often react quite positively to training in CPR, and equally positively to training in the use of the AED (automatic external defibrillator). If anything, the overall psychologic adaptation ability of many

high-risk patients seems to *improve* after their spouses are instructed in performance of CPR and in the operation of AEDs (Cummins et al, 1985). Thus, there is little evidence to support objections of health care providers against teaching family members CPR. We probably ought to be routinely recommending CPR training—*especially* to the *right* people (Goldberg, 1989)!

A word of caution is in order. Anxiety and depression may increase in certain high-risk cardiac patients when CPR is taught to family members, presumably because this intervention makes it more difficult for such patients to deny (or repress) the seriousness of their illness (Dracup et al, 1986). This is *not* to say that CPR should not be taught to family members of such patients, but only to emphasize the *ongoing* need for open communication and encouragement of high-risk patients and their families with the health care team to discuss their feelings related to CPR and the specter of sudden death.

Layperson CPR: How Quickly They Forget

One of the problems involved in teaching CPR to the lay public is the rapidity with which cognitive and psychomotor skills are forgotten. Although *immediate* retention of skills following BLS instruction may be excellent, a disappointingly small number of lay individuals are able to correctly perform one-person CPR according to AHA standards when retested 6 months later (Weaver et al, 1979). When one considers how infrequently lay individuals are called on to perform CPR in a real-life situation, this result should not be unexpected.

Simplification of CPR for the Lay Public

In an attempt to improve retention of skills by the lay public, guidelines of the standards for performance of CPR have been simplified. Lay individuals need no longer concern themselves with delivering external chest compressions at a precise rate as they had been advised in the past.* Instead a *range* (between 80 and 100 chest compressions per minute) is now the standard. In addition, lay persons are no longer taught two-person CPR. As noted above, it is extremely uncommon for out-of-hospital cardiac arrest to occur in the presence of two or more lay individuals who are trained in CPR. Utilization of a two-rescuer sequence by lay individuals adds complexity to the task and could be counterproductive if skills in CPR had not been maintained. In reality, the victim might be better served when the most knowledgeable person on the scene

---

*Prior to 1986, the recommended rate for delivery of external chest compressions during basic life support was 60 per minute.

initiates one-rescuer CPR, and additional witnesses direct their efforts at ensuring that an EMS unit is promptly summoned. Practically speaking, long-term survival of a victim of out-of-hospital ventricular fibrillation depends less on whether one- or two-rescuer CPR is administered, and much more on whether trained professionals capable of defibrillating arrive in a timely manner.

A problem that sometimes arises is what to do if you are the sole witness to a cardiopulmonary arrest that occurs in an area where help is unlikely to be forthcoming *unless you leave the patient to seek assistance.* If the patient is pulseless, should you:

1. Continue to administer one-rescuer CPR? . . . or
2. Stop one-rescuer CPR and run (to the nearest telephone or residence) for help???

There is no ideal solution to this problem. Leaving the patient to seek assistance means that CPR will be stopped until you return. The longer you are gone, the less chance for meaningful survival. If the patient is in asystole, the chance for meaningful survival is virtually nil regardless of what is done. However, if the patient is in ventricular fibrillation, the *only* realistic chance for survival will be to get the patient defibrillated. *CPR alone will not save the patient.* In this case, the longer you wait to seek assistance, the less the chance (however small) for recovery. Therefore if there has been no response (after about 1 minute) to initial attempts at one-rescuer CPR and there is no indication that help will soon arrive, it may be preferable to stop CPR and run for assistance (to the nearest telephone or residence) in the hope you can contact the EMS system within a minute or so, return to the patient, restart CPR, and sustain the patient until help (in the form of a defibrillator) arrives or it may be preferable to contact EMS as soon as you establish unresponsiveness and pulselessness.

On the other hand, if a pulse is present (and/or returns) and the patient remains in respiratory arrest, performance of rescue breathing may be lifesaving. In this case, *remain with the patient and continue rescue breathing!*

The Physiologic Response

Despite the vast number of lay individuals who have undergone CPR training, relatively little information is available on the physiologic response of the rescuer who performs CPR and the safety of this procedure. This issue is particularly important considering the relatively older age of persons most likely to witness an out-of-hospital cardiac arrest.

A study by Hoeyweghen et al (1991) on a group of subjects with a mean age of 30 compared cardiovascular and ventilatory parameters during prolonged CPR performance and maximal exercise testing. During CPR, systolic blood pressure and heart rate achieved approximately 75% of the levels attained during maximal exercise testing. Overall, CPR performance was viewed as an aerobic effort that produced cardiorespiratory changes, which were well tolerated in the study population. The most common complaints voiced during CPR performance related to the uncomfortable position assumed (causing knee and low back pain) rather than to any difficulty in the amount of physical exertion. A similar type of study by Manfre et al (1987) in older subjects (mean age 61) with a history of coronary artery disease was similarly comforting in

suggesting that the intensity of effort required to perform chest compressions was generally well within their cardiovascular capability. *Most lay individuals who are able to successfully complete a CPR training course appear to be physically able to safely perform these skills in the event that the need arises.*

Mouth-to-Mouth Resuscitation: An Extinct Art?*

The setting is all too familiar. A cardiac arrest is called in the far reaches of your hospital. You run to the bedside and find yourself among the first to arrive. Neither respiratory therapy nor the code team (or crash cart) are yet on the scene. Health care providers are feverishly putting on monitor leads, obtaining IV access, getting a bedboard under the patient, and performing external chest compressions . . . *and no one is breathing for the patient.* And the patient is blue. Knowing looks pass back and forth from those in attendance . . . *and no one is breathing for the patient.* As precious seconds (which seem like hours) pass by, *you reflect on your options.*

You could:

1. Perform mouth-to-mouth resuscitation.
2. Wait a little longer and hope that help (in the form of someone with a bag-valve mask) arrives.
3. Perform mouth-to-mouth resuscitation.
4. Yell for a nurse.
5. Look for a medical student and have him/her perform mouth-to-mouth resuscitation.
6. Busy yourself with the ECG monitor.
7. Wait a little longer.
8. Let the patient die.
9. Perform mouth-to-mouth resuscitation.

In the 1990s, the practice of performing mouth-to-mouth resuscitation in a medical environment is at risk of becoming an extinct art (Lawrence, 1985). Fear of AIDS has overcome everything else. Even elderly ladies and gentlemen who have not ventured out of nursing homes for years are not receiving rescue breathing because of the possibility that they somehow contracted "the disease."

Our survey of over 200 critical care nurses corroborates the prevalence of these fears (Grauer, Green, Cavallaro, 1990). Sixty-four percent of the nurses stated they would *not* routinely administer mouth-to-mouth resuscitation if an Ambu bag was unavailable. Ninety-one percent would not administer mouth-to-mouth resuscitation if they were aware that the victim had AIDS. Although 92% of the responders knew what a pocket mask was, only 48% indicated that pocket masks were readily available in their facility for use during a cardiac arrest.

Several important points can be made from these responses. Although 36% of responders indicated that they still routinely administer mouth-to-mouth resuscitation when an Ambu bag

---

*Reproduced (and adapted) with permission from Grauer K, Kravitz L: On Mouth-to-Mouth. *J Am Bd Fam Prac* 1:55-56, 1987.

is unavailable, this number drops to 9% with prior knowledge that the victim has AIDS. These results are consistent with those of Raviglione et al (1988), who showed that, in general there was a less aggressive and invasive approach to resuscitation of patients with AIDS who suffer cardiac arrest compared with patients without AIDS, despite the fact that patients with AIDS who arrest tend to be much younger. This is particularly important considering how much more common a respiratory mechanism for cardiopulmonary arrest is in patients with AIDS than in patients without this disease (Raviglione et al, 1988). The problem is likely to increase, given a current prevalence of up to 6% of HIV infection in unselected patients presenting to some emergency departments (Kelen et al, 1989). Even in areas of the country where the prevalence of HIV infection is less (due to a lower incidence of IV drug abuse and homosexuality in the population), health care providers are still likely to encounter HIV sero-positive patients in the emergency department when least expected (Sturm, 1991).

Ironically, reluctance to perform mouth-to-mouth resuscitation seems to be less of a problem with out-of-hospital cardiac arrest. Most events that occur outside the hospital take place in the home. Lay person witnesses in this setting most often know the victim well and are frequently aware of their medical history. If lay person witnesses know CPR, they usually administer it promptly.

> Disagreeable physical characteristics such as the presence of dentures, vomitus, blood, and the breath of alcohol are found in a *majority* of victims of out-of-hospital cardiac arrest. The presence of such disagreeable physical characteristics does not seem to detract from the willingness of knowledgeable lay bystanders to perform CPR, especially when such bystanders are related to the victim who arrests (McCormack et al, 1989).

Delay in providing respiratory support is also less of a problem in hospital emergency departments and intensive care units. While reluctance to perform mouth-to-mouth resuscitation among health care providers is still prevalent in these areas, the crash cart is usually nearby and the personnel in attendance so familiar with emergency cardiopulmonary care that the time for control of the airway is frequently minimal. In contrast, the problem of achieving airway control in other medical environments (on regular wards, in waiting rooms, out-patient clinics, and medical offices) is significant. Reluctance to perform mouth-to-mouth resuscitation in these settings has reached epidemic proportions. Considering that respiratory equipment (and the crash cart) is often just *too* many minutes away, prompt administration of rescue breathing must be looked on as the essential first step in the lifesaving process.

The facts are these:
1. Although the HIV (AIDS) virus is present in saliva, no transmission of infection during mouth-to-mouth resuscitation has ever been documented (Health and Public Policy Committee, 1988; ECC Committee of the AHA, 1989; Cummins, 1989). Isolation of HIV virus from saliva is much less common than isolation of the virus from blood, so that even seemingly high-risk saliva exposure situations such as biting are felt to be exceedingly unlikely to transmit infection from HIV virus if the skin is not broken by the bite (Lifson, 1988).

2. Intact skin forms the primary defense barrier preventing transmission of blood-borne HIV infection during CPR. Transmission of HIV virus would be more likely if the rescuer had open wounds or sores in or around the mouth or on the hands, or had direct contact with the victim's blood, or with vomitus or saliva that contains blood. However, if skin and mucous membranes of the rescuer remain intact, the risk of transmission of HIV virus by performance of CPR is exceedingly small (ECC Committee of the AHA, 1989).

3. The epidemiology of HIV infection is similar to that of hepatitis B virus infection. The risk of hepatitis B virus transmission in health care settings far exceeds that for HIV virus transmission. While experience with AIDS is still fairly limited, more than 15 years of experience in management has been accumulated with hepatitis B virus infection. No transmission of infection during mouth-to-mouth resuscitation has ever been documented for hepatitis B (MMWR, 1985; ECC Committee of the AHA, 1989).

4. Although final answers are not yet in, it appears that the potential ("theoretical") risk of transmission of AIDS by mouth-to-mouth resuscitation is extremely small (Lifson, 1988).

We suggest the following:

1. If a patient arrests outside the hospital and you do not perform CPR, the chances are good that no one else will. If the cause of the arrest is purely respiratory (such as drowning or drug overdose), prompt administration of rescue breathing could be lifesaving. *Breathe* for the patient.

> The American Heart Association suggests that rescuers faced with the prospect of performing mouth-to-mouth resuscitation on a patient with an unknown health history be "guided by individual moral and ethical values" (Cummins, 1989). We interpret this to mean that rescuers should do what they think best in the situation, realizing that the patient may be saved by prompt mouth-to-mouth resuscitation, and will probably die without it (Grauer, Green, Cavallaro, 1990).

2. If a patient arrests in a hospital setting and you know help (and a bag-valve mask) is on the way, it may be reasonable to wait a few moments for their arrival. Ventricular tachycardia/fibrillation is the most common cause of cardiopulmonary arrest in this setting. Defibrillation is the treatment of choice. Putting off management of the airway for a few moments (although

less than ideal) probably will not adversely affect outcome in most instances. However, if help in the hospital is late in arriving and the patient is not being ventilated, *breathe* for the patient.

3. If nothing in the available history of the patient even remotely suggests that he/she might have AIDS, hepatitis B, herpes, active tuberculosis, or meningococcal meningitis, do not even wait the few moments. If the patient is not being ventilated and a bag-valve mask unit is not available at the bedside, *breathe* for the patient.

4. Consider more widespread use of the *pocket mask*. This underutilized, inexpensive device has been shown to be far superior to bag-valve mask systems in ventilating the patient in respiratory arrest (Harrison et al, 1982; Elling and Politis, 1983). Because the mask eliminates direct contact between rescuer and victim, the risk of disease transmission is dramatically lessened. The device may be made even safer by adding a *one-way valve* to the mask (so that air expired by the victim is directed away from the rescuer). Greater availability of this inexpensive airway adjunct in medical settings where cardiac arrest may occur (for example, nursing stations on all floors, waiting rooms, medical offices) would go a long way toward alleviating the problem.

5. Anticipate. Consider keeping a pocket mask (preferably with a one-way valve) or bag-valve mask unit at the bedside of those patients at particularly high risk of coding.

6. Do not let the patient die of hypoxemia.

What If You KNOW the Patient Has AIDS?

As suggested by the results of our survey, the likelihood of enticing a health care provider to administer mouth-to-mouth resuscitation to a victim of cardiopulmonary arrest who is *known* to have AIDS is extremely small. As a result, having a bag-valve-mask or pocket mask at the bedside of such patients is probably the only realistic way to ensure adequate ventilation in the event of cardiopulmonary arrest.

The attitude of many health care providers toward resuscitation of AIDS victims all too often seems to be, *"Why bother?"*

The facts are these:
1. Pulmonary infection, usually with PCP (*Pneumocystis carinii*) is a major cause of morbidity and mortality among patients with AIDS. Although survival until hospital discharge is almost negligible among AIDS patients who undergo CPR after cardiopulmonary arrest, this is *not* necessarily the case for AIDS patients with respiratory

failure who require mechanical ventilation but who do not actually arrest (Raviglione et al, 1988).

In a study by Efferen et al (1989), no less than 64% of AIDS patients who required intubation for a first episode of PCP survived to leave the hospital. Twenty-five percent of AIDS patients who required intubation for their second episode of PCP survived to leave the hospital. The mean duration of survival for such patients in their study was 9.4 months, suggesting that the overall long-term prognosis of patients who survive intubation for ventilatory failure secondary to PCP pneumonia is not unlike that of AIDS patients who do not develop respiratory failure.

2. Patients with AIDS who suffer cardiopulmonary arrest tend to be significantly younger than patients without AIDS who arrest. AIDS patients are also usually healthy prior to developing their disease. Hope for development of new treatments *must* remain ever present.

As a result, we suggest that:

1. Patients with AIDS who develop cardiopulmonary arrest in the hospital deserve intensive attempts at resuscitation unless they have expressed wishes to the contrary in a validly executed advance directive. Ventilatory adjuncts (i.e., bag-valve mask units, pocket masks) should be routinely placed at the bedside of hospitalized AIDS patients, especially when there is known pulmonary infection.

In the absence of suitable ventilatory adjuncts, if fear of acquiring infection prevents the rescuer from administering mouth-to-mouth resuscitation, *performing external chest compressions is better than doing nothing.* A primary cardiac arrest victim usually still has oxygenated blood in his or her system, and performance of chest compressions may help circulate some of this blood (Cummins, 1989). However, after one or two cycles of CPR the oxygen will be used up, and further compressions will be of little value.

2. *The goal is to have discussed code status with AIDS patients **prior** to the occurrence of cardiopulmonary arrest!* Considering the exceedingly poor long-term prognosis for AIDS patients once they suffer cardiopulmonary arrest, it is essential for such discussion to take place as early as possible in the course of the disease (Raviglione et al, 1989). Ideally this will be *prior* to hospitalization at a time when the patient is still mentally competent.

The purpose of initiating a discussion with *all* AIDS patients about their code status at a relatively early point in the course of their disease is to encourage their active participation in this decision. Such discussion must be undertaken with a caring and positive attitude (i.e., *hope always exists for development of new treatments; we are not giving up*) while conveying information about the chance for long-term survival in realistic terms.

3. Considering the constantly improving long-term survival statistics for AIDS patients who do recover from an episode of PCP pneumonia (1989), the attitude of the health care team must remain positive.

References

American Heart Association Subcommittee on Emergency Cardiac Care: Standards and guidelines for cardiopulmonary resuscitation (CPR) and emergency cardiac care (ECC), *JAMA* 255:2905-2992, 1986.

Cummins RO, Eisenberg MS, Moore JE, Hearne TR, Andresen E, Wendt R, Litwin PE, Graves JR, Hallstrom AP, Pierce J: Automatic external defibrillators: clinical, training, psychological, and public health issues, *Ann Emerg Med* 14:755-760, 1985.

Cummins RO: Infection control guidelines for CPR providers, *JAMA* 262:2732-2733, 1989.

Dracup K, Guzy PM, Taylor SE, Barry J: Cardiopulmonary resuscitation (CPR) training: consequences for family members of high-risk cardiac patients, *Arch Intern Med* 146:1757-1761, 1986.

Dracup K, Heanly DM, Taylor SE, Guzy PM, Breu C: Can family members of high-risk cardiac patients learn cardiopulmonary resuscitation? *Arch Intern Med* 149:61-64, 1989.

Efferen LS, Nadarajah D, Palat DS: Survival following mechanical ventilation for pneumocystis carinii pneumonia in patients with the acquired immunodeficiency syndrome: a different perspective, *Am J Med* 87:401-404, 1989.

Elling R, Politis J: An evaluation of emergency medical technicians' ability to use manual ventilation devices, *Ann Emerg Med* 12:765-768, 1983.

The Emergency Cardiac Care Committee of the American Heart Association: Risk of infection during CPR training and rescue: supplemental guidelines, *JAMA* 262:2714-2715, 1989.

Goldberg RJ, Gore JM, Love DG, Ockene JK, Dalen JE: Layperson CPR—are we training the right people? *Ann Emerg Med* 13:701-704, 1984.

Goldberg RJ: Training of family members of high-risk cardiac patients in cardiopulmonary resuscitation: skills performance and need for physician recommendations, *Arch Intern Med* 149:25-26, 1989.

Grauer K, Green E, Cavallaro D: Less publicized aspects of cardiac arrest: a survey of caregivers at the bedside, *Fam Pract Recert* 12:32-46, 1990.

Harrison RR, Maull KL, Keenan RL, Boyan CP: Mouth-to-mask ventilation: a superior method of rescue breathing, *Ann Emerg Med* 11:74-76, 1982.

Health and Public Policy Committee, American College of Physicians. The Infectious Diseases Society of America: The acquired immunodeficiency syndrome (AIDS) and infection with the human immunodeficiency virus (HIV), *Ann Intern Med* 108:460-469, 1988.

Hoeyweghen RJV, Verbruggen G, Rademakers E, Bossaert LL: The physiologic response of CPR training, *Ann Emerg Med* 20:279-282, 1991.

Kelen GD, DiGiovanni T, Bisson L, Kalainov D, Siverston KT, Quinn TC: Human immunodeficiency virus infection in emergency department patients: epidemiology, clinical presentations, and risk to health care workers: the Johns Hopkins experience, *JAMA* 262:516-522, 1989.

Lawrence PJ: Ventilation during cardiopulmonary resuscitation: which method? *Med J Aust* 143:443-447, 1985.

Lifson AR: Do alternate modes for transmission of human immunodeficiency virus exist? a review, *JAMA* 259:1353-1356, 1988.

Mandel LP, Cobb LA: CPR training in the community, *Ann Emerg Med* 14:669-671, 1985.

Manfre MJ, Treijs A, Linkfield B, Depping B, Mallis G: Hemodynamic, metabolic, and symptomatic responses in patients with cardiac disease who perform chest compressions during CPR, *J Cardiopulm Rehab* 7:346-348, 1987.

McCormack AP, Damon SK, Eisenberg MS: Disagreeable physical characteristics affecting bystander CPR, *Ann Emerg Med* 18:283-285, 1989.

Piazza M, Chirianni A, Picciotto L, Guadagnino V, Orlando R, Cataldo PT: Passionate kissing and microlesions of the oral mucosa: possible role in AIDS transmission, *JAMA* 261:244-245, 1989.

Raviglione MC, Battan R, Taranta A: Cardiopulmonary resuscitation in patients with the acquired immunodeficiency syndrome: a prospective study, *Arch Intern Med* 148:2602-2605, 1988.

Recommendations for preventing transmission of infection with human T-lymphotropic virus type III/lymphadenopathy-associated virus in the workplace, *MMWR* 34:681-696, 1985.

Sturm JT: HIV prevalence in a midwestern emergency department, *Ann Emerg Med* 20:276-278, 1991.

Weaver FJ, Ramirez AG, Dorfman SB, Raizner AE: Trainees' retention of cardiopulmonary resuscitation: how quickly they forget, *JAMA* 241:901-903, 1979.

CHAPTER 11

SUDDEN CARDIAC DEATH

SECTION A

OUT-OF-HOSPITAL CARDIAC ARREST

Sudden cardiac death (SCD) has been defined as unexpected death of cardiac etiology occurring either immediately or within 1 hour of the onset of symptoms (Eisenberg et al, 1981). It claims the lives of almost a half million individuals in the United States each year. Although most of these victims have significant coronary artery disease, in many the disease is silent, and sudden death is the first manifestation in an otherwise healthy adult (Goldstein et al, 1986).

In a sense, the very term "sudden cardiac death" has become almost obsolete. Initially the designation was applied synonymously with the occurrence of out-of-hospital ventricular fibrillation, as the latter event was almost uniformly fatal—hence, sudden "death." Today this is no longer the case. Overall outcome for patients with out-of-hospital cardiac arrest has improved tremendously. In many communities where advanced emergency medical service (EMS) systems exist, the rate of successful resuscitation and ultimate discharge home has more than doubled during the past decade. In Seattle, Washington, for example, response time from dispatch until arrival of a basic life support team averages less than 3 minutes, and a paramedic unit capable of administering ACLS arrives 4 minutes later. As a result, up to 60% of cases of ventricular fibrillation are successfully resuscitated on the scene, and more than 25% survive to leave the hospital (Cobb and Werner, 1982; Eisenberg et al, 1990). In addition to their advanced EMS system, more than a third of the population now knows CPR (compared to only 5% a decade ago). Thus, Seattle has become the prototype community for delivery of BLS and ACLS, and being victim to an out-of-hospital cardiac arrest there is no longer synonymous with mortality. The same holds true in other areas of the country where community interest in CPR is high, and advanced EMS systems exist.

Predicting Survival: The ACLS Score

The likelihood of survival from out-of-hospital cardiac arrest depends on *fate factors* (which for the most part are

unalterable and relate to the patient's individual characteristics or to chance) and on *program factors* (which relate to characteristics of the EMS system operating in the geographic area where the arrest occurs). Although often taken for granted, the quality and availability of EMS systems vary tremendously in different parts of the country. Whereas little can be done to alter "fate" factors (patient age, prior medical condition, precipitating cause of the arrest, and whether the arrest is witnessed), focused attention on improving "program factors" (such as the type and quality of the EMS system) can strongly impact on the likelihood of survival (Eisenberg et al, 1987).

An example of an unalterable fate factor is the underlying disease process. Thus the patient who develops ventricular fibrillation secondary to massive pulmonary embolism or rupture of a ventricular aneurysm is likely to be unsalvageable regardless of how efficient resuscitation techniques of the available EMS system are. Beyond the underlying disease process, *four* additional factors appear to be most important in determining survival. These four factors have been incorporated by Eisenberg into a mnemonic known as the "**A-C-L-S**" Score:

A- *Was the **A**rrest witnessed?*
C- *What was the initial **C**ardiac rhythm documented by the paramedics on arrival?*
L- *Was **L**ay-bystander CPR performed?*
S- *How long did it take for help to arrive (i.e., **S**peed of paramedic response time)?*

The first factor (**A**) depends on fate, the last (**S**) on the characteristics of the EMS program—and the middle two (**C** and **L**) are a combination of fate and program factors.

Eisenberg et al (1981) examined the importance of each of these factors in a review of 611 cases of out-of-hospital cardiac arrest (defined as a pulseless condition confirmed by paramedics). For arrests that were witnessed (**A**), 28% of 380 patients were ultimately discharged from the hospital. In contrast, only 3% of 231 victims of unwitnessed cardiac arrest survived. When the mechanism of the arrest (the initial **C**ardiac rhythm) was ventricular tachycardia or fibrillation, 28% of 389 patients survived, compared to a dismal 3% survival in the 222 patients for whom the initial documented rhythm was asystole. In those 168 patients for whom a lay bystander performed CPR (L), a 32% survival rate was seen. When CPR was delayed until arrival of the EMTs, that figure dropped to 14%. Finally, when paramedics were able to respond with ACLS in less than 4 minutes (Speed), 56% of patients were saved. Survival decreased to 35% when response time was between 4 to 8 minutes, and to only 17% if response time exceeded 8 minutes.

Mechanisms of Out-of-Hospital Cardiac Arrest

From the above, it can be seen that the initial mechanism of an arrest is an extremely important determinant of survival. Statistically, about two thirds of patients arresting outside the hospital are initially found in ventricular fibrillation. An additional 5% to 10% are in ventricular tachycardia when the rescue team arrives, and the remainder are in a bradyarrhythmia (including asystole). Prognosis is by far best for those patients found in ventricular tachycardia. The large majority of these individuals can be successfully resuscitated on the scene, and up to two thirds of them will be ultimately discharged from the hospital (Myerburg et al, 1982). In contrast, patients initially found in a bradyarrhythmia or asystole have a dismal prognosis with a minuscule ultimate survival rate. Outcome of patients initially found in ventricular fibrillation is intermediate between these two groups.* The data collected by Myerburg et al from Miami during the 3-year period from 1975 to 1978 demonstrated a 23% long-term survival rate for 220 such patients with out-of-hospital ventricular fibrillation. Slightly higher figures have been obtained from Seattle (Greene, 1990).

> Recent years have seen the maximal long-term survival rate for victims of *witnessed* out-of-hospital ventricular fibrillation plateau at between 25% to 30% in communities with advanced EMS systems (Eisenberg et al, 1990).

In discussing the mechanism of out-of-hospital cardiac arrest, the obvious question to raise is how can one be sure that the initial cardiac rhythm documented by the EMS unit on the scene is truly the *precipitating* mechanism of the arrest. *The answer is that one cannot.* In the Miami experience, this was assumed to be the case because data were included only from episodes in which the onset of cardiac arrest was witnessed, EMS personnel were summoned without delay, and arrival on the scene was documented to have occurred within 4 minutes of summons. Nevertheless, it is still quite possible that at least some of the bradyarrhythmias represented a *secondary* rather than primary mechanism of arrest in which asystole or EMD succeeded ventricular fibrillation as time from patient collapse until arrival of the EMS unit elapsed.

Similarly, ventricular tachycardia could have preceded development of ventricular fibrillation. That this probably occurs much more commonly than is generally appreciated is suggested by several observations. SCD survivors who have a second cardiac arrest while being monitored in the hospital often demonstrate ventricular tachycardia as the initial rhythm of their recurrence (Josephson et al, 1980). In addition, patients sustaining cardiac arrest during Holter monitoring frequently demonstrate ventricular tachycardia of variable duration as the precipitating mechanism of arrest (Pratt et al, 1983; Kempf and Josephson, 1984; Milner et al, 1985). *Ventricular tachycardia* (rather than ventricular fibrillation) may well be the primary (precipitating) mechanism of many *(if not most)* cardiac arrests (Buxton, 1986).

> The significance of the clinical finding that ventricular tachycardia is really a common precipitating mechanism of cardiac arrest lies with the much better chance for successfull resuscitation if this is the initial rhythm found on arrival of the EMS unit. The reason ventricular tachycardia has been documented so infrequently in previous studies of out-of-hospital cardiac arrest may be due to the time it takes for help to arrive. During these critical minutes, ventricular tachycardia probably deteriorates to ventricular fibrillation in many cases. *Were it possible for emergency care providers to get to the scene sooner (when ventricular tachycardia is still present), survival from out-of-hospital cardiac arrest would doubtlessly improve.* Considering the previously mentioned plateau in survival rates for victims of *witnessed* out-of-hospital ventricular fibrillation, *reducing the time until delivery of definitive care (defibrillation) will hold the key for any future improvement in survival.*

SVT as a Precipitating Cause of Cardiac Arrest

In addition to ventricular fibrillation, ventricular tachycardia, and bradycardia/asystole, there may be yet another mechanism responsible for precipitating cardiac arrest in a small but significant percentage of susceptible individuals. Surprising data from Wang et al (1991) suggest that in as many as 5% of victims of out-of-hospital cardiac arrest, a *supraventricular tachyarrhythmia* is the precipitating cause of collapse.

> Supraventricular tachyarrhythmias responsible for cardiac arrest in the study by Wang et al included atrial fibrillation (with and without an accessory pathway) and AV nodal reentrant tachycardia (i.e., PSVT). While PSVT will almost always be well tolerated when it occurs in an otherwise healthy individual with normal ventricular function, this may not be the case if it occurs in an older patient with underlying coronary artery disease and/or impaired contractility. It is easy to imagine how abrupt development of a tachycardia (at 200 or more beats per minute) in such a patient might precipitate angina and/or sudden hemodynamic decompensation—even if the tachycardia was supraventricular. Alternatively, it may be that a vasomotor factor (rather than the rapid rate per se) is the precipitating mechanism of cardiovascular collapse in

---

*Among the group with ventricular fibrillation, prognosis may vary according to the *amplitude* of the fibrillatory waveform. Thus, patients with **fine ventricular fibrillation** (defined as an amplitude of ≤0.2 mm for the greatest peak-to-peak deflection in any sinusoidal wave) tend to be unattended for a significantly longer period of time prior to arrival of EMS personnel, and consequently have a much poorer prognosis than patients initially found in **coarse ventricular fibrillation** (Weaver et al, 1985).

certain patients with SVT who develop hemodynamic decompensation (Leitsch et al, 1992; Rothenberg, 1992).

Awareness of the potential causative role of supraventricular tachycardia in the genesis of cardiac arrest has obvious and important clinical implications. Clearly, contemplated diagnostic evaluation and treatment considerations may be very different if the precipitating tachyarrhythmia is supraventricular rather than ventricular. One might also anticipate a much better long-term prognosis with treatment for patients with a readily identifiable supraventricular etiology for their event. Thus, although supraventricular tachycardia will *not* be a common cause of out-of-hospital cardiac arrest, it may be helpful to keep it in mind as a possibility for selected patients.

The Immediate Post-Resuscitation Rhythm

The poor prognostic implications of bradyarrhythmias carry over to the *immediate postresuscitation rhythm* (i.e., the *first* rhythm seen *after* conversion out of ventricular fibrillation). For patients initially discovered in ventricular fibrillation, conversion to an organized rhythm with a heart rate greater than 100 beats/min is associated with greater than 40% long-term survival (Nagel et al, 1975). In contrast, long-term survival is only 5% when the initial postresuscitation rhythm is bradycardia. Patients in whom the heart rate immediately following conversion from ventricular fibrillation is between 60 and 100 beats/min have an intermediate prognosis. Thus, *the faster an organized postconversion rhythm is, the better the chance for ultimate survival.*

Slow idioventricular rhythm* (IVR) has generally been included with the bradyarrhythmias. As such, it is commonly associated with an exceedingly poor prognosis when seen in the setting of cardiac arrest. Slow IVR is a relatively infrequent primary (precipitating) mechanism of out-of-hospital cardiac arrest (Warner et al, 1985). In contrast, slow IVR is seen much more often as a post-defibrillation rhythm. Surprisingly, prognostic implications of slow IVR in this context are not nearly as dismal as when the rhythm occurs as the primary mechanism of the arrest.

> Hoffman et al (1987) have shown that development of slow IVR following defibrillation of out-of-hospital ventricular fibrillation is actually associated with a good ultimate outcome in a substantial number of patients *even in the absence of a pulse!* They postulate that in such patients slow IVR probably represents a *transient recovery (or transition) rhythm* in which supraventricular pacemakers are temporarily suppressed by the defibrillating shock. Resumption of a more stable (i.e., supraventricular) rhythm associated with a palpable pulse may follow (Hoffman et al, 1987).
>
> Clinically, it is important to be aware of this phenomenon. This is because drugs such as epinephrine may aggravate the situation by precipitating recurrence of ventricular fibrillation (Hoffman et al, 1987). *It is therefore probably best to withhold epinephrine (for at least 30 to 60 seconds) when the rhythm that develops*

in response to defibrillation is slow IVR. Instead, the wisest course of action may be to assure adequate ventilation, perform external chest compression (if pulses are absent), and cautiously observe the patient in the hope that resumption of a supraventricular rhythm with a pulse will soon follow. Epinephrine becomes indicated if pulseless slow IVR persists.

Interpreting the Literature

Interpretation of the voluminous literature on the outcome of out-of-hospital cardiac arrest is difficult. A large overview analysis of the experience in 29 communities (including 8 countries, as well as both rural and urban sites in the United States) demonstrates marked variability in survival rates for out-of-hospital cardiac arrest (Eisenberg et al, 1990). Reasons cited for this variability include the wide discrepancy in definitions used for study parameters (cardiac arrest vs. out-of-hospital ventricular fibrillation, determination of response times, determination if an arrest was "witnessed," etc.), difficulty quantitating (and controlling for) demographic factors of study subjects, and the significant difference in the types of EMS systems involved.

Overall discharge rates following out-of-hospital cardiac arrest range from 2% to 25% (and from 3% to 33% for ultimate survival following out-of-hospital ventricular fibrillation). Highest survival rates are seen with 2-tier EMS systems in which EMTs (and ideally EMT-Ds*) arrive on the scene within several minutes of the arrest to initiate CPR (and ideally to defibrillate), followed shortly thereafter by the arrival of paramedics capable of intubating, establishing IV access, and administering drugs according to ACLS protocol. Survival rates are considerably lower in the three types of 1-tier EMS systems (EMT only, EMT-D only, or paramedic only).

> It is of interest that a major determinate of survival in this large overview analysis was again *time until delivery of definitive care* (defibrillation, and to a lesser extent intubation and drug administration). The key factor for increasing survival was introduction of a second tier into the EMS system, presumably because this step ensures prompt initiation of CPR *and* early defibrillation. This suggests communities truly intent on having a significant impact on survival from out-of-hospital cardiac arrest must invest the time and resources necessary for developing a 2-tier response system for delivery of emergency medical care.

Clinical Implications

Awareness of the primary mechanism for out-of-hospital cardiac arrest provides the rescue team with important (and insightful) prognostic information regarding the chances for successful resuscitation and ultimate survival. This is *not* to say that little attempt should be made to resuscitate a patient who suffers an unwitnessed arrest and

---

*Slow IVR is an organized, regular (or at least fairly regular) cardiac rhythm characterized by QRS widening, absence of P waves, and a heart rate of less than 60 beats/min. *(See Section E of Chapter 3 for more details on slow IVR.)*

---

*Emergency medical technicians (EMTs) who are given the designation EMT-D are able to defibrillate, whereas less specialized EMTs (who do not carry the D designation) are not.

is found in a bradyarrhythmia such as asystole or EMD. On the contrary, rescuers are always obligated to initiate and continue basic and advanced life-support measures until it becomes clear that effective cardiovascular function cannot be restored. Nevertheless, knowledge of the clinical context in which an arrest occurs and appreciation of what the initial cardiac rhythm was *at the time of arrival* of the EMS unit may be extremely helpful to the emergency care provider in determining how aggressively resuscitation efforts should be pursued.

It should be evident from discussion so far that *time is the critical element in cardiac resuscitation.* If a patient is still in ventricular tachycardia at the time *help* (i.e., the defibrillator) arrives, the chances for successful resuscitation are extremely good. The chance for long-term survival is less if the patient is in ventricular fibrillation by the time help arrives, although it may still be as high as 20% to 30%. However, the longer the patient remains in ventricular fibrillation, the less likely it becomes that defibrillation will be successful (Weaver et al, 1984; Eisenberg et al, 1985). By the time ventricular fibrillation has deteriorated to bradycardia (or in those instances when a bradyarrhythmia itself is the primary mechanism of arrest), prognosis is dismal (Greene, 1990).

A recently published 10-year retrospective review of approximately 1,500 patients with out-of-hospital ventricular fibrillation supports these findings (Hargarten et al, 1990). Patients whose cardiac arrest was *witnessed* by paramedics received early defibrillation (within 1 to 2 minutes) and converted to a spontaneously perfusing rhythm 32% of the time following the first countershock attempt. In contrast, when defibrillation was delayed as it was (by a mean time of 5 minutes) for patients with out-of-hospital cardiac arrest not witnessed by paramedics, conversion to a spontaneously perfusing rhythm occurred only 9% of the time following the first countershock attempt. Each minute of delay until debrillation (up to the first 3 minutes) resulted in a significant reduction in the likelihood of converting ventricular fibrillation to a spontaneously perfusing rhythm. *It is clear that delaying defibrillation beyond these first 3 critical minutes dramatically reduces the chances for successful defibrillation of victims of out-of-hospital cardiac arrest.*

For practical purposes then, potentially treatable mechanisms of out-of-hospital cardiac arrest are ventricular tachycardia and ventricular fibrillation. Early defibrillation (or synchronized cardioversion for ventricular tachycardia with a pulse) is the treatment of choice. Institution of lay-bystander CPR is *not* a substitute for this definitive therapy. *CPR by itself (without adjunctive use of drugs such as epinephrine) will not result in adequate perfusion of vital organs such as the heart and brain* (Michael et al, 1984; Sanders et al, 1984). At most, performance of CPR may buy a small amount of time (i.e., preserve potential viability of the patient for 1, or at most 2 minutes) until definitive care can be provided (Cummins et al, 1985; Stueven et al, 1986). However, CPR in and of itself will *not* prevent ultimate deterioration of ventricular tachycardia or ventricular fibrillation to asystole (Enns et al, 1983; Eisenberg et al, 1990).

Preservation of potential viability (i.e, responsiveness to electrical countershock) by CPR may be vitally important (and at times lifesaving) if definitive care arrives in the interim. However, performance of CPR does little (or nothing) if subsequent countershock is not forthcoming (or is excessively delayed). It would therefore seem that an even more important role of CPR in the overall scheme of cardiopulmonary resuscitation is that it teaches the lay public to recognize cardiac arrest sooner. *The sooner cardiac arrest is recognized, the sooner the EMS system will be notified (and activated), and the sooner the patient will receive definitive therapy.*

Knowledge of CPR also teaches the lay public to recognize the signs and symptoms of heart attack sooner. Doing so probably prevents many patients from ever developing ventricular fibrillation because it gets appropriate medical attention (the EMS unit) to the patient sooner. Administration of medication (oxygen, nitroglycerin, morphine, lidocaine, etc.) and early transport to the hospital may prove to be lifesaving because it prevents the cardiac arrest from happening.

Historically, efforts at transporting the victim of cardiac arrest to a defibrillator have not been successful (Eisenberg et al, 1980; Stults et al, 1984). It simply takes too long to get the patient to the hospital. As a result, emphasis has switched to transporting the defibrillator to the scene. This idea first gained support in the 1960s with the advent of mobile coronary care units that carried defibrillators. Initially, physicians were used to staff these units. By the 1970s, a number of communities had begun to use specially trained lay personnel (paramedics) instead of physicians for this purpose. With paramedics providing initial emergency care at the scene, both prompter and wider dispersion of medical services was possible. Early countershock could be delivered to patients with ventricular fibrillation, and survival rates from out-of-hospital cardiac arrest more than doubled (Eisenberg et al, 1980).

In succeeding years, lay personnel with much less extensive training were used to provide emergency care and on-the-scene defibrillation. In communities wihtout paramedics, this meant firemen, policemen, and ambulance drivers received training to become emergency medical technicians (EMTs). With as little as 10 hours of formal instruction, it was shown that such providers could also be taught to accurately identify ventricular fibrillation and effectively defibrillate on the scene (Eisenberg et al, 1980). Even when such personnel were not allowed to do anything other than defibrillate victims of out-of-hospital cardiac arrest (i.e., no intubation and no administration of medication), lives were saved (Stults et al, 1984; Eisenberg et al, 1985).

Automatic External Defibrillators

As an extension of the idea that providing prompter defibrillation for victims of out-of-hospital cardiac arrest improved survival, the *automatic external defibrillator (AED)* was developed. Designed for both the lay public and EMS personnel, this device has become increasingly popular in recent years.

ADVANTAGES OF THE AED

Major advantages of the AED are ease of use, accuracy in diagnosis, reliability in performance, and lifesaving potential. Learning to operate the device is relatively easy. Most lay people accept training with enthusiasm and can be taught to effectively use the AED in as little as 3 hours (Eisenberg et al, 1985; Cummins et al, 1989). All that is required with newer models is to apply two pregelled adhesive pads to the anterior chest of the victim. The machine does the rest. Electrodes attached to the chest pads sense the cardiac rhythm, analyze it, and deliver 200 to 335 joules of electrical energy if ventricular fibrillation is present.

> In earlier models, a breath detector was incorporated into the oral airway to verify the absence of respiration, thus serving as a double check that the victim was truly in cardiopulmonary arrest. However, because agonal respirations may persist despite the presence of ventricular fibrillation, the breath detector has proved to be a double-edged sword. As a result, it has been removed from newer models, thus avoiding the potential situation where the AED might not shock a patient with gasping respiration who was nevertheless in ventricular fibrillation.
>
> Some AED models are less than fully automatic (i.e., they are "semiautomatic"). Semiautomatic AEDs require a greater degree of knowledge and skill by the operator (who must verify the rhythm and the need for defibrillation), and take somewhat longer to deliver the countershock. However, they do provide the added safety feature of requiring the operator to manually depress a "shock button" once defibrillation is decided upon.

Accuracy of the AED in rhythm assessment is encouraging. *Sensitivity* (i.e., detection of ventricular fibrillation) is approximately 80%, and *specificity* (i.e., not inappropriately shocking patients who are not in ventricular fibrillation) approaches 100% (Cummins et al, 1984; 1987).

> The most difficult rhythm for the AED to analyze is *fine* ventricular fibrillation. Practically speaking, failure to recognize (and defibrillate) fine ventricular fibrillation is unlikely to exert a significant effect on survival because of the relative resistance to any form of treatment of this rhythm when it occurs in an out-of-hospital setting (Weaver et al, 1985; 1988).

Device performance and clinical outcome using the AED is comparable to that achieved with manual operation of standard defibrillators (Cummins et al, 1987; Weaver et al, 1988). Additional long-term beneficial features accruing from community-wide implementation of automatic defibrillation into EMS systems include overall expense reduction and improved reliability in performance. As a natural consequence of the computerized analysis system that the machine is programmed with, arrhythmia interpretation (i.e., diagnosis of ventricular fibrillation) is likely to be more consistent than when rhythms are visually interpreted by EMTs on the scene. Similarly, performance variability (once ventricular fibrillation is diagnosed) is likely to be much less with the AED than it is for performance of manual defibrillation by individual EMTs who may have various degress of training and experience.

Use of the AED significantly reduces the time from patient collapse (and presumed onset of ventricular fibril-

lation) until delivery of electrical countershock. With the device, lay individuals who witness an arrest in the home can be taught to administer the first shock in *less* than 2 minutes (Moore et al, 1987). Of perhaps even greater clinical impact is the fact that the AED also enables EMTs *experienced in defibrillation* to deliver the first countershock sooner (by almost a minute) compared to the standard technique of manual defibrillation (Cummins et al, 1987).

> This last observation is particularly important in rural communities where funding and resources (for extensive training and supervision) are often inadequate to provide paramedic programs. Because volunteerism for ambulance services is usually high in such areas while the incidence of out-of-hospital cardiac arrest is quite low, *most EMTs who work in communities with populations under 25,000 will not have an opportunity to test their defibrillation skills in a real situation more often than once every few years* (Stults et al, 1984; Ornato et al, 1984). The obvious advantage of the AED is that it may allow provision of optimal emergency care for out-of-hospital cardiac arrest (i.e., early defibrillation) while minimizing the need for the constant retraining that would be necessary to maintain the skills of individuals who are called on to defibrillate so infrequently. Considering the extremely poor prognosis (*less* than 5% survival) of persons suffering cardiac arrest in rural communities and areas of the country with less well developed EMS systems (Bachman et al, 1986; Eisenberg et al, 1987), instituting some mechanism for expediting emergency defibrillation (i.e., EMT use of the AED) would seem to offer the most realistic chance for improving survival.

An important concern about implementation of EMT-D programs that do not have the luxury of paramedic backup has been regarding the likelihood of *refibrillation* occurring unless antiarrhythmic therapy (with antifibrillatory agents such as lidocaine or bretylium) can be promptly administered. Stutts and Brown (1986) found the incidence of this phenomenon to be 17%. A comforting supplemental finding of their study was that if refibrillation did occur, it usually responded well to additional attempts at defibrillation. This suggests that absence of paramedic backup (i.e., the capability of intubation and drug administration in the field) should *not* deter implementation of EMT programs, and that use of the AED *alone* will provide adequate definitive therapy in most instances of prehospital cardiac arrest that are amenable to treatment. The American Heart Association fully supports incorporation of such early defibrillation programs into a community's EMS system, and acknowledges the critical role that AEDs must play in such programs (Cummins, Thies, and the ECC/ACLS Subcommittee of the AHA, 1990).

USE OF AEDs BY FAMILY MEMBERS

A key issue that remains is determination of the role of the AED in the home. Considering the fact that more than two thirds of cardiac arrests occur in the home, extending availability of the AED to family members and relatives of high-risk cardiac patients would seem to be the ideal way for improving survival from out-of-hospital ventricular fibrillation (Litwin et al, 1987). Unfortunately, achievement of this objective has not yet been borne out in practice. Barriers to home implementation and effective use of the AED by the lay public are numerous and include (Eisenberg et al, 1989):

- A need for the device to be accepted *both* by family members as well as by the patient's personal physician.
- The financial means to afford the device.
- A need for family members to undergo and successfully complete training in operation of the device.
- The need for periodic retraining to ensure retention of (otherwise easily forgotten) skills.
- The need for the cardiac arrest to be *witnessed* by a family member and *recognized* as an event requiring application of the AED.
- The need for the patient to be in ventricular fibrillation at the time the device is applied.
- The need for the family member to follow all operational steps correctly, and for the AED to function properly.
- The need for the post-defibrillation rhythm to be a perfusing one.

The experience reported by Eisenberg et al is sobering (1989). During a 5-year period in which 59 survivors of out-of-hospital cardiac arrest were followed, only 10 patients had a recurrence of cardiac arrest in the home. Of these, the AED was properly applied by a family member on six occasions. In only two of these six occasions was ventricular fibrillation the rhythm at the time the device was applied. Countershock was appropriately delivered in both of these cases, but neither patient responded with a perfusing rhythm. Thus, despite great theoretical benefits, the overall lifesaving potential from home utilization of AEDs may be much more limited than hoped for.

Location of Definitive Care: On-the-Scene or in the Hospital?

The key determinant for ultimate survival of victims of major trauma is the rapidity of transport to a major trauma facility experienced in the care of such patients. This is distinctly different than the case for the victim of out-of-hospital cardiac arrest for whom definitive care *must* be delivered *on the scene* for there to be a meaningful chance for survival (Kellerman et al, 1988; Bonnin and Swor, 1989; Lewis et al, 1990; Greene, 1990).

Rothenberg pooled data from 9 studies in the literature on resuscitation of out-of-hospital cardiac arrest (1990). The review encompassed more than 1,600 patients who arrested in the field and received emergency cardiac care (defibrillation and administration of medication by ACLS protocol) from paramedics. Less than 1% of patients in these 9 studies who were pulseless at the time of arrival in the emergency department were ultimately resuscitated and discharged from the hospital alive with intact neurologic function.

The message is clear. Despite advancements with sophisticated therapeutic modalities and emergency cardiac care, *if paramedics are unable to resuscitate the victim of nontraumatic out-of-hospital cardiac arrest (i.e., restore spontaneous circulation with a palpable pulse) after 20 to 30 minutes of ACLS, it is highly unlikely that transport to an emergency facility will do significantly better* (Rothenberg, 1990).

Despite the sobering result of Rothenberg's review, the *medicolegal issue* of where to terminate resuscitative efforts remains unresolved. Because of the possibility (however small) that victims of out-of-hospital cardiac arrest may subsequently regain spontaneous perfusion, many emergency care physicians are simply not comfortable giving the order (sight unseen) to terminate resuscitation efforts in the field. Instead they advise continuation of CPR and ACLS by EMS units at least until the patient can be transported to a hospital and the situation evaluated personally by a physician in the emergency department (ED).

Although the rationale for this practice is understandable (as it may add to physician comfort by reducing the perceived risk of lawsuit from premature termination of resuscitation), it must be balanced by the tremendous additional cost incurred from hospital-based resuscitation of patients who have little realistic chance of long-term survival. In a study by Gray et al (1991), the mean hospital stay following ED resuscitation of patients who failed prehospital efforts was more than 12 days. None of the patients survived until hospital discharge, and all but one remained comatose throughout the hospitalization. The average cost of their hospital stay was more than $10,000 (and as much as $95,000 for one patient).

In addition, a more than negligible health risk is posed to emergency care providers in rush transit to the hospital. For example, no less than 25 EMTs and paramedics *died* as a direct result of accidents sustained from high-speed ambulance driving during the period from 1983 to 1986. Considering that resuscitation of cardiac arrest by skilled paramedics in the field (with defibrillation, intubation, and administration of medications according to ACLS protocol) is generally quite good, and the difficulty a small paramedic crew experiences trying to continue high-quality CPR and ACLS from the back of a speeding ambulance, it makes sense for skilled paramedics to invest maximal effort in the field toward a full attempt at cardiopulmonary resuscitation. Early transfer of such patients to the hospital might best be reserved for cases in which paramedics are unable to intubate or establish IV access in the field.

In summary, the most important determinant of survival from nontraumatic out-of-hospital cardiac arrest is early defibrillation. Definitive therapy (i.e., defibrillation, intubation, and drug administration) can be effectively delivered by EMS systems with a paramedic tier. The overwhelming majority of cardiac arrest victims who are successfully resuscitated and ultimately discharged from the hospital with intact neurologic function will be saved by application of such definitive therapy in the field. Realistically however, long-term prognosis for victims of out-of-hospital cardiac arrest who cannot be successfully resuscitated by skilled paramedics in the field is dismal. Until such time as policies are developed addressing protocols for termination of resuscitation by nonphysicians in the field, emergency transport (with full CPR in progress) to the ED of pulseless victims not responding to ACLS in the field will probably continue. Hospital-based emergency care providers attending to such victims in the ED should at least be partially comforted by awareness that it will be highly unlikely for them to resuscitate victims of nontraumatic out-of-hospital cardiac arrest if skilled paramedics were unable to do so in the field.

References

Bachman JW, McDonald GS, O'Brien PC: A study of out-of-hospital cardiac arrests in northeastern Minnesota, *JAMA* 256:477-483, 1986.

Bonnin MJ, Swor RA: Outcomes in unsuccessful field resuscitation attempts, *Ann Emerg Med* 17:507, 1989.

Buxton FE: Sudden cardiac death—1986, *Ann Intern Med* 104:716-718, 1986, (editorial).

Cobb LA, Werner JA et al: *Predictors and prevention of sudden cardiac death.* In Hurst JW, editor: *The heart,* New York, 1982, McGraw-Hill.

Cummins RO, Eisenberg MS, Berner L, Hallstrom A, Hearne T, Murray JA: Automatic external defibrillation: evaluations of its role in the home and in emergency medical services, *Ann Emerg Med* 13:798-801, 1984.

Cummins RO, Eisenberg MS: Prehospital cardiopulmonary resuscitation: is it effective? *JAMA* 253:2408-2412, 1985.

Cummins RO, Eisenberg MS, Moore JE, Hearne TR, Andresen E, Wendt R, Litwin PE, Graves JR, Hallstrom AP, Pierce J: Automatic external defibrillators: clinical, training, psychological, and public health issues, *Ann Emerg Med* 14:755-760, 1985.

Cummins RO, Eisenberg MS, Litwin PE, Graves JR, Hearne TR, Hallstrom AP: Automatic external defibrillators used by emergency medical technicians: a controlled clinical trial, *JAMA* 257:1605-1610, 1989.

Cummins RO, Schubach JA, Litwin PE, Hearne TR: Training lay persons to use automatic external defibrillators: success of initial training and one-year retention of skills, *Am J Emerg Med* 7:143-149, 1989.

Cummins RO, Thies W, the ECC/ACLS Subcommittee of the AHA: Encouraging early defibrillation: the American Heart Association and automated external defibrillators, *Ann Emerg Med* 19:1245-1248, 1990.

Eisenberg MS, Bergner L, Hallstrom A: Out-of-hospital cardiac arrest: improved survival with paramedic services, *Lancet* 1:812-815, 1980.

Eisenberg MS, Copass MK, Hallstrom AP, Blake B, Bergner L, Short FA, Cobb LA: Treatment of out-of-hospital cardiac arrest with rapid defibrillation by emergency medical technicians, *N Engl J Med* 302:1379-1393, 1980.

Eisenberg MS, Hallstrom A, Bergner L: The ACLS score—predicting survival from out-of-hospital cardiac arrest, *JAMA* 246:50-52, 1981.

Eisenberg MS, Cummins RO, Hallstrom AP, Hearne T: Defibrillation by emergency medical technicians, *Crit Care Med* 13:921-922, 1985.

Eisenberg MS, Cummins RO, Moore J, Hallstrom AP, Hearne T, Litwin P: Use of automatic external defibrillators in the home *Crit Care Med* 13:946-947, 1985, (abstract).

Eisenberg MS, Cummins RO, Ho MT: *Code Blue: cardiac arrest and resuscitation,* Philadelphia, 1987, WB Saunders.

Eisenberg MS, Moore J, Cummins RO, Andriesen E, Litwin PE, Hallstrom AP, Hearne T: Use of the automatic external defibrillator in homes of survivors of out-of-hospital ventricular fibrillation, *Am J Cardiol* 63:443-446, 1989.

Eisenberg MS, Horwood BT, Cummins RO, Reynolds-Haertle R, Hearne TR: Cardiac arrest and resuscitation: a tale of 29 cities, *Ann Emerg Med* 19:179-186, 1990.

Enns J, Tween WA, Donen N: Prehospital cardiac rhythm deterioration in a system providing only basic life support, *Ann Emerg Med* 12:478-481, 1983.

Goldstein S, Medendorp SV, Landis JR, Wolfe RA, Leighton R, Ritter G, Vasu CM, Archeson A: Analysis of cardiac symptoms preceding cardiac arrest, *Am J Cardiol* 58:1195-1198, 1986.

Gray WA, Capone RJ, Most AS: Unsuccessful emergency medical resuscitation-are continued efforts in the emergency department justified? *N Engl J Med* 325:1393-1398, 1991.

Greene HL: Sudden arrhythmic cardiac death—mechanisms, resuscitation, and classification: the Seattle perspective, *Am J Cardiol* 65:4B-12B, 1990.

Hargarten KM, Stueven HA, Waite EM, Olson DW, Mateer DR, Aufderheide TP, Davin J: Prehospital experience with defibrillation of coarse ventricular fibrillation: a ten-year review, *Ann Emerg Med* 19:157-162, 1990.

Hoffman JR, Stevenson LW: Postdefibrillation idioventricular rhythm—a salvageable condition, *West J Med* 146:188-191, 1987.

Josephson ME, Horowitz LN, Spielman SR, Greenspan AM: Electrophysiologic and hemodynamic studies in patients resuscitated from cardiac arrest, *Am J Cardiol* 46:948-955, 1980.

Kellerman AL, Staves DR, Hackman BB: In-hospital resuscitation following unsuccessful pre-hospital advanced cardiac life support: "heroic efforts" or an exercise in futility? *Ann Emerg Med* 17:589-594, 1988.

Kempf FC, Josephson ME: Cardiac arrest recorded on ambulatory electrocardiograms, *Am J Cardiol* 53:1577-1582, 1984.

Leitch JW, Klein GJ, Yee R, Leather RA, Kim YH: Syncope associated with supraventricular tachycardia: an expression of tachycardia rate or vasomotor response? *Circulation* 85:1064-1071, 1992.

Lewis LM, Ruoff B, Rush C, Stothert JC: Is the emergency department resuscitation of out-of-hospital cardiac arrest victims who arrive pulseless worthwhile? *Am J Emerg* 8:118-120, 1990.

Litwin PE, Eisenberg MS, Hallstrom AP, Cummins RO: The location of collapse and its effect on survival from cardiac arrest, *Ann Emerg Med* 16:787-791, 1987.

Michael JR, Guerci AD, Kochler RC, Shi AY, Tsitlik J, Chandra N, Niedermeyer E, Rogers MC, Traystman RJ, Weisfeldt ML: Mechanisms by which epinephrine augments cerebral and myocardial perfusion during cardiopulmonary resuscitation in dogs, *Circulation* 69:822-835, 1984.

Milner PG, Platia EY, Reid PR, Griffith LSC: Ambulatory electrocardiographic recordings at the time of fatal cardiac arrest, *Am J Cardiol* 56:588-592, 1985.

Moore JE, Eisenberg MS, Cummins RO, Hallstrom A, Litwin P, Carter W: Lay person use of automatic external defibrillation, *Ann Emerg Med* 16:669-672, 1987.

Myerburg RJ, Kessler KM, Zaman L, Conde CA, Castellanos A: Survivors of prehospital cardiac arrest, *JAMA* 247:1485-1490, 1982.

Nagel EL, Liberthson RR, Hirshman JC, Nussenfeld SR: *Emergency care.* In Prineas JK, Blackburn H, editors: *Sudden coronary death outside hospital, Circulation* 52 (Suppl 3):216-218, 1975.

Ornato JP, McNeill SE, Craren EJ, Nelson NM: Limitation on effectiveness of rapid defibrillation by emergency medical technicians in a rural setting, *Ann Emerg Med* 13:1097-1099, 1984.

Pratt CM, Francis MJ, Luck JC, Wyndham CR, Miller RR, Quinones MA: Analysis of ambulatory electrocardiograms in 15 patients during spontaneous ventricular fibrillation with special reference to preceding arrhythmic events, *J Am Coll Cardiol* 2:789-797, 1983.

Rothenberg MA: Failed pre-hospital resuscitation-is there hope of success in the ED? *ACLS Alert* 1:21-23, 1988.

Rothenberg MA: Failed pre-hospital resuscitation-is the jury finally in? *ACLS Alert* 3:61-64, 1990.

Rothenberg MA: Adenosine may not be safe. *ACLS Alert* 5:61-63, 1992.

Sanders AB, Meislin HW, Ewy GA: The physiology of cardiopulmonary resuscitation: an update, *JAMA* 252:3283-3286, 1984.

Stueven H, Troiano P, Thompson B, Mateer JR, Kastenson EH, Tonsfeldt D, Hargartern K, Kowalski R, Aprahamian C, Darin J: Bystander/first responder CPR: ten years experience in a paramedic system, *Ann Emerg Med* 15:707-710, 1986.

Stults KR, Brown DD, Schug VL, Bean JA: Prehospital defibrillation performed by emergency medical technicians in rural communities, *N Engl J Med* 310:219-223, 1984.

Stults KR, Brown DD: Refibrillation managed by EMT-Ds: incidence and outcome without paramedic back-up, *Am J Emerg Med* 4:491-495, 1986.

Wang Y, Scheinman MM, Chien WW, Cohen TJ, Lesh MD, Griffin JC: Patients with supraventricular tachycardia presenting with aborted sudden death: incidence, mechanism, and long-term follow-up, *J Am Coll Cardiol* 18:1711-1719, 1991.

Warner LL, Hoffman JR, Baraff LJ: Prognostic significance of field response in out-of-hospital ventricular fibrillation, *Chest* 87:22-28, 1985.

Weaver WD, Copass MK, Bufi D, Ray R, Hallstrom AP, Cobb LA: Improved neurologic recovery and survival after early defibrillation, *Circulation* 69:943-948, 1984.

Weaver WD, Cobb LA, Dennis D, Ray R, Hallstrom AP, Copass MK: Amplitude of ventricular fibrillation waveform and outcome after cardiac arrest, *Ann Intern Med* 102:53-55, 1985.

Weaver WD, Hill D, Fahrenbruch CE, Copass MK, Martin JS, Cobb LA, Hallstrom AP: Use of the automatic external defibrillator in the management of out-of-hospital cardiac arrest, *N Engl J Med* 319:661-666, 1988.

SECTION B

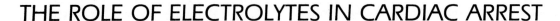

THE ROLE OF ELECTROLYTES IN CARDIAC ARREST

The potential role of hypokalemia in arrhythmogenesis and/or precipitation of cardiac arrest is intriguing (Grauer and Gums, 1988). Although conflicting reports exist in the literature, a majority of studies seem to suggest an increased incidence in both frequency and complexity of ventricular arrhythmias among patients with diuretic-induced hypokalemia (Holland et al, 1981; Podrid, 1990). The effect appears to be most marked in patients with underlying heart disease (Papademetriou et al, 1983). Most studies also suggest an inverse relationship between serum potassium levels and ventricular ectopy during the acute phase of myocardial infarction (Nordrehaug et al, 1985). Unfortunately, spontaneous variability in PVC frequency, less than optimal methodology (i.e., an absence of studies using long-term Holter monitoring for PVC quantitation), and the near impossibility of controlling for multiple variables make it difficult to draw definite conclusions about the true relation between PVC frequency in nonsustained ventricular arrhythmias and hypokalemia (Podrid, 1990).

More can be said about the relation between hypokalemia and malignant ventricular arrhythmias. Sustained VT and V Fib are both significantly more likely to occur in patients with hypokalemia who are admitted to the intensive care unit for acute ischemic heart disease (angina or infarction). A study by Hulting suggests that the effect is dose-related, with the risk of developing V Fib within the first 12 hours of hospital admission for suspected acute infarction increasing more than fourfold when serum potassium is <3.5 mEq/L compared to when serum potassium is ≥3.9 mEq/L (Hulting, 1981). In this same study, patients with borderline serum potassium values (i.e., between 3.5 to 3.8 mEq/L) still had more than a twofold increase in V Fib compared to when values were clearly within the normal range (Hulting, 1981). The risk of developing VT also appears to be dose-dependent, with up to a fivefold increase in the occurrence of VT in patients with acute ischemic heart disease and a serum potassium <3.0 mEq/L (Hulting, 1981; Solomon and Cole, 1981).

It is of interest that among survivors of out-of-hospital ventricular fibrillation, serum potassium values obtained immediately following resuscitation are significantly lower than levels obtained from a matched group of ambulatory controls with comparable underlying heart disease who are on similar medications including diuretics (Thompson and Cobb, 1982; Salerno et al, 1987). This suggests that the hypokalemia commonly observed following resuscitation is not simply a reflection of potassium depletion from diuretic use prior to the arrest (Thompson and Cobb, 1982; Grauer and Gums, 1988). Instead, it is much more likely that hypokalemia in this setting occurs as a direct

result of the arrest rather than its precipitating cause (Salerno, 1988).

Available evidence suggests that catecholamines play a pivotal role in hypokalemia-induced arrhythmogenesis (Thompson and Cobb, 1982; Grauer and Gums, 1988; Salerno et al, 1987; Salerno, 1988). The mechanism is probably related to stress. Enhanced secretion of endogenous epinephrine is the natural accompaniment of acutely stressful conditions such as trauma, surgery, stroke, cardiac arrest, myocardial infarction, and intense emotional states (Lauler, 1986). In the laboratory, infusion of epinephrine to healthy volunteers in concentrations comparable to those produced by such conditions significantly lowers serum potassium, often by as much as 1.0 mEq/L (Brown et al, 1983; Kaplan, 1984). Serum potassium falls within minutes of beginning catecholamine infusion, and remains low for 1 to 2 hours after the infusion is stopped. If subjects are pretreated with diuretics for several days prior to catecholamine infusion, serum potassium levels are lowered even further (Brown et al, 1983; Brown, 1985; Vincent et al, 1985).

It is thought that the reduction in serum potassium from catecholamine infusion is specifically mediated by β-2 adrenergic receptors (Brown et al, 1983; Lauler, 1985; Brown, 1985; Vincent et al, 1985). Evidence supporting this theory is that cardioselective β-blockade (i.e., blockade of β-1 adrenergic receptors) does not prevent the drop in serum potassium levels, whereas nonselective β-blockade (i.e., of both β-1 and β-2 adrenergic receptors) with agents such as propranolol does. Thus stress-related hypokalemia does not appear to be the result of actual potassium depletion from the body, but *rather to a shift of this cation from the extracellular to the intracellular compartment.*

Two additional factors to consider in assessing the role of hypokalemia on arrhythmogenesis are the effect of β-blockers and the potential interaction hypokalemia may have on other antiarrhythmic agents. Hypokalemia from the extra- to intracellular shift of potassium produces a hyperpolarization (i.e., a greater negativity) of the resting membrane potential of cardiac cells. This increases the upstroke velocity of the initial portion (i.e., phase 0) of the action potential and speeds up conduction velocity of the cardiac impulse, an effect that may at least partially counteract the therapeutic action of antiarrhythmic agents such as quinidine, disopyramide, lidocaine, and others (Podrid, 1990).

Nonselective β-blockade blunts the catecholamine-induced drop in serum potassium. This may at least partially explain the beneficial effect of nonselective β-blockade during the acute phase of myocardial infarction during the post-infarction period. However, it does not explain why a similar beneficial effect is also found with the use of certain selective β-blockers (Grauer and Gums, 1988). Presumably, other pharmacologic effects of β-blockers are operative such as sympathetic blockade, a decrease in oxygen consumption, their antiarrhythmic effect, antiplatelet action, or membrane stabilizing effect.

Clinical implications of these experimental findings are uncertain. However, the following statements can be made:

1. Hypokalemia is commonly found in patients following resuscitation from cardiac arrest.
2. Hypokalemia in this setting most often results from a *shift* of potassium from the extracellular to the intracellular compartment. This shift is most likely related to *increased catecholamines* (from stress-related endogenous secretion or exogenous administration of epinephrine used in management of the arrest).
3. The presence of hypokalemia may predispose susceptible individuals to developing malignant ventricular arrhythmias (such as VT or V Fib), especially in the setting of acute ischemia (from angina or infarction) in patients with underlying heart disease.
4. Preexisting hypokalemia (i.e., from excessive diuretic use) is likely to aggravate the degree of hypokalemia produced by cardiac arrest.
5. Antiarrhythmic agents (such as lidocaine or procainamide) are likely to be less effective in treating ventricular arrhythmias in the presence of hypokalemia.

Based on the above, it seems reasonable to assume that the risk of developing malignant ventricular arrhythmias in the setting of acute infarction or in the post-resuscitation period may be lessened by maintaining a serum potassium level that is well within the normal range, and ideally ≥4.0 mEq/L (Podrid, 1990).

The final factor to consider is the role of **magnesium.** It has become increasingly clear that magnesium and potassium are closely interrelated in their clinical actions. The essence of this relationship can be summarized by the following statements:

6. The likelihood of successful resuscitation from cardiac arrest is positively correlated to normomagnesemia, and negatively correlated to hypomagnesemia (Cannon et al, 1987).
7. Adequate body stores of magnesium (intracellular and extracellular) are needed to maintain adequate body stores of potassium.
8. The presence of hypomagnesemia can produce all of the clinical manifestations of hypokalemia, including arrhythmias.

9. *Adequate potassiium repletion is often difficult* (if not impossible) *unless magnesium has been replaced first* (Graber et al, 1981; Gums, 1987).

Thus it appears that *the risk of developing malignant ventricular arrhythmias* (such as VT or V Fib) *is increased not only by the presence of hypokalemia, but also by hypomagnesemia,* especially in the setting of acute ischemia in patients wih underlying heart disease (Rasmussen et al, 1986; Kafka et al, 1987). This may explain the beneficial therapeutic (antiarrhythmic) effect of magnesium in treatment of torsade de pointes, digitalis toxicity, and other ventricular arrhythmias including cardiac arrest (Perticone et al, 1986; Tzivoni et al, 1988; Rasmussen et al, 1988; Craddock et al, 1991; Tobey et al, 1992).

Unfortunately, serum magnesium levels are not an optimal indicator for evaluating magnesium homeostasis. Patients may be depleted in total body magnesium despite having serum levels that fall within the normal range (Gums, 1987). This is because serum levels reflect *extracellular* magnesium, whereas the overwhelming majority of body magnesium is found within the *intracellular* compartment. As a result, empiric magnesium therapy may sometimes exert a beneficial therapeutic effect on certain arrhythmias even though serum concentrations of magnesium may be normal (Perticone et al, 1986; Tzivoni et al, 1988; Rasmussen et al, 1988; Kulick et al, 1988).

In summary, we emphasize that certain electrolyte disorders (i.e., hypokalemia, hypomagnesemia) may play a surprisingly important primary or secondary role in development of cardiac arrhythmias (and/or in the occurrence of cardiac arrest), especially in patients with underlying cardiac disease. Prudent evaluation and management of patients with acute cardiac emergencies should therefore include assessment of serum electrolytes and consideration of magnesium and/or potassium replacement when appropriate.

Empiric magnesium therapy may have a role in emergency treatment, even in patients with normal serum magnesium levels! We therefore suggest consideration of empiric magnesium administration for patients who fail to respond to conventional measures, and/or who have one or more factors predisposing them to magnesium depletion.

Additional discussion on the role of magnesium in emergency cardiac care and our suggestions for dosing and for use as an antiarrhythmic agent are found in Chapters 14 (under Magnesium) *and 16* (under Torsade de Pointes).

References

Brown MJ, Brown DC, Murphy MB: Hypokalemia from beta 2-receptor stimulation by circulating epinephrine, *N Engl J Med* 309:1414-1419, 1983.

Brown MJ: Hypokalemia from beta 2-receptor stimulation by circulating epinephrine, *Am J Cardiol* 56:3D-9D, 1985.

Cannon LA, Heiselman DE, Dougherty JM, Jones J: Magnesium levels in cardiac arrest victims: relationship between magnesium levels and successful resuscitation, *Ann Emerg Med* 16:1195-1199, 1987.

Craddock L, Miller B, Clifton G, Krumbach B, Pluss W: Resuscitation from prolonged cardiac arrest with high-dose intravenous magnesium sulfate. *J Emerg Med* 9:469-476, 1991.

Graber TW, Yee AS, Baker JF: Magnesium: physiology, clinical disorders, and therapy, *Ann Emerg Med* 10:49-57, 1981.

Grauer K, Gums J: Ventricular arrhythmias, part II: special concerns in evaluation, *J Am Bd Fam Pract* 1:201-206, 1988.

Grauer K, Gums J: Ventricular arrhythmias, conclusion: new agents, additional treatment modalities, and overall approach to the problem, *J Am Bd Fam Pract* 1:267-273, 1988.

Gums JG: Clinical significance of magnesium: a review, *Drug Intell Clin Pharm* 21:240-246, 1987.

Holland OB, Nixon JV, Kuhnert L: Diuretic-induced ventricular ectopic activity, *Am J Med* 70:762-768, 1981.

Hulting J: In-hospital ventricular fibrillation and its relation to serum potassium, *Acta Med Scand* (Suppl)647:109-116, 1981.

Kafka H, Langevin L, Armstrong PW: Serum magnesium and potassium in acute myocardial infarction: influence on ventricular arrhythmias, *Arch Intern Med* 147:465-469, 1987.

Kaplan NM: Our appropriate concern about hypokalemia, *Am J Med* 77:1-4, 1984.

Kulick DL, Hong R, Ryzen E, Rude RK, Rubin JN, Elkayam U, Rahimtoola SH, Bhandari AK: Electrophysiologic effects of intravenous magnesium in patients with normal conduction systems and no clinical evidence of significant cardiac disease, *Am Heart J* 115:367-372, 1988.

Lauler DP: Stress hypokalemia, *Conn Med* 49:209-213, 1985.

Nordrehaug JE, Johannessen KA, von der Lippe G: Serum potassium concentration as a risk factor of ventricular arrhythmias early in acute myocardial infarction, *Circulation* 71:645-649, 1985.

Papademetriou V, Fletcher R, Khatri IM, Freis ED: Diuretic-induced hypokalemia in uncomplicated systemic hypertension: effect of plasma potassium correction on cardiac arrhythmias, *Am J Cardiol* 52:1017-1022, 1983.

Perticone F, Adinolfi L, Bonaduce: Efficacy of Magnesium sulfate in the treatment of torsade de pointes, *Am Heart J* 112:847-849, 1986.

Podrid PJ: Potassium and ventricular arrhythmias, *Am J Cardiol* 65:33E-44E, 1990.

Rasmussen HS, Aurup P, Hojberg S, Jensen K, McNair P: Magnesium and acute myocardial infarction: transient hypomagnesemia not induced by renal magnesium loss in patients with acute myocardial infarction, *Arch Intern Med* 146:872-874, 1986.

Rasmussen HS, Cintin C, Aurup P, Breum L, McNair P: The effect of intravenous magnesium therapy on serum and urine levels of potassium, calcium, and sodium in patients with ischemic heart disease, with and without acute myocardial infarction, *Arch Intern Med* 148:1801-1805, 1988.

Salerno DM, Singer RW, Elsperger J, Ruiz E, Hodges M: Frequency of hypokalemia after successfully resuscitated out-of-hospital cardiac arrest compared to that in transmural acute myocardial infarction, *Am J Cardiol* 59:84-88, 1987.

Salerno DM: Postresuscitation hypokalemia in a patient with a normal prearrest serum potassium level, *Ann Intern Med* 108:836-837, 1988.

Solomon RJ, Cole AG: Importance of potassium in patients with acute myocardial infarction, *Acta Med Scand* (Suppl)647:87-93, 1981.

Thompson RG, Cobb LA: Hypokalemia after resuscitation from out-of-hospital ventricular fibrillation, *JAMA* 248:2860-2863, 1982.

Tobey RC, Birnbaum GA, Allegra JR, Horowitz MS, Plosay JJ: Successful resuscitation and neurologic recovery from refractory ventricular fibrillation after magnesium sulfate administration, *Ann Emerg Med* 21:92-96, 1992.

Tzivoni D, Banai S, Schuger C, Benhorin J, Keren A, Gottlieb S, Stern S: Treatment of Torsade de pointes with magnesium sulfate, *Circulation* 77:392-397, 1988.

Vincent HH, Man in't Veld AJ, Boomsma F, Schalekamp MA: Prevention of epinephrine-induced hypokalemia by nonselective beta blockers, *Am J Cardiol* 56:10D-14D, 1985.

SECTION C

WHAT IF THE PATIENT DIES?

Despite our best efforts, many (if not most) patients brought to the Emergency Department (ED) in cardiac arrest will not be resuscitated. *Our job does not end with an unsuccessful resuscitation effort.* The responsibility to talk to the family remains.

Few members of the health care team have ever received more than minimal formal training in how to deal with surviving family members of a victim of out-of-hospital cardiac arrest. This task is all the more difficult when the victim was previously well and the arrest was unexpected. An interesting study by Parrish et al surveyed the feelings of surviving family members on their care after learning that their loved one had been declared dead in the ED (1987). Although many were satisfied with the warmth, sympathy, and reassurance received from the ED staff, more than one quarter of the surviving family members rated their treatment as no more than "average." Considering that the family may "weigh for months the words and emotions of the ED staff, and review for a lifetime the happenings of the day" (Parrish et al, 1987), the importance of optimizing the initial interaction between the health care team and the family after the death of a loved one cannot be overemphasized.

Major concerns among dissatisfied family members in Parrish's survey were:

1. Not being kept informed during the waiting period while resuscitation was in progress.
2. Overintensive resuscitation efforts by the ED staff without regard for the family's wishes.
3. Never getting a chance to talk to the physician who treated their loved one (or not realizing that the ED staff person who they talked to was the treating physician).
4. Not understanding (or never receiving) explanation of the prehospital and hospital care given to their loved one.
5. Improper handling of the victim's personal belongings.
6. Not having a method for getting questions answered *after* leaving the hospital.
7. The high financial cost of the resuscitation effort, and the insensitivity they perceived certain members of the ED staff had about the burden this cost might impose on surviving relatives.

Solutions suggested by Parrish et al are simple *(Table 11C-1)*.

Table 11C-1

Suggested Approach for Addressing Concerns of the Family of the Victim of Out-of-Hospital Cardiac Arrest*
1. **Be sure a hospital representative** (such as an ED support team member, nursing supervisor, social worker, religious representative) **spends time with the family** *while* **the resuscitation is still in progress.** During this time, update the family as often as possible on the progress of the resuscitation effort.
2. **Involve the family as much as possible in decisions about the intensity of the resuscitation effort.** (Admittedly it may be difficult from a medicolegal viewpoint to pursue anything less than an all-out resuscitation effort in the ED without written documentation of a prior decision to do otherwise. Nevertheless, it may be helpful to be aware of the potential for resentment when intense resuscitation efforts are pursued in elderly and/or debilitated patients despite family wishes to do otherwise.)
3. **Be sure the treating physician addresses the family at the earliest possible moment.** Make it clear to the family that the physician they have talked to is the physician who was directly involved in the resuscitation effort of their loved one.
4. **Offer appropriately explicit details of the victim's prehospital and hospital care.** Although this information may not be needed or wanted by some family members, it is immensely important to others in helping to understand and *accept* the death of their loved one. Be sure to allow family members an opportunity to express their feelings and/or to ask questions.
5. **Check on the family's religious affiliation, and offer to contact the appropriate representative for consultation or final religious blessing.**

Continued.

Table 11C-1

Suggested Approach for Addressing Concerns of the Family of the Victim of Out-of-Hospital Cardiac Arrest*—cont'd

6. **Contact the victim's family physician at the earliest opportunity**—and let the family know you have done so.

7. **Handle the victim's personal belongings with care and respect.** It is easy to envision how "bloody shoes in a brown paper bag (may be) enough to cause haunting memories of the ED experience"*

8. **Be sure a mechanism exists in your institution for answering questions raised by surviving family members *after* they leave the hospital.** Family members may understandably forget to ask certain questions during the initial shock of the acute event. Providing a mechanism for follow-up—either by phone or in writing—assures they will have adequate opportunity to have their concerns addressed. (*Social service* consultation is often invaluable in this regard.)

9. **Be aware of the long-term financial cost a resuscitation effort may impose on surviving family members.**

10. **Offer the family an opportunity to view the deceased.**

*Adapted from Parrish et al, 1987.

The last item in *Table 11C-1* deserves special comment. While admittedly painful, acute viewing of the deceased undeniably establishes the reality of death. Long-term acceptance of this reality by the family seems to be facilitated compared to those families who do not view the deceased. In addition, denial may be lessened and the bereavement period shortened by viewing.

Slightly more than half of the surviving family members in Parish's study chose to view the deceased. Although some later regretted this decision, they were in the minority. We support the recommendation of Parish et al to provide the option for viewing with appropriate education and preparation of the family about the experience and its implications prior to having them make this decision.

> A final point to consider regards involvement of the family during transport to the hospital. If at all possible, it may be desirable to have a close family member ride along in the ambulance. Doing so may serve several purposes. It may save time by providing an opportunity for the EMS crew to obtain important historical information. It also allows the family to experience first hand "all-out" efforts to save their loved one. Finally, if the patient does not survive the ambulance trip, it may be easier for the family to accept their loss if they were with their loved one at the time the patient expired.

In summary, awareness of the needs of bereaved family members with extra attention to providing compassion and emotional support can be instrumental in easing the pain and suffering brought on by the unexpected death of a loved one. *A little extra caring (and empathy) may go a long way.*

On another level, a little extra attention to the needs of bereaved family members may go a long

way toward preventing (or *at least reducing*) the likelihood of an eventual law suit brought about by angry relatives who may be grieving from the loss, upset about the process, and looking for a way (or someone on whom) to express their frustration.

What If the Patient Dies *Before* the Family Is Notified?

Sudden, unexpected death may occur *before* family members are notified of the patient's condition. If this is the case, contact family members as soon as possible. Rather than informing them over the phone about the patient's death, *we favor delaying this information until the family arrives at the hospital.* Instead, we favor telling the family that the patient has been admitted to the ED in an extremely serious condition—and that they should come immediately.

> At this point, the principles outlined in Table 11C-1 can be applied. Recruit assistance from a hospital representative (such as a nursing supervisor, social worker, and/or appropriate religious representative). Quickly usher the family to a private location as soon as they arrive at the hospital. Sit them down. *Sit down yourself.* Introduce yourself. Indicate your role in the resuscitation effort.* Avoid trite sayings such as, "she's gone," or "he met his maker." Instead, recount in explicit detail the events leading up to the patient's arrest, and prehospital as well as in-hospital efforts at resuscitation (Rothenberg, 1992).
>
> Don't apologize for the patient's death (i.e., by saying, "I'm sorry"). Instead, emphasize how everything possible that

---

*The importance of having the physician in charge of the resuscitation effort talk to the family cannot be overemphasized.

could be done was done. Allow time for questions, and be sure a mechanism is in place for answering any questions that may arise *after* the family leaves the hospital. At the earliest opportunity, notify the victim's family physician of the patient's demise—and let the family know you have done so. And finally, be sure to offer the family an opportunity to view the deceased if they so desire (after suitably preparing them for what they will see—including detailed description of any IV lines, ET tubes, and/or monitoring devices that may still be in place).

Family Participation During CPR: An Option?

Traditionally it has been standard policy in most EDs to exclude close family members from the treatment room during attempted resuscitation of cardiac arrest victims. *Is this always the best policy?*

The assumption of many (most?) medical care providers that family members do not want to participate in the resuscitation effort of a loved one may not be valid. On the contrary, a majority of family members surveyed in a study by Doyle et al (1987) indicated a definite preference to be present during CPR.

Of the 47 respondents in the study who completed and returned a retrospective survey, 44 (94%) indicated that if given the opportunity, they would choose to be present again. More than two thirds of these respondents believed their presence not only facilitated the grieving process (and their ad-

justment to the loss of their loved one), but that it also was *beneficial* to the dying family member. More than one third went as far as emphatically declaring it to be their *right* to be present during resuscitation of their loved one.

Reasons commonly given for excluding family members from the resuscitation room are that lay individuals might be horrified by the nature of the resuscitation effort being performed on their loved one, that family members might try to interfere with resuscitation, that observation by others may reveal apparent weaknesses and failures in medical care (and/or increase the risk of subsequent lawsuit), and that the resuscitation team might become uneasy and lose concentration and objectivity.

Data in the literature in support of these assumptions is lacking. In general, lay individuals have become familiar with the resuscitation process through graphic portrayal in the movies or on television. Moreover, this study by Doyle et al suggests that a policy allowing *selected* family members to be present during resuscitation of their loved one may be beneficial in facilitating the grieving process as well as in increasing the perception of a substantial number of family members that they are in some way helping their loved one who is undergoing resuscitation. We support the concluding statement by Doyle et al that "there appears to be no reason for continuation of policies that exclude family members from the resuscitation room" *(Table 11C-2).*

Table 11C-2

Suggested Approach for Providing the Option for Close Family Members to Be Present During Resuscitation of a Loved One*
1. **Consider a policy allowing close family members to be present during resuscitation of their loved one if they so desire.**
2. **Be sure that one or more members from the health care team** (i.e., nursing supervisor, physician, social worker, religious representative, etc.) **meet with the family member(s) in the waiting room *beforehand.*** Briefly describe all events that have taken place up to this point.
3. **Ask the close family member(s) if they want to witness the resuscitation effort.** If so, describe the code scene that they are about to see in detail including information on the appearance of their loved one (i.e., presence of IV lines, NG tube, urinary catheter, intubation equipment, etc.). Indicate anticipated actions (i.e., defibrillation, performance of additional invasive procedures, etc.). Determine if the family member still wants to be present.
4. **Encourage the family member(s) to *talk* to their loved one during resuscitation.** Allow them (if possible) to *touch* their loved one (but be sure to emphasize the importance of not interfering with the resuscitation effort).
5. **Reserve the option of asking family members to *temporarily* leave the resuscitation room if additional invasive procedures need to be performed** (or at the discretion of the resuscitation team if certain aspects of resuscitation need to be discussed in private).
6. **Be sure a health care designee** (i.e., nursing supervisor, social worker, religious representative) **remains with the family member(s) at all times.** Provide a chair (if desired), and allow family members to enter and leave the resuscitation room as they choose. Let them know it is OK for them to leave before the resuscitation effort is over.

Continued.

Table 11C-2

Suggested Approach for Providing the Option for Close Family Members to Be Present During Resuscitation of a Loved One*—cont'd

7. **Be sure the patient undergoing resuscitation is covered** (with a sheet or towels) **as much as possible during the resuscitation process.**

8. **Do not prolong the resuscitation because of the presence of a family member.** A number of perceptive family members in Doyle's study felt that the resuscitation effort on their loved one may have been excessively prolonged for their benefit. Doing so is unnecessary.

9. If (once) **a decision is made by the physician in charge to terminate CPR because of *unresponsiveness* to resuscitation efforts, immediately inform family members of this decision.** After this decision is made, pronounce the patient, stop life support measures, turn lights down, and allow (encourage) family members to remain with the body (in the company of a religious representative or other health care designee if desired) for as long as they wish. If no post-mortem (autopsy) study is to be performed, IV lines and other tubes may then be removed.

*Adapted from Doyle et al, 1987.

References

Parrish GA, Holdren KS, Skiendzielewski JJ, Lumpkin OA: Emergency department experience with sudden death: a survey of survivors, *Ann Emerg Med 16:792-796, 1987.*

Doyle CJ, Post H, Burney RE, Maino J, Keefe M, Rhee KJ: Family participation during resuscitation: an option, *Ann Emerg Med 16:673-675, 1987.*

Rothenberg MA: Handling the psychological challenges of CPR (based on a presentation by Dr. Richard Swanson at the April, 1992 Emergency Cardiac Care Update Conference in Seattle, Washington). *ACLS Alert 5:69-71, 1992.*

IN-HOSPITAL CARDIAC ARREST

Most individuals who suffer cardiac arrest outside the hospital have underlying coronary artery disease. In contrast, in-hospital cardiac arrest is frequently the common terminal event for a variety of end-stage disease processes. Cardiac arrests occur in 1% to 2% of all patients admitted to the hospital (Lowenstein et al, 1986). Among those who die, cardiopulmonary resuscitation is attempted about one third of the time (Bedell et al, 1983; Schiederemyer, 1988). Overall survival for in-hospital cardiac arrest is somewhat poorer than for arrest that occurs outside the hospital. This has been attributed to the fact that hospitalized patients are usually sicker and carry a poorer prearrest prognosis than ambulatory individuals. Across the board, about half of the patients who arrest in the hospital are initially resuscitated, one third are still alive the next day, and 15% survive to leave the hospital (Bedell et al, 1983; Scaff et al, 1984; McGrath, 1987; Roberts et al, 1990; Tortolani et al, 1990).

Factors Influencing Survival

Survival rates for in-hospital resuscitation do *not* appear to be significantly influenced by *where* in the hospital the arrest occurs. Instead, *time until discovery* is a much more critical factor in determining whether the resuscitation effort will be successful (Bedell et al, 1983; Roberts et al, 1990). Although patients who arrest in the emergency department and intensive care unit often do better than those arresting on a general ward, this is probably because such patients are more often monitored and discovered sooner after collapse. For the same reason, the *time of day* that an arrest occurs is not thought to be important except for the fact that arrests occurring during early morning hours are more likely to go a longer period of time until discovery (Gulati et al, 1983; Scaff et al, 1984). Were there some way to monitor a greater number of patients (or better predict who was going to have an arrest), survival from resuscitation during early morning hours on general wards would doubtlessly improve.

An important factor in predicting outcome from in-hospital cardiac arrest is *duration* of the code. Among 241 patients in the study by Bedell (1983) for whom cardiac arrest lasted longer than 15 minutes, 95% died. No one survived when the arrest lasted longer than 30 minutes. In contrast, 56% of patients survived to leave the hospital when resuscitation was accomplished in less than 15 minutes.

Equally poor statistics have been seen by others for survival after prolonged resuscitation (Scaff et al, 1984; Hendrick et al, 1990; Tortolani et al, 1990). Although some patients are brought back initially, ultimate survival is extremely rare.

Thus, **it may be reasonable for the emergency care provider to consider terminating resuscitation efforts in *adults* as code duration approaches 30 minutes,** especially if there have been no signs that a patient is responding. (A notable exception to this generality is the arrest victim who is *hypothermic*, for whom a code should never be called until adequate core rewarming has been achieved. Other less commonly encountered exceptions in which prolonged resuscitation may be warranted despite patient unresponsiveness include victims of a lightning strike, electrocution, or barbiturate overdose.)

The likelihood of ultimate survival for patients who arrest more than once during a given hospital stay is extremely small (Debard, 1981; Scaff et al, 1984). Careful thought must therefore be given to whether a patient should be recoded a second or third time if an initial resuscitation is successful.

Finally, with respect to personnel directing the code, whether housestaff or attending physicians are in charge appears to be not nearly as important as whether emergency care providers are trained in ACLS (Scaff et al, 1984). In a study by Lowenstein et al (1986), survival from in-hospital cardiac arrest nearly doubled following such training.

Precipitating Mechanisms of In-Hospital Cardiac Arrest

As is the case for out-of-hospital events, ventricular fibrillation is thought to be an extremely common precipitating mechanism of in-hospital cardiac arrest. This is especially true for patients seen during the first few hours of acute myocardial infarction when ventricular fibrillation is most likely to arise. As alluded to earlier, in noninfarcting patients, ventricular tachycardia probably precedes many *(if not most)* episodes of ventricular fibrillation. The importance of acute care monitoring lies with detecting potentially lethal arrhythmias such as ventricular tachycardia *before* deterioration to ventricular fibrillation occurs.

As is the case for out-of-hospital cardiac arrest, ventricular fibrillation and sustained ventricular tachycardia are the precipitating mechanisms most amenable to treatment. In general, most patients arresting in the hospital as a result of either of these rhythms who can be resuscitated will respond promptly to appropriate electrical therapy (with unsynchronized countershock or synchronized cardioversion for ventricular tachycardia). In a study by Roberts et al (1990) on in-hospital cardiopulmonary resuscitation, patients not responding to three or more attempts at defibrillation or cardioversion rarely survived. Despite potential beneficial effects of epinephrine in the arrested heart, patients requiring this medication during the course of their resuscitation also almost uniformly died (Roberts et al, 1990).

Next to ventricular tachycardia/fibrillation, *primary respiratory arrest* may be the most common precipitating mechanism of in-hospital cardiac arrest (Debard, 1981; Bedell et al, 1983). This is important because discovery of the patient at the time of respiratory arrest *before cardiac arrest has occurred* is an easily treatable problem in a hospital setting. Management of the airway by rescue breathing, ventilation with airway adjuncts, and/or intubation is usually all that is needed. In contrast, by the time the EMS unit arrives on the scene of a respiratory arrest that occurred outside the hospital, the rhythm has usually deteriorated to ventricular fibrillation or asystole.

Special mention should be made of *asystole* as a mechanism of in-hospital cardiac arrest. While prognosis for asystole is never good, the outlook for patients with this rhythm may not be quite as bleak when asystole is seen in a hospital setting as when it occurs on the outside (McGrath, 1987; Tortolani et al, 1989; Hendrick et al, 1990). Again, this may be attributable to the shorter time until discovery of the arrest. In addition, the pathogenesis of asystole may differ for the two conditions. Asystole occurring on the outside is most often a *preterminal* event that develops following prolonged cardiopulmonary arrest and deterioration from ventricular fibrillation. Structural damage is frequently present, which renders the myocardium unresponsive to therapy (Coon et al, 1981; Niemann et al, 1985). In contrast, asystole occurring with in-hospital cardiac arrest may sometimes result from massive parasympathetic discharge. As such, it is less likely to be associated with irreversible structural damage, and may on occasion respond to atropine or high-dose epinephrine (Coon et al, 1981).

Pre-Arrest and Post-Arrest Variables Predictive of Prognosis

Although somewhat different results have been obtained from the various studies in the literature, a number of *pre-arrest* variables have been found helpful in predicting prognosis from in-hospital cardiac arrest. One of the most insightful of these studies was performed by Bedell et al (1983) in which the following five *pre-arrest* variables were found to be predictive:

1. Pneumonia
2. Hypotension (systolic blood pressure of less than 100 mm Hg for at least 1 day *before* the arrest)
3. Renal failure
4. Cancer (excluding skin cancer)
5. Homebound life-style *before* hospitalization

In Bedell's study of 294 patients who suffered in-hospital cardiac arrest, long-term survival after the arrest was *only* 5% if any of the above five factors were present beforehand. In contrast, long-term survival was 66% when none of these fac-

tors were present prior to the arrest. While it may not be surprising that patients in her study who had hypotension, renal failure, or cancer fared poorly following cardiac arrest, the finding that none of the 58 patients who had pneumonia before the arrest survived was indeed unexpected. It is also insightful to note the association between preadmission ambulatory status and ultimate survival following cardiac arrest.

Subsequent studies have corroborated the generally poor prognostic implications of pre-existing pneumonia (McGrath, 1987; Hendrick et al, 1990), renal failure (McGrath, 1987; Roberts et al, 1990), cancer (Taffet et al, 1988), and homebound life-style prior to hospitalization (Urberg and Ways, 1987). They also suggest a number of additional poor prognostic indicators including pre-existing heart failure (Roberts et al, 1990), recent myocardial infarction (Roberts et al, 1990), and sepsis (Taffet et al, 1988). Thus, *available evidence all points toward the importance of pre-existing health status/severity of underlying disease as a strong predictive factor of the chance for survival following in-hospital cardiac arrest.*

A predictive factor impossible to control for is the underlying cause of a sudden, unexpected cardiac arrest. Unfortunately, the true precipitating cause of in-hospital cardiac arrest often remains unknown. While long-term prognosis will not be improved by discovery of untreatable disease processes (such as metastatic cancer), future events could well be prevented if there was a way to better understand and anticipate those clinical disorders most likely to cause sudden, unexpected cardiac arrest.

Routine autopsy studies reveal unexpected findings in as many as 15% of patients who die during the course of hospital admission (Cameon et al, 1980). An interesting autopsy report by Bedell and Fulton (1986) revealed that by far the two most common *unexpected* diagnoses among patients suffering cardiac arrest in the hospital were diseases that have remained clinically elusive for centuries: *pulmonary embolism* and *ischemic bowel with infarction*. In their study, these two diseases accounted for 89% of all major missed diagnoses discovered at autopsy. Although mortality from each of these disorders tends to be high regardless of what interventions are made, early detection and treatment (i.e., anticoagulation of pulmonary embolism; surgery and antibiotics for ischemic bowel) might be life-saving in selected cases if the diagnosis could be discovered in time. Consideration of these two clinical entities in the evaluation of critically ill hospitalized patients with uncertain diagnoses may therefore be helpful in reducing the chance of future cardiac arrest and death.

Important prognostic information regarding the likelihood of ultimate survival is also provided by the patient's clinical condition on the day *following* the arrest. Patients who are alert and off pressor agents by 24 hours after CPR is performed have a greater than 90% chance of living to be discharged from the hospital. In contrast, long-term survival is less than 20% for patients who are still comatose or on pressor drugs the day after. Only 1 of the 52 patients in Bedell's study (1983) who were still in coma at this time lived to leave the hospital, and that patient remained lethargic until succumbing 2 months later.

Prediction of the degree of neurologic recovery following resuscitation from cardiac arrest is often difficult. It is clear that survivors of cardiac arrest who rapidly regain consciousness tend to have good neurologic recovery and low mortality

(Bertini et al., 1989). In contrast, patients who do not rapidly regain consciousness generally have a poorer long-term prognosis and are much more likely to have major problems with neurologic recovery. With respect to survivors of out-of-hospital cardiac arrest, *time delay* (i.e., the time elapsed from loss of consciousness until delivery of ACLS) appears to be a key factor in determining the likelihood that a patient will regain consciousness by the time they arrive in the hospital. Delay in initiation of BLS may also lessen the chance of neurologic recovery in survivors (Lee et al., 1989). However, a recent study by Bertini et al (1989) suggests that post-arrest clinical assessment of neurologic function does not become a reliable prognostic indicator of final outcome (in terms either of neurologic recovery or of survival) until *at least 48 to 72 hours* have elapsed after resuscitation. *Active supportive care in an intensive care unit may therefore be justified (and necessary) for at least this period of time following resuscitation regardless of how limited neurologic recovery initially appears to be from bedside clinical assessment.*

The Role of *Age* as a Pre-Arrest Variable

The importance of *age* as a predictive prognostic factor is only now becoming clear. Earlier studies suggested that age was not important in predicting the likelihood of ultimate survival from in-hospital resuscitation (Bedell et al, 1983; Gulati et al, 1983; Scaff et al, 1984). More recent studies on in-hospital resuscitation conflict with these earlier results and suggest that as a group, long-term prognosis of older patients* is poorer than for younger patients (McGrath, 1987; Taffet et al, 1988; Murphy et al, 1989). Considering the much greater prevalence and severity of underlying disease in older individuals, this finding is not unexpected.

Regardless of the true overall effect of age on ultimate survival, this factor by itself should *never* be used to exclude a patient from consideration for resuscitation. Even if prognosis is poorer in general for older individuals (as it appears to be), many elderly patients are nevertheless successfully resuscitated. Moreover, proper consideration must be given to the *perceived* "quality of life," a perception that is highly individualized. It is important to realize that some elderly patients are extremely satisfied with a sedentary, seemingly uneventful existence that might be meaningless and boring to younger individuals. Other factors being equal, such individuals may still be appropriate candidates for resuscitation despite their advanced age. *As alluded to above, pre-existing health status/severity of underlying disease appears to be a much more important predictive prognostic factor than chronologic age per se.*

These points notwithstanding, suggestion in the more recent literature that older patients generally do significantly poorer following in-hospital cardiac arrest may be useful (in conjunction with other factors) to assist these patients, their families, and their treating physicians to arrive at a more informed and appropriate decision regarding DNR status. Rather than depending on chronologic age as a definitive criterion for determining resuscitation status, the advanced age of a patient might better be used as a "trigger" to induce the treating

physician to discuss code status and the patient's *realistic* chances of survival *before* the arrest occurs (Schiedermeyer, 1988).

Even though advanced age does appear to be an adverse prognostic factor for survival from *in-hospital* cardiac arrest (as noted above), this is *not* necessarily true for out-of-hospital cardiac arrest. Such patients, *even if elderly*, are less likely to have other severe underlying diseases than are patients who arrest in the hospital. As a result, chances for long-term survival are surprisingly good if the precipitating mechanism of the arrest is ventricular fibrillation and EMS units capable of defibrillating arrive promptly on the scene. As borne out in a recent study by Longstreth et al (1990), as many as 24% of elderly patients (70 years of age or older) with out-of-hospital cardiac arrest from ventricular fibrillation may be resuscitated and ultimately survive to leave the hospital.

Regarding resuscitation in the elderly, Longstreth et al (1990) go on to caution against the following self-fulfilling prophecy: "If those performing the resuscitation do not believe that it will benefit the elderly, resuscitative efforts might be less than maximal, and the success rate accordingly low."

Patient Recollection of the Arrest

Most survivors of cardiac arrest do not recall anything of the event itself. A few in Bedell's study remembered receiving a "hard bang on the chest." All had a sore chest the next day. Some recalled the "look of terror in the eyes of the doctors and nurses" who worked to revive them. Only one described a "near-death" experience. For him the arrest was "peaceful, beautiful, and accompanied by angels over my head. It would have been an easy death."

How Well Are the Survivors?

A prevalent fear among hospitalized patients is that they will be successfully resuscitated, only to lead a long-lingering life in a vegetative state. Although this may occur, it appears to be much less common than is generally thought. The study by Bedell et al (1983) is again insightful. Thirty-eight of the 41 patients in her study who survived to leave the hospital had an intact mental status at the time of discharge. Two of the survivors were demented, but had been so before the arrest. Only one survivor developed a grossly impaired mental status as a direct result of the arrest. Thus it appears that *most patients who survive cardiac arrest in the hospital remain mentally intact* (Hendrick et al, 1990). Those who become comatose or mentally impaired following a resuscitation effort usually go on to die within the next few days. Rarely do such patients live to leave the hospital. Awareness of this information may be comforting to patients whose greatest fear is indefinite persistence in a vegetative state.

---

*"Older" (i.e., *elderly*) has been variously defined in studies on cardiopulmonary resuscitation as between 60 to 70 years of age or older.

Psychologically, most of the survivors in Bedell's study were depressed at the time of discharge. Within 6 months, this depression had almost uniformly lifted! Physically, all of the survivors reported a decrease in functional capacity. For some this simply meant that although they could still pursue the same activities as before the arrest, they had to do them slower. However, of the 38 mentally intact survivors, 5 of 9 who were previously employed retired, 10 became newly homebound, and 5 required new institutionalization. In many cases the investigators felt the degree of impairment to be out of proportion to the extent of organic disease. More than half of the survivors seemed to limit their physical activities because of fear. The message is clear. *Survivors of cardiopulmonary resuscitation need continued encouragement and support from health care providers in order to maximize functional recovery.*

Deciding about DNR Status

A final take-home message from Bedell's study comes from the survey she conducted on the 38 mentally competent survivors. These individuals were asked if they would want to be resuscitated again in the event of a second cardiac arrest. Initially 21 of the 38 patients answered affirmatively, 16 preferred to be made DNR *(Do Not Resuscitate)*, and 1 patient was ambivalent. Six months later, over 90% of these patients held firm to their initial request. This suggests that most competent patients have thought about cardiopulmonary resuscitation, and that many (if not most) of these individuals have definite feelings about what they would like to be done should they arrest.

Unfortunately, all too often the patient is *not* involved in such decisions. In a follow-up study by Bedell et al (1986), discussion with the patient regarding resuscitation status was undertaken *before* DNR orders were written in only 22% of 389 cases. A major reason given for this was that 76% of the patients in Bedell's study were mentally incompetent and therefore unable to participate in the decision-making process at the time DNR status was determined. However, when one considers that an average of 7 days passed before resuscitation status was addressed, and that the overwhelming majority of patients (89%) were mentally competent at the time of admission, the need for health care providers to *routinely* inquire about a patient's wishes for resuscitation *early* in the hospitalization is evident.

More detailed discussion on deciding about DNR status (including how to elicit the patient's true desires regarding resuscitation) is presented in Chapter 18 on Medicolegal Aspects.

Can Cardiac Arrest Be Prevented?

We conclude this section by reviewing the results of a recent soul-searching study performed by Bedell et al (1991) in a university teaching hospital. The authors evaluated the cases of all patients who underwent cardiopulmonary resuscitation over a 1-year period in an attempt to determine the immediate precipitating cause of the arrest. *An **iatrogenic complication** was found to be the direct cause of cardiac arrest in 14% of cases!* The principal causes of iatrogenic cardiac arrest in their study are summarized in *Table 11D-1.*

Table 11D-1

Causes of Iatrogenic Cardiac Arrest
Errors of Commission • **Complications from performing a procedure** • **Errors in the use of medications** (especially inappropriate dosing of digoxin or other antiarrhythmic medications and failure to recognize marked QT interval prolongation) **Errors of Omission** • **Insufficient recognition of and/or response to:** —Fluid and electrolyte balance —Relevant laboratory data —ECG findings —Clinical signs and symptoms (especially failure to recognize new-onset dyspnea/tachypnea—and to consider development of heart failure or pulmonary embolus as the cause)
Adapted from Bedell et al, 1991

Of particular concern was the finding that 64% of the iatrogenically-induced arrests "might have been prevented by stricter attention to the patient's history, findings on physical examination, and laboratory data." Most of the patients with iatrogenically-induced cardiac arrest were successfully resuscitated, and overall mortality was less than that from cardiac arrest not due to iatrogenic causes. Nevertheless, mistakes proved to be fatal in a significant percentage of patients.

The most common potentially preventable causes of iatrogenic cardiac arrest in the study by Bedell et al were associated with:

1. Medication errors (especially failure to recognize development of digitalis toxicity, and failure to recognize and act on QT interval prolongation that ultimately resulted in torsade de pointes).

2. Suboptimal attention to clinical signs and symptoms (especially to the possible causes of new-onset dyspnea/tachypnea).

Bedell et al respond to the question of why iatrogenic illness occurs (even in a setting in which patients are carefully monitored!) by suggesting that it may "be a price we pay for medical progress" (i.e., patients living longer on much more complicated therapeutic regimens than in the past).

Unfortunately, the sad reality is that *"mistakes are inevitable in medicine."* In a study by the authors of this quote (Wu et al, 1991), physicians who accepted responsibility for their mistakes *and openly discussed the mistake* (as appropriate with colleagues, faculty, the affected patient, and/or the patient's family) were significantly more likely to experience a constructive change in their practice. *Credit must be given to health care providers who have the courage to admit their mistakes, and who learn from these mistakes* (Lundberg, 1991).

References

Bedell SE, Delbanco TL, Cook EF, Epstein FH: Survival after cardiopulmonary resuscitation in the hospital, *N Engl J Med* 309:569-576, 1983.

Bedell SE, Pelle D, Maher PL, Cleary PD: Do-not-resuscitate orders for critically ill patients in the hospital: how are they used and what is their impact? *JAMA* 256:233-237, 1986.

Bedell SE, Fulton EJ: Unexpected findings and complications at autopsy after cardiopulmonary resuscitation (CPR), *Arch Int Med* 146:1725-1728, 1986.

Bedell SE, Deitz DC, Leeman D, Delbanco TL: Incidence and characteristics of preventable iatrogenic cardiac arrests, *JAMA* 265:2815-2820, 1991.

Bertini G, Margheri M, Giglioli C, Cricelli F, De Simone L, Taddel T, Marchionni N, Zini G, Gensini GF: Prognostic significance of early clinical manifestations in postanoxic coma: a retrospective study of 58 patients resuscitated after prehospital cardiac arrest, *Crit Care Med* 17:627-633, 1989.

Cameron HM, McGoogan E, Watson H: Necropsy: a yardstick for clinical diagnoses, *Br Med J* 281:985-988, 1980.

Coon GA, Clinton JE, Ruiz E: Use of atropine for brady-asystolic prehospital cardiac arrest, *Ann Emerg Med* 10:462-467, 1981.

Debard ML: Cardiopulmonary resuscitation: analysis of six years experience and review of the literature, *Ann Emerg Med* 10:408-416, 1981.

Gulati RS, Bhan GL, Horan MA: Cardiopulmonary resuscitation of old people, *Lancet* 2:267-269, 1983.

Hendrick JMA, Pijls NJH, van der Werf T, Crul JF: Cardiopulmonary resuscitation on the general ward: no category of patients should be excluded in advance, *Resuscitation* 20:163-171, 1990.

Lee SK, Vaagenes P, Safar P, Stezoski SW, Scanlon M: Effect of cardiac arrest time on cortical cerebral blood flow during subsequent standard external cardiopulmonary resuscitation in rabbits, *Resuscitation* 17:105-117, 1989.

Longstreth WT, Cobb LA, Fahrenbruch CE, Copass MK: Does age affect outcomes of out-of-hospital cardiopulmonary resuscitation? *JAMA* 264:2109-2110, 1990.

Lowenstein SR, Sabyan EM, Lassen CF, Kern DC: Benefits of training physicians in advanced cardiac life support, *Chest* 89:512-516, 1986.

Lundberg GD: Promoting professionalism through self-appraisal in this critical decade (editorial), *JAMA* 265:2859, 1991.

McGrath RB: In-house cardiopulmonary resuscitation-after a quarter of a century, *Ann Emerg Med* 16:1365-1368, 1987.

Murphy DJ, Murray AM, Robinson BE, Campion EW: Outcomes of cardiopulmonary resuscitation in the elderly, *Ann Intern Med* 111:199-205, 1989.

Niemann JT, Adomien GE, Garner D, Rosborough JP: Endocardial and transcutaneous cardiac pacing, calcium chloride, and epinephrine in postcountershock asystole and bradycardias, *Crit Care Med* 13:599-604, 1985.

Roberts D, Landolfo K, Light RB, Dobson K: Early predictors of mortality for hospitalized patients suffering cardiopulmonary arrest, *Chest* 97:413-419, 1990.

Scaff B, Munson R, Hastings DF: Cardiopulmonary resuscitation at a community hospital with a family practice residency, *J Fam Prac* 18:561-565, 1984.

Schiedermeyer DL: The decision to forgo CPR in the elderly patient, *JAMA* 260:2096-2097, 1988.

Taffet GE, Teasdale TA, Luchi RJ: In-hospital cardiopulmonary resuscitation, *JAMA* 260:2069-2072, 1988.

Tortolani AJ, Risucci DA, Powell SR, Dixon R: In-hospital cardiopulmonary resuscitation during asystole-therapeutic factors associated with 24-hour survival, *Chest* 96:622-626, 1989.

Tortolani AJ, Risucci DA, Rosati RJ, Dixon R: In-hospital cardiopulmonary resuscitation: patient, arrest and resuscitation factors associated with survival, *Resuscitation* 20:115-128, 1990.

Urberg M, Ways C: Survival after cardiopulmonary resuscitation for an in-hospital cardiac arrest, *J Fam Prac* 25:41-44, 1987.

Wu AW, Folkman S, McPhee SJ, Lo B: Do house officers learn from their mistakes? *JAMA* 265:2089-2094, 1991.

SECTION E

SURVIVORS OF CARDIAC ARREST: OPTIONS FOR MANAGEMENT

As we discussed in Section D of this chapter, overall survival from *in-hospital cardiac arrest* is generally poorer than for out-of-hospital cardiac arrest. This has been attributed to the more extensive underlying disease that patients who arrest in the hospital usually have. For many of these individuals, in-hospital cardiac arrest marks the terminal event of any number of end-stage disease processes. Prospects for long-term survival are understandably poor because they hinge on reversal of the extent and severity of these underlying diseases.

In contrast, victims of *out-of-hospital cardiac arrest* tend not to have nearly as many underlying disease processes. As a result, their potential for restoration to an active lifestyle following successful resuscitation is much greater. It is on this group of individuals that we focus our attention in this section, exploring the options for management and prospects for long-term survival.

Perspective on Out-of-Hospital Cardiac Arrest

The overwhelming majority of adults (middle-aged or older) who are victims of out-of-hospital cardiac arrest have underlying coronary artery disease (CAD). In up to 20% of these individuals, cardiac arrest is the first (and unfortunately last) manifestation of CAD (Cobb et al, 1980; Kannel et al, 1975). Surprisingly, acute myocardial infarction (AMI) is the actual cause of the cardiac arrest in *less* than one third of such cases (Myerburg et al, 1982).*

The prognosis from out-of-hospital cardiac arrest in

---

*Although much less common, out-of-hospital cardiac arrest may also occur in adolescents and younger adults. Rather than CAD, many of these individuals have some other type of structural heart disease—of which hypertrophic cardiomyopathy (formerly known as IHSS) appears to be the most common form (Grauer and Gums, 1988; Drory et al, 1991; Weiss et al, 1991; Safranek et al, 1992). In addition to congenital abnormalities, other important causes to consider include myocarditis (which may result from acute viral infection), conduction system abnormalities, drowning, and drug-related phenomena. The latter group includes overdose (especially from cocaine—but also from alcohol, barbiturates, and narcotics), mixed drug ingestion, and toxin exposure (i.e., from carbon monoxide).

Although not generally appreciated, drug-related phenomena appear to be an increasingly important cause of the syndrome of sudden death in young patients. Clinically, awareness of this fact may lead to appropriate early consideration of potentially beneficial therapeutic interventions (such as administration of naloxone or charcoal, and proper evacuation of the stomach) when a teenager or young adult presents to the emergency department in a state of cardiac arrest (Weiss et al, 1991; Safranek et al, 1992).

Due to space constraints, discussion in the rest of this Section is limited to consideration of adults (over 30 to 40 years of age) who suffer out-of-hospital cardiac arrest.

adults over 30 to 40 years of age depends greatly on whether acute infarction is the inciting mechanism. This is because ventricular electrical instability is a common phenomenon during the early hours of AMI. Most deaths from AMI result from primary ventricular fibrillation that develops within these first few hours after the onset of symptoms. Electrical instability associated with AMI is a transient phenomenon, however, and it generally resolves with evolution of the infarct.

> Clinically, it is of interest that the occurrence of ventricular fibrillation during the early hours of acute infarction does not seem to affect long-term survival. Patients who have an otherwise uncomplicated course demonstrate an equally good prognosis as those with uncomplicated AMI who never had ventricular fibrillation (Bigger and Coromilas, 1983; Lo and Nguyen, 1987; Tofler et al, 1987). As a result, little (or no) additional workup need be done *because* of the episode of ventricular fibrillation if it occurred in association with AMI (within hours of the onset of symptoms), and the patient goes on to recover uneventfully.

In contrast, adults who develop out-of-hospital cardiac arrest that is not associated with AMI most often do not have any obvious inciting cause. As a result, it is hard to explain why their cardiac arrest occurred, and equally difficult to intervene in a manner that will reduce the risk of recurrence. Management of such individuals therefore poses a true clinical dilemma. Left alone, the rate of recurrence for a second episode of cardiac arrest approaches 30% during the year following the initial episode and 50% by the second year (Bigger, 1984; Lo and Nguyen, 1987). Ventricular ectopy is exceedingly common in these patients; when Holter monitoring is performed after the acute episode, extremely frequent and complex ventricular ectopy with runs of ventricular tachycardia is the rule (Myerburg et al, 1982). Suppression of this ventricular ectopy with antiarrhythmic drugs is usually attempted. Although total elimination of PVCs would seem to be the ideal end point of such therapy, this goal is an unrealistic (if not impossible) one to achieve. Moreover, *even if PVCs could be completely eliminated,* current knowledge suggests that this does *not* guarantee such patients will be at less risk of developing a lethal arrhythmia such as sustained ventricular tachycardia or ventricular fibrillation (Ruskin et al, 1983; Grauer and Gums, 1988; Miller and Josephson, 1990). Paradoxically, a small (but significant) percentage of patients with malignant ventricular arrhythmias are actually placed at *higher* risk of sudden death by empiric treatment with antiarrhythmic agents, *even in cases when the frequency and complexity of their ventricular ectopy is significantly reduced by such treatment* (Ruskin et al, 1983). Clearly, determination of the optimal approach to management of these patients is no easy task.

General Assessment of Patients with Ventricular Arrhythmias

Full discussion of evaluation and management of patients with ventricular arrhythmias extends well beyond the scope of this book. *(Our views on the subject have been presented elsewhere:* Grauer and Gums, 1988; Skluth, Grauer, and Gums, 1989; Hatch and Grauer, 1993.) Nevertheless, brief review may prove insightful and provide a framework from which the approach to management of survivors of out-of-hospital cardiac arrest can be better understood. What follows is our consolidation of key principles in assessment of patients with ventricular arrhythmias. We then conclude the section by returning to the clinical dilemma posed by the survivor of out-of-hospital cardiac arrest and explore options available in management.

1. ***Classify the arrhythmia.*** Ventricular arrhythmias can be classified into one of the following three categories:
   a. ***Benign*** *ventricular arrhythmias*
   b. ***Potentially lethal*** *ventricular arrhythmias*
   c. ***Lethal*** *ventricular arrhythmias*

In general, it will be easy to determine the type of ventricular arrhythmia that a patient has according to this classification. We have found doing so tremendously facilitates our task in deciding on an optimal approach to evaluation and management of these patients *(Table 11E-1).*

Table 11E-1

Classification of Ventricular Arrhythmias*			
TYPE OF ARRHYTHMIA:	**Benign**	**Potentially Lethal**	**Lethal**
Prevalence	≈30% of ventricular arrhythmias	≈65% of ventricular arrhythmias	<5% of ventricular arrhythmias
Risk of Sudden Death	Minimal (which is why these arrhythmias are called "benign")	Moderate to high	Very high (which is why these arrhythmias are called "lethal")
Underlying Heart Disease	Absent!!!	Present	Present (Note—*AMI is the cause only* ≈1/3 *of the time!*)
Arrhythmias Commonly Seen	PVCs usually *not* frequent or complex; nonsustained VT is rare	PVCs may be frequent and complex	PVCs almost always frequent and complex; runs of sustained VT are common
Clinical Presentation	—Incidental finding on routine exam —Symptoms (i.e., palpitations)	—Incidental finding —Symptoms —Screening by the physician (i.e., found on Holter, etc.)	—Syncope —Cardiac arrest
Reasons to Consider Treatment	—To relieve symptoms (if present)	—To relieve symptoms (if present) —To try to reduce the risk of sudden death *(unproven!!!)*	—To reduce the risk of sudden death
Therapeutic Measures	—Identify and treat extracardiac factors or exacerbating causes of PVCs —Reassurance —Anxiolytics —Antiarrhythmic drugs (esp. β-blockers)	—Identify and treat extracardiac factors or exacerbating causes of PVCs —Conventional antiarrhythmic drugs	—Identify and treat extracardiac factors or exacerbating causes of PVCs —Conventional antiarrhythmic drugs —Investigational drugs —PES studies —AICD/surgery

*Adapted from Grauer and Gums (1988) and Hatch and Grauer (1993).

As can be seen from Table 11E-1, presence of *underlying heart disease* (i.e., CAD, heart failure, cardiomyopathy, or valvular heart disease other than mitral valve prolapse) is the criterion that distinguishes benign ventricular arrhythmias from those that are potentially lethal or lethal.

Note also from Table 11E-1 that lethal ventricular arrhythmias are by far the least common form. They are found in less than 5% of patients who have ventricular arrhythmias. Lethal ventricular arrhythmias are distinguished from those that are only "potentially lethal" by the hemodynamic instability (i.e., syncope, cardiac arrest) they produce.

2. **Consider the clinical setting.** *The significance of ventricular arrhythmias depends on the clinical setting in which they occur.* Even if ventricular arrhythmias are exceedingly frequent and complex (including runs of nonsustained ventricular tachycardia), in the absence of underlying heart disease, they tend to be associated with an excellent long-term prognosis. This explains the importance of determining the presence of underlying heart disease in evaluation of patients with ventricular ectopy.

In contrast, in the setting of acute ischemia or infarction, even isolated PVCs (if *new* in onset) may potentially "trigger" malignant ventricular arrhythmias (sustained ventricular tachycardia or ventricular fibrillation). This is the reason for considering treatment and/or prophylaxis with lidocaine for patients with suspected AMI.

3. *Look for possible* **extracardiac factors** *and/or* **exacerbating causes** *of ventricular ectopy (Table 11E-2).* It is far more effective (and safer) to treat ventricular ectopy that is due to one of these causes by measures such as avoidance of stimulants, stress reduction, or medication targeted at the underlying cause of ventricular ectopy (i.e., nitrates or calcium channel blockers for ischemia, diuretics, ACE-inhibitors, or

Table 11E-2

Extracardiac Factors and Exacerbating Causes of Ventricular Arrhythmias*

Extracardiac Factors:
—Stimulants (i.e., caffeine, nicotine, alcohol, diet pills, over-the-counter cough/cold remedies containing sympathomimetics)
—Stress
—Insufficient sleep

Exacerbating Causes:
—Metabolic abnormalities (i.e., hypokalemia, hypomagnesemia)
—Coronary artery disease (i.e., angina pectoris, coronary artery spasm, or silent ischemia)
—Congestive heart failure

*Adapted from Grauer and Gums (1988) and Hatch and Grauer (1993).

digoxin for heart failure, etc.), than to use empiric antiarrhythmic therapy.

In an interesting study by Hallstrom et al (1986) of more than 300 survivors of out-of-hospital cardiac arrest, **smoking** was found to be a strong predictive risk factor for arrhythmia recurrence. The authors speculate that smoking may directly affect myocardial vulnerability to development of ventricular fibrillation in patients with established CAD, and suggest that smoking cessation may offer at least as much protection from sudden death recurrence as many pharmacologic interventions. *Reference to this study may prove helpful in motivating patients with underlying CAD and ventricular arrhythmias to stop smoking.*

4. **Before** *beginning antiarrhythmic therapy,* **be sure you know WHY you want to treat the patient.** There are *only* two reasons to treat patients with ventricular arrhythmias:
   a. *To try to make them* **feel** *better*
   b. *To try to make them* **live** *longer*

These are the *ONLY* two reasons to treat patients with PVCs. It has *never* been shown that patients with *chronic* benign or potentially lethal ventricular arrhythmias can be made to live any longer by treatment with antiarrhythmic drugs. Moreover, antiarrhythmic drugs are expensive, associated with significant adverse effects in a substantial number of patients with long-term use, require close follow-up monitoring, and in 5% to 10% of cases may actually exacerbate the very arrhythmias they are being used to treat (*proarrhythmic* effect).

In view of the above, it would seem that the *ONLY* justifiable reason for considering treatment of patients with benign ventricular arrhythmias is *symptom relief* (that is, **if** the patient has symptoms!). An *empiric* trial of antiarrhythmic therapy *may* be reasonable for selected asymptomatic patients who have potentially lethal ventricular arrhythmias—*BUT only if (and for as long as) the treatment is not worse than the disease.* If at any time treatment *becomes* "worse than the disease" (i.e., if significant adverse effects develop to the drugs used), the balance may then shift in favor of withdrawing antiarrhythmic therapy.

In contrast, patients with lethal ventricular arrhythmias are at extremely high risk of sudden death, and treatment can improve prognosis. The dilemma is in deciding what the optimal treatment course will be for a particular patient.

Finally, it should be emphasized that "all bets are off" in the acute care setting. Patients with acute ischemic heart disease (i.e., angina, AMI) who develop new-onset ventricular ectopy should be treated. Lidocaine is the usual agent of choice in this situation. (*See Section E on the Use of Lidocaine in Chapter 12*).

5. *Remember the meaning of the word* **empiric.** Empiric antiarrhythmic treatment is a *"trial and error" process* without guarantee of success and with the potential for producing undesirable side effects.

Standard monitoring techniques (Holter monitoring and exercise testing) are also somewhat empiric in that their reproducibility for assessing the frequency and severity of ventricular arrhythmias is less than ideal. The situation is complicated further by the tremendous *spontaneous* (or *chance*) variation in PVC frequency and severity (even when baseline conditions remain constant) and the fact that a reduction in ventricular ectopy does *not* necessarily correlate with a reduction in the likelihood of developing a lethal ventricular arrhythmia. Thus, even under the best of possible circumstances of empiric therapy (i.e., good patient tolerance to the drug chosen without significant side effects), it may be extremely difficult by standard monitoring techniques for the clinician to determine if a particular antiarrhythmic agent is truly effective in controlling the arrhythmia, and if such control is truly effective in reducing the risk of sudden death (Grauer, 1993).

6. ***Consider the alternatives.*** As noted above, patients with benign or potentially lethal ventricular arrhythmias do not necessarily benefit from (and may be harmed by) antiarrhythmic therapy. Therefore, such patients need not necessarily be treated.

Similarly, patients who develop primary ventricular fibrillation during the early hours of AMI do not necessarily need (or benefit from) long-term antiarrhythmic therapy as long as their arrhythmias resolved and their hospital course was otherwise uneventful.* Many of these individuals can be managed in a similar manner as other patients who recover from AMI that was not complicated by primary ventricular fibrillation.

In contrast, patients with *lethal ventricular arrhythmias* not associated with AMI comprise a group at extremely high risk of recurrent cardiac arrest. Empiric antiarrhythmic treatment is no longer viewed as an optimal (or even acceptable) alternative approach for the management of such patients (Brooks et al, 1991). Instead, strong consideration should be given to referral of these patients to a center with facilities and an interest in comprehensive evaluation and management of malignant ventricular arrhythmias.

Not only is empiric antiarrhythmic therapy unproven, but it is potentially hazardous. This unfortunate reality was well demonstrated in a 15-year longitudinal study performed by Hallstrom et al (1991) of more than 900 consecutive survivors of out-of-hospital cardiac arrest from ventricular fibrillation that was not associated with AMI. After adjusting for confounding variables, empiric antiarrhythmic treatment (with either quinidine or procainamide) was found to significantly reduce long-term survival. Of interest, empiric treatment with β-blockers in patients able to tolerate these agents improved long-term survival in the study. Thus, it would appear that extreme caution is warranted in the evaluation and management of survivors of out-of-hospital cardiac arrest. Purely empiric treatment with IA antiarrhythmic agents (such as quinidine or procainamide) is not advisable. Consideration may be given to empiric use of oral β-blocker therapy (if there are

no contraindications)—but optimal management probably entails electrophysiologic evaluation with treatment based on the results of such studies.

Our discussion in the remainder of this chapter briefly reviews methods for evaluation and modalities of treatment for patients with **lethal ventricular arrhythmias** that are *not* associated with AMI.

Options for Treatment of Lethal Ventricular Arrhythmias

Programmed electrophysiologic stimulation (PES) studies, surgical techniques (including endocardial electrophysiologic mapping), and implantation of the automatic cardioverter/defibrillator are all excellent modalities for treatment of selected patients with lethal ventricular arrhythmias. They clearly are more sensitive than Holter monitoring for determining the population at highest risk of recurrence from sudden cardiac death (Kim, 1987; Brooks et al, 1991). They are also decidedly more effective than empiric antiarrhythmic therapy in preventing such recurrences, and should be considered for selected patients when possible (Skale et al, 1986). Unfortunately, these procedures are costly, invasive, and require specialized centers with highly skilled personnel for their implementation. As such, they are unfortunately still not accessible to many survivors of out-of-hospital cardiac arrest.

PROGRAMMED ELECTROPHYSIOLOGIC STIMULATION (PES) STUDIES

Perhaps the major difficulty in managing survivors of out-of-hospital cardiac arrest is in determining a suitable endpoint of therapy. For obvious reasons, recurrence of sudden death is not an acceptable endpoint. This is the most important drawback of empiric antiarrhythmic therapy—namely the lack of an objective way to know if (and to what extent) the patient is protected from recurrence of their lethal arrhythmia. Even near total elimination of ventricular ectopy on Holter monitoring is no guarantee of clinical efficacy in preventing recurrent ventricular tachycardia or ventricular fibrillation (Lo and Nguyen, 1987; Morganroth, 1988; Miller and Josephson, 1990).

Use of *programmed electrophysiologic stimulation (PES) studies* may resolve this dilemma by providing a reproducible and objective endpoint for antiarrhythmic therapy. Application of the procedure entails passage of an intravenous electrode catheter into the right ventricle under fluoroscopic guidance, followed by introduction of one or more ventricular extrastimuli at various points in the cardiac cycle. The objective is to try to induce ventricular tachycardia in the laboratory. The ability to reproducibly induce this arrhythmia in this controlled setting appears to be an excellent indicator of which patients are at greatest risk of

---

*As we discuss in Section B of Chapter 12 on Acute Myocardial Infarction, long-term oral β-blocker therapy should be considered for such patients as a fairly well-tolerated form of treatment that may help reduce the risk of sudden death and recurrent infarction.

its spontaneous occurrence (Lo and Nguyen, 1987; Freedman et al, 1988; Miller and Josephson, 1990). For those patients in whom induction of sustained ventricular tachycardia is no longer possible following administration of an antiarrhythmic agent, recurrence of the arrhythmia becomes much less likely when the drug is continued on a long-term basis (Swerdlow et al, 1983; Kim, 1987; Lo and Nguyen, 1987). Partial suppression of arrhythmia inducibility by an antiarrhythmic drug with reduction in the rate of ventricular tachycardia and the degree of symptoms may also improve prognosis (Waller et al, 1987).

PES studies are surprisingly safe, and death is an exceedingly *rare* complication. However, they are invasive, time-consuming, expensive, and not universally available. In addition, they are unsuccessful in finding an effective drug in more than one third of cases (Kim, 1987; Kuchar et al, 1988; Miller and Josephson, 1990). Thus, although they may be extremely helpful in the management of selected patients with lethal ventricular arrhythmias, other modalities of treatment may be needed to achieve optimal control.

SURGERY FOR REFRACTORY VENTRICULAR ARRHYTHMIAS

Surgery has taken on an increasingly important role in the treatment of survivors of out-of-hospital cardiac arrest. Given that coronary artery disease is so common in these individuals, coronary artery bypass grafting (CABG) may control arrhythmias in some of these patients simply by treating the underlying ischemic disease.

Surgical therapy for ventricular arrhythmias is not without risk, and an operative mortality of 10% or more may be expected with most procedures (Ferguson and Cox, 1990; Scheinman, 1990). As a result, refractoriness to medical therapy is the primary indication for surgical treatment of lethal ventricular arrhythmias. Conditions such as ventricular aneurysm or endocardial scarring may be the anatomic substrate for recurrent episodes of ventricular tachycardia. Utilization of intraoperative electrophysiologic mapping may allow precise localization of an arrhythmogenic focus. If such a focus is found, surgical ablation by endocardial resection and/or cryothermia may control the arrhythmias in up to 90% of cases, frequently without the need for additional antiarrhythmic therapy (Miller and Josephson, 1990; Ferguson and Cox, 1990; Scheinman, 1990).

A final surgical option that may be considered is cardiac transplantation. Although viewed as an experimental procedure as recently as a few years ago, significant advances in immunosuppression, patient selection, management of complications, and myocardial preservation have resulted in a dramatic increase in the utilization of the procedure. Availability in donor hearts remains the major factor limiting the number of transplants performed. Success of the operation continues to improve, and most experienced centers now report survival rates at 1 year of between 80% to 100% (Schroeder and Hunt, 1987). Consideration for cardiac transplantation may therefore be a viable option for a small number of selected patients with end-stage cardiomyopathy and life-threatening ventricular arrhythmias refractory to other forms of treatment.

AUTOMATIC IMPLANTABLE DEFIBRILLATOR

Perhaps the most exciting advance in the treatment of patients with lethal ventricular arrhythmias is the ever increasing use of the *automatic implantable defibrillator (AID)*. Since its conception by Mirowski and the first human implantation in 1980, the AID has undergone significant evolution and improvement in design (Mirowski, 1985). The current device consists of a pulse generator that weighs approximately 250 g and is implanted in the abdomen. Two defibrillating electrodes that also serve as sensors are positioned in the superior vena cava and over the apex of the heart. Newer models include a bipolar right ventricular electrode that allows R-wave synchronization and cardioversion (i.e., automatic implantable *cardioverter*-defibrillator or *AICD*). The device has a lifespan of up to 3 years and the capability of delivering 100 to 150 shocks over this time (Manolis et al, 1989).

> Conceptually, the AID functions essentially as a pacemaker. However, instead of sensing bradyarrhythmias and pacing, it senses tachyarrhythmias and cardioverts or defibrillates, depending on the rhythm detected.

Survival rates for patients who have received implantable defibrillators have been truly remarkable. Two-year mortality from sudden death is reduced to less than 10%, compared to the 40% to 50% expected mortality for patients with lethal ventricular arrhythmias who are left untreated (Tchou et al, 1988; Kelly et al, 1988; Manolis et al, 1989; Brooks et al, 1991). Survival rates with the AICD are all the more amazing when one considers the tremendously high risk nature of recipients who have generally been resistant to all other forms of antiarrhythmic therapy. An additional advantage of the device is that it does not significantly affect life-style or impair functional status in most patients, whereas antiarrhythmic drugs often produce undesirable side effects with long-term use (Tchou et al, 1988).

> Patients who receive an AICD are sometimes also continued on antiarrhythmic drugs in an attempt to reduce the number of shocks that the machine must deliver. Ventricular arrhythmias are partially suppressed by medical therapy. Implantation of the AICD provides "backup insurance" for *breakthrough* episodes of ventricular tachycardia or ventricular fibrillation that otherwise would have been fatal. Availability of the AICD also provides backup in case drugs need to be stopped because of toxicity or suspected proarrhythmia.

As of 1989, more than 5,000 units had been implanted worldwide (Manolis et al, 1989). An additional 4,000 units were implanted in 1990 (Brooks et al, 1991). It may be anticipated that use of the device will continue to become even more widespread in the future.

Most recently, extensively programmable devices have been developed that include combinations of antitachycardia pacemakers, bradycardia pacemakers, and defibrillators—*all* in the same implantable unit (Kutalek and Michelson, 1991; Brooks et al, 1991). Sophisticated algorithms capable of identifying and classifying pathologic tachyarrhythmias, and then *individualizing* treatment based on this analysis hold promise of truly revolutionizing the therapeutic approach to patients with lethal ventricular arrhythmias.

References

Bigger JT, Coromilas J: *Identification of patients at risk for arrhythmic death: role of Holter ECG recording.* In Josephson ME, editor: *Sudden cardiac death, cardiovascular clinics, vol 15,* Philadelphia, 1983, FA Davis.

Bigger JT: Antiarrhythmic treatment: an overview, *Am J Cardiol* 53:8B-16B, 1984.

Brooks R, McGovern BA, Garan H, Ruskin JN: Current treatment of patients surviving out-of-hospital cardiac arrest, *JAMA* 265:762-768, 1991.

Cobb LA, Werner JA, Trobaugh GB: Sudden cardiac death, *Mod Conc Cardvivasc Dis* 49:31-36, 1980.

Drory Y, Turetz Y, Hiss Y, Lev B, Fisman EZ, Pines A, Kramer MR: Sudden unexpected death in persons under 40 years of age, *Am J Cardiol* 68:1388-1392, 1991.

Ferguson TB, Cox JL: *Surgical treatment of cardiac arrhythmias.* In Parmley WW, Chatterjee K, editors: *Cardiology,* Philadelphia, 1990, JB Lippincott.

Freedman RA, Swerdlow CD, Soderholm-Difatte V, Mason JW: Prognostic significance of arrhythmia inducibility or noninducibility at initial electrophysiologic study in survivors of cardiac arrest, *Am J Cardiol* 61:578-582, 1988.

Grauer K, Gums J: Ventricular Arrhythmias:
Part I- Prevalence, significance, and indications for treatment, *J Am Bd Fam Prac* 1:135-142, 1988.
Part II- Special concerns in evaluation, *J Am Bd Fam Prac* 1:201-206, 1988.
Part III- Benefits and risks of antiarrhythmic therapy, *J Am Bd Fam Prac* 1:255-266, 1988.
Part IV- New agents, additional treatment modalities, and overall approach to the problem, *J Am Bd Fam Prac* 1:267-273, 1988.

Grauer K: *Holter monitoring.* In Pfenninger JL, editor: *Office procedures for primary care,* St Louis, 1993, Mosby–Year Book.

Hallstrom AP, Cobb LA, Ray R: Smoking as a risk factor for recurrence of sudden cardiac arrest, *N Engl J Med* 314:271-275, 1986.

Hallstrom AP, Cobb LA, Yu BH, Weaver WD, Fahrenbruch CE: An antiarrhythmic drug experience in 941 patients resuscitated from an initial cardiac arrest between 1970 and 1985, *Am J Cardiol* 68:1025-1031, 1991.

Hatch RL, Grauer K: Cardiac arrhythmias. In Taylor R, editor: Family medicine: principles and practice, ed 4, New York, (in press), Springer-Verlag.

Kannel WB, Doyle JT, McNamara PM, Quickenton P, Gordon T: Precursors of sudden coronary death: factors related to incidence of sudden death, *Circulation* 51:606-613, 1975.

Kelly PA, Cannom DS, Garan H, Mirabal GS, Harthorne JW, Hurvitz RJ, Vlahakes GJ, Jacobs ML, Ilvento JP, Buckley MJ, Ruskin JN: The automatic implantable cardioverter-defibrillator: efficacy, complications and survival in patients with malignant ventricular arrhythmias, *J Am Coll Cardiol* 11:1278-1286, 1988.

Kim SG: The management of patients with life-threatening ventricular tachyarrhythmias: programmed stimulation or holter monitoring (either or both?), *Circulation* 76:1-5, 1987.

Kuchar DL, Garan H, Ruskin JN: Electrophysiologic evaluation of antiarrhythmic therapy for ventricular tachyarrhythmias, *Am J Cardiol* 62:39H-45H, 1988.

Kutalek SP, Michelson EL: Cardiac pacing and antiarrhythmic devices: antitachycardia and antifibrillatory devices:
Part I- Arrhythmia detection and antitachyarrhythmia pacing, *Mod Conc Cardiovasc Dis* 60:7-12, 1991.
Part II- Electrical cardioversion and defibrillation, *Mod Conc Cardiovasc Dis* 60:13-18, 1991.

Lo YSA, Nguyen KPV: Electrophysiologic study in the management of cardiac arrest survivors: a critical review, *Am Heart J* 114:596-606, 1987.

Manolis AS, Rastegar H, Estes NAM: Automatic implantable cardioverter defibrillator: current status. *JAMA* 262:1362-1368, 1989.

Miller JM, Josephson ME: Ventricular arrhythmias. In Parmley WW, Chatterjee K, editors: *Cardiology,* Philadelphia, 1990, JB Lippincott.

Mirowski M: The automatic implantable cardioverter-defibrillator: an overview, *J Am Coll Cardiol* 6:461-466, 1985.

Morganroth J: Evaluation of antiarrhythmic therapy using holter monitoring, *Am J Cardiol* 62:18H-23H, 1988.

Myerburg RJ, Kessler KM, Zaman L, Conde CA, Castellanos A: Survivors of prehospital cardiac arrest, *JAMA* 247:1485-1490, 1982.

Ruskin JN, McGovern B, Garan H, DiMarco JP, Kelly E: Antiarrhythmic drugs: a possible cause of out-of-hospital cardiac arrest, *N Engl J Med* 308:1302-1306, 1983.

Safranek DJ, Eisenberg MS, Larsen MP: The epidemology of cardiac arrest in young adults, *Ann Emerg Med* 21:1102-1106, 1992.

Scheinman MM: *Catheter Ablation for Cardiac Arrhythmias.* In Parmley WW, Chatterjee K, editors: *Cardiology,* Philadelphia, 1990, JB Lippincott.

Schroeder JS, Hunt S: Cardiac transplantation: update 1987, *JAMA* 258:3142-3145, 1987.

Skale BT, Miles WM, Hegar JJ, Zipes DP, Prystowsky EN: Survivors of cardiac arrest: prevention of recurrence by drug therapy as predicted by electrophysiologic testing or electrocardiographic monitoring, *Am J Cardiol* 57:113-119, 1986.

Skluth H, Grauer K, Gums J: Ventricular arrhythmias: an assessment of newer therapeutic agents, *Postgrad Med* 85:137-153, 1989.

Swerdlow CD, Winkle RA, Mason JW: Determinants of survival in patients with ventricular tachyarrhythmias, *N Engl J Med* 308:1436-1442, 1983.

Tchou PJ, Kadri N, Anderson J, Caceres JA, Jazayeri M, Akhtar M: Automatic implantable cardioverter defibrillators and survival of patients with left ventricular dysfunction and malignant ventricular arrhythmias, *Ann Int Med* 109:529-534, 1988.

Tofler GH, Stone PH, Muller JE, Rutherford JD, Willich SN, Gustafson NF, Poole WK, Sobel BE, Willerson JT, Robertson T, Passamani E, Braunwald E, and the MILIS Study Group: Prognosis after cardiac arrest due to ventricular tachycardia or ventricular fibrillation associated with acute myocardial infarction (The MILIS study), *Am J Cardiol* 60:755-761, 1987.

Waller TJ, Kay HR, Spielman SR, Kutalek SP, Greenspan AM, Horowitz LN: Reduction in sudden death and total mortality by antiarrhythmic therapy evaluated by electrophysiologic drug testing: criteria of efficacy in patients with sustained ventricular tachyarrhythmia, *J Am Coll Cardiol* 10:83-89, 1987.

Weiss LD, Janasiewicz S, Perper JA, Verdile VP, Yealy DM, Menegazzi JJ: Non-traumatic prehospital sudden death in young patients: an urban EMS experience, *Prehosp Dis Med* 6:315-320, 1991.

CHAPTER 12

ACUTE MYOCARDIAL INFARCTION

INTRODUCTION AND OVERVIEW
APPROACH TO INITIAL EVALUATION:
Use of the History, Initial ECG, and Cardiac Enzymes

The area of emergency cardiac care that has probably undergone the most change since the second edition of our book was published is evaluation and management of acute myocardial infarction. At that time, thrombolytic therapy was just coming into its own. Although still in a continual state of evolution, acute reperfusion with thrombolytic therapy has become firmly established as the standard of care against which other therapeutic measures are compared.

The subject of acute myocardial infarction is sufficiently large to merit development of a book of its own. Limited by space constraints, we restrict our comments here to discussion of issues in evaluation and management that we feel are most relevant to emergency care providers.

Acute management is an especially controversial issue. **No consensus exists.** Protocols vary from state to state, city to city, and hospital to hospital. *Sometimes it seems like they even vary from cardiologist to cardiologist within the same group and practicing in the same hospital!* Moreover, the protocols change from month to month, week to week, *and sometimes even from one day to the next.* In recognition of this tremendous variability in practice tendencies, the American College of Cardiology and American Heart Association have compared their task of developing guidelines for treatment of acute myocardial infarction to "shooting at a moving target" (ACC/AHA Task Force, 1990).

With these thoughts in mind, we present an overview of the subject in this chapter. We have done so by summarizing what is known from our review of the literature and assimilation of the data, and by consolidating this information into a practical clinical approach to each treatment issue. The suggestions that follow admittedly reflect our personal bias. However, our goal in developing this chapter is not that you necessarily agree with each of our viewpoints, but rather to provide a well-referenced framework that will hopefully assist you in developing the most appropriate approach to the problem for your particular clinical setting.

INTRODUCTION

Despite an almost 50% reduction in mortality over the past 25 years, coronary artery disease remains the leading cause of death in the United States today. It accounts for more than 500,000 deaths each year (ACC/AHA Task Force, 1990). Well over 5 million Americans have clinically evident coronary artery disease (ACC/AHA Task Force, 1990). It is likely that a comparable number have clinically undetectable disease (i.e., silent ischemia) that places them at similar risk of cardiac-related morbidity and mortality (Grauer, 1990).

Acute myocardial infarction (AMI) occurs in an estimated 750,000 Americans each year (ACC/AHA Task Force, 1990). Although a majority of patients have an uneventful hospital course and are discharged within 7 to 14 days, the ever-present threat of complications during the early phase of AMI demands constant vigilance and a readiness to intervene at any moment. Examining the role of emergency care providers in evaluation and management of these patients is the purpose of this chapter.

As recently as 1980, the etiology of AMI was unclear. Autopsy studies performed prior to that time often failed to reveal thrombosis at the site of infarction, suggesting a cause other than acute thrombotic occlusion of a coronary artery as the precipitating event. Such autopsy studies were usually performed a day or more after the patient's death (and therefore at least 1 to 2 days after the infarct). Earlier examination of coronary anatomy by cardiac catheterization during the initial hours of acute infarction was virtually unheard of prior to 1980 because of the fear of inducing a potentially lethal complication. DeWood et al (1980) demonstrated that cardiac catheterization is not contraindicated during the early hours of AMI. On the contrary, this procedure is often essential for diagnostic and therapeutic purposes, and it is frequently performed by cardiologists during the initial phase of AMI. As a result of numerous angiographic procedures, it has become clear that sudden thrombotic occlusion of a major coronary artery is in fact the primary cause of AMI in the overwhelming majority of cases.

Catheterization within the first 4 hours of infarction almost always reveals total or near-total (>95%) occlusion of a coronary vessel (DeWood et al, 1980). The reason previous investigators failed to detect this is that spontaneous lysis of clot begins almost immediately. By 12 to 24 hours following an infarct, total occlusion of the infarct-related artery (IRA) is present in only 65% of cases. Unfortunately, the process of myocardial necrosis has usually progressed too far by this time for spontaneous lysis to exert an appreciable beneficial effect on prognosis. Nevertheless, our improved understanding of the pathophysiologic mechanism for acute infarction has provided the impetus for reperfusion therapy which has now become the standard of care.

Prognostic Determinants of Acute MI

OBJECTIVES OF THIS CHAPTER

Practically speaking, the three most important determinants of acute and long-term prognosis in patients with myocardial infarction are: (1) the amount of myocardium damaged by the acute event (and residual left ventricular function); (2) the amount of myocardium at risk of damage from a future event (i.e., the amount of *ischemic* myocardium; and (3) the presence and severity of ventricular arrhythmias. Arrhythmias are most important early in the course, with the incidence of *primary* ventricular fibrillation being many times greater during the first few hours of the infarction than during the rest of the hospital stay (Hancock, 1986). Yet even today, most people fail to seek emergency care as promptly as they should. Delays of several hours ("to see if the chest pain goes away") remain all too common. As a result, primary ventricular fibrillation *prior* to the patient's arrival in the hospital remains the most common cause of death from AMI.

Once in the hospital, intensive care monitoring and antiarrhythmic therapy have virtually eliminated the acute risk of mortality from ventricular arrhythmias. Extent of the infarct now assumes the most important role in determining survival. Simply stated, *the greater the amount of myocardium affected, the less likely it is that adequate hemodynamic function can be maintained—and the higher the mortality.*

As the amount of nonfunctioning myocardium approaches 35% to 40%, the chances of developing pump failure become increasingly greater. Unfortunately, despite advances in virtually all other aspects of management, treatment of cardiogenic shock (once the full-blown syndrome has set in) remains unsatisfactory. Ventricular fibrillation is the usual preterminal event. It is important to appreciate that development of ventricular fibrillation in the setting of cardiogenic shock is the *result* of extensive myocardial damage *(secondary* ventricular fibrillation) rather than a primary reflection of electrical instability

from the infarct itself. *Secondary ventricular fibrillation resulting from cardiogenic shock is rarely amenable to pharmacologic therapy.* In order to reduce mortality from AMI once the patient has reached the hospital, efforts must therefore be directed at limiting infarct size and preserving as much potentially viable myocardium as possible.

The adequacy of left ventricular function depends on the residual amount of functioning myocardium. Because myocardial damage is *cumulative,* prognosis is generally much better after a first infarction than after a second or third infarction. This observation was highlighted in a study by Moss and Benhorin (1990) in which 1-year mortality following a first infarction was 6.2%, compared to a 13.0% 1-year mortality in patients with at least one previous infarction. As a result, special attention should be focused on the estimated 60% to 80% of patients with AMI who are having their first infarction. Hospital management is less likely to be complicated in this group (because of the greater likelihood that left ventricular function will be preserved). After discharge, extra efforts can then be directed at *secondary prevention* including risk factor modification, use of aspirin and treatment with a β-blocker or calcium channel blocker (as appropriate). Special attention should also be directed at assessing the amount of myocardium that is still at risk after AMI. The extent of myocardial ischemia assumes major importance as a prognostic indicator in the immediate post-infarction period, and the weeks and months that follow shortly thereafter.

The potential treatment measures for AMI that we cover in this chapter are shown in *Table 12A-1.* In addition to discussion of **Standard Treatment Measures** (our focus in Section B of this chapter), **Antiarrhythmic Therapy** (our focus in Sections B and E of this chapter, as well as in Section E in Chapter 11 on Sudden Cardiac Death), and **Reperfusion/Interventional Therapy** (our focus in

Table 12A-1

Potential Treatment Measures for AMI
Standard Treatment Measures -Pain control (i.e., use of morphine sulfate) -Oxygenation -Pharmacologic therapy (nitrates, β-blockers, calcium channel blockers)
Antiarrhythmic Therapy -Use of lidocaine, procainamide, β-blockers, or other agents
Reperfusion Therapy -Antiplatelet agents (i.e., aspirin) -Heparin anticoagulation -Thrombolytic therapy (i.e., tPA, streptokinase, APSAC, or other agents)
Interventional Therapy -Angioplasty -Acute bypass surgery

Section C of this chapter), we'll also address **Special Treatment Considerations** (such as autonomic nervous system dysfunction, clinical significance of the AV blocks in AMI, unstable angina, right ventricular infarction, etc.) in Section D. In an attempt to consolidate the material covered and place it into a practical, clinical perspective, we conclude this chapter in Section F with an **Illustrative Case Study on the Evaluation and Management of AMI.** Before delving into these treatment issues, however, we feel it important to first emphasize a number of practical considerations in the diagnosis of patients with suspected acute infarction.

Evaluation of Patients with Suspected Acute Infarction

PITFALLS IN DIAGNOSIS OF AMI

Because of the high risk of potentially lethal ventricular arrhythmias during the early hours of acute infarction, accurate diagnosis with close observation in a protective environment and treatment when appropriate is the essential first step toward minimizing mortality. Several points merit the special attention of the emergency care provider entrusted with making the diagnosis of AMI:

1. Presenting symptoms of AMI may be atypical or totally absent.
2. The initial ECG of patients with AMI is often nondiagnostic, and may be entirely normal.
3. Despite their drawbacks, *the history, physical examination, and the initial ECG remain the most important evaluative parameters* for making the decision of whether to admit a patient with acute chest pain to the hospital.

The importance of emphasizing pitfalls in recognition of AMI is the clinical reality that this diagnosis is still missed in practice by emergency care providers. Insight into the frequency that this diagnosis is missed was provided in a study by Lee et al (1987) of over 3,000 patients who presented with a complaint of chest pain to an ED. Less than 15% of these patients developed AMI, underscoring the finding of other studies that most patients who present to an ED with chest pain will *not* be infarcting. Of the 447 patients who did develop AMI in this study, the diagnosis was missed in approximately 1% of cases. Of particular concern was the finding that 26% of those patients who were inappropriately discharged from the ED (in whom the diagnosis was missed) died within 72 hours. This was more than *double* the mortality of patients with AMI who were admitted to the hospital. Thus, although the overall *rate* of missed diagnosis was relatively low (approximately 1%), potential clinical implications of missing the diagnosis were severe. Perhaps the most important take-home message of the study, however, was the finding that almost

half of those infarctions that were missed could have been recognized by improved ECG interpretation skills (and more careful comparison of acute tracings to previous ECGs), and/or paying more attention to the patients' historical account of their chest pain.

ATYPICAL (OR ABSENT) PRESENTING SYMPTOMS

There is little question that the previously healthy middle-aged individual with cardiac risk factors who complains of the sudden onset of severe substernal chest pain radiating up to the neck and down the left arm needs immediate admission to the coronary care unit. All too often, however, the history is much less typical. For example, patients with inferior (diaphragmatic) infarction may present with only epigastric discomfort or seemingly mild signs of gastrointestinal upset. Not infrequently, these symptoms are partially or even totally relieved by belching or a "GI cocktail." In other instances, a purely referred pattern of pain may be noted. Thus the patient may describe pain isolated to either arm, either shoulder blade, the neck and/or jaw *without* the slightest indication of chest discomfort. At least 25% of the time, AMI is entirely "silent" or only associated with vague symptoms (such as malaise or myalgias) that are *not at all* suggestive of ischemic heart disease (Margolis et al, 1973; Van der Does et al, 1980; Zarling et al, 1983, Kannel et al, 1984; Yano et al, 1989). The absence of typical cardiac chest pain is particularly likely to occur in patients with diabetes mellitus (due to decreased pain sensation from neuropathy) and in the elderly (Solomon et al, 1989; Niakan et al, 1986). In the latter group, a change in mental status (i.e., confusion or disorientation), an arrhythmia, dizziness, syncope, stroke, dyspnea, or the insidious development of congestive heart failure may be the only clue to AMI. It is of interest that long-term prognosis of patients with such silent (or otherwise unrecognized) infarctions is at least as serious as for patients with AMI and typical chest pain (Kannel et al, 1984; Yano et al, 1989).

The incidence of silent AMI appears to increase progressively with increasing age. In a study by Muller et al (1990) of elderly patients with AMI, 29% of study subjects between the age of 65 to 74 years old had a silent infarction (i.e., AMI *without* any chest pain). The percentage of elderly individuals with silent infarction increased to 50% for those between 75 to 85 years of age, and up to 75% for those over 85 years of age! Awareness of the surprisingly high prevalence of silent infarction in the elderly is especially important in view of the much greater mortality associated with AMI in older patients (Rich et al, 1992). Clinically, appreciation of the fact that the most common presenting symptom of painless AMI in an elderly population is *shortness of breath* (with or without associated congestive heart failure) may help greatly to improve our ability to recognize AMI in this age group (Aronow, 1989; Muller et al, 1990).

At the other end of the spectrum, one should not forget about the *possibility* of AMI in younger individuals (in their 20s or 30s!). This consideration becomes especially important for young adults who may be abusers of cocaine.

> Because cocaine blocks central reuptake of the neurotransmitters dopamine and norepinephrine, abuse of this drug typically produces excessive adrenergic discharge with sympathetic activation. This commonly results in tachycardia, hypertension, and arterial vasoconstriction. The latter effect may occasionally be sufficiently intense to induce coronary artery spasm and/or AMI (especially of the non-Q-wave type) in young adults with previously normal coronary arteries (Kossowsky et al, 1989).

Young adults who present to the ED with a history of new-onset chest pain *must* therefore be taken seriously (and have an ECG ordered)—*especially* when the possibility of cocaine abuse exists.

THE ROLE OF THE INITIAL ECG

The importance of the initial ECG in evaluation of patients with suspected acute infarction cannot be overemphasized (Grauer, 1992a). In addition to its diagnostic utility, the initial ECG provides prognostic information and is one of the major determinants of a patient's suitability for thrombolytic therapy.

Patients likely to benefit most from thrombolytic therapy are those who are treated early and those who have larger infarctions (Bar et al, 1987). The initial ECG is extremely helpful in identifying such patients *(Table 12A-2)*. In general, anterior infarctions are larger than inferior or isolated lateral infarctions. Patients with marked ST segment elevation in multiple leads, especially when accompanied by marked ST segment depression (i.e., reciprocal

Table 12A-2

AMI Patients Likely to Benefit Most from Thrombolytic Therapy
• **Patients Treated Early in the Course of AMI** *(especially within the first 2 to 4 hours of infarction)*
• **Patients with Evidence of Larger Infarction as Suggested by the Initial ECG:**

MORE BENEFIT:	LESS BENEFIT:
-Anterior AMI	-Inferior or lateral AMI
-Marked ST elevation	-Minimal ST segment changes
-Marked reciprocal ST depression	
-No Q waves (or small q waves)	-Large Q waves already present

(Adapted from Bar et al, 1987)

changes) in multiple leads are more likely to have larger infarctions than patients with only minimal ST segment changes (although admittedly the degree of ST segment change also depends on when in the course of infarction the ECG was obtained). Finally, the presence and relative size of Q waves at the time of the initial ECG provides a rough indication of the extent of myocardial damage. It is important to emphasize, however, that early development of Q waves does *not* necessarily indicate definite necrosis (i.e., irreversibly damaged myocardium), since extensive ischemia may occasionally produce Q waves due to transient conduction delay in the ischemic zone of the infarct (Bar et al, 1987). Even when Q waves do reflect myocardial necrosis, this does not rule out the potential for benefit from thrombolytic therapy. It simply implies that the amount of benefit from thrombolytic therapy is likely to be less than if Q waves were absent on the initial ECG, or if Q waves were extremely small.

> Inferior infarctions account for nearly half of all cases of AMI. Although they are generally thought to be smaller in size and associated with a better prognosis than anterior infarctions, this is not always the case. Complete AV block develops in more than 10% of patients with acute inferior infarction, and is associated with a surprisingly high in-hospital mortality of at least 20% (Berger and Ryan, 1990: Clemmensen et al, 1991). Other patients with acute inferior infarction believed to have more extensive infarction and consequently a poorer prognosis include those with ST segment depression in the anterior precordial leads (suggesting acute posterior involvement and/or concommitant anterior ischemia) and those with evidence of associated right ventricular infarction (Berger and Ryan, 1990). These high-risk subgroups may prove to be excellent candidates for consideration of thrombolytic therapy (with much to benefit) *despite* the inferior location of their infarction.

Important prognostic information is provided by the initial ECG. The finding of an *unremarkable* initial ECG (either a normal tracing, one with only minor nonspecific ST-T wave abnormalities, or one without significant change from previous tracings) at the time of admission in patients with AMI is a strong predictor of a relatively benign hospital course (Brush et al, 1985; Lee et al, 1985; Slater et al, 1987). In contrast, the presence of acute ST segment changes (either ST segment elevation or depression), diagnostic Q waves, or an intraventricular conduction defect on the initial ECG is associated with a fairly high incidence of complications. Other factors predictive of a high-risk hospital course include ongoing chest pain at the time of admission, pulmonary rales, persistent sinus tachycardia, and/or PVCs on the initial 12-lead ECG (Fuchs and Scheidt, 1981; Crimm et al, 1984). Surveillance in a coronary care unit is usually preferable for individuals with any of these findings. In their absence and when the initial ECG is unremarkable, observation in a step-down (telemetry) unit is a reasonable course of action for those patients in whom the history dictates the need for hospital admission.

Finally, the initial ECG may be helpful in suggesting that the patient had a prior myocardial infarction. As we have already noted, early mortality with AMI is almost doubled in patients with a history of prior infarction (Moss and Benhorin, 1990).

DRAWBACKS OF THE INITIAL ECG

It is important to appreciate that the initial ECG of a patient with AMI may fail to reveal findings suggestive of the diagnosis. There are a number of reasons for this (Grauer and Curry, 1992; Grauer, 1992b):

1. A lag time of hours (or even days) may exist before diagnostic electrocardiographic changes become evident.
2. Changes may be subtle (i.e., nonspecific ST-T wave abnormalities, loss of R wave amplitude, development of seemingly "insignificant" q waves).
3. The ECG may be one of *transition* (obtained at a time when ST segments have returned to the baseline just after the period of ST segment elevation and just before the period of T wave inversion).
4. ECG changes of AMI may be obscured by a *competitive* condition (bundle branch block, left or right ventricular hypertrophy, pulmonary disease pattern, early repolarization, electrolyte disorders, Wolff-Parkinson-White syndrome) or by previous infarction.
5. A previous ECG may not be available for comparison.
6. The infarction may be taking place in an "electrically silent" area of the heart (the apex, right ventricle, or posterobasal portion of the left ventricle).

The initial ECG is most helpful in diagnosis when it is clearly abnormal. The absence of diagnostic changes, however, in no way rules out the possibility of acute infarction. In such instances, history becomes the pivotal factor for deciding whether to admit the patient to the hospital. Considering the potential for life-threatening arrhythmias during the early hours of infarction, it is usually wiser to err on the side of caution (and admit the patient to the hospital) if there is any doubt about the diagnosis.

> Echocardiography has been advocated by some as an alternative diagnostic study for evaluating patients with new-onset chest pain but no evidence of AMI or ischemia on their initial ECG. While this test has a high sensitivity for detection of AMI (of up to 90%), its specificity is disappointing (50% or less) due to the difficulty distinguishing between the regional asynergy of chronic coronary artery disease and AMI (Peels et al, 1990). Moreover, inclusion of echocardiography as an emergent diagnostic modality for patients with new-onset chest pain would not only require adequate echocardiographic facilities, but round-the-clock availability of echocardiographic technicians to perform the test as well as skilled interpreters ready to render an immediate reading. Most hospitals in the country do *not* offer this availability at the present time.
> After the decision to admit the patient to the hospital has

been made, however, echocardiography may prove invaluable in evaluation of selected patients with AMI by providing a noninvasive measure of left ventricular function and allowing detection of complications (such as right ventricular infarction, ventricular septal defect, acute valvular regurgitation, aortic dissection, pericarditis, pericardial effusion, aneurysm formation, the presence of mural thrombi, etc.) that might otherwise be exceedingly difficult to identify (Popp, 1990). Early recognition of such complications may be extremely important in view of the ever increasing use of thrombolytic therapy.

THE ROLE OF CARDIAC ENZYMES

The occurrence of AMI is characteristically accompanied by elevations in serum concentrations of cardiac enzymes. In general, the larger the infarct, the greater the rise in cardiac enzymes. The earliest change is usually noted with CK* (creatine kinase), which begins to rise within 3 to 6 hours of the onset of AMI, peaks at 10 to 18 hours, and returns to normal by 3 to 4 days. LD† (lactic dehydrogenase) rises later (usually by 24 to 48 hours), peaks in 3 to 6 days, and then gradually returns to normal over 8 to 14 days.

Unfortunately, CK elevations may be significantly delayed and not show any increase at the time of presentation. In addition, numerous other conditions may falsely elevate cardiac enzymes, including skeletal muscle injury from trauma or injection, prolonged immobility (as may be seen in victims of drug overdose or incapacitated elderly patients), primary liver disease, hepatic congestion (from congestive heart failure), shock, seizures, myocarditis, pulmonary embolism, hypothyroidism, hemolysis, anemia, certain neoplasms, and electrical countershock. Differentiation of these conditions from AMI can usually be made reliably by obtaining cardiac isoenzyme studies. However, because such determinations may require 1 to 2 days to be processed, they are generally of little assistance to the emergency care provider faced with making the "on-the-spot" decision of whether to admit a patient with chest pain to the hospital. Moreover, since the time course for elevation of cardiac isoenzymes is similar to that for the standard studies, falsely negative (normal) readings may be obtained if blood is sampled too early.

Our feeling is that standard cardiac enzyme studies (CK and LD) should *not* play any role in making the decision of whether to admit a patient with chest pain to the hospital. Normal studies provide a false sense of security (since they in no way rule out infarction), while abnormal studies may be due to any of the causes listed above. History, physical examination, and the initial ECG should be the principal parameters assessed in the emergency department (Seager, 1980; Lee et al, 1985; Nowakowski, 1986, Grauer, 1992b; Grauer and Curry, 1992). If these do not confidently exclude the possibility of an acute ischemic

---

*CK was formerly designated CPK (creatine phosphokinase).
†LD was formerly designated LDH.

event (AMI, unstable angina), the patient should be admitted to the hospital (at least to a telemetry unit). It is at this point that cardiac enzymes (and isoenzymes) become invaluable in confirming AMI and in providing a rough estimation of infarct size.

LD isoenzymes need *not* be routinely obtained on all patients. As already noted, LD levels often do not rise until 24 to 48 hours in the course of AMI. In contrast, CK levels are almost always elevated early in the course of AMI. Thus, LD enzymes and isoenzymes need not be drawn in patients presenting within the first few hours of the onset of symptoms. If serial ECGs and CK values are normal in such individuals, acute infarction has not occurred. On the other hand, LD isoenzymes may prove *invaluable* for evaluation of patients who delay seeking medical attention for 1 or more days in whom ECG and CK studies may no longer be diagnostic.

Many of the topics covered in the rest of this chapter are discussed in detail elsewhere in Volume I and Volume II of this book. Consequently, we limit our comments here to aspects of care most relevant to evaluation and management of AMI, and refer the reader to those sections where more material may be found.

References

American College of Cardiology/American Heart Association Task Force: Guidelines for the early management of patients with acute myocardial infarction, *Circulation* 82:664-707, 1990.

Aronow WS: New coronary events at four-year follow-up in elderly patients with recognized or unrecognized myocardial infarction, *Am J Cardiol* 63:621-622, 1989.

Bar FW, Vermeer F, De Zwaan C, Ramentol M, Braat S, Simoons ML, Hermens WT, Van Der Laarse A, Verheugt FWA, Krauss XH, Wellens HJJ: Value of admission electrocardiogram in predicting outcome of thrombolytic therapy in acute myocardial infarction: a randomized trial conducted by the Netherlands Interuniversity Cardiology Institute, *Am J Cardiol* 59:6-13, 1987.

Berger PB, Ryan TJ: Inferior myocardial infarction: high-risk subgroups, *Circulation* 81:401-411, 1990.

Brush JE, Brand DA, Acampora D, Chalmer B, Wackers FJ: Use of the initial electrocardiogram to predict in-hospital complications of acute myocardial infarction, *N Engl J Med* 312:1137-1141, 1985.

Clemmensen P, Bates ER, Califf RM, Hlatky MA, Aronson L, George BS, Lee KL, Kereiakes DJ, Gacioch G, Berrios E, Topol EJ, and the TAMI Study Group: Complete atrioventricular block complicating inferior wall acute myocardial infarction treated with reperfusion therapy, *Am J Cardiol* 67:225-230, 1991.

Crimm A, Severance HW, Coffey K, McKinnis R, Wagner GS, Califf RM: Prognostic significance of isolated sinus tachycardia during first three days of acute myocardial infarction, *Am J Med* 76:983-988, 1984.

DeWood MA, Spores J, Notske R, Mouser LT, Burroughs R, Golden MS, Lang LT: Prevalence of total coronary occlusion during the early hours of transmural myocardial infarction, *N Engl J Med* 303:897-902, 1980.

Fesmire FM, Percy RF, Wears RL, MacMath TL: Initial ECG in Q wave and non-Q-wave myocardial infarction, *Ann Emerg Med* 18:741-746, 1989.

Fuchs R, Scheidt S: Improved criteria for admission to cardiac care units, *JAMA* 246:2037-2041, 1981.

Grauer K: Silent myocardial ischemia: dilemma or blessing? *Am Fam Phys* 42(suppl):13S-28S, 1990.

Grauer K: Expanding applications of the 12-lead ECG in suspected acute infarction, *Am Fam Phys* (suppl): 46:55S-76S, 1992a.

Grauer K: A practical guide to ECG interpretation, St Louis, 1992b, Mosby–Year Book.

Grauer K, Curry RW: Clinical electrocardiography: a primary care approach, ed 2, Cambridge, Mass, 1992, Blackwell Scientific.

Hancock EW: Ischemic heart disease: acute myocardial infarction. In Rubenstein E, Federman DD (eds): New York, 1986, Scientific American Medicine.

Kannel WB, Abbott RD: Incidence and prognosis of unrecognized myocardial infarction: an update on the Framingham study, *N Engl J Med* 311:1144-1147, 1984.

Kossowsky WA, Lyon AF, Chou SY: Acute non-Q wave cocaine related myocardial infarction, *Chest* 96:617-621, 1989.

Lee TH, Cook F, Weisberg M, Sargent RK, Wilson C, Goldman L: Acute chest pain in the emergency room: identification and examination of low-risk patients, *Arch Intern Med* 145:65-69, 1985.

Lee TH, Rouan GW, Weisberg HC, Brand DA, Acahpora D, Stasiulewicz C, Walshon J, Terranoua G, Gottlieb L, Goldstein WB: Clinical characteristics and natural history of patients with acute myocardial infarction sent home from the emergency room, *Am J Cardiol* 60:219-224, 1987.

Margolis JR, Kannel WS, Feinleib M, Dawbaer TR, McNamara PM: Clinical features of unrecognized myocardial infarction—silent and symptomatic: eighteen year follow-up: the Framingham Study, *Am J Cardiol* 32:1-7, 1973.

Moss AJ, Benhorin J: Prognosis and management after a first myocardial infarction, *N Engl J Med* 322:743-753, 1990.

Muller RT, Gould LA, Betzu R, Vacek T, Pradeep V: Painless myocardial infarction in the elderly, *Am Heart J* 119:202-204, 1990.

Niakan E, Harati Y, Rolak LA, Comstock JP, Rokey R: Silent myocardial infarction and diabetic cardiovascular autonomic neuropathy, *Arch Intern Med* 146:2229-2230, 1986.

Nowakowski JF: Use of cardiac enzymes in the evaluation of acute chest pain, *Ann Emerg Med* 15:354-360, 1986.

Peels CH, Visser CA, Kupper AJ, Visser FC, Roos JP: Two-dimensional echocardiography for immediate detection of myocardial ischemia in the emergency room, *Am J Cardiol* 65:687-691, 1990.

Popp RL: Echocardiography, *N Engl J Med* 323:165-172, 1990.

Rich MW et al: Is age an independent predictor of early and late mortality in patients with acute myocardial infarction? *Am J Med* 92:7-13, 1992.

Seager SB: Cardiac enzymes in the evaluation of chest pain, *Ann Emerg Med* 9:346-349, 1980.

Slater DK, Hlatky MA, Mark DB, Harrell FE, Pryor DB, Califf RM: Outcome in suspected acute myocardial infarction with normal or minimally abnormal admission electrocardiographic findings, *Am J Cardiol* 60:766-770, 1987.

Solomon CG et al: Comparisons of clinical presentation of acute myocardial infarction in patients older than 65 years of age to younger patients: the multicenter chest pain study experience, *Am J Cardiol* 63:772-776, 1989.

Van der Does E, Lubsen J, Pool J: Acute myocardial infarction: an easy diagnosis in general practice? *J Royal Col Gen Prac* 30:405-409, 1980.

Yano K, MacLean CJ: The incidence and prognosis of unrecognized myocardial infarction in the Honolulu, Hawaii heart program, *Arch Intern Med* 149:1528-1532, 1989.

Zarling EJ, Sexton H, Milnor P: Failure to diagnose acute myocardial infarction: the clinicopathologic experience at a large community hospital, *JAMA* 250:1177-1181, 1983.

SECTION B

STANDARD TREATMENT MEASURES AND ANTIARRHYTHMIC THERAPY

Interpreting the Literature: The Pros and Cons of Meta-Analysis

By necessity, recommendations for management of AMI cannot be rigid. There are simply too many variables and viewpoints to allow a uniform approach that would be suitable for all patients. Unfortunately, help from the literature is not always forthcoming. This is because many treatments and interventions in cardiovascular disease demonstrate only modest (i.e., 15% to 25%) statistical improvement on clinical outcomes as important as mortality or myocardial infarction (Yusuf et al, 1988). The difficulty in confirming treatment efficacy with such modest clinical benefits results from the fact that *hundreds* of study subjects will usually be needed to demonstrate a statistically significant positive response to therapy. Sufficiently large trials performed in a single study center are hard to come by. Smaller trials (of 100 to 200 subjects or less) are much more prevalent, but may be misleading, as their sample size is often too small to detect a less than 25% reduction in mortality that would have easily achieved statistical significance in a larger study (Yusuf et al, 1988).

Another problem is the potential for small trials to "build in" selection bias. Imagine, for example, that 10 small trials are performed on a brand new drug. Imagine that 6 of the 10 studies show no benefit from the drug, and that 3 of the studies even suggest an adverse outcome! The 10th study demonstrates a 20% reduction in mortality. Which of the 10 studies is most likely to be written up and submitted to a journal? to be accepted for publication? *(Would you expect investigators from each of the 9 trials that failed to show a favorable outcome to even submit their manuscripts for review?)* Given that 3 of the studies demonstrated an *adverse* outcome, it could be that the overall effect of the drug in question was actually *detrimental* (and carried an unfavorable risk-benefit profile) *despite the possibility that the single small trial with positive results might be the ONLY one published!* While this scenario is purely hypothetical, it highlights the risk inherent in readily accepting (and potentially altering practice patterns) from positive results obtained from a single small trial.

In an attempt to address the problem posed by uncertain (and sometimes contradictory) results from multiple smaller trials, the technique of **meta-analysis** was developed. With this technique, clinical investigators meticulously review the literature in a search for all relevant trials on a particular treatment issue. Data is then *pooled*, allowing extremely large numbers (in the *thousands*) of study subjects to be included in the analysis. By pooling data in this manner, meaningful (and statistically significant) conclusions can sometimes be reached that were not at all evident from individual analysis of any of the smaller trials.

The technique of meta-analysis is not without problems. Inclusion and exclusion criteria often differ substantially from one trial to the next because of different study sites (which are sometimes in different countries!), protocols, and patient characteristics. As a result, it is probably best to adopt a conservative approach to interpreting data from pooled trials, accepting conclusions *only* when results are dramatic. Despite this drawback, use of the meta-analysis technique has been instrumental in providing much of the documentation for supporting the scientific rationale for many of our standard treatments for cardiovascular disease.

Specific Treatment Issues

In the sections that follow we review what is known from the literature on specific treatment issues for management of AMI. Reference is made to the findings of large meta-analysis trials when appropriate. We attempt to incorporate this information into a practical, clinical approach to the patient with suspected acute infarction, and then conclude the chapter by working through a case study in Section F.

OXYGEN THERAPY

The most basic treatment recommendation for AMI regards oxygen therapy. Provision of supplemental oxygen by nasal cannula (at 2 to 4 L/min) is routinely recommended for all patients with suspected infarction (ACC/AHA Task Force, 1990). Although such treatment probably has little effect on the arterial oxygen content of otherwise normal individuals, it may significantly improve oxygenation of an ischemic myocardium in the patient with hypoxemia from pulmonary congestion. Even in the absence of pulmonary congestion or other complications, it seems that some patients do develop modest hypoxemia early during the course of AMI (ACC/AHA Task Force, 1990). The mechanism of this hypoxemia is not entirely clear, but it probably relates to a relative ventilation-perfusion mismatch (Fillmore et al, 1970). As a result, supplemental oxygen should never be withheld in the initial treatment of patients suspected of having acute infarction. Retention of CO_2 will not be a problem in the acutely ill patient who is being closely monitored, so that it will be safe to administer supplemental oxygen even to patients with severe chronic obstructive pulmonary disease.

PAIN RELIEF

Angiographic studies have demonstrated that relief of chest pain often accompanies restoration of flow (i.e., reperfusion) to an acutely occluded coronary artery. This clinical observation strongly supports the concept that the chest pain of AMI at least partially reflects *ongoing ischemia* in potentially viable myocardium, rather than simply being the end result of completed myocardial necrosis (ACC/AHA Task Force, 1990). It also supports the rationale for choosing anti-ischemic therapy to treat such chest pain, and for making a concerted effort to render the patient completely pain free as soon as possible.

It follows that failure to completely relieve ischemic chest pain suggests that potentially viable myocardial tissue remains at risk of necrosis. Continued chest pain may also result in tachycardia and further release of endogenous catecholamines. This in turn may increase cardiac work and the oxygen demand on an already ischemic myocardium. A faster heart rate causes disproportionate shortening of the diastolic interval (during which the coronary arteries are perfused), ultimately compromising blood flow even more. Thus a vicious cycle is set up where ischemic chest pain engenders physiologic changes that result in more chest pain. All of these effects may be aggravated when chest pain is accompanied by a significant *anxiety* component.

In view of the above pathophysiologic considerations, one may select from among four types of medication to treat the chest pain of acute ischemic heart disease. Synergism is obtained from using several of these agents at the same time, and this is the approach most commonly followed:

1. Analgesic agents (i.e., morphine)
2. Anti-ischemic agents (i.e., nitroglycerin, β-blockers, calcium channel blockers)
3. Thrombolytic agents (i.e., tPA, streptokinase, APSAC, or others)
4. Anxiolytic agents (i.e., diazepam or other benzodiazepines)

> The persistence of chest pain in patients with suspected AMI has definite prognostic significance. In a study by Fesmire and Wears (1989), the incidence of life-threatening complications was increased almost *fourfold* in patients whose chest pain persisted until (or recurred during) the initial ED evaluation compared to patients with suspected AMI whose chest pain had resolved prior to arrival in the ED. *Chest pain associated with acute ischemic heart disease should always be treated (and relieved) as soon as possible.*

MORPHINE SULFATE

Morphine sulfate is a potent analgesic agent that also allays anxiety and exerts beneficial hemodynamic effects in the patient with pulmonary congestion. By increasing venous capacitance and inducing mild arterial vasodilatation, the drug reduces *both* preload and afterload and thus improves cardiac performance. In addition, circulating catecholamines are reduced (decreasing the tendency toward arrhythmias) as a result of the drug's analgesic and anti-anxiety effect.

Morphine may be administered in 2- to 5- mg IV increments every 5 to 30 minutes according to the patient's symptoms and clinical response. Although excessive use of the drug may result in bradycardia, hypotension, oversedation, nausea, or respiratory depression, these undesirable effects can usually be avoided by cautious dosing. Respiratory depression can be reversed with 0.4 mg of naloxone (Narcan), while vagotonic actions are easily treated in most instances by placing the patient in Trendelenburg position, fluid infusion and/or 0.5 to 1 mg of IV atropine sulfate *(see Chapter 2).*

Despite the trend in recent years to use less morphine than in the past, it should be emphasized that this drug is easy to titrate, generally safe, and extremely effective in relieving the chest pain associated with AMI. It should be strongly considered for use in this situation, especially if chest pain fails to resolve with other measures (i.e., anti-ischemic, thrombolytic, or anxiolytic agents).

> Some clinicians choose to withhold morphine from patients with acute infarction who are treated with thrombolytic therapy because they feel it may "mask" the principal clinical sign of reperfusion (relief of chest pain). Considering the potential adverse pathophysiologic effects that continued chest pain may have on an ischemic myocardium, this practice is not advised (ACC/AHA Task Force, 1990). *Chest pain associated with acute infarction should always be treated (and relieved) as soon as possible.*

> Clinically, it is sometimes difficult to judge the efficacy of analgesic measures in relieving chest pain. Verbal responses from problematic patients (i.e., stoic individuals or those with a strong element of denial) are particularly hard to interpret. Asking the patient to grade chest pain *severity* on a **10 point number scale** (where 0 reflects no pain, and 10 reflects maximal pain severity) often resolves the difficulty. Even though stoic individuals and those with denial will still tend to downgrade the severity of their chest pain, it will usually be possible to determine whether chest pain is still present (and if so, whether it is improving) from their response on the number scale.

NITROGLYCERIN

Nitroglycerin has resurfaced as a treatment of choice for relief of the chest pain associated with AMI. Although its predominant action is to increase venous capacitance (decrease preload), nitroglycerin also reduces afterload by arteriolar vasodilatation and improves coronary artery blood flow by a direct vasodilatory effect on epicardial coronary vessels. Thus the drug offers the distinct clinical advantage of *relieving ischemic chest pain by treating its cause.*

> Nitroglycerin produces a series of favorable hemodynamic effects in the setting of AMI, especially in patients with pulmonary congestion. The reduction in preload decreases left ventricular end-diastolic pressure, which in turn lowers pulmonary venous pressure (and alleviates pulmonary congestion). Another benefit resulting from the reduction in *left ventricular end-diastoic pressure* is improved perfusion of the subendocardium and improved collateral flow, effects that may limit the size of the peri-infarction ischemic zone.* Improved myocardial perfusion enhances contractility, leading to an increase in cardiac output.
>
> In contrast, the potent vasodilator (and afterload reducer) nitroprusside does not favor blood flow to the subendocardium and peri-infarction ischemic zone, which is why it is much more likely than nitroglycerin to produce coronary "steal."

Meta-analysis on more than 2,000 patients involved in trials on the use of IV nitroglycerin in AMI suggest at least a trend toward decreased mortality (Yusuf et al, 1988). The drug seems to work best when given *early* in the course of AMI to patients with moderate-to-large size infarctions. As a result, many clinicians favor *prophylactic* use of IV nitroglycerin (i.e., use in patients with AMI even in the *absence* of chest pain) in an attempt to limit infarct size.

Two additional indications for nitroglycerin in the setting of AMI are associated hypertension and heart failure / pulmonary edema *(Table 12B-1).* A distinct advantage of the drug is that an IV infusion can usually be administered and titrated to optimal clinical effect *without* the need for invasive hemodynamic monitoring as long as the patient is closely observed. Should marked hypertension persist despite use of IV nitroglycerin at appropriate doses, Swan-Ganz monitoring, IV β-blockers, and/or sodium nitroprusside may be needed.

> Nitroglycerin can be administered in variety of ways. Sublingual or spray forms are rapid in onset (within 2 to 5 min),

---

*The **subendocardial** area of the heart is especially susceptible to ischemia. This is because the vascular supply of the subendocardial area (which arises from *epicardial* coronary vessels) must perfuse a relatively long distance (through ventricular myocardium) until it finally arrives at the endocardial layer. Patients with congestive heart failure and/or ischemia commonly manifest an elevated end-diastolic pressure. This further impedes subendocardial blood flow by a mechanical effect due to the increased resistance to flow produced by this elevated end-diastolic pressure (i.e., increased "back pressure" that opposes the *gradient* to blood flow from epicardial vessels to the deep subendocardial layer).

and are usually tried first (often by the patient) at the onset of chest pain. Although it may be reasonable to follow this with topical administration (with nitroglycerin paste or ointment) in patients who are only mildly symptomatic, the persistence of severe chest pain beyond several minutes in a patient with suspected AMI should be viewed as an indication for starting an IV infusion of the drug. Doing so allows moment-to-moment dose titration and provides the best opportunity for rapid and complete pain relief as well as hemodynamic control.* *Failure to respond to sublingual, spray forms, or topical nitroglycerin is NOT predictive of the subsequent response to IV nitroglyercerin!*

The recommended starting dose of IV nitroglycerin is in the range of 10 μg/min. The infusion rate may be gradually increased every few minutes until chest pain is controlled, provided that the patient does not become hypotensive (i.e., systolic blood pressure should not drop below 90 mm Hg). Although there is no absolute upper dosage limit, infusion rates should generally not exceed 200 μg/min, because adverse effects (especially hypotension) are much more likely to occur at this higher dosage range.

When nitroglycerin is used *prophylactically* (i.e., in an attempt to *limit infarct size* in patients who are no longer having chest pain), an infusion rate of between 50 to 100 μg/min is usually selected and empirically continued for 24 to 48 hours. Alternatively, parameters that may be used to determine the optimal rate for prophylactic infusion of nitroglycerin are a lowering of mean arterial blood pressure by at least 10% (with maintenance of systolic blood pressure at 90 to 110 mm Hg or greater), and avoidance of excessive tachycardia (i.e., heart rate should not exceed 110 beats/min).

> Although headache is commonly seen with nitroglycerin usage, it will usually not be so severe as to require discontinuation of the drug. Headache tends to be less marked with IV administration of the drug than with oral or sublingual preparations; it often becomes less severe (and better tolerated) with time, and may be at least partially relieved by acetaminophen. Reduction of the rate of infusion (at least temporarily) is sometimes needed if headache is severe.

In general, nitroglycerin is a safe drug to administer to patients with suspected AMI. Nevertheless, a number of precautions should be observed. The drug should not be used in patients who are hypovolemic or hypotensive. It must be used with extreme caution in patients who have a borderline blood pressure (with systolic readings between 90 to 100 mm Hg), or who have acute right ventricular infarction, since hemodynamics may be further compromised in such individuals. Reflex tachycardia is common and may be blunted by addition of β-blockers (provided that the patient is not in heart failure). Occasionally during nitroglycerin infusion paradoxical *brady-*

---

*Be sure to wipe off any remaining nitroglycerin paste *before starting an IV infusion of the drug.*

Table 12B-1

Suggested Approach for the Use of Nitroglycerin for Patients with Suspected AMI

INDICATIONS
-Initial treatment of choice for acute ischemic chest pain.
-Hypertension associated with AMI
-Heart failure/pulmonary edema
-Limitation of infarct size in patients with AMI (as a *prophylactic* measure even in the absence of chest pain)

NITROGLYCERIN FORMULATIONS
Sublingual or nitroglycerin spray:
-Rapid onset (2 to 5 min)
-Usually the first form of nitroglycerin to be tried (often by the patient)

Topical (paste or ointment):
-May be tried after sublingual or spray forms in relatively stable patients with acute ischemic chest pain. However, if chest pain persists, remove any remaining paste/ointment and begin infusion of IV nitroglycerin.

IV nitroglycerin:
-Treatment of choice for severe acute ischemic chest pain
-Failure to respond to sublingual, spray forms, or topical nitroglycerin is NOT predictive of the response to IV nitroglycerin.
-Begin infusion at 10 μg/min. Gradually titrate dose upward as needed (and tolerated) for desired clinical effect.
-Avoid doses above 200 μg/min if at all possible.
-Consider doses of between 25 to 100 μg/min when used *prophylactically* (to treat patients with suspected AMI in the absence of chest pain). Empirically continue the infusion for 24 to 48 hours. Consider reducing the dose at night (to prevent development of tolerance).

Other formulations (i.e., patch, buccal, oral):
-Usually not indicated for treatment of *acute* ischemic chest pain

PRECAUTIONS
-Use with extreme caution in patients with low or borderline blood pressure (i.e., 100 mm Hg systolic or less), hypovolemia, and/or suspected acute right ventricular infarction.
-Consider incorporation of a nitrate-free interval into the dosing schedule.

cardia will be seen in association with marked hypotension. If this occurs, the drug should be immediately stopped and the patient placed in Trendelenburg position. Administration of IV fluid and atropine are indicated if hypotension and bradycardia persist. Finally, it should be appreciated that the phenomenon of **nitrate tolerance** is real, and may develop in some patients who are receiving IV nitroglycerin after as little as 12 to 24 hours, especially when a high dose and constant rate of infusion is used (AHFS Drug Information, 1990).

It is important to differentiate between nitrate *tolerance* (i.e., an initially beneficial response to nitrates, with a gradual need for higher and higher doses of drug to maintain the beneficial response) and *resistance* (i.e., the patient *never* responded at all to nitroglycerin). Discontinuation of IV nitroglycerin for as

little as 12 hours will usually restore nitrate responsiveness in patients who develop tolerance to the drug. In such cases, incorporation of a *"nitrate-free" interval* (of *at least* 8 to 10 hours) may prevent tolerance from developing again. Another vasodilator/antianginal medication (such as a calcium channel blocker) may be added during this nitrate-free interval to ensure 24-hour control of symptoms.

Clinically, the phenomenon of nitrate tolerance appears to be much more of a problem for patients receiving long-term nitrate therapy (with patch, oral, and/or sustained sublingual formulations of the drug). It is for this reason that "round-the-clock" dosing (i.e., at 4 to 6 hour intervals) is no longer recommended with chronic use. Instead, there should be routine incorporation of a *nitrate-free interval* into the dosing schedule—at least for patch, oral, and sustained sublingual formulations of the drug (AHFS Drug Information, 1990).

> Because of variable blood levels and a relatively short duration of action, *paste forms* of nitroglycerin are less likely to foster development of tolerance. Practically speaking, one can probably do equally well administering nitroglycerin paste "round-the-clock" (i.e., every 6 hours) as three times a day (with inclusion of an 8 to 10 hour nitrate-free interval).
>
> In contrast, the much more constant drug levels produced by *patch formulations* of the drug *necessitate* removal (either at night or during the day) for a nitrate-free interval in order to ensure maximal responsiveness to the effects of the drug.
>
> Although development of tolerance is probably less of a problem for patients receiving a low-dose (i.e., prophylactic) IV nitroglycerin infusion, consideration might be given to reducing the dose at night (so as to provide for a *"relatively nitrate-free"* interval).

OTHER ANALGESIC AGENTS

Anxiolytic agents such as oral **diazepam** (Valium) or other benzodiazepines should be considered as an adjunctive analgesic measure, especially when a significant anxiety component complicates the chest pain of AMI. *Awareness that one may be having a heart attack is an acute anxiety-producing situation.* A vicious cycle is often created in which chest pain is exacerbated by this anxiety, and the anxiety is further exacerbated by the increase in chest pain. Short-term administration of a potent anxiolytic agent is *not* addictive in this situation, and may be extremely effective in breaking the cycle. Physiologic benefits that may accompany the reduction of anxiety and chest pain in this setting include decreased myocardial oxygen consumption, decreased preload and/or afterload, and a beneficial antiarrhythmic effect due to the reduction in sympathetic tone (Côté et al, 1974; Gillis et al, 1974; Lown and Verrier, 1976)

> It is important to emphasize that anxiolytic agents are much less likely to be given in the setting of acute ischemic chest pain if the order is written for "prn" use. Many health care providers seem to retain preconceived notions about the inappropriate use of these drugs. Rather than depending on the patient to ask for medication (or on the health care team to dispense it when written as a "prn" order), it may therefore be preferable to write for a *fixed-dosage schedule*—especially for selected, acutely anxious patients with new-onset chest pain.

> Discussion on the use of other anti-ischemic agents (β-blockers and calcium channel blockers) for relieving chest pain is deferred until later in this section; use of thrombolytic agents for this purpose is addressed in Section C.

ANTIARRHYTHMIC THERAPY
General Comments on the Use of Lidocaine for Suspected AMI

Lidocaine is the antiarrhythmic agent of choice for treatment of ventricular ectopy associated with AMI. The principal objective for using lidocaine in the setting of acute ischemia and/or infarction is to reduce the likelihood of developing potentially life-threatening ventricular arrhythmias (sustained ventricular tachycardia or primary ventricular fibrillation).

The threshold for developing malignant ventricular arrhythmias is reduced by ischemia and infarction. Although the mechanism for these arrhythmias is multifactorial and complex in nature, *reentry* is felt to comprise a major component (Hancock, 1990). Occurrence of PVCs at a vulnerable period in the cardiac cycle may "trigger" development of reentrant ventricular tachyarrhythmias which may then degenerate to ventricular fibrillation. The rationale for considering treatment of PVCs in patients with suspected AMI is to reduce (or eliminate) this "trigger" for reentry.

A number of key factors are involved in the decision of whether to use lidocaine to treat patients with suspected AMI. Difficulties arise as a result of the following facts:

1. *Treatment with lidocaine is not benign.* In addition to a series of well-known neurologic adverse effects, lidocaine may cause hypotension, seizures, and potentially fatal asystole.
2. Treatment with lidocaine has *not* been shown to reduce mortality.
3. Potential indications for drug administration (i.e., lidocaine treatment vs prophylaxis, prevention of primary vs secondary ventricular fibrillation) are confusing.
4. Lidocaine pharmacokinetics are somewhat complex, and no consensus exists on the optimal protocol for administration.

> Full discussion of lidocaine pharmacokinetics (and the specifics of dosing for administering the drug) is deferred until Section E of this chapter. We focus discussion here on review of the basic principles of treatment, and then summarize this information in *Table 12B-2.*

Primary vs Secondary Ventricular Fibrillation

Appreciation of the difference between primary and secondary ventricular fibrillation is essential for understanding the rationale of treatment recommendations for lidocaine in patients with suspected AMI. *Primary* ventricular fibrillation refers to the acute electrical instability that develops as a direct consequence of the infarction. It is most often seen within the first few hours of infarction and becomes rare after 24 hours. *Prevention of primary ventricular fibrillation is the principal objective of antiarrhythmic therapy in patients with AMI.* In contrast, secondary ventricular fibrillation typically occurs a number of days after the onset of symptoms as a result of (i.e., *secondary* to) development of cardiogenic shock. Secondary ventricular fibrillation is usually a pre-terminal rhythm. As one might expect, it is generally resistant to antiarrhythmic therapy.

Use of Lidocaine as *Treatment* for Suspected AMI

Patients who appear to be most at risk of developing primary ventricular fibrillation with AMI include those seen early (within the first few hours of the onset of symptoms) who demonstrate *new-onset* ventricular ectopy that is frequent and/or associated with *repetitive* forms (i.e., couplets, salvos, and runs of ventricular tachycardia). Administration of lidocaine to such patients is still generally recommended (ACC/AHA Task Force, 1990). It should be emphasized that all PVCs do *not* necessarily need to be eliminated for lidocaine to exert a protective effect in this setting. Reduction in frequency, and in the most dangerous PVC forms (couplets, salvos, and especially longer runs of ventricular tachycardia) may suffice.

Use of lidocaine in this manner to suppress (or at least reduce) the frequency and complexity of manifest ventricular ectopy in patients with acute ischemic heart disease syndromes (such as unstable angina or suspected AMI) is referred to as lidocaine *treatment*. This is in contrast to the *prophylactic* use of lidocaine in which the drug is administered to patients with suspected AMI who do not have PVCs, or who only have rare, isolated PVCs. Whether to use lidocaine prophylactically for patients with suspected AMI remains an extremely controversial issue.

Use of *Prophylactic* Lidocaine for Suspected AMI

Meta-analysis of 14 randomized trials in the literature involving more than 9,000 patients with AMI supports the premise that treatment with lidocaine reduces the incidence of ventricular fibrillation (by 30 to 35%). However, it has never been shown that this reduction in the incidence of ventricular fibrillation translates into improved survival

(MacMahon et al, 1988; Hine et al, 1989). On the contrary, treatment with lidocaine appears to *increase* the incidence of fatal asystole (from 0.2 to 0.4%) compared to patients with AMI who are not given prophylactic lidocaine (Yusuf et al, 1988). Thus, under certain circumstances (i.e., when the drug is given during the monitored hospital phase of AMI), mortality may actually be increased in patients who are treated prophylactically with lidocaine (Hine et al, 1989).

Unfortunately, there are problems interpreting data from these studies. The overall event rate (i.e., the incidence of ventricular fibrillation) was surprisingly low among the 9,000 patients in the meta-analysis (less than 2%). This suggests that as a whole, patients enrolled in these studies comprised a relatively low risk group. Considering that the greatest risk (by far) of developing primary ventricular fibrillation in association with AMI is during the initial 1 to 2 hours after the onset of symptoms, delay of even a few hours beyond this point could significantly reduce the potential for benefit from prophylactic antiarrhythmic therapy (and might also account for the low incidence of primary ventricular fibrillation in the studies). Statistically, many more *thousands* of patients would probably be needed to demonstrate a beneficial effect on mortality in a study with such a low baseline rate of ventricular fibrillation.

Other problems complicating interpretation of these studies include the vastly different protocols used (with significant variation in dosing protocols and mixture of prehospital trials using IM lidocaine with in-hospital trials using IV bolus and infusion therapy); incomplete data on the cause of mortality (ventricular fibrillation, asystole, or other); and incomplete data on the outcome of patients in whom the diagnosis of AMI was not confirmed, with limited duration of follow-up after admission to the hospital.

In summary, no definite conclusion can be drawn at this time from existing literature regarding the issue of whether prophylactic lidocaine is helpful or harmful when given to patients with suspected AMI. In practice, because such treatment has *not* been shown to save lives, an increasing number of clinicians seem to have moved *away* from prophylactic use of the drug, and many appear somewhat less inclined to use lidocaine as treatment. Rather than endorsement of any particular policy, we feel it more important to *individualize* the decision of whether to use lidocaine, basing it on careful consideration of the pros and cons of such treatment, an understanding of relevant pharmacokinetics of the drug, and the goals of therapy in the context of each clinical setting. *(See Table 12B-2 and Section E of this chapter for our suggested approach for using lidocaine for patients with suspected AMI.)*

Factors to Consider in Deciding Whether to Use Lidocaine to Treat Patients with Suspected AMI

DEFINITIONS

Lidocaine *Treatment*—Use of the drug to treat frequent or complex PVCs in patients with suspected AMI.

Lidocaine *Prophylaxis*—Use of the drug prophylactically in patients with suspected AMI who *do not* have PVCs (or who only have rare, isolated PVCs).

Primary Ventricular Fibrillation—Ventricular fibrillation that develops as a direct consequence of the electrical instability that is seen during the earliest hours of acute infarction. It is rare after 24 hours.

Secondary Ventricular Fibrillation—Ventricular fibrillation that develops later (usually after several days) as a result of (i.e., *secondary* to) cardiogenic shock. It is usually a *preterminal* rhythm (i.e., antiarrhythmic therapy is generally ineffective).

PRINCIPAL OBJECTIVE OF ANTIARRHYTHMIC THERAPY

-Prevention of potentially life-threatening ventricular arrhythmias (sustained ventricular tachycardia, *primary* ventricular fibrillation).

INDICATIONS FOR ANTIARRHYTHMIC THERAPY

- *New-onset* frequent and/or repetitive ventricular ectopy (i.e., couplets, salvos, or runs of ventricular tachycardia) in patients with suspected AMI.*
- Possibly as antiarrhythmic prophylaxis for patients suspected of AMI†
- Prevention/treatment of patients with reperfusion arrhythmias (following acute angioplasty or thrombolytic therapy)

THE PROS AND CONS OF LIDOCAINE TREATMENT

PROS—Primary ventricular fibrillation occurs in 5% to 10% of patients with AMI. Use of lidocaine appears to reduce this risk.

CONS—Use of lidocaine may be associated with adverse effects (disorientation, confusion, dysarthria, seizures, etc.) including a slight increased risk of fatal asystole. Prophylactic use of the drug has never been shown to improve survival from AMI.

SUGGESTIONS FOR OPTIMAL USE OF LIDOCAINE

For Lidocaine TREATMENT:

- Strongly consider treating patients with suspected AMI who manifest *new-onset* frequent and/or repetitive ventricular ectopy.
- Don't "chase" every PVC. Reduction in PVC frequency and minimization of repetitive forms is probably the most reasonable (and realistic) endpoint of therapy.
- Try not to exceed an infusion rate of 2 mg/minute (or at least minimize the duration of time that the patient is given the drug at higher infusion rates).
- Be particularly cautious in treating (or avoid treating):
  -Patients at greatest risk of developing lidocaine toxicity (i.e., the elderly, those with heart failure or liver disease, patients of lighter body weight, etc.) in whom the use of lower infusion rates (of 1 to 2 mg/min—or less!) becomes especially important
  -Patients with pre-existing conduction disturbances or bradyarrhythmias (i.e., bundle branch block, AV block)

For Lidocaine PROPHYLAXIS:

- Strongly consider lidocaine prophylaxis for patients who receive thrombolytic therapy.
- Patients with suspected AMI who are treated with IV β-blockers probably do *not* need lidocaine prophylaxis.
- Limit consideration of lidocaine prophylaxis to those patients at greatest risk of developing primary ventricular fibrillation:
  -Patients seen soon after the onset of symptoms (especially if seen within the first 6 hours)
  -Patients with a history and/or ECG that is strongly suggestive of AMI
  -Patients under 70 years of age
- Lidocaine prophylaxis in an otherwise stable patient need not be continued beyond 12 to 24 hours.
- The benefits of lidocaine prophylaxis are uncertain. As a result, it is perfectly reasonable to adopt a policy of *careful observation* of patients with suspected AMI (rather than routine institution of lidocaine prophylaxis)†

*It should be emphasized that use of lidocaine in this setting constitutes antiarrhythmic *treatment* (and *not* prophylaxis!).
†Lidocaine prophylaxis remains a controversial issue!

Antiarrhythmic Treatment: *If Lidocaine Doesn't Work*

As already discussed, the presence of *new-onset* frequent and/or repetitive ventricular ectopy in patients with acute ischemia or infarction increases the risk of developing primary ventricular fibrillation. Antiarrhythmic treatment is recommended for such patients, and lidocaine is preferred as the drug of choice.

> In addition to antiarrhythmic therapy, careful attention must *always* be given to detection and treatment of other factors that might produce or exacerbate ventricular arrhythmias. These include continued ischemia and/or chest pain, uncontrolled anxiety, worsening heart failure, hypoxemia, acid-base disturbances, and electrolyte abnormalities (especially hypokalemia or hypomagnesemia). If present, alleviation of these other factors is likely to be much more effective than antiarrhythmic therapy in suppressing ventricular ectopy.

Should frequent and complex ventricular ectopy persist despite attention to potentially exacerbating factors and optimal dosing with lidocaine, additional antiarrhythmic therapy should be considered. **Procainamide** is generally recommended as the second drug of choice (AHA ACLS Text, 1986; Hancock, 1990). Increments of 100 mg may be administered IV over a 5-minute period, until either the arrhythmia is controlled, a total loading dose of 1 gram has been given, or untoward side effects appear (i.e., hypotension or widening of the QRS complex). This may be followed by a continuous procainamide infusion of 2 to 4 mg/min (1 to 2 mg/min in patients with renal impairment). Procainamide loading can also be accomplished by infusing 500 to 1,000 mg over a 30- to 60-minute period *(See Chapter 14.).*

> Procainamide offers the distinct advantage of availability in both an IV and oral form. This facilitates transition to oral therapy in preparation for discharge of patients who will need long-term antiarrhythmic therapy. Additional advantages of procainamide are that the drug is also effective in treatment of supraventricular arrhythmias—and that this drug is likely to be even more effective than lidocaine for treatment of ventricular arrhythmias that are not induced by acute ischemia (Wesley et al, 1991).

Alternatively, administration of an **IV β-blocker** may provide effective antiarrhythmic therapy, especially for patients whose arrhythmia is likely to reflect ongoing ischemia and/or excessive sympathetic tone (i.e., in patients with anterior infarctions who are tachycardic and/or hypertensive).

> Administration of IV β-blockers reduces the incidence of primary ventricular fibrillation in patients with AMI *(as we will discuss momentarily in the section on IV β-blockers in this chapter).* The sooner in the course that the drug is given, the greater the chance for clinical benefit. Patients treated with an IV β-blocker early in the course of AMI probably do *not* need prophylactic lidocaine (Conti, 1989).

Use of **bretylium** has also been suggested as an alternative for treatment of frequent and/or repetitive PVCs in the setting of AMI. However, because of the drug's initial sympathomimetic effect (which may actually *exacerbate* ventricular ectopy), its potentially delayed onset of action in the treatment of ventricular tachycardia (which may require 10 to 20 minutes before working), and its tendency for producing hypotension, use of bretylium may be problematic. As a result, the drug might best be reserved for treatment of malignant ventricular arrhythmias that have not responded to other measures, or for use as an antifibrillatory agent in the setting of cardiac arrest to treat refractory ventricular fibrillation *(see Chapter 2).*

Recently, attention has been drawn to the use of **amiodarone** for emergency treatment of malignant ventricular arrhythmias. While it is generally recommended that more conventional antiarrhythmic therapy be tried first (i.e., lidocaine, procainamide, and β-blockers), rapid IV loading of amiodarone may prove to be lifesaving in selected cases refractory to other measures *(see Chapter 2).*

> Treatment with **thrombolytic agents** is usually not thought of as antiarrhythmic therapy. Nevertheless, it is of interest that use of thrombolytic therapy during the early hours of AMI has been shown to exert a protective effect against development of secondary ventricular fibrillation (Volpi et al, 1990). The mechanism accounting for this protective effect is twofold: reduction of infarct size as a result of successful reperfusion, and decreased ability to support the "substrate" (i.e., potential for reentry) of ventricular tachyarrhythmias (Peter and Helfant, 1990). Thus prevention of secondary ventricular fibrillation is yet another reason for strongly considering early administration of thrombolytic therapy in patients with AMI.

Consideration of Magnesium

Consideration of magnesium for use as an antiarrhythmic agent in the setting of acute ischemic heart disease merits special attention. Serum magnesium levels have been shown to drop in AMI, as well as in response to other stressful conditions (Abraham et al, 1986). Rather than a decrease in overall body content of this cation, the mechanism accounting for the fall of serum magnesium in the setting of AMI may relate to a *transient shift* in the balance between intra- and extracellular cation concentration. Myocardial tissue magnesium levels are also altered in AMI (flux of potassium and magnesium ions from injured myocardial cells ?). Considering the inverse relationship that has been shown to exist between intracellular magnesium and potentially lethal ventricular arrhythmias in such patients, the importance of optimizing intramyocardial magnesium levels is clear (Abraham et al, 1986; Tzivoni and Keren, 1990).

An interesting study by Abraham et al (1987) demonstrated that prophylactic administration of magnesium sulfate (as a *single* 2.4 g IV dose infused over 20 minutes at the time of admission) significantly reduced the incidence of potentially lethal ventricular arrhythmias in patients with AMI during the first 24 hours of their hospital stay. Although one third of the patients in their study experienced flushing during magnesium infusion, this did not necessitate discontinuation of the drug (and perhaps could have been avoided by a slower rate of infusion). Significant adverse effects from magnesium infusion did not occur.

A similar beneficial effect from prophylactic magnesium sulfate infusion for patients with AMI was seen by Shecter et al (1990). In a randomized, double-blind, placebo-controlled trial, those patients who received magnesium (infused in a total amount of 22 g over 48 hours!) had a significantly lower in-hospital mortality compared to placebo controls (2% vs 17%—p <0.01). Baseline hypomagnesemia was *not* common in the study. Moreover, mortality in the control group occurred principally from cardiogenic shock and/or EMD, suggesting that rather than a pure antiarrhythmic effect, the mechanism of action of magnesium administration in the setting of AMI may be due more to a "cardioprotective" effect (reduced tendency to developing coronary spasm? decreased platelet aggregability? improved stability of transmembrane potentials with resultant reduction in myocardial cell excitability?).

An overview incorporating results from five other randomized trials (involving more than 1,000 patients) on the use of IV magnesium in patients with suspected AMI suggests a comparable favorable response to prophylactic administration of this cation—with an overall reduction in mortality of *up to 60%* compared to placebo (Teo et al, 1991). More recently, similar beneficial results have been obtained from prophylactic IV magnesium administration to a randomized group of more than 2,000 patients with suspected AMI (Woods et al, 1992). Clearly, use of prophylactic magnesium infusion for patients with AMI is still in the investigative stage, and additional, larger prospective studies are needed to confirm these exciting and provocative results. Nevertheless, we anticipate that the future may well see increased (? routine) use of magnesium as a prophylactic (antiarrhythmic ?) and/or treatment measure for patients with AMI.

Additional discussion on the use of magnesium in emergency cardiac care is found in Section B of Chapter 11 on Sudden Cardiac Death, Chapter 2 (which reviews suggestions for dosing), and in Section C of Chapter 16 (under discussion of treatment of Torsade de Pointes).

β-BLOCKER THERAPY

AMI is a source of intense physiologic and psychologic stress that is associated with a generalized increase in sympathetic activity and circulating catecholamine levels. This may result in a number of adverse effects on the heart including tachycardia, arrhythmogenesis, hypertension, and an increase in cardiac contractility (that may lead to an increase in myocardial oxygen consumption). β-block-

ers may prove useful in treatment of patients with AMI by counteracting a number of these effects.

Efficacy of β-Blocker Therapy

Pooled data from more than 25 trials (on more than 20,000 patients) have conclusively shown that oral β-blocker therapy initiated in the days to weeks following AMI reduces mortality (by 20% to 25%) during the first few years of the post-infarction period. The incidence of nonfatal reinfarction and sudden cardiac death is also reduced during this period (Yusuf et al, 1988).

β-blockers also appear to lower mortality when administered *acutely* during the course of AMI. Pooled data from nearly 30 randomized trials (on more than 25,000 patients) suggest an overall reduction in mortality of between 10% to 15% during the first week of AMI (Yusuf et al, 1988; ACC/AHA Task Force, 1990).

Especially favorable results were obtained with acute use of β-blockers in the prospective, double-blind, placebo-controlled Göteborg trial. In this study, 1,395 patients presenting with suspected or definite AMI received either IV metoprolol (3 IV injections totalling 15 mg) or placebo as soon as possible after admission to the hospital (Hjalmarson, 1984). Less than 7% of the patients who were given the drug were unable to tolerate it. Oral therapy (100 mg of metoprolol b.i.d.) was started in the others. Overall mortality was decreased by 36% after 90 days (compared to placebo-treated patients), and remained low when treatment was continued over the first year after the infarct. In addition, chest pain (and the need for analgesic drugs), ventricular arrhythmias, infarct size, and hospital stay were all decreased in those given IV metoprolol acutely compared to the placebo group. In particular, the incidence of venricular fibrillation was dramatically reduced in the metoprolol-treated group. Only 6 episodes of ventricular fibrillation occurred in patients treated with this IV β-blocker compared to 41 episodes of ventricular fibrillation that occurred in patients who were treated with placebo (Ryden et al, 1983).

Mechanism of Action

Despite this evidence that oral and intravenous β-blocker therapy reduce mortality from myocardial infarction both acutely and in the post-infarction period, the mechanism accounting for these favorable results remains open to question. The effect appears to be *multifactorial (Table 12B-3)* due to a combination of sympathetic blockade, decreased myocardial workload and oxygen consumption, antiarrhythmic activity, improved collateral blood flow, and decreased platelet aggregation (Lichstein, 1985; Campbell et al, 1986; Conti, 1989). High levels of circulating catecholamines associated with AMI exert positive chronotropic and inotropic effects on the heart that increase demand (myocardial oxygen consumption) on an already ischemic myocardium. This may lead to extension of the infarct and generation of ventricular arrhythmias. By decreasing heart rate and contractility, β-blockers lessen metabolic demand. Flow to ischemic areas is improved because the reduction in contractility lowers left ventricular end-diastolic pressure, thus enhancing perfusion to the subendocardium.* The reduction in heart rate also improves coronary flow because it results in an increase in *diastolic* time (during which the coronary arteries are perfused).† β-blockers exert an antiarrhythmic effect (which at least in part is due to sympathetic blockade) that reduces the incidence of ventricular arrhythmias and protects against development of 1° ventricular fibrillation. Finally these drugs appear to favorably alter platelet aggregability.

Table 12B-3

Proposed Mechanisms of Action for the Beneficial Effect of β-Blockers with AMI
-Sympathetic blockade (reduction in level of circulating catecholamines)
-Decreased myocardial workload (from slowing of heart rate and reduction of blood pressure)
-Decreased myocardial oxygen consumption (from decreased contractility)
-Antiarrhythmic effect (with reduction in the incidence of 1° ventricular fibrillation)
-Improved blood flow to ischemic areas (i.e., the subendocardium)
-Favorable effect on platelet aggregation

Selection of Patients Most Likely to Respond to IV β-Blockers

Table 12B-4 summarizes key points to keep in mind when considering the use of IV β-blockers in the setting of AMI. As noted above, these drugs *are* effective. The beneficial effect of IV β-blocker therapy appears to be most marked (up to a 25% reduction in mortality) when the drug is begun *early* in the course of AMI (i.e., within the first 24 to 48 hours of the infarct, and ideally within the first 3 to 6 hours), and when priority for treatment is given to sicker patients with more extensive infarction (Yusuf et al, 1988;

---

*As mentioned earlier, a reduction in left ventricular end-diastolic pressure favors blood flow to the subendocardium because it lessens mechanical resistance ("back pressure") to perfusion of blood through ventricular myocardium.

†*Systolic* time (during which the ventricles contract) is of a relatively constant duration; it is only minimally affected by changes in heart rate. In contrast, the duration of *diastolic* time (during which ventricular relaxation occurs) is much more variable and likely to be affected by changes in heart rate. Since the coronary arteries are perfused during diastole, bradycardia (which lengthens the cardiac cycle) will increase the time for coronary flow by prolonging the period of diastole. A deleterious effect of tachycardia is that it produces the opposite effect.

Gregoratos, 1990). Patients especially likely to benefit are those with clinical signs suggestive of *sympathetic overactivity* such as hypertension and/or tachycardia. Acute *anterior* infarction is much more likely to produce such signs than acute inferior infarction (which is more commonly associated with signs of parasympathetic overactivity such as bradycardia and hypotension).

Table 12B-4

Key Points to Consider in the Use of IV β-Blockers with Acute MI
Conditions Most Likely to Respond to IV β-Blocker Therapy
-Acute anterior infarction with clinical evidence of sympathetic overactivity (i.e., tachycardia and/or hypertension)
-Tachyarrhythmias or chest pain that is likely to be due to *excessive sympathetic tone* (and which may have been refractory to standard therapy)
-Extensive AMI when patients are treated *early* in the course (ideally within 6 hours of the onset of infarction)
Contraindications to the Use of IV β-Blockers*
-Bronchospasm
-Significant bradycardia (i.e., heart rate less than 50 to 60 beats/min)
-Hypotension (i.e., blood pressure less than 90 to 100 mm Hg)
-Pulmonary edema
*In most cases IV β-blocker therapy is well tolerated and can be used safely even if there are bibasilar rales (provided that other evidence of heart failure is absent, a systolic blood pressure of at least 100 mm Hg is maintained, and heart rate remains over 60 beats/min).

Another situation in which IV β-blocker therapy may be beneficial is for treatment of refractory tachyarrhythmias (ventricular or supraventricular) when the underlying cause of the arrhythmia is excessive sympathetic stimulation. In such cases standard antiarrhythmic therapy with lidocaine, procainamide, or bretylium may have been ineffective because it failed to address the underlying cause of the problem—excess circulating catecholamines. Similarly, selected patients with chest pain refractory to standard treatment measures (i.e., nitroglycerin, morphine, calcium channel blockers) sometimes respond dramatically to relatively small doses of IV β-blockers when excessive sympathetic activity underlies the patient's symptomatology *(Table 12B-4)*.

Suggestions/Precautions in Dosing of β-Blockers with AMI

In this country, the β-blocker most commonly selected for IV administration in the setting of AMI is **metoprolol.** Although the drug is generally well tolerated and the incidence of significant adverse effects is relatively low, administration of IV β-blockers *acutely* to patients with AMI still carries with it the potential risk of producing hypotension, bradyarrhythmias, and/or myocardial depression. As a result, caution is urged if this intervention is contemplated. Depending on the clinical setting, the health care provider's level of comfort and degree of expertise, local practice, and specialist availability, such caution may take the form of careful observation in an intensive care unit, consultation with a cardiologist, and/or invasive hemodynamic monitoring. Fortunately, because the half-life of IV metoprolol is short, even if adverse effects do occur, they usually resolve fairly rapidly (within 30 minutes).

IV β-blockers such as metoprolol should *not* be given to patients with bronchospasm, significant bradycardia, hypotension, or pulmonary edema *(Table 12B-4)*. Except for these contraindications, the drug can usually be used safely *even* if there are bibasilar rales (provided that other evidence of congestive heart failure is absent, a systolic blood pressure of greater than 100 mm Hg is maintained, and heart rate remains over 60 beats per minute).

Standard dosing recommendations for **IV metoprolol** are to administer three 5 mg IV boluses every 2 to 5 minutes for a total loading dose of 15 mg *(Table 12B-5)*. Initial dosing with smaller increments of the drug (1 to 2 mg IV) is sometimes used to minimize the chance of an untoward reaction. If patient tolerance is good, 3 to 5 mg IV boluses may be repeated every 5 to 10 minutes until the total 15 mg IV loading dose has been administered. *Oral dosing* should then be started (50 mg to be given 15 minutes after the last IV bolus, followed by 50 mg orally q6h for 2 days, and then 100 mg orally q12h for at least 3 months).

Table 12B-5

β-Blocker Preparations for IV and Oral Use with AMI and in the Post-Infarction Period

METOPROLOL (Lopressor):
 IV Dose—5 mg IV boluses repeated q2-5 min × 3 (= a total of 15 mg).
     —Initial dosing with smaller increments (1 to 2 mg IV) may minimize untoward reactions. If patient tolerance is good, 3 to 5 mg IV boluses may then be repeated q5-10 min until the recommended 15 mg IV loading dose has been administered.
 Oral Dose (for 2° prevention of myocardial infarction)—Oral metoprolol may be started at a dose of 50 mg given 15 minutes after the last IV bolus, followed by 50 mg PO q6h for 2 days, and then 100 mg PO q12h.
 	
 ESMOLOL (Brevibloc):
 IV Dose—Administer a 500 μg/kg loading dose over 1 min, followed by a 25 μg/kg/min IV infusion. Rebolus the drug and increase the IV infusion rate by 25 to 50 μg/kg/min q5 min until the desired effect is achieved.
     —Most patients achieve a therapeutic response at infusion rates of 100 to 200 μg/kg/min.
     —The maximum infusion rate is 300 μg/kg/min.
 	
 PROPRANOLOL (Inderal):
 IV Dose—1 mg by *slow* IV administration q5 min (up to a total of 5 mg)
 Oral Dose (for 2° prevention of myocardial infarction)—40 to 60 mg Tid, Qid
 	
 TIMOLOL (Blocadren):
 Oral Dose (for 2° prevention of myocardial infarction)—10 mg Bid
 	
 ATENOLOL (Tenormin):
 Oral Dose (for 2° prevention of myocardial infarction)—50 mg Qd

Other β-blockers may also be used intravenously in an attempt to reduce mortality in patients with AMI, although they have not been as extensively studied as metoprolol for this indication *(Table 12B-5).*

> **IV esmolol** offers the advantage of having an even shorter half-life (less than 10 minutes) than metoprolol, resulting in a return toward baseline hemodynamic measurements within 15 minutes of stopping the drug (Kirshenbaum et al, 1988). Esmolol is dosed by administering a 500 μg/kg loading dose over 1 minute, followed by a 25 μg/kg/min IV infusion. Additional IV boluses are given every 5 minutes as the rate of the infusion is increased (by 25 to 50 μg/kg/min) until the desired effect is obtained. Most patients achieve a therapeutic response to esmolol at infusion rates of 100 to 200 μg/kg/min. The maximum recommended dose is 300 μg/kg/min.

Oral β-Blocker Therapy

Oral β-blocker therapy should be considered for patients who survive the initial phase of AMI. Treatment should be started *early* (ideally within the first few days of infarction), and probably continued (if tolerated) for *at least 2 years* (ACC/AHA Task Force, 1990). Patients who are likely to benefit most from long-term oral β-blocker therapy are those who suffered more extensive infarction with one or more complications, but who do not have contraindications (such as bronchospasm or heart failure) to this class of drug. In contrast, patients who recover uneventfully after their first infarction who retain good ventricular function, do not have angina or ventricular arrhythmias, and who do not develop ischemia on predischarge exercise testing have an excellent prognosis regardless of whether they receive long-term β-blocker therapy (ACC/AHA Task Force, 1990).

Choices for long-term oral β-blocker therapy as a *secondary* prevention measure (against *recurrence* of infarction) include the *non-selective* agent **propranolol** (used in a dose of 180 to 240 mg/day in the studies), and the β-1 selective agents **metoprolol** (used in a dose of 100 mg Bid in the studies) and **timolol** (used in a dose of 10 mg Bid in the studies). Empiric use of lower doses of these drugs, or of other β-1 selective agents such as **atenolol** (at a dose of 50 mg Qd) may be reasonable in an attempt to improve tolerance *(Table 12B-5).*

> The theoretical benefit of *nonselective* β-blockade (i.e., blockade of β-2 adrenergic receptors with consequent blunting of transient, catecholamine-induced hypokalemia) may be clinically relevant (Grauer and Gums, 1988), but is unproven. Consideration of this theoretical benefit should be balanced against the poorer tolerance and patient acceptance of long-term oral therapy with nonselective β-blockers.
>
> Unfavorable effects on lipid metabolism (i.e., increased cholesterol and decreased HDL levels) are unfortunately associated with long-term therapy using all of the β-blockers indicated above. Although adverse lipid effects are not seen with β-blockers that have ISA (intrinsic sympathomimetic activity) such as pindolol (Viskin) or acebutolol (Sectral), nor with the

alpha-beta blocker labetalol (Normodyne, Trandate), beneficial effects on post-infarction mortality have not been demonstrated for these agents. As a result, these drugs have not been recommended for this purpose (ACC/AHA Task Force, 1990).

Clinical Assimilation of the Studies

Analysis of the data on the use of oral β-blockers after AMI can be deceptive. As already noted, *overall mortality* is decreased by 20-25% during the first few years after infarction. Looking at the same data another way indicates that mortality was only decreased from 9.8% to 7.6% by treatment among the nearly 4,000 patients in the Beta-Blocker Heart Attack Trial (1982). Viewed in this manner, the efficacy of treatment does not appear to be nearly as great, and suggests the need to treat approximately 100 patients in order to potentially benefit just two or three of them. Considering the adverse effects commonly associated with long-term oral β-blocker therapy (fatigue, depression, insomnia, etc.), and the overall good prognosis of patients with otherwise uncomplicated infarction (especially if the infarction was small and inferior in location), it's easy to understand why enthusiasm has waned among many clinicians for the routine use of oral β-blocker therapy as a secondary prevention measure after recovery from an otherwise uncomplicated infarction.

In contrast, despite the intuitive logic (and strong supportive data) in favor of using IV β-blockers early in the course of AMI for patients with clinical evidence of sympathetic overactivity (tachycardia and hypertension), many clinicians still appear reluctant to initiate this therapy. *We strongly recommend consideration of IV β-blocker therapy for such patients.*

Use of IV β-Blockers with Cardiac Arrest

Traditionally, IV β-blockers have not been used as first-line therapy for treatment of ventricular arrhythmias associated with cardiac arrest. Nevertheless, these drugs may prove invaluable in management when such arrhythmias occur in patients with AMI who clearly demonstrate evidence of sympathetic overactivity *prior* to their cardiac arrest (i.e., anterior site of infarction, pre-arrest tachycardia or hypertension). In such cases, we strongly suggest consideration of IV β-blocker therapy *with* lidocaine as treatment of the arrest, and as prophylactic treatment to help prevent recurrence of ventricular fibrillation after return of spontaneous circulation. In selected patients with refractory ventricular fibrillation or recurrent ventricular tachycardia, IV β-blocker therapy will occasionally prove to be life-saving after all other agents (lidocaine, procainamide, bretylium) have failed. *(Metoprolol, esmolol, or propranol may be used for this purpose in the dosage suggested in Table 12B-5.)*

> A final clinical point to keep in mind is that administration of IV β-blocker therapy during the initial hours of AMI provides at least partial protection against development of primary ventricular fibrillation. As a result, such patients may not need to be considered for prophylactic antiarrhythmic treatment with lidocaine since they probably are already protected (Conti, 1989).

CALCIUM CHANNEL BLOCKERS

Calcium channel blockers are extremely effective agents in the management of many cadiovascular disorders including supraventricular tachyarrhythmias, hypertension, and the various types of angina (stable chronic angina, unstable angina, and vasospastic angina). Beneficial effects of these agents are thought to result from multiple actions including coronary vasodilatation, improved collateral flow to ischemic areas, afterload reduction, decreased myocardial oxygen consumption, heart rate slowing and suppression of supraventricular arrhythmias (for verapamil and diltiazem), and prevention of intracellular calcium overload during ischemic episodes (Gregoratos, 1990; Messerli, 1990; Kern, 1992).

> Calcium mobilization is a key step in platelet activation (Mehta, 1985). Recent evidence suggests that calcium antagonists in therapeutically achieved concentrations may significantly inhibit platelet activation by a variety of mechanisms on a microcellular level including impairment of thromboxane A2 generation and formation of oxygen free radicals from injured cells (Mehta et al, 1991; Mehta et al, 1992).

Additional beneficial effects that may be seen with long-term use of calcium channel blocking agents include reversal of left ventricular hypertrophy in patients with hypertension (Liebson, 1990) and regression of coronary artery narrowing in some patients with ischemic heart disease (Kobler et al, 1989; Lichtlen et al, 1990). Considering all of these favorable cardiovascular effects, one might ex-

pect calcium antagonists to be equally beneficial in the treatment of patients with AMI. However, despite widespread use of calcium channel blockers in clinical practice (and the very frequent prescription of these drugs to patients *during* and *after* AMI), existing data are conflicting and have *not* conclusively demonstrated benefit from these drugs in the clinical setting of AMI (Hlatky et al, 1988; ACC/AHA Task Force, 1990; Messerli, 1990).

Comparison of Available Calcium Channel Blockers

At the time of this writing, four calcium channel blockers have been approved in this country for treatment of coronary artery disease: nifedipine, diltiazem, verapamil, and nicardipine.* Future years will doubtlessly see many additions to this list.† Although all drugs in this class share the common property of reducing transmembrane flux of calcium ions across "slow" (i.e., calcium-dependent) channels, the three prototype agents (nifedipine, diltiazem, and verapamil) each have very different chemical structures and consequently manifest some different pharmacologic and clinical effects.

> All calcium channel blockers are smooth muscle vasodilators. As a class, the drugs are effective antihypertensive and antianginal agents. Clinical differences among the agents arise principally from the degree of coronary and arterial vasodilatation they produce, as well as from differing effects on conduction tissue and left ventricular contractility.

Comparison of the cardiovascular effects of the prototype calcium channel blocking agents is shown in *Table 12B-6*. Dosing recommendations for selected calcium chan-

---

*Although we do not discuss nicardipine separately, this drug exerts similar cardiovascular effects as nifedipine (Table 12B-6), has similar indications, and merits similar precautions.
†Isradipine and felodipine are more recently released calcium channel blockers that have been approved for use in hypertension. As members of the dihydropyridine class of calcium channel antagonists, they exert similar clinical effects as nifedipine.

Table 12B-6

Cardiovascular Effects of the Prototype Calcium Channel Blocking Agents					
Drug	Coronary Dilatation	Peripheral Arterial Dilatation	AV Nodal Depression	SA Nodal Depression	Net Clinical Effect on LV Contractility
Nifedipine	+	+++	0	0	↑/0
Diltiazem	+	++	+	++	↓(?)
Verapamil	+	+	++	+	↓↓

nel blockers follow in *Table 12B-7*. Appreciation of differences in the clinical effects shown in the table may help explain some of the rather surprising results obtained from clinical studies in the literature. It also provides a rationale for our suggested approach to the use of these agents in the peri-infarction period.

Nifedipine

Of the three prototype calcium channel blockers, the dihydropyridine **nifedipine** is the most potent vasodilator. To a large extent, this accounts for its side effect profile, which primarily consists of flushing, dizziness, headache, and/or reflex tachycardia. In addition, up to 15% of patients who take the drug on a long-term basis develop a type of peripheral edema that usually does not respond well to treatment with diuretics. Although this edema is *not* a reflection of new-onset heart failure (it is thought to reflect vasodilatation at the *capillary* level), it may complicate long-term management of patients who *already* have heart failure by making it harder to monitor for exacerbation of their disease.

> A *sustained-release* form of nifedipine is available **(Procardia XL—Nifedipine GITS)**. By attenuating the peak and trough levels produced with the short-acting form of the drug, long-term compliance is improved and the incidence of reflex tachycardia (as well as other adverse effects) may be substantially reduced. These features could prove advantageous if a calcium channel blocker is desired for post-infarction treatment of a patient with impaired left ventricular function (although long-term studies are lacking at this time regarding use of the sustained-action preparation for this purpose).

Clinically, nifedipine differs from verapamil and diltiazem in that it exerts virtually no depressant effect on the AV node. As a result, it is the calcium channel blocking agent of choice for patients with bradycardia or conduction system disturbances. In long-term management of coronary artery disease, the reflex tachycardia it produces may be minimized by addition of a β-blocker, resulting in an overall synergistic antianginal effect with combination therapy. Development of reflex tachycardia is more likely to be deleterious when it occurs in the setting of acute ischemia, and this may account for disappointing results in the literature that have been seen with use of nifedipine in patients with evolving AMI.

Nifedipine exerts a potent negative inotropic effect in vitro. Clinically this effect is largely negated by the compensatory reflex tachycardia it produces. In contrast, diltiazem and verapamil each exert a negative inotropic effect in the clinical setting, especially in patients with underlying left ventricular dysfunction. As a result, nifedipine is favored when a calcium channel blocker is desired for treatment of ischemic heart disease in patients known to have impaired left ventricular function.

Use of **sublingual nifedipine** has become popular as a treatment of hypertensive urgency in an office or emergency department setting. Administration of the drug in this manner may be ideal in such situations because it is rapidly absorbed, effective in lowering blood pressure, and does not require the moment-to-moment titration and monitoring of nitroprusside.

In the setting of AMI, however, we feel sublingual nifedipine is *contraindicated*. Because the extent of the antihypertensive effect to sublingual nifedipine is not predictable, marked (and potentially dangerous) hypotension may occasionally be precipitated, further exacerbating ischemia (Shettiger and Lougani, 1989). As a result, we feel use of IV nitroglycerin (initially), IV β-blockers, or IV nitroprusside (if the patient is resistant) are all far more preferable to sublingual nifedipine for treatment of marked hypertension that occurs in association with AMI.

Verapamil

Verapamil is the calcium channel-blocking agent that exerts the most potent depressant effect on the AV node. As a result, it is extremely effective in the treatment of reentrant supraventricular tachyarrhythmias. By the same token, the drug must be used cautiously in patients with bradycardia, conduction system disturbances, and/or sick sinus syndrome.

The strong negative inotropic effect of verapamil is its greatest drawback. As a result, the drug is clearly contraindicated for use in patients with impaired left ventricular function.

Diltiazem

Diltiazem is intermediate in its hemodynamic profile to nifedipine and verapamil *(Table 12B-6)*. As a result (and because of its favorable side effect profile), this calcium channel blocking agent is preferred by many for treatment of acute and chronic ischemic heart disease. Although diltiazem is not as potent a vasodilator as nifedipine, it appears to be an equally effective antianginal agent. It has less of a depressant effect on the AV node than verapamil, but is nevertheless effective in long-term management of supraventricular tachyarrhythmias. It also exerts a depressant effect on the SA node, and must therefore be used with caution in patients with bradycardia and/or sick sinus syndrome.

Although the depressant effect of diltiazem on contractility is not as marked as that of verapamil, a number of studies have demonstrated the potential of diltiazem to exacerbate heart failure if the drug is used in patients with impaired left ventricular function *(See below.)*.

> It is important to appreciate the difference between *systolic* and *diastolic* dysfunction when discussing the potential effect of calcium channel blockers on contractility, especially in patients who already have a degree of impaired left ventricular function. Overall, heart failure most commonly results from **systolic dysfunction,** in which cardiac chambers are typically dilated and poorly contractile. Volume overload and pulmo-

Table 12B-7

Dosing of Selected Calcium Channel Blocking Agents		
Drug	**Initial Dose (mg)**	**Usual Maximal Dose/Day**
Nifedipine	10 mg PO Tid	90-120 mg/day
Procardia XL	30 mg PO Qd	60-90 mg/day
Nicardipine	20 mg PO Tid, Qid	160 mg/day
Isradapine	2.5 mg PO Bid	20 mg/day
Felodipine	2.5 to 5.0 mg PO Qd	20-40 mg/day
Diltiazem	30-60 mg PO Tid, Qid (or an equivalent amount of sustained release forms of the drug)	360 mg/day
Verapamil	80 mg PO Tid (or 240 mg Qd of sustained release forms of the drug)	360-480 mg/day

nary congestion follow. Medical treatment of this form of heart failure (due to systolic dysfunction) consists of diuretics, vasodilators (especially ACE-inhibitors), nitrates (to reduce preload), and in the chronic setting digitalis (for its positive inotropic effect).

In contrast, contractility is preserved (and sometimes even *increased*) with **diastolic dysfunction.** Rather than development of left ventricular dilatation, concentric hypertrophy (leading to a *decrease* in actual chamber cavity size) is the usual end result. Thus, the principal problem with this form of heart failure is *inadequate ventricular filling.* Agents that increase contractility (such as digitalis) are contraindicated because they further impair ventricular filling. Diuretics, nitrates, and vasodilators may all be used, but caution is essential to ensure that these drugs do not exacerbate the condition by making the patient hypovolemic. Medical treatment for pure diastolic dysfunction consists of *negatively inotropic agents.* Thus verapamil, diltiazem, and/or β-blockers are all drugs of choice for treatment of heart failure due to diastolic dysfunction.

Clinically, heart failure that develops acutely as the result of AMI is almost invariably due to systolic dysfunction (impaired contractility in the area of infarction). It is important to realize, however, that as many as one third of all patients with *chronic* congestive heart failure (especially elderly patients with long-term hypertension) have a significant component of diastolic dysfunction (Kessler, 1988). Recognition of such individuals (i.e., by echocardiography*) has obvious clinical implications in view of dramatically different treatment considerations for systolic and diastolic dysfunction.

---

*Echocardiography is an invaluable noninvasive diagnostic tool for evaluation of patients with heart failure. In addition to providing insight to the possible underlying cause of heart failure (i.e., valvular disease, cardiomyopathy), it usually allows the clinician to determine if systolic or diastolic dysfunction is present.

Efficacy of Calcium Channel Blockers in Treatment of AMI

Up until recently, data from at least 28 randomized trials (involving more than 19,000 patients) on the use of calcium channel blockers in AMI had not shown a beneficial effect. If anything, results from a number of these studies suggested a trend toward *increasing* mortality (Yusuf et al, 1988; Held et al, 1989). Although the reason for these disappointing results is not completely clear, it may be related to an increase in oxygen consumption from precipitation of reflex tachycardia in an ischemic patient (as may occur with nifedipine), or a direct negative inotropic effect (from verapamil or diltiazem) in a patient in whom the infarct-related artery is totally occluded (Messerli, 1990).

Careful examination of selected studies suggest that certain special subsets of patients may benefit from the use of certain calcium channel blockers in the peri-infarction period. The best known of these trials is the Multicenter Diltiazem Reinfarction Study (Gibson et al, 1986).

In this study, administration of **diltiazem** in a dose of 90 mg every 6 hours (begun 24 to 72 hours after the onset of infarction), was shown to be effective in preventing early reinfarction and severe angina in patients with *non-Q wave infarction.* Patients at highest risk of reinfarction were those who continued to have post-infarction angina associated with ischemic ECG changes. This was the group who appeared to benefit most from post-infarction use of diltiazem (Gibson et al, 1987; Skolnick and Frishman, 1989). Unfortunately, adverse effects (i.e., bradyarrhythmias such as 1° AV block, sinus bradycardia, and prolonged sinus pauses) were increased in the treated group, and long-term benefit (beyond the first few weeks of the post-infarction period) from diltiazem was not demonstrated.

A larger, randomized, double-blind, placebo-controlled trial of over 2,400 survivors of AMI examined the *long-term* effect of diltiazem on mortality and reinfarction (Multicenter Diltiazem Postinfarction Trial Research Group, 1988).

> Patients enrolled in this trial (known as the MDPIT study) received either diltiazem (in a dose of 60 mg every 6 hours) or placebo while still hospitalized (within 3-15 days of the onset of infarction). Patients were followed for a mean period of 2 years. Overall mortality in the study was not reduced by treatment with diltiazem. However, subgroup analysis demonstrated a definite benefit with treatment following AMI in patients who had normal ventricular function. In contrast, mortality was *increased* by diltiazem treatment in patients with evidence of left ventricular dysfunction (diagnosed either clinically or by pulmonary congestion on chest X-ray).
>
> Analysis in the group of patients with an ejection fraction of *less* than 40% revealed a 21% risk of developing clinical heart failure if they were treated with diltiazem, compared to a 12% risk if they were given placebo (p = 0.004). In contrast, the risk of developing clinical heart failure was only 4% among patients with an ejection fraction of 40% or greater *regardless* of whether or not they received diltiazem (Goldstein et al, 1991).
>
> Additional subgroup analysis in this study among patients with non-Q-wave infarction again demonstrated a reduction in the incidence of reinfarction.

The most recent study demonstrating a beneficial effect from treatment of AMI patients with calcium channel blockers is the DAVIT II Trial (Danish Study Group on Verapamil in Myocardial Infarction, 1990).

> DAVIT II was a follow-up trial of DAVIT I (1984). In the previous trial, administration of verapamil in the early post-infarction period did not reduce overall mortality after 6 months. However, retrospective analysis of the period between day 22 and 180 revealed a significantly lower mortality in the group treated with verapamil compared to placebo.
>
> As a result of the 1984 study, the protocol for DAVIT II was developed with the goal of determining whether treatment with **verapamil** (in a dose of 120 mg three times a day) begun in the second week after AMI could improve prognosis at 12 to 18 months after infarction. A total of nearly 1800 patients were enrolled in the randomized, double-blind, placebo-controlled multicenter DAVIT II Trial. Among those patients who did not develop heart failure while in the coronary care unit, *major event rates* (i.e., death or reinfarction) at 18 months were decreased by 26% from 19.7% in the placebo group to 14.6% in the verapamil-treated group (p = 0.01). In contrast, among study subjects who did develop clinical heart failure while in the coronary care unit, major event rates at 18 months were significantly higher (approximately 24%) *regardless* of whether or not verapamil was taken.

Thus it appears that treatment of survivors of AMI with verapamil (in a dose of 360 mg/day begun 1 to 2 weeks after infarction) is "cardioprotective" (reducing mortality and the rate of reinfarction) at 18 months provided that there was no evidence of clinical heart failure during the hospital stay. How to "cardioprotect" AMI patients during the first week of the post-infarction period, whether to use a β-blocker or verapamil (or both) as cardioprotection in the post-infarction period, and whether other calcium antagonists might also be cardioprotective if started 1 to 2 weeks after infarction are questions that remain to be answered (Messerli, 1990).

> It is possible that the reason earlier studies in the literature (on the use of calcium channel blockers in AMI) failed to show a benefit (and were sometimes deleterious) is because of the much greater likelihood that the infarct-related artery was still completely occluded at the time drug therapy was initiated. As a result, there may have been little to gain (since the vessel was still occluded) and much to lose (development of reflex tachycardia/increased oxygen consumption from nifedipine, negative inotropic effect with diltiazem or verapamil) from early initiation of drug therapy (Messerli, 1990). Continued recanalization naturally occurs with time, which may account for the improved response to calcium antagonists when they are started later (*after* the first week) instead of earlier. In support of this theory is the data from the DAVIT I Study which showed a *greater* mortality during the first week in patients who were treated with verapamil (Skolnick and Frishman, 1989), and the Multicenter Diltiazem Reinfarction Study (Gibson et al, 1986) and MDPIT Trial (1988) which specifically demonstrate benefit for patients with non-Q-wave (i.e., "incomplete") infarction.
>
> It should also be remembered that most of the cohorts of patients in studies on the use of calcium antagonists in AMI were not treated with thrombolytic therapy. Early reperfusion of the infarct-related artery (by thrombolytic therapy) may well enable calcium antagonists to exert a much more positive effect than was seen in the earlier studies for the same reason cited above. Calcium antagonists may exert an additional benefit in this setting by preventing reocclusion (which may be precipitated by spasm?) of vessels opened by thrombolytic therapy. (ACC/AHA Task Force, 1990).
>
> Finally, use of an intravenous calcium channel blocking agent (IV diltiazem) has now been approved.* It is possible that the adverse effect of oral and sublingual calcium antagonists is related to the variations in absorption, distribution, and clearance that are inherent with the use of such preparations. Administration of the drug by continuous IV infusion should largely resolve this problem, and may therefore be more beneficial for treatment of acute ischemic syndromes (Jaffe, 1992). Clearly, additional trials on the use of calcium antagonists in patients with AMI will have to be performed in the current thrombolytic era (utilizing both oral and intravenous formulations) before the true role of these agents in this setting can be determined.

In an attempt to assimilate findings in the literature and put them into a clinical perspective, we summarize our suggested approach to the use of calcium channel blocking agents in patients with acute ischemic heart disease in *Table 12B-8*.

---

*See Chapter 14 for further discussion on the use of IV Diltiazem.

Table 12B-8

Suggested Approach to the Use of Calcium Channel Blocking Agents in Patients with Acute Ischemic Heart Disease

-Use calcium channel blocking agents freely (in addition to nitrates) in treatment of patients with unstable angina. Consider diltiazem as a drug of choice (most favorable side effect profile) unless the patient is bradycardic (in which case nifedipine or nicardipine would be preferred), or having runs of supraventricular tachyarrhythmias (in which case verapamil may be more effective).
  -With diltiazem, begin low (with 30 mg) for the first 1-2 doses, and then rapidly increase the dose to 60-90 mg PO q6h as needed for control of chest pain.

-Consider diltiazem for patients with AMI who have persistent chest pain *not* relieved by IV nitroglycerin in appropriate doses. (Realize that IV β-blockers may be more effective than diltiazem in this setting.)

-In patients without evidence of impaired left ventricular function, consider diltiazem (in addition to nitrates) for treatment of angina in the postinfarction period, especially after non-Q-wave infarction).

-Consider beginning verapamil (in a dose of 360 mg/day) as a cardioprotective agent (either alone and/or with a β-blocker) in the early postinfarction period (between day 7-15) in patients who do not demonstrate any clinical evidence of heart failure.

-Be extremely cautious using diltiazem in patients with impaired left ventricular function (i.e., ejection fraction of *less* than 40%). Avoid verapamil entirely in such patients. Consider nifedipine (perhaps in the sustained-release form) or nicardipine as preferred calcium channel blocking agents for such patients.

-Avoid using sublingual nifedipine for treatment of hypertensive urgency in patients with acute ischemic heart disease. IV nitroglycerin (and/or an IV β-blocker) is the treatment of choice for significant hypertension in the setting of AMI.

-Avoid nifedipine (and nicardipine) in patients with acute ischemic heart disease who demonstrate resting tachycardia.

-Be open to the possibility that calcium channel blockers may well prove to be much more effective in the management of AMI in the era of thrombolytic therapy (since prevention of vasospasm may be an important mechanism of maintaining patency after reperfusion with thrombolytic therapy!)

-Be open to future developments regarding the use of IV diltiazem for the treatment of acute ischemic heart disease syndromes (See Chapter 14).

References

Abraham AS, Rosenmann D, Meshulam Z, Zion M, Eylath U: Serum, lymphocyte and erythrocyte potassium, magnesium and calcium concentrations and their relation to tachyarrhythmias in patients with acute myocardial infarction, *Am J Med* 81:983-988, 1986.

Abraham AS, Rosenmann D, Kramer M, Balkin J, Zion MM, Farbstien H, Eylath U: Magnesium in the prevention of lethal arrhythmias in acute myocardial infarction, *Arch Intern Med* 147:753-755, 1987.

American College of Cardiology/American Heart Association Task Force: Guidelines for the early management of patients with acute myocardial infarction, *Circulation* 82:664-707, 1990.

American Heart Association: Textbook of advanced cardiac life support, ed 3, Dallas, 1987, The Association.

Beta-Blocker Heart Attack Trial Research Group: A randomized trial of propranolol in patients with acute myocardial infarction. I—Mortality results, *JAMA* 247:1707-1714, 1982.

Bigger JT, Weld FM, Rolnitzky LM: Which postinfarction ventricular arrhythmias should be treated? *Am Heart J* 103:660-666, 1982.

Bigger JT, Coromilas J: Identification of patients at risk for arrhythmic death: role of Holter ECG recording. In Josephson ME (ed): Sudden cardiac death, cardiovascular clinics, Philadelphia, 1983, FA Davis Company.

Bigger JT: Antiarrhythmic treatment: an overview, *Am J Cardiol* 53:3B-16B, 1984.

Campbell CA, Przyklenk K, Kloner RA: Infarct size reduction: a review of the clinical trials, *J Clin Pharmacol* 26:317-329, 1986.

Conti RC: Drug therapy of patients with acute myocardial infarction in the era of thrombolysis, *Mod Conc Cardiovasc Dis* 58:19-24, 1989.

Côté P, Gueret P, Bourasa MG: Systemic and coronary hemodynamic effects of diazepam in patients with normal and diseased coronary arteries, *Circulation* 50:1210-1216, 1974.

The Danish Study Group on Verapamil in Myocardial Infarction: Verapamil in acute myocardial infarction, *Eur Heart J* 5:516-528, 1984.

The Danish Study Group on Verapamil in Myocardial Infarction: Effect of verapamil on mortality and major events after acute myocardial infarction (The Danish Verapamil Infarction Trial II- Dvait II), *Am J Cardiol* 66:779-785, 1990.

Ferguson JJ, Diver DJ, Boldt M, Pasternak RC: Significance of nitroglycerin-induced hypotension with inferior wall acute myocardial infarction, *Am J Cardiol* 64:311-314, 1989.

Fesmire FM, Wears RL: The utility of the presence or absence of chest pain in patients with suspected acute myocardial infarction, *Am J Emerg Med* 7:372-377, 1989.

Fillmore SJ, Shapiro M, Killip T: Arterial oxygen tension in acute myocardial infarction: serial analysis of clinical state and blood-gas changes, *Am Heart J* 79:620-629, 1970.

Gibson RS, Boden WE, Theroux P, Strauss HD, Pratt CM, Gheorghiade M, Capone RJ, Crawford MH, Schlant RC, Kleiger RE, Young PM, Schechtman K, Perryman MB, Roberts R, and the Diltiazem Reinfarction Study Group: Diltiazem and reinfarction in patients with non-Q wave myocardial infarction: results of a double-blind, randomized, multicenter trial, *N Engl J Med* 315:423-429, 1986.

Gibson RS, Young PM, Boden WE, Schechtman K, Roberts R: Prognostic significance and beneficial effect of diltiazem on the incidence of early recurrent ischemia after non-Q-wave myocardial infarction: results from the Multicenter Diltiazem Reinfarction Study, Am J Cardiol 60:203-209, 1987.

Gillis RA, Thibodeaux H, Barr L: Antiarrhythmia properties of chlordiazepoxide, *Circulation* 49:272-282, 1974.

Goldstein RE, Boccuzzi SJ, Cruess D, Nattel S, the Adverse Experience Committee, and the Multicenter Diltiazem Postinfarction Research Group: Diltiazem increases late-onset congestive heart failure in postinfarction patients with early reduction in ejection fraction, *Circulation* 83:52-60, 1991.

Grauer K, Gums J: Ventricular arrhythmias. Part II: Special concerns in evaluation, *J Am Bd Fam Pract* 1:201-206, 1988.

Gregoratos G: Management of uncomplicated acute myocardial infarction. In Parmley WW, Chatterjee K (eds): Cardiology: physiology, pharmacology, diagnosis, Philadelphia, 1990, JB Lippincott Company.

Held PH, Yusuf S, Furberg CD: Calcium channel blockers in acute myocardial infarction and unstable angina: an overview, *Br Med J* 299:1187-1192, 1989.

Hine LK, Laird N, Hewitt P, Chalmers TC: Meta-analytic evidence against prophylactic use of lidocaine in acute myocardial infarction, *Arch Int Med* 149:2694-2698, 1989.

Hancock EW: Ischemic heart disease: acute myocardial infarction. In Rubenstein E, Federman DD (eds): Scientific American Medicine, New York, Section I. Chapter X: 1990.

Hjalmarson A: Early intervention with a beta-blocking drug after acute myocardial infarction, *Am J Cardiol* 54:11E-13E, 1984.

Hlatky MA, Cotugno HE, Mark DB, O'Connor C, Califf R: Trends in physician management of uncomplicated acute infarction: 1970 to 1987, *Am J Cardiol* 61:515-518, 1988.

Jaffe AS: Use of intravenous diltiazem in patients with acute coronary artery disease, *Am J Cardiol* 69:25B-29B, 1992.

Kern MJ: Perspective: the cellular influences of calcium antagonists on systemic and coronary hemodynamics, *Am J Cardiol* 69:3B-7B, 1992.

Kessler K: Heart failure with normal systolic function, *Arch Int Med* 148:2109-2111, 1988.

Kirshenbaum JM, Kloner RF, McGowan N, Antman EM: Use of an ultrashort-acting beta-receptor blocker (esmolol) in patients with acute myocardial ischemia and relative contraindications to beta-blockade therapy, *J Am Coll Cardiol* 12:773-780, 1988.

Kirshenbaum JM: Nonthrombolytic intervention in acute myocardial infarction, *Am J Cardiol* 64:25B-28B, 1989.

Kober G, Schneider W, Kaltenbach M: Can the progression of coronary sclerosis be influenced by calcium antagonists? *J Cardiovasc Pharmacol* 13 (suppl 4): S2-S6, 1989.

Lichstein E: Why do beta-receptor blockers decrease mortality after myocardial infarction? *JACC* 6:973-975, 1985.

Lichtlen PR, Hugenholtz PG, Rafflenbeul W, Hecker H, Jost S, Deckers JW, and the INTACT Group Investigators: Retardation of angiographic progression of coronary artery disease by nifedipine, Lancet 335:1109-1113, 1990.

Liebson PR: Clinical studies of drug reversal of hypertensive left ventricular hypertrophy, *Am J Hypertens* 3:512-517, 1990.

Lown B, Verrier RL: Neural activity and ventricular fibrillation, *N Engl J Med* 294:1165-1170, 1976.

MacMahon S, Collins R, Peto R, Koster RW, Yusuf S: Effects of prophylactic lidocaine in suspected acute myocardial infarction: an overview of results from the randomized, controlled trials, *JAMA* 260:1910-1916, 1988.

McEvoy GK: AHFS drug information, Bethesda, Md, 1990, Am Soc Hosp Pharmacists.

Mehta JL: Influence of calcium-channel blockers on platelet function and arachidonic acid metabolism, *Am J Cardiol* 55:158B-168B, 1985.

Mehta P, Nicolini FA, Mehta JL: Influence of extracellular calcium on superoxide radical generation in cholesterol-poor and cholesterol-rich neutrophils: Effect of slow-channel calcium blockers, *Clin Res* 39:459A, 1991.

Mehta JL, Nicolini FA, Donnelly WH, Nichols WW: Platelet-leukocyte-endothelial interactions in coronary artery disease, *Am J Cardiol* 69:8B-13B, 1992.

Messerli FH: "Cardioprotection"—not all calcium antagonists are created equal, *Am J Cardiol* 66:855-856, 1990.

Mitchell JM, Wheeler WS: The golden hours of the myocardial infarction: nonthrombolytic interventions, *Ann Emerg Med* 20:540-548, 1991.

Moss AJ: Secondary prevention with calcium channel-blocking drugs in patients after myocardial infarction: a critical review, *Circulation* 75 (suppl V): V148-V153, 1987.

The Multicenter Diltiazem Postinfarction Trial Research Group: The effect of diltiazem on mortality and reinfarction after myocardial infarction, *N Engl J Med* 319:385-392, 1988.

Peter CT, Helfant RH: Postinfarction ventricular tachycardia and fibrillation: reassessing the role of drug therapy and approach to the high risk patient, *J Am Coll Cardiol* 16:531-532, 1990.

Roberts R: Recognition, diagnosis and prognosis of early reinfarction: the role of calcium channel-blockers, *Circulation* 75 (suppl V): V139-V147, 1987.

Ryden L, Ariniego R, Arnman K, Herlitz J, Hjalmarson A, Holmberg S, Reyes C, Smedgard P, Svedberg K, Vedin A, Wangstein F, Waldenstrom A, Wilhelmsson C, Wedel H, Yahamoto M: A double-blind trial of metoprolol in acute myocardial infarction: effects on ventricular tachyarrhythmias, *N Eng J Med* 308:614-618, 1983.

Shechter M, Hod H, Marks N, Behar S, Kaplinsky E, Rabinowitz B: Beneficial effect of magnesium sulfate in acute myocardial infarction, *Am J Cardiol* 66:271-274, 1990.

Shettigear VR, Lougani R: Adverse effects of sublingual nifedipine in acute myocardial infarction, *Crit Care Med* 17:196-197, 1989.

Skolnick AE, Frishman WH: Calcium channel blockers in myocardial infarction, *Arch Intern Med* 149:1669-1677, 1989.

Teo KK, Yusuf S, Collins R, Held PH, Peto R: Effects of intravenous magnesium in suspected acute myocardial infarction: overview of randomized trials, *BMJ* 303:1499-1503, 1991.

Tofler GH, Stone PH, Muller JE, Rutherford JD, Willich SN, Gustafson NF, Poole WK, Sobel BE, Willerson JT, Robertson T, Passamani E, Braunwald E, and the MILIS Study Group: Prognosis after cardiac arrest due to ventricular tachycardia or ventricular fibrillation associated with acute myocardial infarction (The MILIS Study), *Am J Cardiol* 60:755-761, 1987.

Tzivoini D, Keren A: Suppression of ventricular arrhythmias by magnesium, *Am J Cardiol* 65:1397-1399, 1990, (editorial).

Volpi A, Cavalli A, Franzosi MG, Maggioni A, Mauri F, Santoro E, Tognoni G: One-year prognosis of primary ventricular fibrillation complicating acute myocardial infarction, *Am J Cardiol* 63:1174-1178, 1989.

Volpi A, Cavalli A, Santoro E, Tognoni G: Incidence and prognosis of secondary ventricular fibrillation in acute myocardial infarction—evidence for a protective effect of thrombolytic therapy, *Circulation* 82:1279-1288, 1990.

Wesley RC, Resh W, Zimmerman D: Reconsideration of the routine and preferential use of lidocaine in the emergent treatment of ventricular arrhythmias, *Crit Care Med* 19:1439-1444, 1991.

Wilber DJ, Olshansky B, Moran JF, Scanlon PJ: Electrophysiological testing and nonsustained ventricular tachycardia: use and limitations in patients with coronary artery disease and impaired ventricular function, *Circulation* 82:350-358, 1990.

Willems AR, Tijssen JGP, van Capelle FJL, Kingma JH, Hauer RNW, Vermeulen FEE, Brugada P, van Hoogenhuyze DCA, Janse MJ, and the Dutch Ventricular Tachycardia Study Group: Determinants of prognosis in symptomatic ventricular tachycardia or ventricular fibrillation late after myocardial infarction, *J Am Coll Cardiol* 16:521-530, 1990.

Woods KL, Fletcher S, Roffe C, Haider Y: Intravenous magnesium sulfate in suspected acute myocardial infarctions: results of the second Leicester Intravenous Magnesium Intervention Trial (LIMIT-2), *Lancet* 339:1553–1558, 1992.

Yusuf S, Wittes J, Friedman L: Overview of results of randomized clinical trials in heart disease. Part I: Treatments following myocardial infarction, *JAMA* 260:2088-2093, 1988.

Yusuf S: The use of beta adrenergic blocking agents, IV nitrates, and calcium channel blocking agents following acute myocardial infarction, *Chest* 93:25S-28S, 1988.

Yusuf S, Wittes J, Friedman L: Overview of results of randomized clinical trials in heart disease: Part II: Unstable angina, heart failure, primary prevention with aspirin, and risk factor modification, *JAMA* 260:2259-2263, 1988.

SECTION C

REPERFUSION AND ACUTE INTERVENTIONAL THERAPY

Thrombolytic Therapy

CONSENSUS CONCEPTS

By far, the most controversial area in the management of AMI regards the use of thrombolytic therapy. Despite our expectation that debate on various aspects of thrombolytic therapy will continue, we find it encouraging that a general consensus seems to be emerging on many of the most important issues:

1. *Thrombolytic therapy works.* Regardless of which particular thrombolytic agent is used (streptokinase, APSAC, rt-PA, urokinase, or some other agent), administration of thrombolytic therapy during the *early* hours of AMI to appropriately selected patients will:
   - Reestablish flow to the **infarct-related artery (IRA)** in a significant percentage of patients.
   - Limit infarct size (and thus preserve—or at least *minimize* deterioration of) ventricular function.
   - Reduce the incidence of AMI-associated lethal ventricular arrhythmias.
   - Improve short-term and long-term prognosis in patients with a beneficial response.

Much more important than debate about which particular thrombolytic agent is selected is *making the decision to strongly consider use of **some** thrombolytic agent—as soon as possible*—for appropriately selected patients with AMI.

---

2. *The reason thrombolytic therapy works is that it reestablishes flow to the IRA.* It is now generally accepted that the cause of AMI in the overwhelming majority ($\geq$90%) of cases is sudden, *total occlusion* of a coronary vessel. Virtually all clinical manifestations and/or complications of AMI are the result (either directly or indirectly) of this sudden total occlusion to coronary flow. Knowing this facilitates our basic approach to management, which is to try to reverse the *precipitating* cause of the infarct (i.e., *to reestablish flow to the IRA*) in the hope of reducing infarct size.

3. *Time* is the most critical (*limiting*) factor regarding the administration of thrombolytic therapy (and the hoped for benefits from such therapy). With respect to the course of an acute evolving infarction— ***"Time is muscle"!*** Therefore:

The sooner in the course of AMI that thrombolytic therapy can be administered, the larger the amount of myocardium that can potentially be salvaged.

It is from this tenet that the concept of a ***"window of opportunity"*** has evolved. The "window" refers to a time period during which reestablishment of flow is most likely to be able to salvage myocardium. Although definitions vary, most authorities in the field seem to set their usual *upper limit* for this period at 6 hours (since the process of myocardial necrosis is almost always complete by this time), and reperfusion of otherwise *uncomplicated* cases of AMI after 6 hours is unlikely to substantially affect ultimate infarct size. Considering the usual delay of patients with new-onset chest pain in seeking medical attention (an average of *1-3 hours!*), and the unavoidable time required to mobilize resources and institute therapeutic measures, the period remaining in which to assess the patient and decide on their potential suitability for acute intervention (i.e., thrombolytic therapy and/or angioplasty) is often quite limited indeed.

4. *Rapid assessment and prompt institution of treatment are the KEY components of success.* Everything possible must be done to expedite the process. Thus, *ALL* patients who present with a history of new-onset chest pain should be immediately attended to—they *ALL* should have an ECG performed STAT (i.e., within *minutes* of their arrival)—and the ECG must be read *"equally STAT"* by the clinician entrusted to their care. Based on information from a brief history, rapid physical examination, and interpretation of the initial ECG, an assessment can then be made regarding the likelihood of AMI and the potential suitability of the patient for thrombolytic therapy.

5. *Regardless* of whether or not thrombolytic therapy is administered, *other appropriate treatment measures should be initiated as soon as possible once a preliminary diagnosis of acute ischemic heart disease/suspected AMI is made.*

In addition to our discussion of the specific treatment measures covered in Section B, several points should be emphasized regarding the management of patients with AMI who are treated with thrombolytic therapy. First, *every effort must be made to completely **relieve chest pain** as early as possible in the process.* IV nitroglycerin, β-blockers, calcium antagonists, and/or morphine should *NEVER* be withheld for fear that giving these agents might "mask" the principal clinical indicator of reperfusion (i.e., relief of chest pain).

Second, **lidocaine prophylaxis** should probably be considered for all patients who receive thrombolytic therapy. Although reperfusion arrhythmias usually do not deteriorate to sustained ventricular tachycardia or ventricular fibrillation, routine administration of lidocaine may help provide an additional measure of protection against this possibility.

Finally, **aspirin** should be given to *ALL* patients with acute ischemic heart disease/suspected AMI as soon as this diagnosis is made (provided there are no contraindications to the use of this drug). Neither thrombolytic therapy nor heparization preclude the use of aspirin in this setting, and the addition of aspirin appears to be synergistic when combined with other treatment.

6. *Acute* (i.e., at the time of presentation) *cardiac catheterization is not required to make the diagnosis of AMI, nor for making the decision to institute thrombolytic therapy.* History (of *new-onset* chest pain) and *definitive* ECG changes suffice for this purpose. Furthermore, cardiac catheterization immediately *after* completion of thrombolytic therapy is *not* essential to demonstrate recanalization (i.e., restoration of coronary flow) in patients who are otherwise doing well clinically (i.e., normotensive and without chest pain or clinical evidence of persistent ongoing ischemia).

The reason cardiac catheterization is not routinely recommended immediately after completion of thrombolytic therapy in patients who are otherwise doing well clinically is that intervention at this time (i.e., with angioplasty) has *not* been shown to improve prognosis, and it may be harmful (i.e., increased bleeding complications, need for emergency surgery).

7. In contrast, *further investigation and/or treatment measures* (i.e., urgent catheterization, angioplasty, emergency bypass surgery, etc.) *may be needed* for patients who remain unstable (and/or have persistent chest pain) *after* completion of thrombolytic therapy.

8. *Thrombolytic therapy does not solve the problem.* Although reestablishment of coronary flow (by clot dissolution) may be invaluable in limiting infarct size and preserving ventricular function, *thrombolytic therapy does little to reverse the underlying atherosclerotic process.* As a result, efforts to prevent reocclusion (i.e., short-term heparin and continued use of aspirin) *and* full evaluation with consideration for a more definitive revascularization procedure once the patient's condition has stabilized must be included in the management plan.

CLINICAL ASSIMILATION OF MAJOR CONCLUSIONS FROM THE LITERATURE

Thrombolytic therapy works. Data from an ever increasing number of studies (on well over 100,000 patients!) overwhelmingly support the use of this intervention in patients with AMI. Unfortunately, assimilation of information from this seemingly endless stream of clinical trials is complicated by the multitude of study protocols (using different doses of the different thrombolytic agents), varying patient populations (obtained from multiple sites in many different countries), and the use of different clinical endpoints.

Insight into a particular trial is often provided by the type of clinical endpoint selected. The most definitive findings have been obtained from trials that use **recanalization** as their endpoint (as documented by cardiac catheterization performed immediately before *and* immediately after administration of thrombolytic therapy). Unfortunately, performance of such trials not only requires catheterization twice during the early course of AMI, but also unnecessarily delays institution of thrombolytic therapy (because the patient must be catheterized *before* the drug can be given). As a result, true recanalization trials are no longer commonly done (Tiefenbrunn and Sobel, 1989).

Other trials choose **patency rate** at a *later point* in the process as their endpoint (determined from a single catheterization performed hours to several days or weeks *after* thrombolytic therapy). By definition such studies do *not* document complete occlusion of a coronary artery before thrombolytic therapy is begun. Consequently, results are much harder to interperet because they unavoidably include an unknown percentage of patients with acute ischemic syndromes other than AMI (i.e., "incomplete" thrombotic occlusion from unstable angina or a "stuttering course" infarction). This is especially true when patency rates are defined by results of cardiac catheterization performed more than 24 hours after thrombolytic therapy, since *spontaneous reperfusion* (by the body's own inherent thrombolytic mechanism) has already occurred at this time in up to one third of cases (DeWood et al, 1980).

The last type of endpoint used in trials of thrombolytic therapy is purely **clinical** in nature, and based on parameters such as reinfarction rate, anginal recurrence rate, late mortality, and/or objective determination of ultimate ventricular function. Although easier to carry out, such studies do not provide information regarding reperfusion rates, and much larger numbers of patients are needed to demonstrate meaningful results compared to a placebo control group.

Rather than recount the specific protocols and results from each of the major trials on thrombolytic therapy, we have opted instead to synthesize the most important clinical findings.

CHOICE OF THROMBOLYTIC AGENT

At the present time, three thrombolytic agents are in common use in the United States: streptokinase, APSAC (**A**nisoylated **P**lasminogen **S**treptokinase **A**ctivator **C**omplex), and rt-PA (**r**ecombinant **t**issue-**P**lasminogen **A**ctivator). Clinical characteristics of these agents are compared in *Table 12C-1.*

Table 12C-1

Comparison of Selected Thrombolytic Agents			
	Streptokinase (Streptase/Kabikinase)	**APSAC** (Antistreplase/Eminase)	**rt-PA** (Alteplase/Activase)
Elimination half-life	20-80 minutes (although clinical effects last longer)	90 minutes (although clinical effects last longer)	6-8 minute first phase half-life—and a 50 minute elimination half-life
Dose	1.5 million units infused over 30-60 minutes	30 units infused over 2-5 minutes	100 mg infused over 3 hours (10 mg initially, 50 mg over the next hour, and 20 mg over each of the next 2 hours)*
Expected reperfusion rate	50-60%**	50-70%**	60-80%
Hypotensive effect	+ +	+ +	+
Allergic reactions	Yes	Yes (APSAC contains streptokinase!)	No
Antigenic reactions	Yes! -Caution if pt had recent strep infection -Do *not* readminister STK for ≥6-9 mo	Yes! -Caution if pt had recent strep infection -Do *not* readminister APSAC for ≥6-9 mo	No -Ab do not develop since rt-PA is not a foreign protein
Cost	~$100-200	~$1,700	~$2,200-2,500
Miscellaneous points	-Efficacy greatest if administered within first few hrs -Slightly lower risk of cerebral hemorrhage than for APSAC or rt-PA (?) -IV heparin may help to maintain patency of the IRA	-Dosing regimen is the most convenient! -IV heparin may help to maintain patency of the IRA	-Short half-life advantageous if a bleeding complication develops -Most effective at opening IRA -More "clot specific" (at least theoretically) -IV heparin essential; MUST be started before end of infusion!

*Some studies suggest more rapid infusion of rt-PA (i.e., over ≤90 min) may increase reperfusion rate to ≥80%-90%
**Reperfusion rates obtained with streptokinase and APSAC are best when the drug is initiated within the first *few* hours of the onset of symptoms.

Streptokinase

Streptokinase is a bacterial protein produced by the Lancefield group C strains of β-hemolytic streptococci (Heras et al, 1988). It was the first agent to be widely used for treatment of AMI after introduction of the thrombolytic era in the late 1970's. Early studies on *intracoronary (IC)* use of streptokinase demonstrated superior recanalization rates (of approximately 75%) compared to 50% or less

with IV administration of the drug (Rentrop, 1985; Tiefenbrunn and Sobel, 1989). At the present time, however, the issue of IC administration has almost become academic since only a minority of hospitals in this country maintain both the facilities and staffing to provide round-the-clock catheterization capability. Moreover, use of thrombolytic protocols with IV administration of drug enables earlier initiation of treatment (since acute catheterization is no longer necessarily required), with the result that comparable reperfusion rates may now be obtained with IV forms of thrombolytic agents.

Streptokinase is decidedly more effective if administered early (i.e., within the first 3 hours of the onset of symptoms). For example, in the large GISSI-1 Trial, an almost 50% reduction in mortality was achieved when streptokinase was started within the first hour of the onset of symptoms. (Gruppo Italiano, 1986).

> The usual dose of streptokinase is 1.5 million units infused over a 30 to 60 minute period. Because the drug is a foreign protein, antibody formation is common. As a result, allergic reactions and/or antibody-mediated resistance may occur. In most cases, reactions are not severe with the initial dose, but may become so with subsequent dosing (Tiefenbrunn and Sobel, 1989). In particular, antibody titers sufficiently high to neutralize at least 50% of a standard dose of the drug have been found in up to 90% of patients screened 4 to 8 months after receiving the drug (Jalihal and Morris, 1990). Consequently, if readministration is contemplated at any time during the subsequent 9 months, another (non-streptokinase-containing) thrombolytic agent should be selected. Similarly, a non-streptokinase-containing agent may be preferred for patients suspected of having a recent streptococcal infection (Muller and Topol, 1990). Use of steroids and/or diphenhydramine may help reduce the incidence of allergic reactions (when given prophylactically), or help with treatment if a reaction occurs.
>
> Because hypotension commonly occurs with the use of IV streptokinase, blood pressure must be closely monitored during drug administration (Tiefenbrunn and Sobel, 1989; Rowe et al, 1989). The drug may need to be discontinued on occasion if hypotension persists despite reducing the rate and/or temporarily stopping the infusion.

Clots are lysed by the action of the proteolytic enzyme *plasmin*. Thrombolytic agents all induce thrombolysis by directly or indirectly producing plasmin from *plasminogen*. Because streptokinase binds to and activates *circulating* plasminogen, its mechanism of action is generalized. Not only does it lyse the clot, but it also depletes body stores of certain circulating plasma proteins (including fibrinogen and other procoagulant factors). As a result, use of streptokinase produces a *systemic lytic state* (i.e., it is *not* clot-selective). Although the elimination half-life of streptokinase is no more than 80 minutes, clinical effects last significantly longer because of an indirect action (from depletion of circulating fibrinogen/pro-coagulant factors and increased concentrations of fibrinogen degradation products that potentiate anticoagulation by inhibiting fibrin polymerization). Clinically, this accounts for the persistent anticoagulant effect of streptokinase, and the much less urgent need (than for rt-PA) to supplement its activity with IV heparin after administration of the drug is completed. Thus, in the large GISSI-2 and International Study Group Trials (which included over 20,000 patients), the addition of heparin (beginning 12 hours after streptokinase administration and continued throughout the hospital stay) did *not* improve clinical outcome, and may have resulted in a slightly increased incidence in the number of bleeding complications (Gruppo Italiano, 1990; International Study Group, 1990).

> If supplementation of the effect of IV streptokinase is desired, the PTT should be checked after completion of drug infusion, and every four hours thereafter. IV heparin may be started (at an infusion rate of 1,000 units/hour) once the PTT falls to between two and three times of its control value.

The principal advantage of streptokinase is cost, with the agent being significantly cheaper than both APSAC and rt-PA *(Table 12C-1)*. Therefore when cost is a factor, a good case can be made for selecting streptokinase if the patient is seen *early* in the course (i.e., within the first 3 hours), provided that the blood pressure is stable and there has been no previous exposure to the drug within the previous 9 months.

> Although additional confirmatory studies are needed, preliminary data from the large ISIS-3 Trial suggests a slight but significant increase in the incidence of cerebral hemorrhage with the use of either APSAC or rt-PA compared to IV streptokinase (Check, 1991).

APSAC

APSAC is an acylated inactive complex of streptokinase and human lys-plasminogen. This second generation thrombolytic agent clinically acts as a "sustained release" form of streptokinase with enhanced bioavailability at the site of clot and a prolonged duration of action (of several hours) following IV bolus administration of the drug (Tiefenbrunn and Sobel, 1989).

Reperfusion rates following administration of APSAC appear to be intermediate between those achieved with IV streptokinase and IV rt-PA (in the range of between 50-70%), with greatest success rates when the drug is given within 4 hours of the onset of symptoms (Anderson, 1989; ACC/AHA Task Force, 1990). Reocclusion rates are low, and appear to be somewhat less than for other thrombolytic agents (Anderson, 1989).* These features, and particularly the *ease of administration* of the drug make it an attractive alternative agent for thrombolytic therapy.

> The usual dose of APSAC is 30 units administered as an IV bolus over 2 to 5 minutes. Because the drug is a streptokinase-containing compound, precautions for use (including the potential for allergic and antigenic reactions and the tendency to produce hypotension) are similar to those for administration of IV streptokinase. The drug is slightly cheaper than rt-PA, but substantially more expensive than streptokinase.

rt-PA

Tissue-type plasminogen activator (t-PA) is a protein that is naturally produced by human tissues including

---

*Although use of IV heparin is not specifically recommended to maintain patency following administration of IV APSAC, a majority of patients in the clinical studies have received heparin for this purpose (Med Letter, 1990).

vascular endothelium and uterus (Heras et al, 1988). Initially it was isolated from cultures of human melanoma cells, but is now synthetically produced by genetic *recombinant* DNA technology (i.e., **rt**-PA). Earlier studies used a formulation consisting primarily of *double-chained* rt-PA. Shortly after completion of the TIMI-1 Trial, a new product consisting predominantly of *single-chained* rt-PA was developed. Recent studies (and current clinical practice) almost uniformly use the single-chain formulation, although a double-chain form (duteplase) was selected for use in the ISIS-3 Trial.*

The mechanism by which rt-PA induces thrombolysis differs from that of streptokinase and APSAC. Affinity for circulating plasminogen is low. Instead, rt-PA requires fibrin for its activation. In the presence of thrombus (i.e., fibrin), rt-PA combines with *clot-bound* plasminogen and activates its conversion to plasmin, which then lyses the clot. Circulating plasmin is rapidly inactivated by other circulating blood factors, limiting the degree of the systemic lytic effect.

> Although rt-PA has been touted as a "clot-specific" thrombolytic agent (that should therefore be less likely to induce systemic bleeding complications), this claim has not been fully borne out in clinical practice. Rather than the almost unattainable goal of true "clot specificity", rt-PA appears to be *fibrin specific* (Chamberlain, 1989). However, since fibrin is present not only in thrombi, but also in hemostatic plugs, the risk of bleeding complications is not necessarily reduced.

The currently used (predominantly single-chained) rt-PA formulation is most often administered as an initial 10 mg IV bolus (given over 2-3 mintues), followed by a 50 mg infusion over the next hour, and 20 mg IV infusions over the 2 succeeding hours (for a ***total dose*** of 10 + 50 + 20 + 20 = **100 mg** over 3 hours). Reperfusion rates achieved with this regimen average between 70-80%, and are superior to those obtained with other thrombolytic agents (Tiefenbrunn and Sobel, 1989).

> The obvious disadvantage of a 3-hour dosing protocol is the relatively long time required for infusion of the drug, and the need for constant monitoring during this period. As a result, other dosing regimens with rt-PA have been tried, and preliminary results are exciting. Neuhaus et al (1989) reported on a "front-loading" regimen in which the 100 mg dose is given over 90 minutes. This resulted in a recanalization rate of *greater than 90%* (as determined by catheterization performed at 90 minutes) *without* any increase in the incidence of reocclusion or bleeding complications. Other investigators have attempted single or multiple bolus regimens of rt-PA, achieving reperfusion rates that are comparable to more conventional

dosing protocols without a significant increase in complications (Tebbe et al, 1989; Tranches et al, 1990; Khan et al, 1990).

Because of the short (6-8 minute) first phase half-life of rt-PA, anticoagulation becomes an *essential* component of the regimen. Thus, IV heparin *must* be started in conjunction with rt-PA administration to maintain vessel patency. Although some centers choose to begin IV heparin at the same time they initiate rt-PA infusion, we favor *delaying heparin* until the rt-PA infusion is almost complete. Doing so allows faster resolution of anticoagulant effect should a bleeding complication develop *during* the period of rt-PA infusion (because the circulating half-life of rt-PA is short and heparin has not been started).

> The short first phase half-life of rt-PA (compared to streptokinase and APSAC) may prove to be a definite advantage if a bleeding complication does develop or if the patient becomes hemodynamically unstable and requires an immediate invasive intervention (such as surgery or intra-aortic balloon counterpulsation).

The beauty of rt-PA is its lack of antigenicity, low incidence of allergic reactions, and minimal hypotensive effect. Its major drawback is cost—a factor that must be balanced according to patient variables (especially time of presentation after onset of symptoms) and medication availability, as well as other intangible clinical factors and/or ethical considerations.

COMPARATIVE CLINICAL TRIALS

Few studies directly compare the thrombolytic effect of rt-PA and steptokinase. Unfortunately those that do have been problematic in design. In addition, there is a need for data directly comparing APSAC and rt-PA.

> The European Cooperative Study (1985) was one of the major earlier comparative trials. Overall, a strong trend was found favoring rt-PA over streptokinase for establishing early patency of the IRA. A strength of the study was early initiation of thrombolytic therapy (within an average time of 3 hours from the onset of symptoms). Because this was a *patency* trial, however, no baseline catheterization was done. As a result, documentation of total occlusion of the IRA is lacking, and definitive conclusions cannot be reached regarding the true reperfusion rate for each drug.
>
> Results from the TIMI-1 Trial are not hindered by this drawback because TIMI-1 was a true *recanalization* study (i.e., total occlusion of the IRA was documented by pre-treatment catheterization, and reperfusion was documented by post-treatment catheterization performed at 90 minutes). However, the mean time until initiation of thrombolytic therapy in this trial was significantly later (an average of almost *5 hours* after the onset of symptoms). Two other potentially problematic aspects of the TIMI-1 protocol were that the double-chained formulation of rt-PA was used, and that catheterization was performed *during* (rather than immediately after) the 3-hour rt-PA infusion (The TIMI Study Group, 1985). Nevertheless, results strongly favored rt-PA for its ability to open the infarct-related vessel. Overall patency of the IRA at 90 minutes was 62% in the group that received rt-PA, compared to only 31%

---

*The circulating half-life of the older, double-chain formulation was slightly longer than the newer single-chain formulation. As a result, a slightly higher dose (100 mg) of rt-PA is now used to obtain equipotency, compared to the 80 mg dose used formerly. Pharmacologic effects of the two formulations are similar, except for a slightly reduced tendency of the single-chain preparation to deplete fibrinogen. In vivo, the cleaving action of plasmin ends up converting a substantial portion of single-chain rt-PA to the double-chain form.

in the group that received streptokinase (p<0.01). As in other studies, streptokinase was decidedly more effective when it was administered sooner (within 4 hours) after the onset of symptoms. Compared to rt-PA, however, streptokinase was consistently less effective in opening the IRA *regardless* of the interval between the onset of symptoms and initiation of treatment.

Other trials have used late patency and clinical end points such as mortality and left ventricular function as the basis for comparison between the thrombolytic agents.

One such late patency trial was performed by White et al. (1989), in which patients with AMI (seen an average of less than 3 hours after the onset of symptoms) were randomly assigned to treatment with either rt-PA or streptokinase. Cardiac catheterization performed 3 weeks later failed to show a significant difference in either left ventricular function (as determined by ejection fraction) or patency of the IRA.

Whether clinically relevant conclusions can be drawn from late patency studies (such as the one by White et al) *is an entirely different question.* Advocates of streptokinase emphasize the importance of the "bottom line"—which for this particular study was the lack of any difference in patency rates and left ventricular function at a point in time 3 weeks after infarction. However, considering that spontaneous reperfusion occurs with time, it is possible that an early difference in opening rates between the two agents could have been "equalized" (negated) by the body's inherent thrombolytic mechanisms during the course of the 3 weeks until catheterization was performed. As a result, advocates of rt-PA question the validity of late patency trials and maintain that the key indicator of the efficacy of thrombolytic therapy is the *early opening rate*. Practically speaking, the *only* way to objectively determine such information in a clinical study is by means of a *recanalization* trial in which total occlusion of the IRA is established beforehand (by initial catheterization), and restoration of flow in the IRA is then documented by follow-up catheterization performed immediately after treatment.

Hope in finding "the answer" had been placed in the eagerly awaited results of two recently performed multicenter, international studies.

A total of more than 20,000 patients were studied in the combined GISSI-2 and International Study Group Trial (Gruppo Italiano, 1990; International Study Group, 1990). Patients were randomly assigned to treatment with either streptokinase or rt-PA (begun within 6 hours of the onset of symptoms). Additional treatment measures included aspirin (in most patients), an IV β-blocker (if there were no contraindications), and *subcutaneous* heparin (in a dose of 12,500 U Bid) beginning 12 hours *after* initiation of thrombolytic therapy. Results failed to reveal a difference in either in-hospital mortality or in the severity of left ventricular damage.

Unfortunately, results of the GISSI-2 and International Study Group Trials are difficult (if not impossible) to interpret because of a fundamental fault in their design: *Subcutaneous (rather than IV) heparin was used, and the heparin was not begun until 12 hours after starting infusion of the thrombolytic agent.* As already emphasized, administration of IV heparin in conjunction with rt-PA is an essential component of any regimen that uses this thrombolytic agent. Early reocclusion of the IRA is much more likely to occur if administration of IV heparin is either withheld or delayed (Bleich et al, 1990). Although administration of aspirin may help reduce the likelihood of reocclusion, it is not nearly as effective in doing so without use of concomitant heparin (Hisa et al, 1990).

In contrast, infusion of IV heparin is not nearly as important for maintaining vessel patency after successful thrombolysis with either streptokinase or APSAC (because of the much longer duration of action of these thrombolytic agents). Thus, despite the extremely large number of patients involved in these multicenter international studies, our feeling is that their results are *not relevant* to the manner in which thrombolytic therapy is used in this country. Results from the large ISIS-3 study that is currently in progress may be equally problematic because administration of IV heparin following thrombolytic therapy (with either streptokinase, APSAC, or rt-PA) is also delayed.

Two additional factors complicating analysis of trials that have compared the efficacy of various thrombolytic agents are: (1) the use of different adjunctive treatment measures in the trials (i.e., inconstant use of aspirin, IV β-blockers, IV nitroglycerin, and/or calcium antagonists); and (2) the considerable difference in mortality rates reported for the *control population* in each of the various studies (Rapaport, 1989). In-hospital mortality rates among placebo controls for many of the earlier studies were in the range of 10-15%. More recent studies have reduced this figure *more than* twofold. However, this may make it difficult to know how to interpret the relative meaning of *percentage* reduction figures given for mortality in the various studies, considering that the percentage reduction is calculated with respect to whatever the baseline mortality of the control group happened to be for that particular study.

In summary, existing data have unfortunately *not* provided a definitive answer as to which thrombolytic agent is best. In general, initial opening rates appear to be higher with the use of rt-PA compared to APSAC or streptokinase (ACC/AHA Task Force, 1990). In conjunction with additional treatment measures (including aspirin, IV β-blockers, IV nitroglycerin, and possibly calcium antagonists for selected patients), *and* prompt institution of IV heparin for patients who receive rt-PA, thrombolytic therapy has been shown to reduce overall in-hospital mortality from AMI by as much as 50% (Topol et al, 1987; Tiefenbrunn and Sobel, 1989). Debate will doubtlessly continue regarding the relative significance of features such as cost, ease of administration, clot "selectivity," incidence of antigenic and allergenic reactions, risk of inducing hypotension, initial opening and late patency rates, and ultimate LV function. However, the KEY point to emphasize at this time is the following:

> Much more import than the particular thrombolytic agent chosen (i.e., streptokinase, APSAC, rt-PA), is *deciding to strongly consider the use of* **some** *thrombolytic agent*—as soon as possible—to appropriately selected patients with AMI.

WHO QUALIFIES FOR THROMBOLYTIC THERAPY?

The selection criteria most commonly used at the present time to determine which patients with new-onset chest pain qualify as potential candidates for thrombolytic therapy are listed in *Table 12C-2*.

Age

In general, enthusiasm is less for administering thrombolytic therapy to older individuals. As a result, many centers arbitrarily set an "upper-age limit" (usually at 75 years) as an exclusion criterion.

The rationale for setting an upper age limit is the progressively increasing risk of developing a major hemorrhagic complication with increasing age (Muller and Topol, 1990). Routine exclusion of elderly patients is a "double-edged sword," however, since both the incidence of AMI, as well as the mortality associated with AMI *also* increase progressively with age. Thus, although less than 20% of the U.S. population is over 65 years old, more than 80% of the mortality from AMI occurs in this age group (Gurwitz et al, 1991). The in-hospital case-fatality rate for a first infarction is less than 5% for patients under 55 years of age, but *more than* 30% for those over 75 (Gurwitz et al, 1991). Overall then, the estimated potential lifesaving benefit from treating elderly patients (over 70 years of age) appears to be significantly greater than that for treating younger patients (Grines and DeMaria, 1990; Yusuf and Furberg, 1991). Thus, despite the clear need for caution in treating older patients, it would seem that chronologic age per se should

Table 12C-2

Qualifying Criteria for the Use of Thrombolytic Therapy in AMI

• **Age <75 Years Old***
-Risk of developing a major hemorrhagic complication progressively increases with increasing age

• **Symptom Onset within 6 Hours**
-History of new-onset (ischemic-sounding) chest pain of *at least* 30 minutes duration that is not relieved by sublingual nitroglycerin
-Symptom onset should be *less than* 6 hours prior to the time of presentation (and ideally less than 3-4 hours).
-Patients with either intermittent chest pain (i.e., "stuttering" infarction) and/or persistent chest pain of *greater than* six hours duration may still be candidates for thrombolytic therapy if the clinical picture suggests that AMI is still in the process of evolving.

• **Definitive Evidence of AMI in Progress**
-*Definitive ECG changes* (i.e., ≥1 mm of ST segment elevation in ≥2 contiguous leads):
   -identifies patients who are most likely to benefit from thrombolytic therapy
   -minimizes chance of misdiagnosing conditions such as acute pericarditis or dissecting aneurysm, and inappropriately treating with thrombolytic therapy
-Strongly consider repeating the ECG if the history is highly suggestive of AMI and the initial tracing fails to show definitive changes
-Strongly consider repeating the ECG if chest pain completely resolves following nitroglycerin to verify that ST segment elevation is still present (i.e., to rule out coronary spasm)
-If readily available, echocardiography may occasionally help diagnose AMI in patients who do not demonstrate definitive ECG changes (although this group of patients are less likely to benefit from thrombolytic therapy)

• **No Absolute Contraindications to Thrombolytic Therapy**
-*See Table 12C-3*

*The cutoff for age should *not* be absolute, however, since the incidence and mortality of AMI *also* increase with age. The decision of whether to treat a patient over 75 may therefore need to be individualized (*See Text.*)

not be a contraindication to the use of thrombolytic therapy. The decision of whether to treat elderly patients (over 70-75 years of age) has to be *individualized*, and might best be based on consideration of "physiologic age," potential risk of developing a bleeding complication, local practice, and other patient related-factors.

Duration of Symptoms

The most fundamental criterion for determining whether a patient is a suitable candidate for thrombolytic therapy depends on the history. The patient should recount a history of new-onset chest pain that suggests possible AMI (i.e., chest pain lasting *at least* 30 minutes, and *not* relieved by sublingual nitroglycerin). As previously emphasized, *the sooner a patient with AMI is treated after the onset of symptoms, the greater the potential benefit from thrombolytic therapy*—with 6 hours currently being the most commonly used *upper limit* for the "window of opportunity".

An important exception to the "6 hour rule" is the patient who presents with either *intermittent* chest pain and/or *persistent* chest pain of *greater* than 6 hours duration. The rationale for considering treatment of such individuals is based on the premise that the presence of chest pain implies the presence of *at least some* myocardial tissue that has not yet become necrotic (i.e., that is *potentially viable*), despite the prolonged duration of symptoms. Patients with this type of history are likely to have an *unstable* coronary syndrome (either unstable angina and/or evolving AMI with a "stuttering" course), and are therefore still likely to benefit from thrombolytic therapy.

> It should be emphasized that selection of an absolute "cutoff time" as an exclusion criterion for administration of thrombolytic therapy is a rather arbitrary process. Difficult to assess patient-related factors (i.e., "stuttering" course of AMI, adequacy of collateral flow) may prolong the period of potential viability and myocardial salvage in a given patient. In addition, there may be uncertainty as the to *true* time of symptom onset in some cases. Even when the *true* time of symptom onset is assured, this will *not* always correlate with the onset of the infarct (See below— *"When Did the Infarct Really Begin?"*). Thus it appears that among patients who present with AMI, a surprisingly large percentage have infarctions of *less* than 6 hours duration *despite* persistence of symptoms for a greater period of time (Beek et al, 1991). In further support of this premise are the results of the large ISIS-2 Trial (involving more than 17,000 patients), in which continued benefit was seen from thrombolytic therapy administered as late as 13-24 hours *after* the onset of symptoms (Second International Study of Infarct Survival Collaborative Group, 1988).

Currently, most clinicians do not *initiate* thrombolytic therapy for patients with AMI whose symptoms began *more than* 6 hours earlier if they are otherwise stable and *pain-free* at the time they are seen. On the other hand, late initiation of thrombolytic therapy (beyond 6 hours) is clearly justified if chest pain persists and there is evidence of ongoing ischemia in a patient whose acute infarction appears to still be evolving (ACC/AHA Task Force, 1990; Muller and Topol, 1990; Grines and DeMaria, 1990).

When Did the Infarct *Really* Begin?

Dependence on the patient's account of the onset of symptoms is clearly a *subjective* method for determining the duration of infarction. Until recently, however, little objective information was available on how reliable the patient's account really was for predicting the onset of AMI.

> Beek et al (1991) examined this issue in a study of 221 consecutive patients who presented with new-onset chest pain and acute ECG changes indicative of AMI. As might be expected, the overwhelming majority of *"early"-presenting patients* (in whom symptom onset was *less* than 6 hours) had only minimally elevated initial CK enzyme readings (of less than twice normal). Surprisingly, 59% of *"late"-presenting patients* with AMI (in whom symptom onset was *greater* than 6 hours) also had only minimally elevated initial CK readings. In addition, many of these "late"-presenting patients with AMI also manifested ECG indicators suggestive of more recent infarction (i.e., ≥2 mm of ST segment elevation, absent or small Q waves).

In view of the importance placed on the patient's history for determining whether to institute thrombolytic therapy, implications of this study are potentially far-reaching. *Patient history of symptom onset IS important*. However, it should NOT be the last word:

Certain patients may *still* be good (or even excellent) potential candidates for thrombolytic therapy *despite* a relatively late presentation (of more than 6 hours after symptom onset)—especially if their initial CK reading is only minimally elevated and their initial ECG suggests acuity (i.e., by marked ST segment elevation, marked reciprocal depression, and minimal or absent Q waves).

Definitive Evidence of AMI in Progress

Electrocardiographically, at least 1 mm of ST segment elevation in *two or more* contiguous leads is required for a patient to qualify as a candidate for thrombolytic therapy.*

There are two principal reasons for the close adherence by most clinicians to this criterion, although admittedly the subject remains controversial:

1. Thrombolytic therapy is *not* benign. It may be particularly dangerous if inadvertently administered to a patient with acute pericarditis with tamponade or acute dissecting aortic aneurysm. Administration of thrombolytic therapy may also prove to be problematic if the cause of chest pain turns out to be an acute

---

*The reason for requiring ST segment elevation in at least *two* contiguous leads is to rule out cases of *single lead* ST segment elevation in leads such as aVL, aVF, III, or V₂. The finding of isolated ST segment elevation in any of these leads most often reflects a normal variant rather than AMI.

abdomen requiring immediate surgical intervention (as may occasionally occur with acute cholecystitis!). Requiring *definitive* ECG changes of AMI (i.e., ST segment elevation) minimizes the chance of misdiagnosis and development of a potentially deleterious (and iatrogenically-induced) consequence from inappropriate thrombolytic therapy.*

2. Patients with AMI who are the most likely to benefit from thrombolytic therapy usually demonstrate marked ST segment elevation in multiple leads (Bar et al, 1987). In general, patients with new-onset chest pain who do not demonstrate ST segment elevation on initial ECG have *not* been shown to benefit from thrombolytic therapy—*even if they do go on to evolve AMI* (Muller and Topol 1990; Martin and Kennedy, 1990; The thrombolysis Early in Acute Heart Attack Trial Study Group, 1990). The significance of this finding becomes all the more important when one considers that approximately 25% to 50% of *all* patients with new-onset chest pain who go on to evolve AMI (especially in the distribution of the circumflex coronary artery) do *not* demonstrate ST segment elevation on their initial ECG (Huey et al, 1988).

> From a practical standpoint, reliance on the presence of definitive ECG findings may greatly simplify decision-making by providing an objective way to identify those AMI patients who have the most favorable *risk-benefit ratio* for receiving thrombolytic therapy (i.e., who potentially have the *most* to gain from receiving thrombolytic therapy, and who are *least* likely to develop a complication because they have something other than AMI as the cause of their symptoms!).

As noted earlier (in Section A), **echocardiography** is a noninvasive procedure that can be performed at the bedside of patients with new-onset chest pain for diagnostic purposes (when definitive ECG changes are either absent or findings are equivocal—Peels et al, 1990). Drawbacks of the procedure include its cost, the need for round-the-clock staff availability to perform the test, and similar availability of clinicians skilled in echocardiography to immediately interpret the results (which are *not* always clear cut). In view of these drawbacks, and the fact that patients who do not demonstrate definitive ECG findings on their initial ECG are much less likely to benefit from thrombolytic therapy, our feeling is that in most cases, emergency echocardiography contributes little to identification of suitable candidates for thrombolytic therapy.

---

*Unfortunately, despite the presence of seemingly "definitive" ECG changes, as many as 15% to 20% of patients with new-onset chest pain may not go on to evolve AMI (Lee et al, 1989).

Two additional points should be emphasized regarding use of the ECG to identify patients with new-onset chest pain who are suitable candidates for thrombolytic therapy:

1. If the initial ECG fails to demonstrate acute changes (and/or shows equivocal findings), and the patient's history is highly suggestive of acute ischemic chest pain (and possible AMI)—**strongly consider repeating the ECG!** AMI is *not* a stable condition. Instead, it is an *evolving* process. New (definitive) ECG changes (that may *now* qualify the patient as an excellent potential candidate for thrombolytic therapy) can develop in as short a period as several minutes.

2. Spasm of an epicardial coronary artery typically produces acute ST segment elevation. Pure coronary spasm (in the absence of acute occluding thrombus formation) may occasionally be the cause of new-onset chest pain. Because patients with pure coronary spasm do *not* benefit from thrombolytic therapy, it is important to rule out this possibility *before* beginning treatment. For those patients whose chest pain completely resolves, coronary spasm can be ruled out by repeating the ECG immediately after administration of nitroglycerin to verify that ST segment elevation is still present.

Contraindications to Thrombolytic Therapy

The major absolute and relative contraindications to thrombolytic therapy are listed in *Table 12C-3*. Most of these are relatively self-evident since they are associated with conditions that predispose the patient to an increased risk of bleeding.

An active bleeding disorder is an obvious absolute contraindication to thrombolytic therapy. Similarly, the risk of developing a potentially disastrous bleeding complication with thrombolytic therapy would be unacceptably high for patients with recent major trauma or surgery, dissecting aortic aneurysm, or a recent cerebrovascular event.

Unfortunately, definitive data are lacking for defining the optimal interval between major surgery or trauma, and the time when thrombolytic therapy may be safely given. The ACC/AHA Task Force (1990) suggests that the absolute contraindications to thrombolytic therapy can be removed after a period of 2 weeks, although some increased risk for developing a bleeding complications probably persists beyond this point (Muller and Topol, 1990).

Patients with a history of a hemorrhagic cerebrovascular accident, or of a *nonhemorrhagic* stroke or TIA within the past 6 months should not receive thrombolytic therapy. As was the case for major surgery or trauma, definitive data are lacking and the decision of whether to institute thrombolytic therapy for a patient with a previous nonhemorrhagic cerebrovascular accident that occurred *more* than 6 months ago has to be individualized.

Hypertension is also listed as an absolute contraindication if blood pressure readings are "excessively" elevated, variously

Table 12C-3

| **Contraindications to the Use of Thrombolytic Therapy in AMI** |
| (Adapted from the ACC/AHA Task Force Report, 1990) |

Absolute Contraindications:

-Active bleeding disorder
-Recent trauma or surgery (i.e., within the previous 2 weeks)
-Suspected aortic aneurysm/acute pericarditis
-Prolonged or traumatic cardiopulmonary resuscitation
-Recent head trauma or known intracranial neoplasm
-Previous allergic reaction to the thrombolytic agent being considered (i.e., streptokinase or APSAC)
-Excessive hypertension (i.e., BP *remains* >180/110 mm Hg)
-History of recent CVA/TIA (i.e., within the previous 6 months), or of a cerebrovascular accident known to be hemorrhagic
-Diabetic hemorrhagic retinopathy or other hemorrhagic ophthalmologic condition
-Pregnancy

Relative Contraindications:

-Relatively recent trauma or surgery (i.e., performed *more than* 2 weeks prior to the time of presentation)
-Long-term history of severe hypertension
-Active peptic ulcer disease (but *without* known GI bleeding)
-History of remote CVA/TIA (i.e., more than 6 months ago)
-Known bleeding diathesis or current use of anticoagulants
-Cardiopulmonary resuscitation of relatively short duration (<10 minutes)
-Significant liver dysfunction
-Prior exposure to streptokinase or APSAC (especially within the preceding 6 to 9 months)*

*Non-streptokinase-containing agents (i.e., rt-PA, urokinase, etc.) may be used again without concern of developing an allergic reaction.

---

defined as a systolic blood pressure of greater than 180 to 200 mm Hg, and/or a diastolic reading of greater than 110 to 120 mm Hg. Hypertension of this degree appears to significantly increase the risk of hemorrhagic stroke in patients with AMI who receive thrombolytic therapy (Muller and Topol, 1990). On the other hand, hypertension that occurs in this setting is often transient and easily controlled with nitroglycerin or other analgesic, antianginal, and/or anxiolytic medication. If blood pressure in a previously normotensive individual is easily controlled by such measures, thrombolytic therapy need *not* necessarily be contraindicated by a single initially elevated reading.

*It should be apparent that the **QUESTION** of whether or not to institute thrombolytic therapy for any particular patient is often NOT a black or white decision!*

To illustrate this point, consider the following two hypothetical cases:

CASE A

A 50 year old man presents within 2 hours after the sudden onset of severe chest pain. Except for the diagnosis of an ulcer that was made a month earlier, the patient is otherwise healthy. His initial ECG is highly suggestive of an extensive *anterior* AMI (marked ST segment elevation in most precordial leads, dramatic reciprocal ST segment depression, and no indication of any Q wave formation).

CASE B

A previously healthy 74 year old man presents with a history of chest pain that began 5½ hours earlier. His initial ECG suggests an inferior AMI. ST segments are elevated approximately 1 mm in each of the inferior leads, and significant Q waves have already formed. Reciprocal ST segment depression in neighboring leads is minimal.

QUESTION: **Would you be in favor of administering thrombolytic therapy to either of these patients?** (HINT: In addition to using Tables 12C-2 *and* 12C-3, you may want to refer back to Table 12A-2 in formulating your answer.)

ANSWER Most clinicians would probably initiate thrombolytic therapy (albeit *cautiously*) for the patient described in Case A *despite* the recent history of peptic ulcer disease. As indicated in Table 12C-3, peptic ulcer disease (in the absence of known GI bleeding) is only a *relative* contraindication to thrombolytic therapy. Considering the patient's age, otherwise healthy status, short duration of symptoms (of *less* than 2 hours!), anterior location of infarction, and ECG indicators of acuity (marked ST segment elevation in multiple leads, dramatic reciprocal changes, and absence of Q waves)—the *tremendous potential benefits* that might accrue from the use of thrombolytic therapy are likely to far outweigh the risk (of developing a bleeding complication) that is posed by the history of recent peptic ulcer disease.

The decision of whether to institute thrombolytic therapy is far more difficult for the patient described in the second example. Nevertheless, the patient in Case B is *less* than 75 years of age, chest pain began *less* than 6 hours earlier, definitive ECG evidence of AMI *is* present (albeit significant Q waves have already formed and the magnitude of ST segment changes appears to be small), and there are ostensibly no contraindications to the use of thrombolytic therapy. Thus, *all* of the qualifying criteria listed in Table 12C-2 *are* satisfied. As a result, many clinicians would probably still favor the use of thrombolytic therapy for the patient in Case B with the hope that doing so might further limit the extent of infarction. Alternatively, we could not fault a decision *against* the use of thrombolytic therapy on the grounds that this patient is much older, has an inferior infarction, and the anticipated benefit from the use of thrombolytic therapy at this point in the evolutionary process is much less.

Site of infarction is an important factor to consider in the decision-making process. As already emphasized, *the larger the infarct, the more the patient is likely to benefit from thrombolytic therapy.* In general, anterior infarctions are larger than inferior infarctions. This accounts for the fact that overall mortality of patients with acute anterior infarction is at least twice that of acute inferior infarction (Muller and Topol, 1990). It also explains why some clinicians do not routinely administer thrombolytic therapy to patients with otherwise uncomplicated inferior AMI (and why they may choose not to treat the patient described in Case B). This view is not universally held, however, and many clinicians do favor the use of thrombolytic therapy for patients who satisfy the qualifying criteria for treatment *regardless* of the site of infarction (ACC/AHA Task Force, 1990).

Recent evidence suggests that patients with inferior AMI can be stratified into a group at highest risk (i.e., who are likely to have more extensive infarction, and who therefore are likely to benefit more from thrombolytic therapy). In most cases, identification of such patients is easily made by recognition of worrisome clinical parameters (i.e., heart failure or hypotension), and/or the presence of ECG findings suggestive of more extensive involvement (i.e., associated 3° AV block, ST segment elevation in *additional* [lateral or right ventricular] leads, or ST segment *depression* in the precordial leads—Bates, 1988; Martin and Kennedy, 1990; Berger and Ryan, 1990). Patients with inferior AMI and any of these clinical or ECG findings should merit equal consideration for thrombolytic therapy as do patients with anterior AMI.

ADDITIONAL PROBLEM **What if the ages of the patients described in Cases A and B were reversed?** *or if instead of 74, the patient in Case A was 76 years old?* **or if it was the patient in Case B who had the history of a recent ulcer?**

ANSWER The number of possible permutations for these case scenarios is endless. Regarding the situations posed above (in the Additional Problem), we would probably still favor *cautious* initiation of thrombolytic therapy for the scenario described in Case A even if the patient was 74 years old. Being 2 years older would probably *not* alter our decision.

In contrast, it would take *very little* to dissuade us from initiating thrombolytic therapy for the scenario initially described for Case B in which qualifying criteria were all just barely met. Thus, the addition of any relative contraindication (such as the history of a recent ulcer) would probably be more than enough to tip the balance against the use of thrombolytic therapy.

> Clearly, the decision of whether to institute thrombolytic therapy for any particular patient must always be *individualized* based on careful consideration of all available information.

RISK OF BLEEDING WITH THROMBOLYTIC THERAPY

The most frequent complication of thrombolytic therapy is bleeding. Although the consequences of developing a bleeding complication can be severe (and potentially disastrous if the bleeding is intracerebral), most episodes fortunately do not result in major sequelae.

More that 80% of all bleeding complications from thrombolytic therapy occur at the site of a vascular puncture (Heras et al, 1988). As a result, most such episodes are relatively easy to control (often simply by local pressure). Surprisingly, the thrombolytic agent per se is generally *not* the direct cause of hemorrhage (Tiefenbrunn and Ludbrook, 1989). Instead thrombolytic agents tend to unmask *preexisting* vascular pathology and/or facilitate continuation of bleeding once it begins. Theoretically, if vascular integrity could be kept intact, the incidence of bleeding would be negligible *re-*

gardless of the presence of other predisposing conditions or the state of circulating clotting factors (Chamberlain, 1989). *Avoidance of unnecessary vascular puncture and other invasive procedures are therefore KEY preventive measures for minimizing the incidence of bleeding complications from thrombolytic therapy.* Thus, insertion of a central line (if needed for hemodynamic monitoring) should be accomplished *before* thrombolytic therapy is begun, and routine arterial blood gas studies should not be drawn on patients who are being considered for treatment.

The other KEY to minimizing the incidence of bleeding complications from thrombolytic therapy is *careful patient selection*. This is especially true with regard to preventing intracerebral hemorrhage, by far the most dangerous form of bleeding complication.

Of the 15% to 20% of bleeding complications from thrombolytic therapy that are not attributable to vascular puncture or performance of an invasive procedure, the majority are due to gastrointestinal hemorrhage or genitourinary bleeding. Less than 1% of bleeding complications result in intracerebral hemorrhage, which is fortunate considering the grave consequences usually associated with this complication.

At the present time, the overall incidence of intracerebral bleeding from thrombolytic therapy is estimated to be between 1-10/1000 patients treated (ACC/AHA Task Force, 1990). Although the higher (150 mg) dose of rt-PA used in the past had been associated with an increased risk of intracerebral hemorrhage, reduction of the dose (to 100 mg) appears to have cut the rate of this complication by half (Califf et al, 1988). Minor differences may still exist between the various thrombolytic agents in the rate of hemorrhagic complications they produce (i.e., slightly higher incidence of systemic bleeding requiring transfusion with streptokinase and APSAC?/slightly higher incidence of intracerebral bleeding with rt-PA?)—albeit interpretation of results from trials in the literature is far from a simple task, and the topic remains controversial. Practically speaking however, *the tendency for any particular thrombolytic agent to produce a systemic bleeding complication appears to depend much more on the presence of patient-specific (predisposing) factors*, than to inherent properties (such as "clot specificity" and fibrinogen depletion) of the thrombolytic agent itself (Tiefenbrunn and Sobol, 1989; Chamberlain, 1989).

Patient-specific factors that seem to predispose to intracerebral hemorrhage include older age, a long-term history of hypertension (and/or hypertension at the time of treatment), and a history of prior cerebrovascular accident.

Individuals with one or more of these factors are likely to be prone to develop weakening of vessel walls in the cerebral microvasculature and/or microaneurysms in which vascular integrity may be impaired and partially supported by fibrin (Tiefenbrunn and Ludbrook, 1989). Administration of a thrombolytic agent to such individuals could induce intracerebral hemorrhage by indiscriminately lyzing "protective" fibrin in the cerebral vasculature at the same time as it is acting on pathologic thrombi in the infarct-related coronary artery.

Although attention to the patient-specific factors cited above is helpful in identifying individuals at highest risk of intracerebral hemorrhage, development of this complication is not completely predictable on the basis of screening for these factors alone. Thus, as many as 40% of cases

of intracerebral bleeding occur in patients *without* any predisposing conditions at all (Grines and DeMaria, 1990). This leaves the clinician with the dilemma of determining whether the potential benefit from thrombolytic therapy for treatment of AMI is truly "worth the risk" of possibly causing a potentially catastrophic (and iatrogenic) complication.

In determining whether the benefit is worth the risk, it should be kept in mind that the incidence of thromboembolic (i.e., *nonhemorrhagic*) stroke as a manifestation of AMI in patients who do *not* receive thrombolytic therapy is also approximately 1%. Cumulative data from several large studies on coronary thrombolysis suggest that "any increment in intracranial bleeding that might be ascribed to treatment with a lytic agent in patients with AMI is *small* and offset by a (comparable) *decrease* in the incidence of thromboembolic stroke" (Tiefenbrunn and Ludbrook, 1989). Admittedly, the consequences of a hemorrhagic stroke are generally more severe than those from a thromboembolic stroke. Nevertheless, it appears that the chance of developing a cerebrovascular event in association with AMI is approximately 1% *regardless* of whether or not thrombolytic therapy is used.

Again—*decisions must be individualized*. In an elderly patient with long-standing hypertension and/or a history of previous stroke, the risk of developing intracerebral hemorrhage from thrombolytic therapy is likely to far outweigh any potential benefit—especially if the AMI is inferior in location and symptom duration before presentation is greater than four hours. In contrast, using thrombolytic therapy to treat a younger patient with convincing ECG evidence of anterior AMI of more recent onset (i.e., ≤3 hours duration) appears to be well worth the small (but unavoidably) increased risk of producing an intracerebral bleeding complication.

Use of Thrombolytic Therapy in Patients Who Have Received CPR

Prolonged cardiopulmonary resuscitation is an absolute contraindication to the use of thrombolytic therapy. There are two principal reasons for this: 1) the significantly increased risk of intrathoracic bleeding that accompanies prolonged CPR (from rib or sternal fractures, pulmonary contusion, and/or pericardial tamponade); and 2) the increased risk of intracerebral hemorrhage (as an end result of hypoxic brain damage, the severity of which is likely to increase exponentially with time—Muller and Topol, 1990). Somewhat surprisingly, the incidence of major bleeding complications has *not* been shown to increase in patients who receive thrombolytic therapy after undergoing CPR of only *brief* (i.e., ≤10 minutes) duration (Topol et al., 1988; Tenaglia et al., 1991). Moreover, those patients with AMI who require CPR appear to comprise a particularly high-risk group with an excellent chance to benefit from thrombolytic therapy Muller and Topol, 1990). Therefore:

The occurrence of cardiac arrest requiring external chest compression of only *brief* duration (i.e., ≤10 minutes), *without* apparent causation of significant trauma from CPR—in a patient who was previously felt to be neurologically intact—should *NOT* be considered a contraindication to thrombolytic therapy.

HOW MANY PATIENTS ACTUALLY *RECEIVE* THROMBOLYTIC THERAPY?

Despite unquestioned benefit from early institution of thrombolytic therapy, the reality of the situation is that relatively few patients with AMI satisfy the inclusion criteria listed in Table 12C-2 and qualify as suitable candidates.

> Insight into this problem was provided from a study performed by Lee et al (1989) involving more than 7,000 patients who presented to an ED with a chief complaint of new-onset chest pain. Of this group, *only 14%* of the patients actually went on to develop AMI, emphasizing the point that *the majority of patients who present to an emergency facility with a chief complaint of new-onset chest pain are not having acute infarction.*
>
> Of the original group (of more than 7,000 patients), *only 23%* satisfied the qualifying criteria for thrombolytic therapy listed in Table 12C-2 regarding age (less than 76 years old), symptom duration (arrival at the hospital within 6 hours of the onset of symptoms), and ECG findings (ST segment elevation in two or more contiguous leads). The overall number of patients to satisfy the criteria would have been even *less* if consideration had also been given to potential contraindications to this treatment.

Other studies have obtained similar results, suggesting that *fewer than 20% of patients with AMI currently qualify for AND actually receive thrombolytic therapy* (Muller and Topol, 1990). Reasons why patients are excluded from consideration for thrombolytic therapy (and the approximate overall relative frequency of these exclusions) are shown in *Table 12C-4.*

It is estimated that *at least* 15% of all patients in this country with AMI who would seem to be "ideal" candidates for thrombolytic therapy (i.e., who satisfy *all* of the qualifying criteria listed in Table 12C-2) are *not* currently receiving this treatment (Muller and Topol, 1990). Thus, *at least* 125,000 patients each year are not currently re-

Table 12C-4

Estimated Percentage of AMI Patients Receiving (or Excluded from Receiving) Thrombolytic Therapy

Estimated percentage of AMI patients who currently receive thrombolytic therapy	≈15-20%
Estimated percentage of AMI patients who are *not* currently receiving thrombolytic therapy	≈80-85%

≈**15%**—Seemingly "ideal" candidates who are not treated

≈**25-30%**—*Excluded* from treatment because of late presentation (>6 hours after symptom onset)

≈**10-15%**—*Excluded* from treatment because of age (>75 years old)

≈**15%**—*Excluded* from treatment because of contraindications to thrombolytic therapy

≈**10%**—*Excluded* from treatment because of equivocal ECG findings (lack of definite ST segment elevation)

≈**80-85%**

Adapted from Muller and Topol, 1990.

---

ceiving optimal care for their acute infarction. Considering the numbers of patients involved, overall mortality from AMI might be reduced as much as 35% (!) if these patients could be treated (Muller and Topol, 1990).

> Efforts must continue to increase the use of thrombolytic therapy—*especially among patients who otherwise appear to be "ideal" candidates for this form of treatment.* A major stumbling block to accomplishing this goal is the reluctance some clinicians still have against prescribing thrombolytic therapy. This reluctance is probably the result of a combination of factors including:
>
> 1. Prevailing local practice (especially in smaller rural communities with smaller hospitals)
> 2. A lack of (or the *perceived* lack of) adequate support staff and facilities for administration of thrombolytic therapy (i.e., less than optimal access to cardiology consultation, less than optimal cardiac catheterization availability, difficulty in arranging transfer to a referral center if the need suddenly arises, etc.)
> 3. A belief that some patients who do "qualify" for thrombolytic therapy are unlikely to benefit enough to justify the risk of treatment (i.e., patients with uncomplicated inferior infarction who are only seen four or more hours after the onset of symptoms)
> 4. Inadequate experience with thrombolytic therapy to feel comfortable with its use
> 5. Medicolegal concerns (that appear to be most prevalent among noncardiologists who are directly involved in the initial evaluation and management of acutely ill patients)

It is important to emphasize that thrombolytic therapy has become a *standard of care* for treatment of *appropriately selected* patients with AMI (ACC/AHA Task Force, 1990). One need *not* necessarily be a cardiologist to initiate treatment of such patients. Nor is it necessary to practice in a large city hospital with round-the-clock catheterization capability. On the contrary, *delaying treatment* for cardiology approval in certain rural settings would be equivalent to depriving a substantial number of otherwise ideally suited candidates from this form of therapy (Henry and deGruy, 1988; Taylor et al, 1990).

Should the Qualifying Criteria Be Expanded?

In view of the fact that 65% to 70% of patients with AMI are excluded from consideration for thrombolytic therapy because of failure to satisfy one or more of the standard qualifying criteria (Tables 12C-2 and 12C-4), it might be reasonable to ask *whether these qualifying criteria could be expanded?*

The most common reason for excluding patients with AMI from consideration for thrombolytic therapy is delayed presentation (*more than* 6 hours after symptom onset). As previously emphasized, AMI may have a "stuttering" course—and the large ISIS-2 Trial *did* demonstrate continued benefit from thrombolytic therapy in a subgroup of patients with AMI who received treatment as late as 13 to 24 hours after the onset of symptoms. One explanation for these results is that achieving patency of the infarct-related vessel could have improved survival by mechanisms other than limitation of infarct size— *even when restoration of flow was delayed beyond 6 hours!* Thus delayed reperfusion may also improve survival by preserving left ventricular contractility—preventing ventricular dilatation and chamber "remodeling" that would otherwise ultimately lead to deterioration of left ventricular function and death from heart failure (Braunwald, 1989). Another explanation is that the patient's account of the onset of symptoms (of chest pain) may not always accurately reflect the true onset of infarction (Beek et al, 1991). Although more data from prospective controlled studies are clearly needed before recommending a change in current practice, it may be that the "window of opportunity" for administration of thrombolytic therapy to *selected* patients with AMI will soon be expanded.

The other major consideration for expanding the impact of thrombolytic therapy regards the age criterion. As emphasized earlier, morbidity and mortality rates are significantly higher when AMI occurs in patients over 70 years of age than when it occurs in younger individuals. Yet despite the potential for at least comparable benefit from medical intervention, proven effective medical treatments (including thrombolytic therapy, use of β-blockers, aspirin, and IV nitroglycerin) are *all* used less often in the elderly than in younger patients (Montague et al, 1991). All too often forgotten is the fact that the average life expectancy of a 65 year old is an additional 16.9 years— and for a 75 year old, an additional 10.7 years. Many of these patients remain active and continue to pursue vigorous and productive lives (Yusuf and Furberg, 1991). Thus, rather than

a strictly defined upper age limit, substantial reduction in overall morbidity and mortality might best be achieved by allowing otherwise healthy elderly patients with evidence of a large AMI to remain eligible for treatment.

SPECIAL CONSIDERATIONS:
Thrombolytic Therapy in the Prehospital Setting

Because of the critical importance of *time until treatment* in determining the clinical response of patients with evolving AMI, the potential impact that could result from initiation of thrombolytic therapy in the prehospital setting is tremendous. Preliminary studies add support to this concept by suggesting that as many as 50% of patients who would be treated by paramedics according to a prehospital protocol could receive thrombolytic therapy *within the first hour of the onset of symptoms*. Implementation of such protocols would dramatically reduce the time until treatment compared to the time usually required when administration of thrombolytic therapy is delayed until hospital arrival (Kennedy and Weaver, 1989; Weaver et al, 1990).

Weaver et al (1990) have shown that prehospital administration of thrombolytic therapy is feasible. Paramedics can be taught in as little as 3 hours to obtain a checklist history (consisting of predetermined inclusion and exclusion criteria for thrombolytic therapy), perform a targeted physical examination, and operate a cellular electrocardiograph machine. The 12-lead ECG recorded on this machine is immediately transmitted to an office-based physician interpreter who can then decide whether treatment is indicated. With training, performance (and transmission) of a cellular 12-lead ECG by paramedics in the field can be accomplished so rapidly that on-scene paramedic time need not be delayed by more than a matter of minutes (Kereiakes et al, 1990; Aufderheide et al, 1992). The end result is that time until treatment is substantially reduced (by up to an hour or more!) because the seemingly unavoidable delays inherent in a system of in-hospital evaluation and treatment are completely bypassed (Weaver et al, 1990; Aufderheide et al, 1992).

Despite its feasibility, and the tremendous potential for benefit to patients with AMI who are promptly identified and treated, questions remain regarding the cost-effectiveness (and the overall risk-benefit ratio) of implementing a system for prehospital administration of thrombolytic therapy. Thus, in the above study by Weaver et al (1990), qualifying criteria for thrombolytic therapy (including ST segment elevation on the cellular ECG) were present in only 4% of the more than 2,400 patients screened by EMS services for a chief complaint of new-onset chest pain. Nevertheless, the prospect of being able to intervene in the prehospital setting is exciting, and further study is eagerly awaited.

Thrombolytic Therapy for AMI After CABG

Although it is clear that acute thrombotic occlusion of a major coronary vessel is the precipitating cause of AMI in more than 90% of cases, much less information is available on the mechanism responsible for AMI in patients who have undergone prior coronary artery bypass graft (CABG) surgery.

An interesting study by Grines et al (1990) examined this issue in a group of 50 patients who had undergone CABG at least one year prior to development of AMI. Acute thrombotic occlusion of the saphenous graft was the most common cause of AMI in the study (occurring in 76% of cases, compared to acute thrombus development in a native coronary vessel in only 16%). However, despite confirmation of acute thrombus development as the precipitating cause of AMI, administration of thrombolytic therapy successfully restored coronary flow in only 25% of cases.

The authors proposed two theories to account for the disappointing reperfusion rates of thrombolytic therapy in these patients: (1) an overwhelmingly large mass of thrombus in the graft could have fostered resistance to thrombolysis; and/or (2) acute obstruction to flow, in association with the absence of side branches (collaterals) in the graft could have produced an environment predisposed to extremely rapid thrombus propagation at a site where delivery of the IV-administered thrombolytic agent was inadequate.

The authors still suggest IV administration of thrombolytic therapy be tried initially in patients with prior CABG who present with AMI. However, they caution that this treatment modality is significantly *less* likely to be successful than when acute thrombolytic occlusion occurs in a native vessel. In such cases, administration of *intragraft* thrombolytic therapy and/or acute angioplasty may be needed to restore graft patency and coronary flow.

USE OF ASPIRIN

In the absence of direct contraindications, administration of aspirin is routinely recommended for *all* patients with new-onset chest pain suggestive of possible AMI (ACC/AHA Task Force, 1990). Aspirin should be started at the *earliest* opportunity (i.e., within *minutes* of seeing the patient) *regardless* of whatever other interventions might be planned.

Perhaps the most insight into the use of aspirin for suspected AMI has been provided by the ISIS-2 Study. In this study, a total of more than 17,000 patients were divided into four groups to compare the effect on mortality of (1) aspirin alone; (2) streptokinase alone; (3) *combined* use of aspirin plus streptokinase; versus (4) placebo controls. Initiation of 160 mg of aspirin on the day of admission and continuation for the next 4 to 5 weeks resulted in an overall reduction in mortality of 21% (Second International Study of Infarct Survival, 1988). In addition, there was a 44% reduction in the incidence of nonfatal reinfarction, and a 36% reduction in the incidence of nonfatal stroke. Aspirin use was not associated with an increased risk of either intracerebral hemorrhage or other major bleeding.

Perhaps the most surprising finding in the ISIS-2 Study was the relative efficacy of aspirin compared to thrombolytic therapy (with IV streptokinase). In view of the fact that the overall mortality reduction in the group of patients who were treated with IV streptokinase was 25%, *the beneficial effect of aspirin alone (started within 24 hours of the onset of symptoms) was almost the same as the overall beneficial effect from thrombolytic therapy!* Although benefit from streptokinase was clearly greatest when this drug was begun early in the course (i.e., within 4 hours of the onset of symptoms), the benefit from aspirin was similar regardless of when during the first 24 hours the drug was started. Finally, *combined* use of aspirin *plus* streptokinase produced a synergistic effect, with an overall reduction in mortality of 42%.

In addition to its beneficial effect for patients with AMI, other studies have demonstrated that use of aspirin (in a dose of 325 mg/day) is also effective in treatment of patients with **unstable angina,** significantly reducing mortality and the risk of progression to AMI (Lewis et al, 1983; Antiplatelet Trialists' Collaboration, 1988).

The message is clear:

Aspirin is by far the most cost-effective agent available for treatment of acute ischemic heart disease (unstable angina or AMI). *Its use is routinely recommended at the earliest opportunity for ALL patients who present with new-onset chest pain of presumed ischemic etiology (provided that there are no specific contraindications to the drug).*

Aspirin is also effective as a *secondary prevention* measure in patients who have had a previous infarction. An overview of more than 10 long-term trials of antiplatelet therapy (involving more than 18,000 patients) suggests that use of aspirin reduced the risk of developing a major vascular event (non-fatal stroke, fatal or non-fatal reinfarction) by approximately 25% (Yusuf et al, 1988). It is of interest that the use of aspirin alone in these studies was equally effective as the combination of aspirin with either dipyridamole or sulfinpyrazone (Yusuf et al, 1988).

As compelling as the evidence in favor of using aspirin for patients with acute ischemic heart disease is, determination of the optimal dose has been far less clear. Aspirin is thought to produce its beneficial effect by blocking formation of thromboxane A2, a potent platelet aggregant and vasoconstrictor. The problem is that use of aspirin in higher doses may also suppress production of prostacyclin, a prostaglandin with antiplatelet and vasodilatory properties. Interference with prostacyclin production could therefore *counteract* the beneficial antiplatelet and vasodilatory effect of thromboxane A2 suppression (Mehta, 1991). Unfortunately, the dose of aspirin required to produce the optimal balance between these vasoactive substances for any given patient remains uncertain.

Secondary prevention trials on the use of aspirin in patients with underlying coronary artery disease have not shown a significant difference in drug efficacy between higher doses (up to 1,500 mg/day) and lower doses of 160 to 325 mg/day (Yusuf et al, 1991). As a result, and because of the much higher incidence of side effects (especially GI intolerance) when higher doses are used, we favor a dose of **160 to 325 mg/day** for treatment of AMI and for secondary prevention.

Because the antiplatelet effect of aspirin is prolonged, it may be that even lower doses (i.e., 75 mg/day)* and/or less frequent administration (i.e., 160-325 mg, 2-3 times/week) would provide adequate cardioprotection with fewer side effects, although the efficacy of treatment with these lower doses has not been studied. Alternatively, use of enteric-coated preparations and/or addition of carafate (1 gm PO Bid—taken at least 1 hour before aspirin) may further reduce the likelihood of gastrointestinal intolerance. It should be emphasized that cardioprotection has not been demonstrated for nonsteroidal antiinflammatory drugs, and these agents should not be substituted for aspirin.

The final point to emphasize is that use of aspirin is recommended for treatment of AMI *regardless* of whatever other interventions might be contemplated. In patients who also receive thrombolytic therapy, use of aspirin is often combined with the thrombolytic agent and IV heparin. Although combining antithrombotic agents in this manner increases the risk of developing a bleeding complication, it also appears to minimize the chance that the infarct-related artery will reocclude. IV heparin is often stopped within 24 to 72 hours after reestablishing coronary flow. In contrast, aspirin prophylaxis (i.e., *secondary* prevention) should be continued indefinitely as long as the drug is well tolerated (ACC/AHA Task Force, 1990).

ANTICOAGULATION

The question of whether to routinely anticoagulate patients with AMI has long been the subject of controversy. Despite numerous trials, the data in favor of full anticoagulation remain inconclusive (Yusuf et al, 1988; ACC/AHA Task Force, 1990). As a result, the use of heparin is usually reserved for specific indications associated with AMI, or as an adjunct to thrombolytic therapy *(Table 12C-5)*.

DVT Prophylaxis

Without prophylactic treatment, deep venous thrombosis (DVT) will develop in as many as one third of patients with AMI (ACC/AHA Task Force, 1990). DVT is especially likely to occur during the first three days of AMI in non-ambulatory patients who are elderly and/or who have associated heart failure or shock. Although early mobilization is clearly the most important preventive measure to institute against development of DVT, initiation of *low-dose, subcutaneous heparin* within 12 to 18 hours of the onset

of symptoms (and continued until the patient is fully ambulatory) has been extremely helpful in reducing the incidence of DVT by more than 80% (ACC/AHA Task Force, 1990). Because of the relatively benign nature of this treatment, subcutaneous heparin (in a dose of 5,000 Units q 12-18 hrs) is therefore routinely recommended for *at least* the first 1 to 2 days in patients with AMI who are not receiving IV heparin for some other indication (ACC/AHA Task Force, 1990).

Treatment of Mural Thrombi

Mural thrombi occur much more commonly than is generally appreciated. Autopsy data from patients with AMI who were not anticoagulated suggest an incidence of between 20% to 60% (Genton and Turpie, 1983), especially among individuals with large anterior AMI, ventricular hypertrophy/cardiomyopathy, congestive heart failure, or ventricular aneurysm. The common feature shared by each of these predisposing conditions is *hypocontractility* (or akinesis) of the anterior wall or apex, with a tendency toward an enlarging apical zone of intraventricular stasis (Fuster and Halperin, 1989). Aspirin alone is not effective in prevention or treatment of mural thrombi that form in association with AMI (Kupper et al, 1989). In contrast, mural thrombi are only rarely associated with uncomplicated inferior AMI.

Patients who develop mural thrombi during the course of AMI are at extremely high risk of systemic embolization. For example, without anticoagulation the risk that a patient with a large anterior AMI will develop a mural thrombus with subsequent cerebral embolization is *at least* 5% (Fuster and Halperin, 1989). This risk is greatest during the immediate post-infarction course (i.e., the first 10 days after AMI), and persists (albeit to a lesser degree) for at least 3 months (Fuster and Halperin, 1989). As a result, full anticoagulation with IV heparin is generally recommended for AMI patients who do not receive thrombolytic therapy if they have evidence of mural thrombi— to be followed by oral coumadin for *at least* 3 to 6 months after infarction (Meltzer et al, 1986; ACC/AHA Task Force, 1990).

Large Anterior AMI: *Empiric Anticoagulation?*

Given the high risk of cerebral embolization faced by patients who have large anterior AMI but who are not treated with thrombolytic therapy, a number of questions arise:

1. Should such AMI patients be routinely screened for the presence of mural thrombi by echocardiography? Would doing so be *cost-effective?*

---

* A recent study by Clarke et al (1991) suggests that maximal sustained inhibition of thromboxane A2 may be achieved by use of a controlled-release formulation containing low-dose aspirin (in the amount of 75 mg)—with only *minimal* suppression of prostacyclin.

Table 12C-5

Suggested Indications for the Use of Heparin in Patients with AMI

• **DVT Prophylaxis of Non-Ambulatory Patients**

-Consider routine treatment of AMI patients who are not to receive thrombolytic therapy or full anticoagulation
    Rx—low-dose subcutaneous heparin (5,000 U q8-12h) for at least the first 1-2 days (or until the patient is fully ambulatory)

• **Treatment of Mural Thrombus**

-Patients with mural thrombi should be fully anticoagulated because of the high risk of cerebral embolization
-Diagnosis can be confirmed by two-dimensional echocardiography
-Diagnosis should be suspected in patients with conditions predisposing to intra-ventricular stasis (i.e., large anterior AMI, heart failure, ventricular aneurysm, ventricular hypertrophy/cardiomyopathy) and in those who present with associated CVA
    Rx—IV heparin or high-dose subcutaneous heparin (to maintain PTT at 1.5-2 × control), followed by oral coumadin (to maintain PT at 1.3-1.5 × control) for at least 3-6 months

• **Empiric/Prophylactic Treatment of Large Anterior AMI**

-Consider empiric/prophylactic anticoagulation for patients with large anterior AMI who are not to receive thrombolytic therapy because of the high risk of developing mural thrombi
-Delaying diagnosis for echocardiographic confirmation may leave such patients unprotected during the period of highest risk
    Rx—IV heparin or high-dose subcutaneous heparin (to maintain PTT at 1.5-2 × control), followed by oral coumadin (to maintain PT at 1.3-1.5 × control) for at least 3-6 months in those patients with documented mural thrombi and/or a large hypokinetic/akinetic area

• **As an Adjunct to Thrombolytic Therapy**

-Full anticoagulation after thrombolytic therapy helps minimize the chance that the infarct-related artery will reocclude (especially following rt-PA infusion)
    Rx—IV heparin (to maintain PTT at 1.5-2 × control) for at least 24-72 hours after reestablishment of coronary flow

• **Other Potential Indication for Anticoagulation**

-Treatment of associated DVT, pulmonary embolism, nonhemorrhagic stroke or TIA, and possibly atrial fibrillation, dilated cardiomyopathy, etc.
    Rx—dose as indicated for specific condition.

---

2. Should AMI patients at highest risk of developing mural thrombi be empirically treated with IV heparin? Or would such empiric treatment unnecessarily increase the *overall* risk of bleeding in a group of patients who do not all have a mural thrombus (and who are *also* already receiving aspirin)?

Although the *sensitivity* of echocardiography for detecting mural thrombi in patients with AMI is far from optimal, the test is completely noninvasive, easily performed at the bedside, and of surprisingly good *specificity* (Popp, 1990). As a result, it may greatly assist in the evaluation of selected patients with large anterior AMI—both for assessment of left ventricular function, as well as for the presence of mural thrombi. In contrast, echocardiography is much less likely to be cost-effective in screening patients with smaller, inferior AMI (especially in the absence of any clinical indication of left ventricular dysfunction).

> It is of interest that the echocardiographic appearance of the thrombus itself may provide additional insight into the risk of systemic embolization. Protruding, mobile and/or rough-surfaced thrombi appear to be significantly more dangerous than sessile, smooth-surfaced thrombi (Visser et al, 1985).

An alternative approach to the problem of anticoagulation is to consider use of IV heparin on an *empiric* basis (i.e., *without* echocardiographic confirmation of mural thrombi)—and/or as a *prophylactic measure*—for selected patients with evidence of large anterior AMI.

Turpie et al (1989) explored this issue in a double-blind, randomized trial of more than 200 patients with anterior AMI. Patients were divided into two groups and treated with *subcutaneous* heparin within 36 hours of the onset of symptoms according to either *low-dose* (5,000 Units q 12 hrs) or *high-dose* (12,500 Units q 12 hrs) regimens. While the PTT was not significantly affected by the low-dose regimen, therapeutic prolongation of the PTT to an average 48 seconds (i.e., between 1.5-2 × control values) was achieved with the high-dose regimen.

At the end of 10 days, echocardiography demonstrated development of left ventricular mural thrombi in 32% of the patients receiving low-dose subcutaneous heparin, compared to only 11% of those receiving high-dose heparin (p < 0.0004). Use of high-dose subcutaneous heparin did not result in an increased incidence of hemorrhagic complications.

Despite the beneficial results obtained by Turpie et al with the use of high-dose subcutaneous heparin, it appears that *continuous IV infusion* of heparin provides superior anticoagulation. Most patients who receive a fixed-dose regimen of 12,500 Units of subcutaneous heparin twice a day demonstrate subtherapeutic heparin levels on the initial day of treatment, and only 50% achieve consistently therapeutic heparin levels on subsequent days (Prins and Hirsh, 1991). Although adjusting the dose of subcutaneous heparin based on the results of PTT monitoring would improve consistency in the heparin levels achieved, it is unlikely that subcutaneous heparin administration would ever be able to attain the consistency achievable with continuous IV infusion of the drug.

Based on these results, it appears to be reasonable to *empirically/prophylactically* anticoagulate patients with clinical evidence of large anterior AMI if they are not to receive thrombolytic therapy (ACC/AHA Task Force, 1990). Patients seen at a point beyond the "window of opportunity" (i.e., *more than* 6 hours after the onset of symptoms) would seem to be ideal candidates to consider for full anticoagulation. Although echocardiography may be helpful in the evaluation of some of these patients, *delaying* treatment until mural thrombi are confirmed echocardiographically might run the risk of leaving the patient unprotected during the most critical period.

Although systemic anticoagulation during hospitalization could be accomplished with *either* IV heparin or high-dose subcutaneous heparin (at sufficient dose to prolong the PTT to 1.5-2 × control values), continuous IV infusion of heparin appears to be preferable because of its more consistent anticoagulant effect (Prins and Hirsh, 1991). Patients with confirmed mural thrombi and/or a large hypokinetic area should then be maintained on oral coumadin (at sufficient dose to prolong the PT to 1.3-1.5 × control values) for *at least* 3-6 months (ACC/AHA Task Force, 1990).

Anticoagulation as an Adjunct to Thrombolytic Therapy

As previously mentioned, the short first phase (6 to 8 minute) half-life of rt-PA makes IV heparin an essential component of any regimen that uses this thrombolytic agent. Use of aspirin alone after rt-PA infusion may be sufficient to minimize the chance of *late* reocclusion of the infarct-related artery. However, use of aspirin alone is clearly less effective in preventing *early* reocclusion (i.e., within the first 24 hours after thrombolytic therapy) than IV heparin (Hsia et al, 1990). In contrast, the longer half-life of streptokinase and APSAC would seem to make immediate anticoagulation following thrombolytic therapy with either of these agents less essential—although it is still common practice to use IV heparin after administration of streptokinase or APSAC in the hope that the likelihood of early reocclusion will be further reduced.

In general, IV heparin is continued for at least 24 to 72 hours after reperfusion with thrombolytic therapy. Ideally, aspirin is begun as early as possible in the course of AMI and continued indefinitely if there are no contraindications.

Other Indications for Anticoagulation

The decision of whether to anticoagulate a patient with AMI is made easy if another potential indication for anticoagulation coincidentally exists. Thus, full anticoagulation should be strongly considered for the patient with AMI who also presents with acute DVT, pulmonary embolism, or a cerebrovascular accident—and possibly for associated atrial fibrillation or dilated cardiomyopathy (Table 12C-5).

Long-Term Anticoagulation After AMI

Following AMI, long-term anticoagulation with coumadin (sufficient to prolong the PT to between 1.5 to 2.0 × control values) has been shown to significantly reduce the incidence of mortality, reinfarction, and cerebrovascular accidents over the ensuing 3 years (Smith et al, 1990). However, long-term use of coumadin has not been shown to be more effective than secondary prevention with aspirin alone for AMI survivors who do not have another specific indication for anticoagulation. As a result, we currently favor the use of aspirin for this indication, since it is cheaper, simpler to administer, and less likely to produce a bleeding complication.

ANGIOPLASTY AND EMERGENCY CARDIAC SURGERY

As emphasized throughout this chapter, a KEY goal in management of AMI is to reestablish flow in the infarct-related artery (IRA). Although thrombolytic therapy is an extremely effective modality for accomplishing this goal, it will not be the *definitive* treatment measure for most patients with AMI because of one or more of the following factors:

1. A majority of patients with AMI either simply fail to qualify for thrombolytic therapy, or do not receive it for some other reason (Table 12C-4).
2. Thrombolytic therapy is not always successful in reestablishing flow to the IRA, even when administered to seemingly "ideal" candidates who satisfy all of the qualifying criteria.
3. Even when thrombolytic therapy is successful and immediately followed by anticoagulation (with IV heparin) and antiplatelet therapy (with aspirin), the risk remains that the IRA will reocclude.
4. The underlying degree of atherosclerosis is not reversed by thrombolytic therapy. A definitive procedure (i.e., angioplasty, bypass surgery) will still be needed in many cases to optimize prognosis.

Percutaneous transluminal angioplasty (PTCA) and coronary artery bypass graft (CABG) surgery represent two additional methods for reestablishing flow and/or maintaining vessel patency of the IRA. Both procedures are potentially lifesaving measures for AMI patients who have not responded to other treatment. Ideally, surgical revascularization is accomplished on an elective (or semielective) basis in hemodynamically stable patients who have survived the acute phase of AMI and are found to have suitable anatomy on predischarge cardiac catheterization. The evaluative approach to such patients clearly extends beyond the scope of this book.

Indications for more immediate surgical intervention—with mobilization of appropriate team members and facilities within four hours (i.e., *emergent* CABG surgery) or 24 hours (i.e., *urgent* CABG surgery)—are less well defined. Practical considerations (i.e., surgical skill and availability, institution experience with the procedure, time requirements for mobilizing resources, risk of increased morbidity and mortality, etc.) often weigh heavily in determining whether to undertake emergency operation. As a result, use of CABG surgery as an *acute* intervention in patients with AMI is generally reserved for patients who fail to respond to conventional treatment measures and thrombolytic therapy. Potential candidates for immediate surgical intervention therefore include patients with persistent chest pain/ischemia and/or hemodynamic instability after failed angioplasty—or unstable patients for whom angioplasty can't be performed (ACC/AHA Task Force, 1990).

In skilled hands, success rates as high as 90% have been reported for acute surgical revascularization of AMI patients who are not in frank cardiogenic shock at the time of operation (Bolooki, 1990).

In contrast to the more limited use of urgent/emergent CABG surgery for patients with AMI, the much greater availability and facility in performing angioplasty has tremendously increased the application of PTCA as an acute revascularization procedure in recent years. In the setting of AMI, angioplasty now has three potential indications: (1) as a *primary* reperfusion procedure; (2) as an *adjunct* to thrombolytic therapy; or (3) as a "rescue" (i.e., *salvage*) procedure. Because of the tremendous importance of timing in identifying suitable candidates for acute revascularization and implementing the procedure, we conclude this section by addressing each of these indications *(Table 12C-6)*.

PTCA as a *Primary* Procedure in AMI

Success rates are remarkably high (up to 90%) when appropriately selected patients receive PTCA as a primary procedure for reestablishing flow to the IRA (Holmes and Vlietstra, 1989). The principal drawback of using PTCA for this indication is the need for round-the-clock staffing and cardiology availability for performing emergency angiography, as well as the need for surgical backup should a lifethreatening complication develop. Use of angioplasty also entails a seemingly unavoidable (and sometimes considerable) delay between patient presentation, diagnosis of AMI, and treatment (including the time for transport of the patient to the hospital and mobilization of staff and facilities for emergency catheterization). Because of the practicality and rapidity with which IV thrombolytic therapy may be initiated, medical (rather than mechanical) thrombolysis remains the most commonly chosen method for *initial* attempts at achieving reperfusion. Nevertheless, in hospitals focused on performing *primary* PTCA as an emergency procedure, this modality offers an extremely effective alternative for reestablishing flow to the IRA during the early hours of AMI (Table 12C-6).

Primary angioplasty may be especially valuable for patients who do not qualify for thrombolytic therapy (because of late presentation or a contraindication), for AMI that occurs in patients who are already hospitalized (and who therefore have ready access to cardiac catheterization in the hospital), and/or when the etiology of new-onset chest pain is unclear (i.e., in patients with ST segment depression or a normal ECG). When the diagnosis is unclear, emergency cardiac catheterization not only reveals the underlying anatomy and confirms the process (of AMI), but through angioplasty it may also provide potentially definitive treatment. As mentioned earlier, PTCA is much more likely to be effective than IV thrombolytic therapy in restoring coronary flow when acute graft occlusion is suspected in a patient with prior CABG surgery. Finally, primary angioplasty may prove to be a lifesaving procedure in the management of critically ill AMI patients who present with hemodynamic instability (i.e., hypotension with pulmonary edema and/or cardiogenic shock). Emergent PTCA (performed within the first 18 hours of the onset of symptoms) is superior to medical treatment and/or the use of intra-aortic balloon counterpulsation (IABC) in this situation, and may improve the chance for survival to as high as 50% (ACC/AHA Task Force, 1990; Klein, 1992).

Table 12C-6

Potential Indications for Percutaneous Transluminal Angioplasty (PTCA) in Patients with AMI

• **PTCA as a *Primary* Procedure**

-When the patient doesn't qualify for thrombolytic therapy (because of late presentation or a contraindication)

-When hospital facilities and cardiology/cardiothoracic support are available and favor use of this intervention as a primary procedure

-When AMI occurs while the patient is in the hospital (i.e., and therefore with ready access to a catheterization laboratory)

-When the etiology of new-onset chest pain is unclear (i.e., performance of acute catheterization for diagnostic purposes, with possible PTCA as treatment)

-For patients with prior CABG surgery in whom acute graft occlusion is suspected

-For selected AMI patients who present in a hemodynamically unstable condition (i.e., hypotensive, in pulmonary edema, and/or cardiogenic shock)

• **PTCA as an *Adjunct* to Thrombolytic Therapy**

-As an *urgent procedure* when despite successful thrombolysis, there is evidence of ongoing ischemia (i.e., persistent ST segment changes, post-infarction angina)

-As a *"semi-elective" procedure* (i.e., a week or more after AMI) in patients who demonstrate proximal high-grade residual stenosis of the IRA on predischarge catheterization, especially when associated with a large area of still viable myocardium and/or evidence of ongoing ischemia (i.e., ST segment changes on resting ECG or on predischarge exercise testing)

• **PTCA as a "Rescue" (i.e., *Salvage*) Procedure**

-For selected AMI patients when IV thrombolytic therapy is not successful in reperfusing the IRA—especially if there is persistent chest pain, hypotension, incipient heart failure, and/or other evidence of ongoing ischemia

-As an urgent/emergent procedure after IV thrombolytic therapy when acute *reocclusion* of the IRA is suspected.

Reperfusion by primary angioplasty in patients with AMI may be complicated by reformation of thrombus and reocclusion of the IRA in as many as one third of cases (Popma and Dehmer, 1989). Most of the time when reocclusion occurs, it does so *early* (i.e., while the patient is still in the catheterization laboratory, or within the ensuing several hours). Immediate redilatation with PTCA, and/or institution of thrombolytic therapy will often be successful in reestablishing and maintaining vessel patency in this situation (Holmes and Vlietstra, 1989; Popma and Dehmer, 1989). More grave complications (i.e., coronary dissection or rupture, thrombus migration with sudden complete occlusion of a coronary artery) are seen infrequently but may necessitate immediate attention (i.e., emergency surgery) when they occur (Bolooki, 1990).

PTCA as an *Adjunct* to Thrombolytic Therapy in AMI

Despite its tremendous efficacy, thrombolytic therapy will not be successful in reperfusing the IRA in 25% to 40% of cases. Even when coronary flow is restored and adjunctive treatment (with aspirin and IV heparin) is immediately started, there is still a 10% to 15% chance that

the IRA will reocclude within the ensuing 24 hours (Tiefenbrunn and Sobel, 1989). Moreover, significant underlying stenosis of the IRA is likely to remain *regardless* of the efficacy of thrombolytic therapy, thus predisposing the patient to recurrent ischemia and/or reocclusion of the IRA (i.e., reinfarction) at a later time.

> In general, the more severe the degree of *underlying* residual stenosis in the IRA, the greater the likelihood that recurrent ischemia and/or reocclusion will occur (Tiefenbrunn and Sobel, 1989).

In an attempt to maximize the opportunity for myocardial salvage and minimize the risk of early reocclusion and post-infarction angina, early catheterization with performance of PTCA had been advocated as an adjunct to thrombolytic therapy for patients with suitable anatomy. Considering that as many as two thirds of those patients who initially achieve reperfusion with thrombolytic therapy remain with a high-grade stenosis of the IRA, the potential impact that a routine investigative strategy (with early catheterization and PTCA if anatomy is suitable) could have is substantial (Topol et al, 1987; the TIMI Study Group, 1989).

Unfortunately, results from several randomized trials have *not* supported this concept. If anything, mortality and reocclusion rates have been *higher* when cardiac catheterization and PTCA are performed *early* (i.e., within 48 hours after administration of thrombolytic therapy) compared to a more conservative strategy in which cardiac catheterization is deferred for at least a week (Topol et al, 1987; the TIMI Research Group, 1988; Tiefenbrunn and Sobol, 1989). In addition, the need for emergency bypass surgery and the incidence of significant bleeding complications are both *greater* in patients who undergo immediate PTCA compared to those who are treated conservatively. Thus despite the intuitive benefit that one might expect from prompt mechanical opening of an occluded IRA, in many cases this vessel simply does not respond well when balloon dilatation is applied early during the course of AMI.

In summary, **there appears to be no indication at the present time for *routine* early catheterization (and PTCA) if thrombolytic therapy is successful** and the patient is otherwise doing well (i.e., asymptomatic, hemodynamically stable, and without evidence of ongoing ischemia). Instead, *"watchful waiting"* appears to be preferable to active intervention in *clinically stable* patients (The TIMI Study Group, 1989).

In contrast, **early catheterization and angioplasty** (if anatomy is suitable) **are definitely indicated** *after thrombolytic therapy* **for patients who become hemodynamically unstable** *and/or demonstrate evidence of* **ongoing ischemia** (i.e., persistent ST segment changes and/or refractory post-infarction angina).

The importance of closely monitoring patients after successful reperfusion with IV thrombolytic therapy is highlighted by results of the TAMI study. Eighteen percent of those patients who remained with high-grade residual stenosis of the IRA after initial reperfusion went on to require an emergency intervention (either PTCA or emergency bypass surgery) because of recurrent symptoms or persistent ischemia during the 1-week period of observation (Topol et al, 1987). Thus a significant percentage of patients with AMI who initially appear to be doing well after thrombolytic therapy may unexpectedly develop the need for emergency catheterization and/or an intervention over the ensuing week. However, in spite of this possibility, the increased risk of complications (bleeding, reocclusion of the IRA, lesion progression requiring bypass surgery) associated with performance of these procedures during the first few days of AMI appears to outweigh any potential benefits that might accrue from *routine* institution of an invasive investigative strategy.

An additional reason why routine early investigation (with cardiac catheterization) and intervention (with angioplasty if deemed appropriate) is *not* an optimal strategy

is that **spontaneous resolution of thrombus in the IRA occurs with time.** Thus, 14% of those patients in the observation group of the TAMI study who initially (on catheterization immediately after thrombolytic therapy) had high-grade stenosis of the IRA deemed suitable for angioplasty, no longer required this procedure when re-evaluated one week later (Topol et al, 1987). One year later, long-term (cumulative) rates for mortality, reinfarction, and need for CABG surgery are no different for AMI patients who were routinely catheterized and received early PTCA (within 48 hours of thrombolytic therapy) compared to patients who were treated in a more conservative manner in which early catheterization and PTCA were only performed for persistent symptoms or ischemia (Rogers et al, 1990).

It is important to emphasize that the risk of developing a complication from cardiac catheterization and/or PTCA becomes much less when these procedures are performed on a more *elective* basis (i.e., a week or more after AMI). Passage of time allows *stabilization* of the IRA. The process of thrombus formation and fibrin lysis is no longer as vigorous after several days, and the vessel wall of the IRA is no longer as susceptible to spontaneous plaque fissure or rupture (Topol et al, 1988). In addition to being safer, delaying cardiac catheterization allows more accurate determination of the true underlying anatomy, and more objective assessment of residual left ventricular function. As a result, one can better predict whether revascularization (by PTCA or CABG surgery) is likely to be beneficial. In general, success rates for PTCA performed after 1 week in appropriately selected candidates exceed 90%, and are superior to success rates achieved when PTCA is performed earlier in the course after thrombolytic therapy (Holmes and Vlietstra, 1989).

PTCA as a "Rescue" (i.e., *Salvage*) Procedure in AMI

As already emphasized, IV thrombolytic therapy will not be successful in reperfusing the IRA 25% to 40% of the time. Because mortality is greater when flow is not reestablished in the IRA, emergency angioplasty is sometimes undertaken as a "rescue" procedure (Topol et al, 1987). The goal of angioplasty in this circumstance is to attempt *salvage* of myocardium that may still be viable. Rescue angioplasty is most likely to be helpful when other indicators of high risk status are also present (i.e., persistent chest pain, ongoing ischemia, hypotension, or incipient heart failure).

Alternatively, reperfusion with IV thrombolytic therapy may be successful initially, only to have the IRA suddenly reocclude. When this situation is suspected, emergency angioplasty may offer the best chance for rapidly reestablishing coronary flow and maintaining patency in the IRA. Emergency bypass surgery may occasionally be indicated if rescue angioplasty fails to reperfuse the IRA, or if coronary anatomy appears to be more conducive to surgical revascularization.

References

AIMS Trial Study Group: Effect of intravenous APSAC on mortality after acute myocardial infarction: preliminary report of a placebo-controlled clinical trial, *Lancet* 1:545-549, 1988.

American College of Cardiology/American Heart Association Task Force: Guidelines for the early management of patients with acute myocardial infarction, *Circulation* 82:664-707, 1990.

Anderson JL, Marshall HW: A randomized trial of intravenous and intracoronary streptokinase in patients with acute myocardial infarction, *Circulation* 70:606-618, 1984.

Anderson JL: Reperfusion, patency and reocclusion with antistreplase (APSAC) in acute myocardial infarction, *Am J Cardiol* 64:12A-17A, 1989.

Antiplatelet Trialists' Collaboration: Secondary prevention of vascular disease by prolonged antiplatelet treatment, *Br Med J* 296:320-331, 1988.

Aufderheide TP, Haselow WC, Hendley GE, Robinson NA, Armaganian L, Hargarten KM, Olson DW, Valley VT, Stueven HA: Feasibility of prehospital r-TPA therapy in chest pain patients, *Ann Emerg Med* 21:379-383, 1992.

Bar FW, Vermeer F, DeZwaan C, Ramentol M, Braat S, Simoons ML, Hermens WT, Van Der Laarse A, Verheugt FWA, Krauss XH, Wellens HJJ: Value of admission electrocardiogram in predicting outcome of thrombolytic therapy in acute myocardial infarction: a randomized trial conducted by the Netherlands Interuniversity Cardiology Institute, *Am J Cardiol* 59:6-13, 1987.

Barbash GI, Roth A, Hod H, Modan M, Miller HI, Rath S, Zahav YH, Keren G, Motro M, Shachar A, Basan S, Agranat O, Rabinowitz B, Laniado S, Kaplinsky E: Randomized controlled trial of late in-hospital angiography and angioplasty versus conservative management after treatment with recombinant tissue-type plasminogen activator in acute myocardial infarction, *Am J Cardiol* 66:538-545, 1990.

Bates ER: Reperfusion therapy in inferior myocardial infarction, *J Am Coll Cardiol* 12:44A-51A, 1988.

Beek AM, Verheugt FWA, Meyer A: Usefulness of electrocardiographic findings and creatine kinase levels on admission in predicting the accuracy of the interval between onset of chest pain of acute myocardial infarction and initiation of thrombolytic therapy, *Am J Cardiol* 68:1287-1290, 1991.

de Belder M, Skehan D, Pumphrey C, Khan B, Evans S, Rothman M, Mills P: Identification of a high risk subgroup of patients with silent ischaemia after myocardial infarction: a group for early therapeutic revascularisation? *Br Heart J* 63:145-150, 1990.

Berger PB, Ryan TJ: Inferior myocardial infarction: high risk subgroups, *Circulation* 81:401-411, 1990.

Bleich SD, Nichols TC, Schumacher RR, Cooke DH, Tate DA, Teichman SL: Effect of heparin on coronary arterial patency after thrombolysis with tissue plasminogen activator in acute myocardial infarction, *Am J Cardiol* 66:1412-1417, 1990.

Bolooki H: Surgical treatment of complications of acute myocardial infarction, *JAMA* 263:1237-1240, 1990.

Braunwald E: Myocardial reperfusion, limitation of infarct size, reduction of left ventricular dysfunction, and improved survival: should the paradigm be expanded? *Circulation* 79:441-444, 1989.

Califf RM, Topol EJ, George BS, Boswick JM, Abbottsmith C, Sigmon KN, Candela R, Masek R, Kereiakes D, O'Neill WW: Hemorrhagic complications associated with the use of intravenous tissue plasminogen activator in treatment of acute myocardial infarction, *Am J Med* 85:353-359, 1988.

Campbell CA, Przyklenk K, Kloner RA: Infarct size reduction: a review of the clinical trials, *J Clin Pharmacol* 26:317-329, 1986.

Chamberlain DA: Unanswered questions in thrombolysis, *Am J Cardiol* 64:34A-40A, 1989.

Check WA: News, *Clin Pharm* 10:486-488, 1991.

Cigarroa RG, Lange RA, Hillis LD: Prognosis after acute myocardial infarction in patients with and without residual anterograde coronary blood flow, *Am J Cardiol* 64:155-160, 1989.

Clarke RJ, Mayo G, Price P, Fitzgerald GA: Suppression of thromboxane A2, but not of systemic prostacyclin by controlled-release aspirin, *N Engl J Med* 325:1137-1141, 1991.

Davies MJ, Thomas AC, Knapman PA, Hangartner JR: Intramyocardial platelet aggregation in patients with unstable angina suffering sudden ischemic cardiac death, *Circulation* 73:418-427, 1986.

DeWood MA, Spores J, Notske R, Mouser LT, Burroughs R, Golden MS, Lang LT: Prevalence of total coronary occlusion during the early hours of transmural myocardial infarction, *N Engl J Med* 303:897-902, 1980.

European Cooperative Study Group for Recombinant Tissue-Type Plasminogen Activator: Randomized trial of intravenous recombinant tissue-type plasminogen activator versus intravenous streptokinase in acute myocardial infarction, *Lancet* 1:842-847, 1985.

Falk E: Morphologic features of unstable atherothrombotic plaques underlying acute coronary syndromes, *Am J Cardiol* 63:114E-120E, 1989.

Fuster V, Halperin JL: Left ventricular thrombi and cerebral embolism, *N Engl J Med* 320:392-394, 1989.

Ganz W, Geft I, Shah PK, Lew AS, Rodriguez L, Weiss T, Maddahi J, Berman DS, Charuzi Y, Swan HJC: Intravenous streptokinase in evolving acute myocardial infarction, *Am J Cardiol* 53:1209-1216, 1984.

Genton E, Turpie AGG: Anticoagulant therapy following acute myocardial infarction, *Mod Conc Cardiovasc Dis* 52:45-48, 1983.

Gray RJ, Sethna D, Matloff JM: Without mechanical complications. In The role of cardiac surgery in acute myocardial infarction, *Am Heart J* 106:728-735, 1983.

Grines CL, DeMaria AN: Optimal utilization of thrombolytic therapy for acute myocardial infarction: concepts and controversies, *J Am Coll Cardiol* 16:223-231, 1990.

Grines CL, Booth DC, Nissen SE, Gurley JC, Bennett KA, O'Connor WN, DeMaria AN: Mechanism of acute myocardial infarction in patients with prior coronary artery bypass grafting and therapeutic implications, *Am J Cardiol* 65:1292-1296, 1990.

Gruppo Italiano Per Lo Studio della Streptochinasi nell'Infarto Miocardioco (GISSI): Effectiveness of intravenous thrombolytic treatment in acute myocardial infarction, *Lancet* 1:397-402. 1986.

Gruppo Italiano Per Lo Studio della Streptochinasi nell'I nfarto Miocardioco (GISSI); Long-term effects of intravenous thrombolysis in acute myocardial infarction: final report of the GISSI study, *Lancet* 2:871-874, 1987.

Gruppo Italiano Per Lo Studio della Sopravvivenza nell'Infarto Miocardioco: GISSI-2: A factorial randomised trial of alteplase versus streptokinase and heparin versus no heparin among 12,490 patients with acute myocardial infarction, *Lancet* 336:65-71, 1990.

Gurwitz JH, Goldberg RJ, Gore JM: Coronary thrombolysis in the elderly? *JAMA* 265:1720-1723, 1991.

Health and Public Policy Committee, American College of Physicians: Thrombolysis for evolving myocardial infarction, *Ann Intern Med* 103:463-649, 1985.

Henry R, deGruy F: Intravenous streptokinase for treatment of acute myocardial infarction in small hospitals, *J Fam Prac* 26:438-442, 1988.

Heras M, Chesebro JH, Gersh BG, Holmes DR, Mock MB: Emergency thrombolysis in acute myocardial infarction, *Ann Emerg Med* 17:1168-1175, 1988.

Holmes DR, Vlietstra RE: Balloon angioplasty in acute and chronic coronary artery disease, *JAMA* 261:2109-2115, 1989.

Hsia J, Hamilton WP, Kleiman N, Roberts R, Chaitman BR, Ross: for the Heparin-Aspirin Reperfusion Trial (HART) Investigators: A comparison between heparin and low-dose aspirin as adjunctive therapy with tissue plasminogen activator for acute myocardial infarction, *N Engl J Med* 323:1433-1437, 1990.

Huey BL, Beller GA, Kaiser DL, Gibson RS: A comprehensive analysis of myocardial infarction due to left circumflex artery occlusion: comparison with infarction due to right coronary artery and left anterior descending artery occlusion, *J Am Coll Cardiol* 12:1156-1166, 1988.

The International Study Group: In-hospital mortality and clinical course of 20,891 patients with suspected acute myocardial infarction randomised between alteplase and streptokinase with or without heparin, *Lancet* 336:71-75, 1990.

The Intravenous Streptokinase in Acute Myocardial Infarction Study Group: A prospective trial of intravenous streptokinase in acute myocardial infarction (ISAM). Mortality, morbidity, and infarct size at 21 days, *N Engl J Med* 314:1465-1471, 1986.

Jalihal S, Morris GK: Antistreptokinase titers after intravenous streptokinase, *Lancet* 335:184-185, 1990.

Kennedy JW, Ritchie JL, Davis KB, Fritz JK: Western Washington randomized trial of intracoronary streptokinase in acute myocardial infarction, *N Engl J Med* 309:1477-1482, 1983.

Kennedy JW, Gensini GG, Timmis GC, Maynard C: Acute myocardial infarction treated with intracoronary streptokinase: a report of the society for cardiac angiography, *Am J Cardiol* 55:871-877, 1985.

Kennedy JW, Weaver WD: Potential use of thrombolytic therapy before hospitalization, *Am J Cardiol* 64:8A-11A, 1989.

Kereiakes DJ, Weaver WD, Anderson JL, Feldman T, Gibler B, Aufderheide T, Williams DO, Martin LH, Anderson LC, Martin JS: Time delays in the diagnosis and treatment of acute myocardial infarction: a tale of eight cities—report from the Pre-Hospital Study Group and the Cincinnati Heart Project, *Am Heart J* 120:773-780, 1990.

Khan MI, Hackett DR, Andreotti F, Davies GJ, Regan T, Haider AW, McFaden E, Halson P, Maseri A: Effectiveness of multiple bolus administration of tissue-type plasminogen activator in acute myocardial infarction, *Am J Cardiol* 65:1051-1056, 1990.

Klein IW: Optimal therapy for cardiogenic shock: the emerging role of coronary angioplasty, *J Am Coll Cardiol* 19:654-656, 1992.

Kupper AJF, Verheugt FW, Peels CH, Galema TW, del Hollander W, Roos JP: Effect of low dose acetyl salicylic acid on the frequency and hematologic activity of left ventricular thrombus in anterior wall acute myocardial infarction, *Am J Cardiol* 63:917-920, 1989.

Laffel GL, Braunwald E: Thrombolytic therapy: a new strategy for the treatment of acute myocardial infarction, *N Engl J Med* 311:710-717, 770-776, 1984.

Lee TH, Weisberg MC, Brand DA, Rouan GW, Goldman L: Candidates for thrombolysis among emergency room patients with acute chest pain. Potential true- and false-positive rates, *Ann Intern Med* 110:957-962, 1989.

Lewis HD, Davis JW, Archibald DG, Steinke WE, Smitherman TC, Doherty JE, Schnaper HW, LeWinter MM, Linares E, Pouget JM, Sabharwal SC, Chester E, DeMots H: Protective effects of aspirin against acute myocardial infarction and death in men with unstable angina: results of a Veterans Administration cooperative study, *N Engl J Med* 309:396-403, 1983.

Logue E, Ognibene A, Marquinez C, Jarjoura D: Elapsed time from symptom onset and acute myocardial infarction in a community hospital, *Ann Emerg Med* 20:339-343, 1991.

Magnani B, for the PAIMS Investigators: Plasminogen Activator Italian Multicenter Study (PAIMS) comparison of intravenous recombinant single-chain human tissue-type plasminogen activator (rt-PA) with intravenous streptokinase in acute myocardial infarction, *J Am Coll Cardiol* 13:19-26, 1989.

Martin G, Kennedy JW: Influence on mortality. In Thrombolytic therapy in the management of acute myocardial infarction, *Mod Conc Cardiovasc Dis* 59:13-18, 1990.

Medical Letter: Anistreplase for acute coronary thrombosis, *Med Letter* 32:15-16, 1990.

Mehta JL: Antithrombotic therapy in chronic coronary artery disease, *Primary Cardiology* 17:24-31, 1991.

Meltzer RS, Visser CA, Fuster V: Intracardiac thrombi and systemic embolization, *Ann Intern Med* 104:689-698, 1986.

Meyer J, Merx W: Sequential intervention procedures after intracoronary thrombolysis: balloon dilatation, bypass surgery, and medical treatment, *Int J Cardiol* 7:281-293, 1985.

Midgette AS, O'Connor GT, Baron JA, Bell J: Effect of intravenous streptokinase on early mortality in patients with suspected acute myocardial infarction: a meta-analysis by anatomic location of infarction, *Ann Intern Med* 113:961-968, 1990.

Montague TJ, Ikuta RM, Wong RY, Bay KS, Teo KK, Davies NJ: Comparison of risk and patterns of practice in patients older and younger than 70 years with acute myocardial infarction in a two-year period (1987-1989), *Am J Cardiol* 68:843-847, 1991.

Muller DWM, Topol EJ: Selection of patients with acute myocardial infarction for thrombolytic therapy, *Ann Intern Med* 113:949-960, 1990.

Naylor CD, Jaglal SB: Impact of intravenous thrombolysis on short-term coronary revascularization rates: a meta-analysis, *JAMA* 264:697-702, 1990.

Neuhaus K, Feuerer W, Jeep-Tebbe S, Niederer W, Vogt A, Tebbe U: Improved thrombolysis with a modified dose regimen of recombinant tissue-type plasminogen activator, *J Am Coll Cardiol* 14:1566-1569, 1989.

Peels CH, Visser CA, Kupper AJ, Visser FC, Roos JP: Two-dimensional echocardiography for immediate detection of myocardial ischemia in the emergency room, *Am J Cardiol* 65:687-691, 1990.

Popma JJ, Dehmer GJ: Care of the patient after coronary angioplasty, *Ann Intern Med* 110:547-559, 1989.

Popp RL: Echocardiography, *N Engl J Med* 323:165-172, 1990.

Prins MH, Hirsh J: Heparin as an adjunctive treatment after thrombolytic therapy for acute myocardial infarction, *Am J Cardiol* 67:3A-11A, 1991.

Rapaport E: Thrombolytic agents in acute myocardial infarction, *N Engl J Med* 320:861-864, 1989.

Reeder GS, Vlietstra RE: Coronary angioplasty: 1986, *MCCD* 55:49-53, 1986.

Rentrop KP, Feit F, Blanke H, Stecy P, Schneider R, Rey M, Horowitz S, Goldman M, Karsch K, Meilman H: Effects of intracoronary streptokinase and intracoronary nitroglycerin infusion on coronary angiographic patterns and mortality in patients with acute myocardial infarction, *N Engl J Med* 311:1457-1463, 1984.

Rentrop KP: Thrombolytic therapy in patients with acute myocardial infarction, *Circulation* 71:627-631, 1988.

Rogers WJ, Baim DS, Gore JH, Brown BG, Roberts R, Williams DO, Chesebro, Babb JD, Sheehan FH, Wacker FJ: Comparison of immediate invasive, delayed invasive, and conservative strategies after tissue-type plasminogen activator: results of the thrombolysis in myocardial infarction (TIMI) phase II—a trial, *Circulation* 81:1457-1476, 1990.

Rowe WW, Simpson RJ, Tate DA, Willis PW, Nichols TC, Noneman JW, Gettes LS, and The University of North Carolina Cardiology Consortium: Nonemergent cardiac catheterization and risk-stratified revascularization following thrombolytic therapy for acute myocardial infarction: a critical analysis of therapy in the community setting, *Arch Intern Med* 149:1611-1617, 1989.

Schlant RC: Thrombolytic therapy of patients with acute myocardial infarction, *JAMA* 264:738-739, 1990.

Second International Study of Infarct Survival (ISIS-2) Collaborative Group: Randomised trial of intravenous streptokinase, oral aspirin, both, or neither among 17,187 cases of suspected acute myocardial infarction: ISIS-2, *Lancet* 2:349-360, 1988.

Sherry S: Tissue plasminogen activator (t-PA): will it fulfill its promise? *N Engl J Med* 333:1014-1017, 1985.

Smith P, Arnesen H, Holme I: The effect of warfarin on mortality and reinfarction after myocardial infarction, *N Engl J Med* 323:147-152, 1990.

Taylor GJ, Mikell F: Intravenous versus intracoronary streptokinase therapy for acute myocardial infarction in community hospitals, *Am J Cardiol* 54:256-260, 1984.

Taylor GJ, Song A, Moses W, Koester DL, Mikell FL, Dove JT, Katholi RE, Wellons HA, Schneider JA: The primary care physician and thrombolytic therapy for acute myocardial infarction: comparison of intravenous streptokinase in community hospitals and the tertiary referral center, *J Am Bd Fam Pract* 3:1-6, 1990.

Tebbe U, Tanswell P, Seifried E, Feuerer W, Scholz KH, Herrmann KS: Single-bolus injection of recombinant tissue-type plasminogen activator in acute myocardial infarction, *Am J Cardiol* 64:448-453, 1989.

Tenaglia AN, Califf RM, Candela RJ, Kereiakes DJ, Barrios E, Young SY, Stack RS, Topol EJ: Thrombolytic therapy in patients requiring cardiopulmonary resuscitation, *Am J Cardiol* 68:1015-1019, 1991.

The Thrombolysis Early in Acute Heart Attack Trial Study Group: Very early thrombolytic therapy in suspected acute myocardial infarction, *Am J Cardiol* 65:401-407, 1990.

The TIMI Study Group: Special report: the thrombolysis in myocardial infarction (TIMI) trial, phase I findings, *N Engl J Med* 312:932-936, 1985.

Tiefenbrunn AJ, Ludbrook PA: Coronary thrombolysis—it's worth the risk, *JAMA* 261:2107-2108, 1989.

Tiefenbrunn AJ, Sobel BE: The impact of coronary thrombolysis on myocardial infarction, *Fibrinolysis* 3:1-15, 1989.

The TIMI Research Group: Immediate vs delayed catheterization and angioplasty following thrombolytic therapy for acute myocardial infarction. TIMI II A results, *JAMA* 260:2849-2858, 1988.

TIMI Study Group: Comparison of invasive and conservative strategies after treatment with intravenous tissue plasminogen activator in acute myocardial infarction: results of the thrombolysis in myocardial infarction (TIMI) phase II trial, *N Engl J Med* 320:618-627, 1989.

Topol EJ, Califf RM, George BS, Kereiakes DJ, Abbottsmith CW, Candela RJ, Lee KL, Pitt B, Stack RS, O'Neill WW, and the Thrombolysis and Angioplasty in Myocardial Infarction (TAMI) Study Group: A multicenter randomized trial of intravenous recombinant tissue plasminogen activator and immediate angioplasty in acute myocardial infarction, *N Engl J Med* 317:581-588, 1987.

Topol EJ, Califf RM, George BS, Kereiakes DJ, Lee KL for the TAMI Study Group: Insights derived from the thrombolysis and angioplasty in myocardial infarction (TAMI) trials, *J Am Coll Cardiol* 12:24A-31A, 1988.

Tranchesi B, Verstraete M, Vanhove MD: Intravenous bolus administration of recombinant tissue plasminogen activator to patients with acute myocardial infarction, *Coronary Artery Disease* 1:83-88, 1990.

Turpie AGG, Robinson JG, Doyle DJ, Mulji AS, Mishkel GJ, Sealey BJ, Cairns JA, Skingley L, Hirsh L, Gent M: Comparison of high-dose with low-dose subcutaneous heparin to prevent left ventricular mural thrombosis in patients with acute transmural anterior myocardial infarction, *N Engl J Med* 320:352-357, 1989.

Urban PL, Cowley M, Goldberg S, Vetrovec G, Hastillo A, Greenspon AJ, Kusiak V, Greenberg R, Walinsky P, Cammarato J: Intracoronary thrombolysis in acute myocardial infarction: clinical course following successful myocardial reperfusion, *Am Heart J* 108:873-878, 1984.

Van de Werf F, Ludbrook PA, Bergmann SR, Tiefenbrunn AJ, Fox KAA, DeGeest H, Verstraete M, Collen D, Sobel BE: Coronary thrombolysis with tissue-type plasminogen activator in patients with evolving myocardial infarction. *N Engl J Med* 310:609-613, 1984.

Visser CA, Kan G, Meltzer RS, Dunning AJ, Roelandt J: Embolic potential of left ventricular thrombus after myocardial infarction: a two-dimensional echocardiographic study of 119 patients, *J Am Coll Cardiol* 5:1276-1280, 1985.

Weaver WD, Eisenberg MS, Martin JS, Litwin PE, Shaeffer SM, Ho MT, Kudenchuk P, Hallstrom AP, Cerqueira MD, Copass MK, Kennedy JW, Cobb LA, Ritchie JL: Myocardial infarction triage and intervention project—phase I: patient characteristics and feasibility of prehospital initiation of thrombolytic therapy, *J Am Coll Cardiol* 15:925-931, 1990.

White HD, Rivers JT, Maslowski AH, Ormiston JA, Takayama M, Hart HH, Sharpe DN, Whitlock RML, Norris RM: Effect of intravenous streptokinase as compared with that of tissue plasminogen activator on left ventricular function after first myocardial infarction, *N Engl J Med* 320:817-821, 1989.

Wilcox RG, von der Lippe G, Olsson CG, Jensen G, Skene AM, Hampton JR: Trial of tissue plasminogen activator for mortality reduction in acute myocardial infarction: Anglo-Scandinavian study of early thrombolysis (ASSET), *Lancet* 2:525-530, 1988.

Yusuf S, Wittes J, Friedman L: Treatments Following Myocardial Infarction. In Overview of results of randomized clinical trials in heart disease, *JAMA* 260:2088-2093, 1988.

Yusuf S, Wittes J, Friedman : Unstable Langina, heart failure, primary prevention with aspirin, and risk factor modification. In Overview of results of randomized clinical trials in heart disease, *JAMA* 260:2259-2263, 1988.

Yusuf S, Furberg CD: Are we biased in our approach to treating elderly patients with heart disease? *Am J Cardiol* 68:954-956, 1991.

SECTION D

SPECIAL TREATMENT CONSIDERATIONS

Autonomic Nervous System Dysfunction with Acute MI

Autonomic nervous system overactivity occurs in a majority of patients during the early minutes and hours of AMI. Autonomic nervous system stimulation may be purely parasympathetic in nature, purely sympathetic, or as is most commonly the case, a combination of the two. In general, parasympathetic overactivity is much more likely to predominate with acute inferior infarction. In contrast, sympathetic overactivity is more likely to predominate with acute anterior infarction. It is important to realize that pharmacologic measures specifically aimed at attenuating parasympathetic or sympathetic overactivity may alter the underlying balance between these two types of autonomic tone.

PARASYMPATHETIC OVERACTIVITY: USE OF ATROPINE

Patients with acute *inferior* infarction frequently demonstrate sinus bradycardia and hypotension (*parasympathetic* overactivity). Atropine sulfate effectively counteracts such increases in vagal tone, as well as accelerating the rate of sinus node discharge. The drug also improves atrioventricular conduction so that it may be effective in the treatment of 2° AV block Mobitz type I (Wenckebach) that occurs in the setting of AMI. However, indiscriminate use of the drug may result in inappropriate acceleration of the sinus rate, hypertension, and induction of ventricular arrhythmias (including ventricular tachycardia or fibrillation). As implied above, this may result from an "unmasking" effect in which the parasympatholytic action of atropine now leaves underlying sympathetic overactivity unopposed. Use of atropine should therefore *never* be taken lightly in the setting of AMI, and the drug is *only* indicated for bradycardic individuals who manifest signs of hemodynamic compromise (i.e., hypotension, PVCs, or chest pain) as a *direct* result of the slow heart rate.

Atropine appears to be most effective at reversing sinus bradycardia and hypotension, and in treating Mobitz I 2° AV block that occurs within the first 6 to 8 hours of acute infarction (ACC/AHA Task Force, 1990). After that time, factors others than vagal overactivity are more likely to come into play, and other forms of treatment (i.e., cardiac pacing) may be needed. Increments of 0.5 mg may be repeated every 5 minutes as needed up to a dose of 2 mg. If the heart rate is excessively slow and the blood pressure extremely low, larger increments of the drug (i.e., 1 mg at a time) may be given more often (i.e., every 2 to 3 minutes) to expedite treatment (up to a total of 3 mg).

It should be emphasized that treatment with atropine is *not* benign, and that the drug should *not* be used to treat a rhythm such as sinus bradycardia if the heart rate is over 40 beats/min and the patient is hemodynamically stable.

(See Section B of Chapter 2 for more information on atropine administration.)

SYMPATHETIC OVERACTIVITY: USE OF β-BLOCKERS

Patients with acute *anterior* infarction frequently demonstrate sinus tachycardia and hypertension (*sympathetic* overactivity). In addition, the sympathetic overactivity that is so commonly present during the early minutes to hours of AMI may well account for the high incidence of primary ventricular fibrillation during this period, and at least partially explain the beneficial response to IV administration of β-blockers. As emphasized earlier in this chapter *(See Section B)*, in the absence of contraindications, administration of IV β-blockers *as early as possible* to patients with AMI should be strongly considered, *especially* for high-risk subgroups of patients (i.e., those having larger infarctions) who manifest clinical evidence of sympathetic overactivity (i.e., anterior site of infarction, tachycardia, hypertension).

Conduction System Disturbances

Atrioventricular (AV) block is a frequent complication of AMI. Prognosis and management vary greatly, depending on the degree of block, the estimated size and location of the infarct, the ventricular response, and the patient's clinical status.

AV BLOCK

AV block most commonly occurs with acute inferior infarction, since the right coronary artery characteristically supplies the AV node. Treatment is generally not necessary for 1° AV block or 2° AV block of the Mobitz I type (Wenckebach), since blood pressure and heart rate usually remain adequate. Even with 3° (complete) AV block from acute *inferior* infarction, insertion of a transvenous pacemaker is not necessarily indicated because such blocks are often transient, respond to atropine when (if) treatment is needed, and are usually associated with a reliable AV junctional escape mechanism (at a rate of 40 to 60 beats/min). Close observation with bedside availability of atropine (and ideally access to an external pacemaker) may be all that is needed.

In contrast, AV block that develops in association with acute anterior infarction carries a much poorer prognosis. Anatomically, this type of block occurs lower in the conduction system (at the level of the His-Purkinje fibers), and is usually of the Mobitz II variety. The QRS complex is typically wider (since it is most often associated with bundle branch block), and the escape mechanism is slower and less reliable. As a result, patients with Mobitz II AV block are much more likely to develop complete AV block (and/or ventricular standstill) than are those with the Mobitz I variety (Scheinman and Gonzalez, 1980). Transvenous pacemaker insertion is mandatory. Atropine may be tried if needed in the interim, but will usually not be effective because of the lower level of the block (which is almost always *below* the bundle of His). Pressor infusion (with isoproterenol, dopamine, or epinephrine) and/or placement of an external pacemaker may provide temporizing treatment until transvenous pacemaker insertion is accomplished.

> Although prognosis of patients who develop complete AV block in association with acute anterior infarction is significantly poorer than that seen when this conduction disturbance develops in association with acute inferior infarction, the latter situation is far from benign. Complete AV block develops in more than 10% of patients with acute inferior infarction. It is especially likely to occur in patients with larger infarctions (i.e., infero-lateral, infero-postero, or associated right ventricular infarctions). About half of these patients gradually develop their block through stepwise progression of their conduction disturbance (from 1°- to Mobitz I 2° AV block- to 3° AV block), while the rest develop their block abruptly (Berger and Ryan, 1990). In-hospital mortality of these patients is surprisingly high (*at least* 20%), suggesting that *overall*, patients who develop 3° AV block (either gradually or abruptly) during the course of acute inferior infarction constitute a high-risk subgroup with a significantly poorer short-term prognosis compared to patients with otherwise uncomplicated acute inferior infarction (Berger and Ryan, 1990; Clemmensen et al, 1991).

BUNDLE BRANCH BLOCK

Bundle branch block is encountered more frequently with acute anterior infarction than with inferior infarction. This is because blood supply to the septum and the bundle branches contained therein is provided mainly by the left anterior descending artery, the vessel that is usually occluded in anterior myocardial infarction. Bundle branch block is estimated to develop in 10% to 15% of patients during the course of hospitalization for AMI. At times it may be difficult to discern whether the block is new and the *result* of infarction, or whether it was present beforehand. In any event, mortality is significantly increased in patients with AMI who are found to have bundle branch block on their admission ECG.

Development of intraventricular conduction defects with AMI is generally felt to be a reflection of extensive myocardial damage. Mortality most often results from power failure rather than from progression of the conduction disturbance to complete AV block (ACC/AHA Task Force, 1990). Consequently, prophylactic pacing will not usually increase survival, although on rare occasions it may benefit patients with bundle branch block and high-degree AV block in the absence of significant heart failure (Hindman et al, 1978).

Controversy still exists regarding the need for pacemaker insertion with unifascicular block and AMI. Ready availability of an external pacemaker may render this controversy academic. There is general agreement, however, that *new onset* bifascicular block, or 2° or 3° AV block in association with bundle branch block, is a *definite* indication for prophylactic pacing in the setting of AMI (ACC/AHA Task Force, 1990).

Invasive Hemodynamic Monitoring

INDICATIONS

Most patients with AMI have either normal hemodynamic indices or pulmonary congestion with only mild to moderate left ventricular failure. More than 90% of such patients survive, and invasive hemodynamic monitoring is not generally needed in these cases.

The mortality rate from AMI rises with increasing degrees of left ventricular failure. Unfortunately, differentiating patients with mild-to-moderate failure from those with severe failure is often difficult to do on clinical grounds alone. Bedside assessment underestimates the degree of hemodynamic compromise at least 15% of the time (Genton and Jaffe, 1986). It is in these patients in whom there is uncertainty about the degree of left ventricular failure,

Table 12D-1

Indications for Invasive Hemodynamic Monitoring in Acute Myocardial Infarction
-Persistent chest pain
-Persistent tachycardia
-Hypertension
-Hypotension
-Significant left ventricular failure
-Suspicion of hemodynamically significant right ventricular infarction
-Use of intravenous inotropic or vasodilator agents for the management of any of the above
-Development of a new systolic murmur (differention of ventricular septal defect from mitral regurgitation)

as well as those in whom significant failure is obvious, that hemodynamic monitoring assumes its greatest importance.

Other indications for invasive hemodynamic monitoring in AMI are indicated in *Table 12D-1*. For example, a patient may manifest tachycardia from persistent chest pain and/or anxiety, hypovolemia (due to inappropriate peripheral vasodilation), sympathetic overactivity, or frank congestive failure. Because of dramatically differing therapeutic implications, determining which of these factors is predominant may be essential to effective management. This may not be possible without invasive monitoring.

MANAGEMENT ACCORDING TO HEMODYNAMIC SUBSETS

The management goal in patients with AMI is to improve ventricular performance while minimizing myocardial oxygen demand. The four most useful parameters to follow in achieving this goal are heart rate, arterial blood pressure (which reflects afterload), left ventricular filling pressure (which reflects preload), and cardiac output. Ideally, left ventricular filling pressure should be maintained between 15 and 18 mm Hg. At this level, cardiac output is optimized by the Starling mechanism. Values above this filling pressure increase the degree of pulmonary congestion, while reductions below this level (i.e., to 5-10 mm Hg) may result in substantially decreased cardiac output.

Classifying patients into clinical subsets according to hemodynamic indices has a number of practical clinical applications, both for prognostic and therapeutic decision making. The five basic subsets are shown in *Table 12D-2*.

Table 12D-2

Clinical Hemodynamic Subsets of Patients with Acute Myocardial Infarction*
Subset I — Patients who are normotensive and have adequate peripheral perfusion.
Subset II — Patients who have pulmonary congestion.
Subset III — Patients who have systolic hypertension.
Subset IV — Patients who have peripheral hypoperfusion but no pulmonary congestion.
Subset V — Patients who have *both* pulmonary congestion and peripheral hypoperfusion (i.e., *"pump failure"*).
*Patients with acute myocardial infarction and significant right ventricular involvement are *not* included in the above classification because of their very different hemodynamic characteristics. *(See the following Section on Right Ventricular Infarction.)*

Subset I

In patients with uncomplicated infarction who are normotensive and have signs of adequate peripheral perfusion (warm skin, sufficient urine output, and clear sensorium), no treatment other than observation is required.

Subset II

Patients with pulmonary congestion (as manifested by an elevated left ventricular filling pressure) require diuretic therapy. Indiscriminate use of diuretic therapy is not without risk, however, since a number of patients considered to have pulmonary congestion clinically (basilar rales) actually have a normal or even low filling pressure on Swan-Ganz catheterization. Administration of furosemide to such patients may result in unnecessary (and potentially dangerous) volume depletion.

Subset III

In patients with systolic hypertension, the addition of vasodilators such as intravenous nitroglycerin or nitroprusside improves cardiac output by lowering the preload and afterload. *Nitroprusside* has a more balanced effect on arteriolar resistance and venous capacitance vessels, and in general is a more potent antihypertensive agent. In contrast, intravenous *nitroglycerin* exerts its predominant effect on venous capacitance vessels, resulting in a significant reduction in preload. It also selectively dilates coronary arteries, and thus offers at least a theoretical advantage in being less likely than nitroprusside to produce "coronary steal." This makes IV nitroglycerin the probable drug of choice in the setting of acute ischemic chest pain. Should marked hypertension persist despite use of IV nitroglycerin (i.e., if diastolic blood pressure remains ≥110 mm Hg), nitroprusside may then be required for its more potent antihypertensive effect. *(See Chapter 14.)*

Subset IV

If there is peripheral hypoperfusion *without* pulmonary congestion, volume infusion rather than pharmacologic therapy becomes the cornerstone of therapy. Left ventricular filling pressure should be increased to a level of between 15 to 18 mm Hg in an attempt to maximize contractility and cardiac output by the Starling mechanism. Once intravascular volume has been restored, hypotension and tachycardia will usually resolve.

Subset V (Cardiogenic Shock)

The final clinical hemodynamic subset is made up of patients with "pump failure" who manifest *both* pulmonary congestion *and* peripheral hypoperfusion. The extreme form (systolic blood pressure under 90 mm Hg, oliguria, and mental confusion) represents the syndrome of *cardiogenic shock*.

Clinical differentiation of patients with pump failure (Stage V) from those with isolated peripheral hypoperfusion (Subset IV) may be difficult. Patients in both groups typically present with tachycardia, hypotension, and a shock-like appearance. Definitive diagnosis can only be made by invasive hemodynamic monitoring (left ventricular filling pressures exceed 20 mm Hg and cardiac output is markedly decreased).

It should be remembered that insertion of a Swan-Ganz catheter is not a benign procedure. In addition to the usual potential complications associated with insertion of any central line, insertion of a Swan-Ganz catheter may also precipitate cardiac arrhythmias, damage cardiac structures, or cause pulmonary infarction or hemorrhage. Risk of developing a complication is increased further because of the hemodynamic instability of these acutely ill patients.

As a result, it may be reasonable (if not clinically prudent) to attempt a **fluid challenge** in *selected* patients as a *diagnostic-therapeutic trial* in the hope of distinguishing between patients with isolated peripheral hypoperfusion (Subset IV) and those with pump failure (Subset V). If *rapid* volume infusion (of 200-1,000 ml of normal saline) results in normalization of peripheral perfusion (improved sensorium, warming of extremities, increased urine output, elevation of blood pressure) *without* worsening of congestive symptoms, the need for invasive hemodynamic monitoring may no longer be present.

The rationale for a fluid challenge rests on the fact that the diagnosis of true pump failure cannot be made unless left ventricular filling pressure is elevated (i.e., ≥15 mm Hg), since hypovolemia itself (from inappropriate vasodilatation, overvigorous diuresis, dehydration, blood loss, etc.) could be the underlying cause of inadequate contractility (ACC/AHA Task Force, 1990). It should further be emphasized that *the volume load of a fluid challenge must be administered over a short period of time* (usually within 10-30 minutes), because slower infusion may result in pulmonary congestion without necessarily elevating left ventricular filling pressure.

If fluid challenge fails and worsening heart failure develops, diagnosis of impending or established cardiogenic shock is strongly suggested. IV furosemide may help in the acute management of pulmonary congestion, but hemodynamic monitoring will almost certainly be needed to assist with further management.

Once cardiogenic shock is diagnosed, attempts at therapy are aimed at optimizing hemodynamic parameters with diuretics (to decrease preload), vasodilators (to decrease preload *and* afterload), and positive inotropic agents such as dopamine, dobutamine, or amrinone (alone or in combination with vasodilators to improve cardiac output). Failure of these conventional measures is an indication for mechanical circulatory assist devices (such as intraaortic balloon counterpulsation) and consideration of cardiac catheterization to better define the underlying problem. A number of patients with heart failure may be saved by prompt surgical revascularization (angioplasty or emergency bypass surgery) and/or repair of mechanical complications of myocardial infarction (such as ventricular septal defect, acute mitral regurgitation from papillary muscle rupture, or left ventricular aneurysm). Despite all these therapeutic interventions, prognosis for patients with pump failure remains dismal, and in-hospital mortality still exceeds 60%.

Right Ventricular Infarction

Due to the lack of a reliable method for diagnosing right ventricular infarction in the past, little attention had been paid to this entity until recently. Development of myocardial scintigraphy, increased use of two-dimensional echocardiography in the acute care setting, and more frequent application of right-sided electrocardiographic monitoring leads have all contributed to improved understanding and more widespread recognition of acute right ventricular infarction. Considering how greatly treatment of AMI may vary depending on whether significant right ventricular infarction is present, the importance of making this clinical distinction becomes obvious.

Isolated right ventricular infarction is rare. However, because the right coronary artery supplies *both* the right ventricle *and* the inferior wall of the left ventricle in most individuals, up to 40% of inferior infarctions also demonstrate some degree of right ventricular involvement (Nixon, 1982; Kulbertus et al, 1985, Yasuda et al, 1990). While in most cases clinical findings and prognosis will both be determined by the degree of left ventricular involvement, right ventricular manifestations do predominate on occasion. In such instances, one would expect to see jugular venous distention with hepatic tenderness and/or enlargement (suggesting right ventricular failure) in the absence of pulmonary congestion (left ventricular failure). A *Kussmaul sign* (distention of the jugular veins during inspiration) may also be present.

> A useful clinical point to remember is that the absence of both jugular venous distention and Kussmaul's sign on physical examination makes it highly unlikely that hemodynamically significant right ventricular infarction is present (Dell'Italia et al, 1983).

MANAGEMENT OF RIGHT VENTRICULAR INFARCTION

Diuresis is an important component of the treatment of patients with AMI and congestive failure from predominant left ventricular involvement *(Subsets II and V of Table 12D-2)*. In contrast, *volume expansion* (rather than diuretic therapy) is the initial treatment of choice for hemodynamically significant right ventricular infarction. Development of right ventricular ischemia and/or infarction typically results in a reduction in right ventricular compliance. Right ventricular end-diastolic filling pressure increases, leading to reduced right ventricular filling and reduced right ventricular stroke volume. As a result, left ventricular filling is impaired, overall cardiac output is decreased, and systemic hypotension may develop (Berger and Ryan, 1990).

The goal of volume infusion with acute right ventricular infarction is to increase contractility of the ischemic right ventricle by invoking the Frank-Starling principle

(See Section A of Chapter 2), with volume expansion being the essential first step for increasing right ventricular stroke volume and left ventricular filling. Decreasing preload (with diuretics or venodilators such as nitroglycerin or morphine) is counterproductive (and potentially dangerous) because it further reduces right ventricular filling.

Management of patients with right ventricular infarction is complex. In addition to cautious volume expansion, many of these individuals also require inotropic and/or vasodilator agents, especially when there is a significant component of associated left ventricular dysfunction (Nixon, 1982; Shah et al, 1985; Genton and Jaffe, 1986; Isner, 1988). Invasive hemodynamic monitoring is commonly needed to ensure optimal treatment.

Patients with acute inferior infarction and significant right ventricular involvement typically have larger infarctions and a poorer overall prognosis than patients who have isolated inferior infarction (Berger and Ryan, 1990). Fortunately a large proportion of the right ventricular dysfunction that is seen acutely is potentially reversible, and normal right ventricular function is evident in most survivors within 1 to 2 weeks following hospital discharge (Yasuda et al, 1990).

Conduction system disturbances (including 2° and 3° AV block) commonly develop with acute right ventricular infarction because the right coronary artery vascularizes *both* the right ventricle and the AV node in 90% of normal individuals. Clinically, AV block associated with acute right ventricular infarction tends to respond less well to atropine than AV block that occurs in association with isolated inferior infarction (Isner, 1988). Optimal treatment entails *sequential* AV pacing (rather than ventricular pacing) because of the hemodynamic need to restore atrioventricular synchrony in order to ensure adequate right ventricular filling.

DIAGNOSIS OF RIGHT VENTRICULAR INFARCTION

Diagnosis of acute right ventricular infarction should be suspected when suggestive clinical signs (as described above) occur in the setting of acute inferior infarction. Utilization of right-sided monitoring leads (particularly a V_4R lead) may provide further supportive evidence (Grauer and Curry, 1992; Grauer, 1992). The finding of a Q wave and ST segment elevation in lead V_4R that exceeds the degree of ST segment elevation in leads V_1-V_3 is both a sensitive and specific clue to the diagnosis (Lopez-Sendon et al, 1985). This is especially true when there is a *rightward* pattern to the ST segment elevation— i.e., when the *degree* of ST segment elevation becomes *greater* as one moves from V_3R to V_4R to V_5R (Kataoka et al, 1990).

The degree of ST segment elevation seen in right-sided precordial leads with acute right ventricular infarction is often subtle and very transient in nature. As a result, it is easy to miss these diagnostic ECG changes unless right-sided precordial leads are obtained *early* in the course of infarction, and ideally at the time the patient is first seen (Isner 1988; Berger and Ryan, 1990).

Other methods for suggesting the diagnosis of acute right ventricular infarction include myocardial scintigraphy and two-dimensional echocardiography (which may show right ventricular enlargement with segmental wall and/or interventricular septal abnormalities). The gold standard for diagnosis is invasive hemodynamic monitoring (which typically demonstrates right atrial and right ventricular end-diastolic pressure elevations that equal or exceed pulmonary capillary wedge pressure).

Clinically, the diagnosis of significant right ventricular involvement should also be suggested if a marked *hypotensive response* is seen after nitroglycerin is given to patients with acute inferior infarction (Ferguson et al, 1989). As noted above, patients with significant right ventricular involvement depend on adequate preload to maintain right ventricular contractility and systemic cardiac output. Any intervention that might compromise right ventricular filling in these patients (i.e., administration of diuretics or venodilators) may therefore precipitate severe hypotension. *If acute right ventricular infarction is suspected, be especially cautious about administration of nitroglycerin!*

SUGGESTED APPROACH TO PATIENTS WITH SUSPECTED ACUTE RIGHT VENTRICULAR INFARCTION

In summary, early recognition of significant right ventricular involvement in patients with acute inferior infarction is essential because of the potentially important prognostic and therapeutic implications this entity may have. Special considerations to keep in mind when acute right ventricular infarction is suspected are summarized in *Table 12D-3.*

Subendocardial (Non-Q-Wave) Infarction

In the past, distinction was made between *transmural* and *subendocardial* myocardial infarction depending on whether or not Q waves developed on the ECG. Since more of the myocardial wall was thought to be involved in the former, prognosis was expected to be correspondingly poorer with this type of infarct. Neither of these tenets are necessarily true. Transmural infarctions do *not* always produce Q waves, while subendocardial infarctions may occasionally do so (Madias et al, 1974). Moreover, *long-term* prognosis for these two entities appears to be quite similar. Although *initial* mortality for transmural infarction may be somewhat greater, subendocardial infarction is a

Table 12D-3

Special Considerations in Patients with Suspected Acute Right Ventricular Infarction

Prevalence:
-Some degree of right ventricular involvement is seen in up to 40% of patients with acute inferior infarction

Prognostic Implications:
-Significant right ventricular involvement in association with acute inferior infarction suggests a larger infarction (and therefore a poorer prognosis) than is seen with isolated inferior infarction

Diagnosis—*A high index of suspicion is needed for diagnosis!*
    Clinically—Look for jugular venous distention, a Kussmaul sign, and hepatic enlargement or tenderness in the absence of signs of left ventricular failure (clear lungs on auscultation, no evidence of pulmonary congestion on chest X-ray)
    Electrocardiographically—Obtain right-sided precordial leads in patients with ECG evidence of acute inferior infarction who are clinically suspected of having significant right ventricular involvement:
        -Look for a Q wave and ST segment elevation (which may be subtle) in lead V_4R, and a *rightward* pattern of ST segment elevation
        -Obtain right-sided monitoring leads as soon as possible in the course of infarction (because ECG changes in these leads are typically short-lived)
    Invasive hemodynamic monitoring—the clinical gold standard for diagnosing acute right ventricular infarction

Treatment:
    Volume infusion—needed to optimize right ventricular filling and contractility
    Venodilators (nitroglycerin, morphine) **and diuretics**—*contraindicated* because they reduce preload and right ventricular filling (unless there is also significant associated left ventricular dysfunction)
    Invasive hemodynamic monitoring—often needed to confirm the diagnosis of acute right ventricular infarction, and to optimize hemodynamic parameters in treatment
    AV sequential pacing—constitutes optimal treatment of conduction system abnormalities that are common with acute right ventricular infarction (and often resistant to treatment with atropine). Preservation of atrioventricular synchrony is essential for ensuring optimal right ventricular filling.

---

more unstable entity associated with a higher incidence of postinfarction angina as well as a higher recurrence rate of infarction during the first few months following hospital discharge (Madias and Gorlin, 1977; Ferlinz, 1990). A reason this may occur is that such infarctions are more often "incomplete" (associated with only *subtotal* occlusion of the infarct-related vessel), and therefore at greater risk of extension (i.e., "completion" of the infarct) in the ensuing days and months (DeWood et al, 1986).*

Current recommendations for management reflect our improved understanding of the usual pathophysiology of this entity (i.e., *subtotal occlusion* of the infarct-related artery in a patient with severe and often multivessel *underlying* coronary disease). In general, these recommendations include:

1. Equally intensive treatment *during* the acute phase of the infarction as for patients with "complete" (Q-wave generating) AMI.
2. Strong consideration of secondary preventive measures *after* hospital discharge (use of diltiazem and/or continued prophylactic aspirin), as well as risk factor modification, cardiac rehabilitation, and other standard medical therapy (including β-blockers if appropriate).

In a dose of 90 mg administered every 6 hours (started 1-3 days after the onset of infarction), *diltiazem* has been shown to be effective in preventing early reinfarction and recurrent angina in patients with non-Q-wave infarction (Gibson et al, 1986; ACC/AHA Task Force, 1990). Unfortunately, long-term benefit from use of diltiazem has not been demonstrated, and the drug exerts an adverse effect in patients with left ventricular dysfunction (ACC/AHA Task Force, 1990). Nevertheless, early use of diltiazem should be strongly considered for patients with non-Q-wave infarction, especially when left ventricular function is normal and there is evidence of continued ischemia (i.e., persistent ST segment depression) and/or angina *(See Section B in this chapter).*

---

* Despite persistence in the literature of the potentially misleading terms *transmural* and *subendocardial*, the anatomically more accurate designations *"Q-wave"* and *"non-Q-wave producing"* appear to be preferable for describing the type of infarction.

3. Strong consideration of *early* cardiac catheterization to define the underlying anatomy and assess the patient's suitability for revascularization (by either angioplasty or coronary bypass surgery).

The goal of early cardiac catheterization and strong consideration of revascularization for suitable candidates is to try to prevent reinfarction (i.e., "completion" of the infarct) from occurring during the early post-hospital (high-risk) period.

Unstable (Preinfarction) Angina

The syndrome of *unstable angina* can be divided into three clinical subsets:

1. Patients with new onset angina.
2. Patients in whom a previously "stable" pattern of angina is now superceded by progressively increasing severity, duration, and/or frequency of attacks despite appropriate medical therapy (*crescendo* angina).
3. Patients with continued anginal pain following recovery from AMI.

Because a significant number of individuals with this syndrome go on to develop AMI (hence the term, *"preinfarction"* angina), prompt recognition and intensive treatment are essential (Rahimtoola, 1985; Munger, 1990). Practically speaking, differentiation between unstable angina and AMI may be extremely difficult (if not impossible) at the time of presentation, especially if the admission ECG is inconclusive. Precipitating mechanisms (progression of atherosclerosis, rupture of an atherosclerotic plaque, platelet aggregation, clot formation, and/or coronary artery spasm) and the extent of underlying disease are similar for both entities (Rackley et al, 1982; Epstein and Pallmeri, 1984; Sherman et al, 1986). The principal difference is that the superimposed clot in the involved vessel is *totally occlusive* with AMI, and *less than* totally occlusive with unstable angina (Falk, 1989). Non-Q-wave AMI is also believed to result from acute total occlusion of a major coronary vessel. However, *rapid spontanous recanalization* (i.e., within minutes to an hour or so) may account for the relatively smaller size of such infarctions compared to the longer lasting total occlusion that is commonly seen with transmural (Q-wave) AMI (Rapaport, 1991).

As a result of the similar underlying pathophysiologic process with Q-wave AMI, non-Q-wave AMI, and unstable angina, initial treatment of these entities for the most part is also very similar. That is, patients who truly have unstable angina should be closely observed in a protective environment with efforts directed at relieving acute ischemic chest pain and reversing the underlying thrombotic process.

Patients with unstable angina should be monitored closely not only for development of cardiac arrhythmias, but also for ST segment changes. Detection of *silent ischemia* (as evidenced by ST segment depression in the absence of chest pain) suggests a group of patients at particularly high risk, especially when episodes of silent ischemia are prolonged (Munger, 1990; Grauer, 1990). Recognition of silent ischemia is important clinically because it indicates the need for more intensive medical treatment, even if chest pain has been completely relieved.

Standard treatment measures for patients with unstable angina include use of aspirin, consideration of anticoagulation and/or thrombolytic therapy, and antianginal medication. Provided there are no contraindications, *aspirin* should be started as soon as possible. When given to patients with unstable angina (in a dose of 325 mg a day), this drug has been shown to significantly reduce mortality and the incidence of AMI (Lewis et al, 1983; Lewis and the VA Cooperative Study Group, 1985). Although higher doses of aspirin have been used, they have not been shown to be more effective (Munger, 1990).

Clinicians should be aware of the practice of *some* cardiovascular surgeons who prefer to withhold aspirin once the decision to operate has been made (in the hope of reducing the amount of perioperative bleeding). However, awareness of this practice should *not* deter (or delay) emergency care providers from administering aspirin at an early point in the evaluative process to patients who present with severe, new-onset chest pain.

Full anticoagulation (with *heparin*) and/or administration of thrombolytic therapy to patients with unstable angina have been suggested as additional measures to (or *instead of*) aspirin. Unfortunately, consensus is lacking regarding the optimal treatment approach. Although heparin (either alone, or in conjunction with aspirin) appears to be more effective in reducing adverse cardiovascular events than aspirin alone in patients with unstable angina, it is also more likely to produce complications from bleeding—especially when heparin is *combined* with aspirin (Théroux et al, 1988). Thus, there appears to be a tradeoff between the beneficial effect of full anticoagulation and the risk of developing a significant bleeding complication.

Whether one opts for use of aspirin alone (our choice in otherwise uncomplicated cases), heparin alone, or aspirin plus heparin depends on many factors. These include patient-specific variables, severity of symptoms and/or the clinician's confidence that the diagnosis is unstable angina, the presence of other conditions that might also benefit from full anticoagulation (such as valvular disease or atrial fibrillation), the patient's likelihood of developing a bleeding complication (i.e., abnormal baseline clotting studies, advanced age, history of alcohol abuse), and the personal preference of the treating clinician.

Infusion of thrombolytic therapy may also prove beneficial when combined with maximal medical therapy of unstable angina, although the benefit appears to be limited to patients with angiographic evidence of intracoronary thrombus (Nicklaus et al, 1989). Practically speaking, this means that the potential benefit of thrombolytic therapy is minimal once the acute syndrome (i.e., chest pain) has resolved, since it is likely that the clot causing the unstable anginal chest pain will have also resolved by this time. Thus, thrombolytic therapy might best be reserved for patients with acute ischemic chest pain who either demonstrate definitive evidence of acute infarction (i.e., ST segment elevation) or angiographically documented intracoronary thrombus in association with *continued* chest pain.

Medical management of the chest pain accompanying unstable angina is similar to that for patients with AMI. Nitrates are usually the first drugs used, and most patients will have already taken one or more sublingual nitroglycerin tablets by the time they arrive at the hospital. If chest pain is not promptly relieved, there should be little hesitation about starting an IV infusion of the drug (to allow more rapid titration to an effective dose).

> It should be emphasized that failure to respond to sublingual or topical forms of nitroglycerin is not predictive of the subsequent response to the IV preparation (Munger, 1990).

In the past, morphine sulfate had been the usual next line of therapy. Use of an intravenous β-blocker and/or calcium channel blocker is now generally preferred after nitroglycerin for treatment of acute ischemic chest pain, especially when the diagnosis is more likely to be unstable angina (Gottlieb and Gerstenblith, 1986; Gottlieb et al, 1986). In most cases, these measures will be effective in relieving acute ischemic chest pain. In the event that they are not, strong consideration should be given to cardiac catheterization (to define the problem) and to more invasive forms of therapy (intracoronary nitroglycerin, thrombolytic therapy, percutaneous transluminal coronary angioplasty, and/or emergency coronary artery bypass grafting). Assist with intra-aortic balloon counterpulsation (IABP) may be needed for patients with persistent chest pain and/or unstable hemodynamics until a definitive revascularization procedure can be performed.

Antiarrhythmic Therapy After the Infarct

As indicated in the introduction of this chapter, the three most important determinants of long-term prognosis following recovery from AMI are:

1. the amount of myocardium damaged by the acute event
2. the amount of myocardium at risk of damage from a future event (i.e., the amount of *ischemic* myocardium)
3. the presence and severity of ventricular arrhythmias.

Interestingly, development of ventricular fibrillation during the early hours of AMI does not seem to affect long-term survival. Patients who have an otherwise uncomplicated course demonstrate an equally good prognosis as those with uncomplicated AMI who never had ventricular fibrillation (Tofler et al, 1987; Volpi et al, 1989). It is only when ventricular arrhythmias persist into the late infarction period (beyond the first 3-5 days) that long-term survival is adversely affected (Bigger et al, 1982; Bigger and Coromillas, 1983). As a result, routine Holter monitoring prior to discharge from the hospital had been

advocated in the past, and antiarrhythmic treatment recommended if frequent and complex ventricular ectopy was found.

Recommendations for optimal treatment of ventricular ectopy occurring after recent infarction are much less certain at the present time. Although it is known that the presence of PVCs following AMI is a definite independent risk factor for increased mortality, it has never been shown that suppression of such PVCs improves survival (Hine et al, 1989; Morganroth and Bigger, 1990). On the contrary, results from the Cardiac Arrhythmia Suppression Trial (CAST) Study suggest that antiarrhythmic treatment of ventricular arrhythmias (with the potent IC antiarrhythmic agents flecainide or encainide) paradoxically *increases* the risk of mortality (The CAST Investigators, 1989). Similarly, a meta-analysis review of the major empiric long-term antiarrhythmic trials conducted after AMI showed an overall *increase* in mortality despite reduction in PVC frequency among those patients who were treated with drugs (Hine et al, 1989). This leaves us with the burden of knowing that survivors of AMI who continue to manifest frequent and complex ventricular ectopy after hospital discharge *are* at increased risk of mortality (i.e., they have *potentially lethal* ventricular arrhythmias*), but that our standard treatment measures have *not* been shown to be effective. *Antiarrhythmic drugs do not reduce mortality in such patients—and they may be harmful!*

> An interesting multicenter study by Willems et al (1990) sought to determine factors predictive of long-term prognosis in patients who developed an episode of either sustained ventricular tachycardia or ventricular fibrillation during the *later stages* of AMI (i.e., 48 hours or more after the onset of symptoms). The following risk factors were found to increase the risk of subsequent mortality among these patients:
>
> 1. Older age (70 years or older)
> 2. Anterior (rather than inferior or lateral) site of infarction
> 3. Associated heart failure
> 4. A history of two or more prior infarctions
> 5. Cardiac arrest at the time of their arrhythmia episode
>
> Among the group of patients in the study at highest risk (i.e., those with several of the above risk factors), 2-year mortality exceeded 50%! In contrast, 2-year mortality was only 12% in patients at lowest risk (i.e., those who were younger, had inferior or lateral infarction, normal left ventricular function, no history of prior infarction, and who had sustained ventricular tachycardia *without* cardiac arrest rather than ventricular fibrillation). Once again, however, despite effective stratification of patients with ventricular arrhythmias into groups at greatest risk, empiric antiarrhythmic therapy did *not* improve long-term survival of the patients in the study.

How then should we proceed in evaluation and management of patients who recover from AMI and *continue* to have ventricular arrhythmias after discharge from the hospital? Although full discussion of this topic extends beyond the scope of this book, a number of basic points

---

* General principles regarding the types of ventricular arrhythmias (*benign, potentially lethal,* and *lethal*) and the clinical implications of each type were discussed in detail in Section E of Chapter 11.

can be made. The key objective of clinical assessment following AMI is to stratify survivors into subgroups that reflect the relative risk of subsequent morbidity and mortality. Age, general health status, previous myocardial insult (i.e., the number of previous infarctions and cumulative damage from these infarctions), hospital course, residual left ventricular function, and the amount of myocardium at risk from a future event (i.e., the amount of *ongoing* myocardial ischemia) are the most important factors in this regard. Integration of these factors into the clinical situation, in conjunction with patient desires and local practice of the treating health care team ultimately determines whether the patient is catheterized, undergoes exercise testing, is treated medically, or is advised to have a revascularization procedure (CABG or angioplasty).

Management decisions regarding ventricular arrhythmias are sometimes resolved during the course of the above evaluative process. For example, if cardiac catheterization, electrocardiographic monitoring (by telemetry or Holter) and/or exercise testing suggest significant ischemia with resultant left ventricular dysfunction, treatment directed at the underlying disorder (i.e., antianginal medication and/or a revascularization procedure) is far preferable (and much more likely to be effective) than antiarrhythmic therapy. The dilemma lies with determining the optimal approach for survivors of AMI who manifest persistent ventricular arrhythmias in the *absence* of a treatable (correctable) underlying cause.

For a short time following the disappointing experience with flecainide and encainide, the CAST Study was continued in the hope that treatment with other antiarrhythmic agents might demonstrate efficacy in reducing the mortality of AMI survivors with persistent ventricular arrhythmias (Morganroth and Bigger, 1990). Moricizine* was the antiarrhythmic used in this second phase of the CAST study (Carnes and Coyle, 1990; Medical Letter, 1990). However, despite correction of problems (in study design and patient selection) that were associated with the initial phase of the CAST study (and which resulted in an exceedingly low mortality rate in placebo-treated patients), treatment of ventricular arrhythmias occurring in AMI survivors with moricizine has yielded equally disappointing results. Although unanswerable questions may still arise as to the relative merits other antiarrhythmic agents (such as quinidine, procainamide, mexiletine, etc.) that were not specifically studied in CAST might have, the inescapable conclusion at this time must be that empiric treatment of ventricular arrhythmias in AMI survivors is not beneficial—and may be harmful.

Given our current state of knowledge, *what should be done?* Is there a cost-effective, practical way to approach these patients? Results from the previously cited study by Willems et al are insightful and suggest that survivors of AMI with persistent ventricular arrhythmias can be stratified according to their relative risk of mortality by application of the simple clinical parameters mentioned above *(Table 12D-4).*

---

*Moricizine is an antiarrhythmic agent with properties intermediate between class IA drugs (such as quinidine) and IC drugs (such as flecainide or encainide).

Table 12D-4

Suggested Approach for Risk Stratification of Patients with Persistent Ventricular Arrhythmias After Recovery from AMI		
	Patients at HIGHER RISK*	**Patients at LOWER RISK**
Patient Age	70 or older	Younger adults
Left Ventricular Function	Poor LV Function: -History of multiple prior infarctions -Anterior location of current infarction -Associated heart failure -Ejection fraction $\leq$35%	Good LV Function: -No prior infarction -Inferior or lateral location of current infarction -No heart failure -Ejection fraction $\geq$50%
Evidence of Ongoing Ischemia (Silent or associated with chest pain)	Present (frequent episodes that are often prolonged)	Absent (or only rare episodes of minimal duration)
Hemodynamic Consequence of Ventricular Arrhythmias	Hemodynamically *unstable* (causing syncope or cardiac arrest)	Hemodynamically *stable* (and often asymptomatic)

Adapted from Willems et al, 1990.
*Patients with some (but not all) of these characteristics are at *intermediate* risk.

Patients at lowest risk in the table have a relatively good prognosis and can probably be managed in a more conservative manner, perhaps as dictated by the nature and severity of symptoms (Willems et al, 1990; Morganroth and Bigger, 1990). This is especially true if arrhythmias detected in such patients are of lesser frequency and complexity (i.e., without significant runs of ventricular tachycardia). In arriving at an individualized approach to management of these patients, it is helpful to keep in mind that *noninvasive assessment* (with Holter monitoring, exercise testing, serum drug levels) and *empiric treatment* are costly, technically problematic, associated with adverse effects, and have *not* been shown to improve prognosis (Morganroth, 1988).

> Use of long-term oral *β-blockers* should be strongly considered for survivors of AMI with persistent ventricular arrhythmias provided there are no contraindications to taking these drugs. Although their antiarrhythmic effect is *not* as potent as for other agents, β-blockers are generally well tolerated, have a low risk of proarrhythmia, and have been shown to reduce mortality by as much as 30% in the first year after AMI (Peter and Helfant, 1990). As a result, they appear to be the first-line antiarrhythmic agent of choice for patients with nonlethal ventricular arrhythmias after AMI (Morganroth and Bigger, 1990).

Patients in Table 12D-4 who are at intermediate or high risk of mortality from ventricular arrhythmias following AMI merit more intensive evaluation. Decisions on management must be individualized, and are based on local availability of the various evaluative techniques, patient desire for such investigation, personal preferences and expertise of the treating health care team, referral availability, and cost considerations.

Traditionally, Holter monitoring has been the initial test performed. In most cases, a 24-hour ambulatory recording provides a general idea of the frequency and severity of the patient's arrhythmia, although *intermittent* episodes of sustained ventricular tachycardia (occurring *less* frequently than once a day) may be easily overlooked by this procedure. Exercise testing provides additional information and insight regarding the likelihood of activity inducing ventricular arrhythmias, but overall is significantly *less* sensitive than Holter monitoring in detecting ventricular arrhythmias. A newer technique for risk stratification is the use of *signal-averaged electrocardiography*, especially when results are interpreted in conjunction with some objective measure of left ventricular function. For example, the presence of *late potentials* on a signal-averaged ECG, in association with impaired left ventricular function (ejection fraction *less* than 35%) identifies a very high risk group of individuals with a mortality rate of greater than 30% in the first year after recovery from AMI (Gomes et al, 1987; Peter and Helfant, 1990).

> ***Signal-averaged electrocardiography*** is a non-invasive diagnostic technique that seeks to determine the presence of delayed, low-amplitude electrical potentials in the terminal portion of the QRS complex. Detection of such *late potentials*

appears to be a relatively sensitive and specific indicator of the "substrate" (i.e., potential for reentry) that supports sustained ventricular tachycardia. Although still an investigational tool and not yet universally available, signal-averaged electrocardiography shows promise of being a much more effective modality for identifying high risk patients than Holter monitoring, especially (as noted above) when results are combined with an objective measure of left ventricular function.

Patients judged to be at higher risk of mortality from ventricular arrhythmias on the basis of non-invasive assessment may be candidates for invasive programmed electrophysiologic (PES) study. As discussed in Section E of Chapter 11, the ability of PES studies to determine an antiarrhythmic regimen that eliminates inducibility of ventricular tachycardia in the laboratory, in conjunction with judicious use of the automatic implantable cardioverter-defibrillator (AICD) offers the best chance for long-term survival of high risk patients who *continue* to manifest malignant ventricular arrhythmias following discharge after AMI (Wilber et al, 1990).

Silent Ischemia After the Infarct

Recently, de Belder et al (1990) examined the prevalence and prognostic implications of silent ischemia in 250 clinically stable patients 1 week after AMI. All underwent submaximal exercise testing prior to discharge from the hospital. *Silent ischemia* (i.e., ST segment depression in the absence of chest pain) occurred in more than 25% of patients, and was nearly *twice* as common as the occurrence of ST segment depression in association with chest pain. Prognosis of patients with ischemic ST segment changes on exercise testing was found to be comparable *regardless* of whether the induced ischemia was silent or accompanied by chest pain (i.e., 5-10% 1-year mortality).

> It is of interest that patients in the study who demonstrated evidence of silent myocardial ischemia had a *12-fold* increased risk of mortality compared to patients with a negative predischarge exercise test. The risk for an adverse prognosis was increased even more if in addition to silent ischemia there was also an abnormal blood pressure response to exercise, or the patient was unable to complete the exercise protocol. In such individuals the risk of mortality was increased *32-fold* compared to patients with a negative predischarge exercise test, corresponding to a 22% 1-year mortality rate.

Thus, silent ischemia is relatively common after acute myocardial infarction, and its presence appears to identify a group of individuals at especially high risk of an adverse prognosis. Moreover, the absence of chest pain on predischarge exercise testing *in no way* ensures a favorable prognosis. Clearly, more intensive evaluation, treatment (i.e., with calcium antagonists and/or other anti-ischemic agents), and consideration for possible intervention (i.e., revascularization with angioplasty, bypass surgery, or other procedures) should be contemplated for post-infarction patients who demonstrate silent myocardial ischemia.

> As emphasized at the beginning of Section A in this chapter, the three most important prognostic determinants of AMI are:

1. Infarct size (i.e., the amount of myocardium damaged by the *acute* event) and residual left ventricular function
2. The amount of myocardium at risk of damage from a *future* event (i.e., the amount of *ischemic* myocardium), and
3. The presence and severity of ventricular arrhythmias

For survivors of the acute event, the principal goal of post-infarction evaluation is risk stratification. Patients at highest risk are likely to need immediate intervention. In contrast, medical therapy (in conjunction with close follow-up) may be more than adequate treatment for patients at intermediate or low risk. Assessment of the extent and degree of ischemia (be it silent or associated with angina) by exercise testing, ambulatory electrocardiographic monitoring, or other techniques) is one key way of determining which patients are at greatest risk (Pepine et al, 1992; Van der Wall et al, 1992).

References

American College of Cardiology/American Heart Association Task Force: Guidelines for the early management of patients with acute myocardial infarction, *Circulation* 82:664-707, 1990.

de Belder M, Skehan D, Pumphrey C, Khan B, Evans S, Rothman M, Mills P: Identification of a high risk subgoup of patients with silent ischaemia after myocardial infarction: a group for early therapeutic revascularisation? *Br Heart J* 63:145-150, 1990.

Beta-Blocker Heart Attack Trial Research Group: A randomized trial of propranolol in patients with acute myocardial infarction: mortality results, *JAMA* 247:1707-1714, 1982.

Berger PB, Ryan TJ: Inferior myocardial infarction: high-risk subgroups, *Circulation* 81:401-411, 1990.

Campbell CA, Przyklenk K, Kloner RA: Infarct size reduction: a review of the clinical trials, *J Clin Pharmacol* 26:317-329, 1986.

Carnes CA, Coyle JD: Moricizine: a novel antiarrhythmic agent, *DICP Ann Pharmacother* 24:745-753, 1990.

The Cardiac Arrhythmia Suppression Trial (CAST) Investigators: Increased mortality due to encainide or felcainide in a randomized trial of arrhythmia suppression after myocardial infarction, *N Engl J Med* 321:406-412, 1989.

Clemmensen P, Bates ER, Califf RM, Hlatky MA, Aronson L, George BS, Lee KL, Kereiakes DJ, Gacioch G, Berrios E, Topol EJ: and the TAMI Study Group: Complete atrioventricular block complicating inferior wall acute myocardial infarction treated with reperfusion therapy, *Am J Cardiol* 67:225-230, 1991.

Dell'Italia LJ, Starling MR, O'Rourke RA: Physical examination for exclusion of hemodynamically important right ventricular infarction, *Ann Int Med* 99:608-611, 1983.

DeWood MA, Stifter WF, Simpson CS, Spores J, Eugster GS, Judge TP, Hinnen ML: Coronary arteriographic findings soon after non-Q-wave myocardial infarction, *N Engl J Med* 315:417-423, 1986.

Falk E: Morphologic features of unstable atherothrombotic plaques underlying acute coronary syndromes, *Am J Cardiol* 63:114E-120E, 1989.

Ferguson JJ, Diver DJ, Boldt M, Pasternak RC: Significance of nitroglycerin-induced hypotension with inferior wall acute myocardial infarction, *Am J Cardiol* 64:311-314, 1989.

Ferlinz J: Acute myocardial infarction: does the lack of Q waves help or hinder? *J Am Coll Cardiol* 15:1208-1211, 1990.

Genton R, Jaffe AS: Management of congestive heart failure in patients with acute myocardial infarction, *JAMA* 256:2556-2560, 1986.

Gibson RS, Boden WE, Theroux P, Strauss HD, Pratt CM, Gheorghiade M, Capone RJ, Crawford MH, Schlant RC, Kleiger RE: Diltiazem and reinfarction in patients with non-Q-wave myocardial infarction: results of a double-blind randomised multicenter trial, *N Engl J Med* 315:423-453, 1986.

Gomes JA, Winters SL, Stewart D, Horowitz S, Milner M, Barreca P: A new noninvasive index to predict sustained ventricular tachycardia and sudden death in the five years after myocardial infarction based on signal-averaged electrocardiogram, radionuclide ejection fraction and holter monitoring, *JACC* 10:349-357, 1987.

Gottlieb SO, Gerstenblith G: Therapeutic choices in unstable angina, *Am J Med* 80(suppl 4C):35-39, 1986.

Gottleib SO, Weisfeldt ML, Ouwang P, Aghuff SC, Baughman KL, Traill TA, Brinker JA, Shapiro EP, Chandra NC, Mellits ED, Townsend SN, Gerstenblith G: Effect of the addition of propranolol to therapy with nifedipine for unstable angina pectoris: a randomized double-blind placebo controlled trial, *Circulation* 73:331-337, 1986.

Grauer K, Curry RW: Clinical electrocardiography: a primary care approach, ed 2, Cambridge, Mass, 1992, Blackwell Scientific.

Grauer K: Silent myocardial ischemia: dilemma or blessing? *Am Fam Phys* 42(suppl):13S-28S, 1990.

Grauer K: A practical guide to ECG interpretation, St Louis, 1992, Mosby–Year Book.

Hindman MC, Wagner GS, JaRo M: The clinical significance of bundle branch block complicating acute myocardial infarction, *Circulation* 58:679-699, 1978.

Hine LK, Laird NM, Hewitt P, Chalmers TC: Meta-analysis of empirical long-term antiarrhythmic therapy after myocardial infarction, *JAMA* 262:3037-3040, 1989.

Hjalmarson A : Early intervention with a beta-blocking drug after acute myocardial infarction, *Am J Cardiol* 54:11E-13E, 1984.

Isner JM: Right ventricular myocardial infarction, *JAMA* 259:712-718, 1988.

Kataoka H, Tamura A, Yano S, Kanzaki K, Mikuriya Y: ST elevation in the right chest leads in anterior wall left ventricular acute myocardial infarction, *Am J Cardiol* 66:1146-1147, 1990.

Kulbertus HE, Rigo P, Legrand V: Right ventricular infarction: pathophysiology, diagnosis, clinical course, and treatment, *MCCD* 54:1-5, 1985.

Lewis HD, Davis JW, Archibald DG, Steinke WE, Smitherman TC, Doherty JE, Schnaper HW, LeWinter MM, Linares E, Pouget JM, Sabharwal SC, Chesler E, DeMots H: Protective effects of aspirin against acute myocardial infarction and death in men with unstable angina: results of a Veterans Administration cooperative study, *N Engl J Med* 309:396-403, 1983.

Lewis HD, Veterans Administration Cooperative Study Group: Unstable angina: status of aspirin and other forms of therapy, *Circulation* 72 (suppl V):V155-V160, 1985.

Lichstein E: Why do beta-receptor blockers decrease mortality after myocardial infarction? *JACC* 6:973-975, 1985.

Lopez-Sendon J, Coma-Canella I, Alcasena S, Sloane J, Gamallo C: Electrocardiographic findings in acute right ventricular infarction: sensitivity and specificity of electrocardiographic alterations in right precordial leads V4R, V3R, V1, V2 and V3, *J Am Coll Cardiol* 6:1273-1279, 1985.

Madias JE, Chahine RA, Gorlin R, Blacklow DJ: A comparison of transmural and nontransmural acute myocardial infarction, *Circulation* 49:498-507, 1974.

Madias JE, Gorlin R: The myth of acute "mild" myocardial infarction, *Ann Med Intern* 86:347-352, 1977.

Medical Letter: Moricizine for cardiac arrhythmias, 32:99-100, 1990.

Morganroth J: Evaluation of antiarrhythmic therapy using holter monitoring, *Am J Cardiol* 62:18H-23H, 1988.

Morganroth J, Bigger JT: Pharmacologic management of ventricular arrhythmias after the cardiac arrhythmia suppression trial, *Am J Cardiol* 65:1497-1503, 1990.

Munger TM: Unstable angina, *Mayo Clin Proc* 65:384-406, 1990.

Nicklas JM, Topol EJ, Kander N, O'Neill WW, Walton JA, Ellis SG, Gorman L, Pitt B: Randomized, double-blind, placebo-controlled trial of tissue plasminogen activator in unstable angina, *J Am Coll Cardiol* 13:434-441, 1989.

Nixon JV: Right ventricular myocardial infarction, *Arch Intern Med* 142:945-947, 1982.

Norwegian Multicenter Study Group: Timolol-induced reduction in mortality and reinfarction in patients surviving acute myocardial infarction, *N Engl J Med* 304:801-807, 1981.

Pepine CJ, Kern MJ, Boden WE: Advisory group reports on silent myocardial ischemia, acute intervention after myocardial infarction, and postinfarction management, *Am J Cardiol* 69:41B-46B, 1992.

Peter CT, Helfant RH: Postinfarction ventricular tachycardia and fibrillation: reassessing the role of drug therapy and approach to the high risk patient, *J Am Coll Cardiol* 16:531-532, 1990.

Rackley CE, Russel RO, Rogers WJ, Mantle JA, Papapietro SE: Unstable angina pectoris: is it time to change our approach? *Am Heart J* 103:154-156, 1982.

Rahimtoola SH: Unstable angina: current status, *MCCD* 54:19-23, 1985.

Rapaport E: Overview rationale of thrombolysis in treating acute myocardial infarction, *Heart Lung* 20:538-541, 1991.

Scheinman MM, Gonzalez RP: Fascicular block and acute myocardial infarction, *JAMA* 244:2646-2649, 1980.

Shah PK, Maddahi J, Berman DS, Pichler M, Swan HJC: Scintigraphically detected predominant right ventricular dysfunction in acute myocardial infarction: clinical and hemodynamic correlates and implications for therapy and prognosis, *J Am Coll Cardiol* 6:1264-1272, 1985.

Sherman CT, Litvack F, Grundfest W, Lee M, Hickey A, Chaux A, Kass R, Blanche C, Matloff J, Morgenstern L, Ganz W, Swan HJC, Forrester J: Coronary angioscopy in patients with unstable angina pectoris, *N Engl J Med* 315:913-919, 1986.

Théroux P, Ouimet H, McCans J, Latour JG, Joly P, Lévy G, Pelletier E, Juneau M, Stasiak J, deGuise P, Pelletier GB, Rinzler D, Waters DD: Aspirin, heparin, or both to treat acute unstable angina, *N Engl J Med* 319:1105-1111, 1988.

Van de Wall EE, Cats VM, Bruschke AVG: Silent myocardial ischemia after acute myocardial infarction, *Am J Cardiol* 69:19B-24B, 1992.

Wilber DJ, Olshansky B, Moran JF, Scanlon PJ: Electrophysiological testing and nonsustained ventricular tachycardia: use and limitations in patients with coronary artery disease and impaired ventricular function, *Circulation* 82:350-358, 1990.

Willems AR, Tijssen JGP, van Capelle FJL, Kingma JH, Hauer RNW, Vermeulen FEE, Brugada P, van Hoogenhuyze DCA, Janse MJ, and the Dutch Ventricular Tachycardia Study Group: Determinants of prognosis in symptomatic ventricular tachycardia or ventricular fibrillation late after myocardial infarction, *J Am Coll Cardiol* 16:521-530, 1990.

Yasuda T, Okada RD, Leinbach RC, Gold HK, Phillips H, McKusick KA, Glover DK, Boucher CA, Strauss HW: Serial evaluation of right ventricular dysfunction associated with acute inferior myocardial infarction, *Am Heart J* 119:816-822, 1990.

Yusuf S, Peto R, Lewis J, Collins R, Sleight P: Beta-blockage during and after myocardial infarction: an overview of the randomized trials, *Prog Cardiovasc Dis* 27:335-371, 1985.

SECTION E

USE OF LIDOCAINE

Lidocaine is the most commonly used antiarrhythmic agent for the emergency treatment of ventricular arrhythmias. Potential indications for the drug include treatment of ventricular arrhythmias associated with AMI, prophylaxis against such arrhythmias *(controversial)*, and management of precipitating rhythms of cardiac arrest (sustained ventricular tachycardia or ventricular fibrillation). Yet despite widespread use of the drug, opinions vary greatly about what constitutes the optimal protocol for administration. While virtually all therapeutic regimens for lidocaine employ an initial loading bolus, the need for one or more additional loading boluses remains open to question. Consensus is also lacking regarding the ideal rate of infusion. Some authorities begin low (at an infusion rate of 1 mg/min) and adjust the infusion rate upward with each subsequent bolus. Others begin high (at an infusion rate of 4 mg/min) and adjust the infusion rate downward. A third group maintains a constant infusion rate of 2 mg/min regardless of whether additional boluses of drug are given.

With such an abundance of treatment protocols to choose from, it is not surprising that many emergency care providers find it difficult to decide on the regimen best suited for a particular patient. This decision is complicated further by consideration of patient variables such as age, weight, use of concomitant drugs, and the presence of AMI, congestive heart failure, or liver disease—since each of these factors may affect lidocaine metabolism.

In addition to the divergence of opinions on lidocaine dosing is a lack of consensus on whether to routinely recommend the drug as prophylaxis for patients suspected of AMI. Finally, controversy surrounds the question of whether lidocaine is an effective antifibrillatory agent. The importance of each of these issues lies with the effect that various specific treatment indications and patient variables may have on drug dosing.

The goal of this section is to clarify essential points on the use of lidocaine. Basic pharmacokinetic principles of the drug are reviewed and clinically applied in an attempt to demonstrate how therapy may be optimized while minimizing the risk of toxicity. We then conclude by adding to our discussion from Section B (on use of lidocaine for prophylaxis/treatment of suspected AMI), and by presenting a rationale for antiarrhythmic use of this agent.

Lidocaine Pharmacokinetics

Lidocaine pharmacokinetics can best be described by reference to a two-compartment model *(Fig. 12E-1)*. In such a model, the smaller *central compartment* consists of the circulating blood volume and highly perfused organs such as the heart and brain. The half-life* of lidocaine in this central compartment is extremely short (less than 10 minutes) because the drug rapidly distributes to other tissues in the body. In so doing it enters the larger *peripheral compartment* which includes poorly perfused tissues of the body such as skin, muscle, and most of the body fat stores. In healthy adults the half-life of lidocaine in this larger compartment is usually 1-2 hours.

---

*The *half-life* of a drug is the amount of time it takes for *half* of the drug to be eliminated.

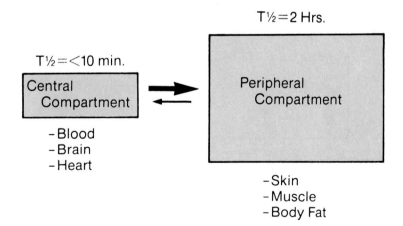

Figure 12E-1.   Pharmacokinetic model for lidocaine.

When a bolus of lidocaine is injected intravenously, it is administered directly into the central compartment (since blood is contained in this compartment). Since the *heart* is also contained within this space, the antiarrhythmic effect of the drug begins almost immediately.

> Note from Figure 12E-1 that the *brain* (as well as the heart) is contained within the central compartment. As a result, the *size* of a loading bolus of lidocaine and the *speed* with which it is administered *must* be controlled, or central nervous system (CNS) toxicity (i.e., seizures) may result.

In view of the short half-life of lidocaine in the central compartment, half of the drug will have already diffused into the peripheral compartment within 10 minutes after giving the initial loading bolus. As a result, the level of drug in the bloodstream will have dropped significantly. PVCs may recur at this time *unless* the serum drug concentration of lidocaine has been maintained within the therapeutic range (2-6 μg/ml) by additional loading boluses.

Lidocaine distribution from the central compartment to the peripheral compartment begins immediately following an IV bolus and continues until a state of equilibrium is established between these two compartments. By giving one or more loading boluses, therapeutic blood levels can be rapidly achieved (so as to maintain an adequate antiarrhythmic effect) until the continuous intravenous infusion has had an opportunity to attain steady state. If one were instead to simply institute a maintenance infusion *without* first giving a loading dose, more than an hour would be needed for serum drug levels to become therapeutic.

This situation is illustrated in the pharmacokinetic simulation shown in *Figure 12E-2*, in which a 75-kg man is begun on a maintenance infusion of 2 mg/min without receiving a loading bolus.

If the same 75-kg man were to receive a 75-mg *loading bolus* of lidocaine (1 mg/kg) *before* starting the 2-mg/min maintenance infusion, therapeutic drug levels of lidocaine would almost immediately be achieved *(Figure 12E-3)*. With the exception of a momentary dip below the therapeutic range (arrow in *Figure 12E-3*), adequate blood levels are maintained until steady state is established.

If one were to follow the initial 75-mg loading bolus with a *second bolus* given a short time later, even the transient "therapeutic hiatus" seen in Figure 12E-3 might be avoided *(Figure 12E-4)*.

If additional loading boluses of lidocaine are given, higher therapeutic levels of drug may be maintained until the eventual *steady state* serum drug level (which in this case is just over 4 μg/ml) is reached *(Figure 12E-5)*. This type of aggressive loading protocol calls for an initial loading dose of 75-mg to be followed by 50-mg boluses every 5 to 10 minutes until a total loading dose of up to 225 mg has been given (i.e., 75 + 50 + 50 + 50 = 225 mg).

One may either keep the infusion rate *constant* at 2 mg/min (as was done in *Figure 12E-5*), or increase the infusion rate by 1 mg/min after each additional loading bolus is given until the maximum rate of 4 mg/min is reached. The problem with the latter protocol is that even in an otherwise healthy 50-year-old man, the presence of any complicating factors that retard lidocaine metabolism

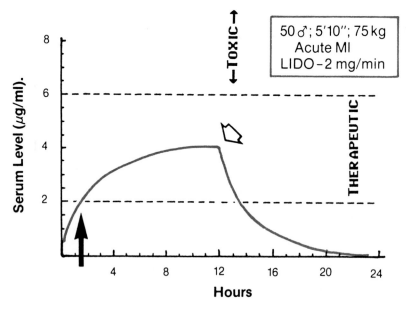

Figure 12E-2.   A 50-year-old man (5 feet, 10 inches, 75 kg) with acute myocardial infarction (AMI) is begun on an IV maintenance infusion of lidocaine at 2 mg/min. No loading dose is given. More than an hour passes before a therapeutic blood level is reached (arrow). The infusion is stopped after 12 hours (open arrowhead). Therapeutic blood levels persist for at least 2 hours after stopping the infusion. (***Therapeutic lidocaine levels*** on this and subsequent figures in this Section are listed as between 2-6 μg/ml).

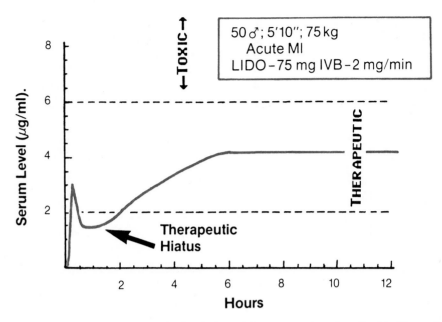

Figure 12E-3. Pharmacokinetic simulation of the same patient described in Figure 12E-2, in this case with administration of a 75-mg IV loading bolus of lidocaine *before* starting the 2 mg/min maintenance infusion. Therapeutic blood levels are reached almost immediately. They then transiently dip into the subtherapeutic range (*therapeutic hiatus*, indicated by the arrow) until a steady state level is established.

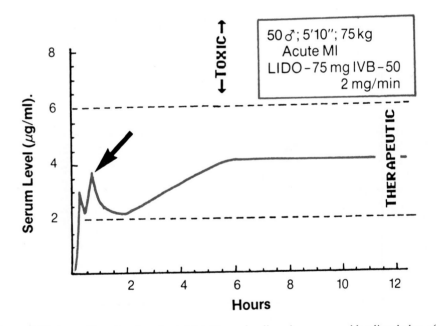

Figure 12E-4. Shortly after the initial 75-mg loading dose, a *second* loading bolus of 50 mg (arrow) is administered to the patient described in Figure 12E-3. Blood levels *never* drop into the subtherapeutic range.

(AMI, shock, congestive failure, or concomitant use of drugs such as propranolol or cimetidine) may be enough to cause the patient to become toxic when higher infusion rates are used *(Figure 12E-6)*.

An important point to emphasize is that pharmacokinetically, *there is no need to increase the rate of the lidocaine infusion during the initial hour of the loading period*—even if "breakthrough PVCs" occur!

Recurrence of PVCs during the 10 to 20 minutes following the loading bolus in Figure 12E-3 is probably *not* a reflection of the maintenance infusion being too slow. Instead it is much more likely to be a result of the drop in the lidocaine blood

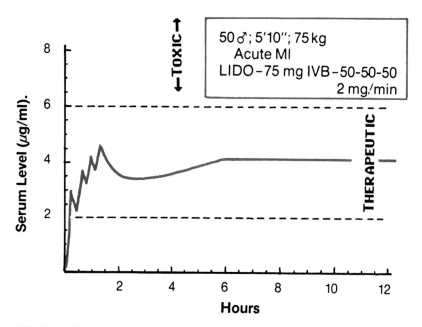

Figure 12E-5. Pharmacokinetic simulation in which the same patient described in Figure 12E-3 receives an initial loading dose of 75 mg, followed by *three* additional 50-mg boluses (for a total loading dose of 225 mg). The maintenance infusion is set at 2 mg/min. The eventual *steady state* drug level is approximately 4 µg/ml.

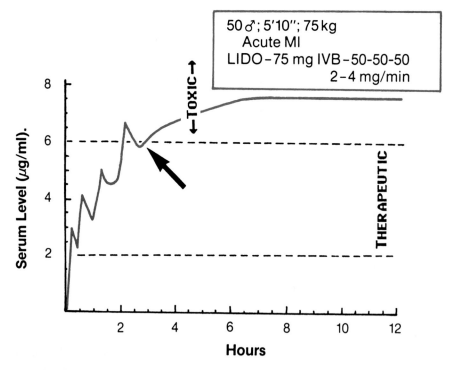

Figure 12E-6. Pharmacokinetic simulation demonstrating that the patient described in Figure 12E-5 would become toxic (arrow) if the rate of infusion was increased (by 1 mg/min increments) after each of the loading boluses.

level that occurs as the drug is redistributed from the central compartment to the peripheral compartment. This drop could be avoided (or at least lessened) by administering one or more additional loading boluses of lidocaine until steady state levels are achieved (as was done in Figures 12E-4 and 12E-5).

Note that the eventual steady state plasma concentration of lidocaine is *not* influenced by the manner in which the patient is loaded. As long as the rate of the maintenance infusion remains constant at 2 mg/min, the *eventual* level of lidocaine in the blood will be the same. Thus it can be seen that the identical steady state level (of just over 4 μg/ml) is ultimately reached for each of the loading protocols we have described (in Figures 12E-3, 12E-4, and 12E-5). *Only* if a serum drug level of greater than 4 μg/ml is required for arrhythmia control would one have to increase the rate of the maintenance infusion to above 2 mg/min.

Suggested Protocol for Lidocaine Administration

Considering the above, a reasonable protocol for administering lidocaine to an adult is to begin with an initial 50- to 100-mg IV *loading bolus* (i.e., 1 mg/kg), while *simultaneously* starting a maintenance infusion at 2 mg/min *(Figure 12E-7)*. The decision of whether to administer additional IV boluses can then be based on the reason for which lidocaine is being given. For example, if the drug is being used purely as a *prophylactic* measure to prevent primary ventricular fibrillation (i.e., in a patient suspected of AMI but *without* ventricular ectopy), additional loading boluses are probably *not* essential. As was seen in Figure 12E-3, administering lidocaine in this manner rapidly achieves a therapeutic blood level, and results in only a *brief* "therapeutic hiatus" (during which lidocaine blood levels drop below the therapeutic range). Alternatively, one might choose to administer a *second* loading bolus (of 50- to 75-mg) within 5 to 10 minutes after the initial bolus (Figure 12E-4). Doing so will probably maintain lidocaine levels within the therapeutic range until steady state is reached without substantially increasing the risk of developing lidocaine toxicity. More aggressive loading protocols (such as the one shown in Figure 12E-5) significantly increase the risk of toxicity, and are probably not warranted *when using lidocaine prophylactically*.

On the other hand, if lidocaine is being used *therapeutically* to treat frequent and complex ventricular ectopy, it

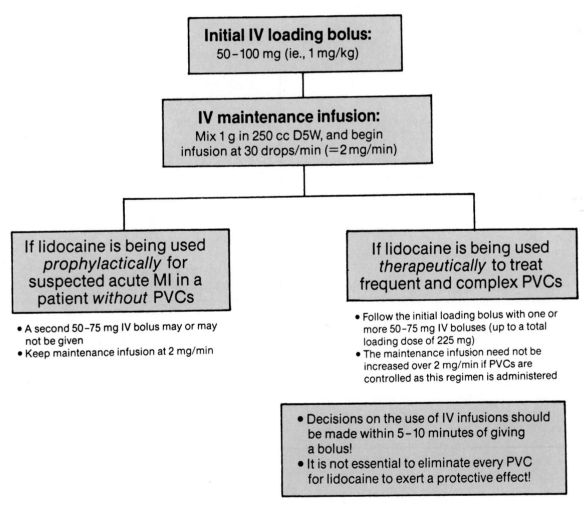

Figure 12E-7. Suggested protocol for lidocaine administration. An IV maintenance infusion is begun *simultaneously* with administration of the initial 50-100 mg IV loading bolus. Additional adjustments in lidocaine dosing are made depending on the *reason* for which lidocaine is being given (i.e., prophylaxis, or treatment of frequent and complex PVCs).

may be preferable to follow the initial loading dose with one or more additional 50- to 75-mg boluses (spaced 5-10 minutes apart) until a total loading dose of up to 225 mg has been given. If ventricular ectopy is controlled as this regimen is administered, the rate of the maintenance infusion need *not* be increased after each bolus.

> Two points about this protocol are deserving of special mention. First, the short half-life of lidocaine in the central compartment makes it essential that adjustments in the rate of the IV infusion be enacted *within 5 to 10 minutes* of giving the IV bolus. Failure to do so will result in dissipation of the effect of the bolus. Thus, if one assumes that the half-life of lidocaine in the central compartment is approximately 10 minutes and a 100-mg IV loading bolus is given, 10 minutes later only half of this amount (i.e., 50 mg) will remain in the central compartment. Were one to delay initiating the maintenance infusion *beyond* this time, the effect of the bolus will have been lost.
>
> The second point to emphasize is that *not every PVC must be treated for lidocaine to exert a protective effect.* The goal of *both* prophylactic and therapeutic administration of lidocaine is, after all, prevention of sustained ventricular tachycardia and ventricular fibrillation. Although in the past efforts were often made to abolish all PVCs, recent evidence suggests this is probably not necessary. A more practical (and much more easily attainable) goal of lidocaine therapy might therefore be to decrease the overall frequency of ventricular ectopy, and to markedly reduce the occurrence of repetitive forms (such as ventricular couplets and salvos)—but not necessarily to eliminate all PVCs.

Pharmacokinetic Points of Interest

A number of questions on the usage of lidocaine may arise from the preceding discussion:

1. Why are loading doses of greater than 1 mg/kg not used?
2. What are the clinical manifestations of lidocaine toxicity?
3. Are there adverse cardiovascular effects that must be kept in mind when the drug is used?
4. How is lidocaine eliminated from the body?
5. When administration of lidocaine is discontinued, can one abruptly stop the infusion, or should it be tapered?
6. What adjustments in administering the drug should be made for the elderly and/or those with congestive heart failure, shock, or liver disease?
7. When should lidocaine be used prophylactically? For how long should the infusion be maintained?
8. Is there a role for lidocaine in the treatment of ventricular fibrillation?

OPTIMAL LOADING DOSE OF LIDOCAINE

The optimal initial loading dose of lidocaine is a 1-mg/kg bolus given intravenously. Despite common usage of the term "bolus" this dose should *not* be injected as rapidly as possible. Instead it should be infused over a 1- to 2-minute period so as not to flood the central compartment with the drug. As mentioned earlier in this section, because the heart is contained within the central compartment the antiarrhythmic effect of a loading dose of lidocaine begins almost immediately. But since the brain is also contained within this same central compartment, too rapid infusion of a loading bolus (or administration of too large a dose) may result in CNS toxicity. Consequently, although doses of greater than 1 mg/kg of lidocaine may achieve steady state levels of the drug more rapidly, they are not recommended because of the unwarranted risk of toxicity.

MANIFESTATIONS OF TOXICITY

In general, lidocaine is an extremely well tolerated antiarrhythmic agent. When adverse effects do occur, they usually involve the central nervous system. Clinical manifestations of CNS toxicity are listed in *Table 12E-1.*

Table 12E-1

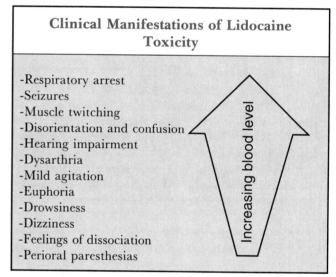

Clinical Manifestations of Lidocaine Toxicity
-Respiratory arrest
-Seizures
-Muscle twitching
-Disorientation and confusion
-Hearing impairment
-Dysarthria
-Mild agitation
-Euphoria
-Drowsiness
-Dizziness
-Feelings of dissociation
-Perioral paresthesias

(Increasing blood level)

The *therapeutic range* of serum drug levels for lidocaine is between 2 and 6 μg/ml. Occasionally, mild signs of lidocaine toxicity (dizziness, feelings of dissociation, and perioral paresthesias) are seen at levels near 5 μg/ml (which is a serum drug concentration that overlaps with the upper limits of the therapeutic range). At other times adverse effects may follow infusion of a loading bolus, particularly if the drug was administered too rapidly. When this is the case, prompt resolution of adverse effects should follow discontinuation of the infusion. In contrast, development of adverse effects at a later stage in dosing (i.e., *after* steady state has been established) is much more suggestive of drug accumulation and impending toxicity. In this instance, the maintenance infusion should be stopped immediately, and if possible a blood level should be drawn to look for toxicity.

The problem with diagnosing lidocaine toxicity is that severe reactions (such as seizures and respiratory arrest) may occasionally occur first *without* warning from any of the milder premonitory symptoms. Thus, a patient convulsing during cardiac arrest may be hypoxic, hypotensive, alkalotic, or toxic from lidocaine. Unfortunately, clinical assessment without laboratory confirmation has not been shown to be accurate in differentiating between these possibilities (Deglin et al, 1980). As a result, cautious dosing and a high index of suspicion are essential, especially when treating patients who are at greater risk of developing toxicity.

ADVERSE CARDIOVASCULAR EFFECTS

Perhaps the most frequently observed adverse cardiovascular effect of lidocaine is hypotension. When this occurs, it is most often due to the too rapid administration of an IV bolus. Momentary placement of the patient in Trendelenburg and reducing the rate of infusion are usually all that are needed to resolve the problem.

Depression of left ventricular function and exacerbation of SA or AV conduction disturbances may occur but are relatively uncommon (especially in patients with normal ventricular function and intact interventricular conduction). In general, lidocaine may be given to such patients without concern about causing new heart failure or precipitating a bradyarrhythmia. In contrast, caution is advised when the drug is administered to patients with severe left ventricular dysfunction or significant impairment of SA or AV nodal conduction (as is the case for patients with sick sinus syndrome, bundle branch block, and second- or third-degree AV block). In such patients, administration of lidocaine may aggravate the conduction disturbance. In addition to slowing the ventricular rate, case reports of asystole following lidocaine administration have been noted (Dunn et al, 1985; Hilleman et al, 1985). Although relatively rare, the potential severity of these reactions warrants caution in selection (and monitoring) of patients who are to receive the drug, particularly if they have preexisting conduction disturbances. Under such circumstances, ready availability of pacemaker therapy may be advisable before lidocaine infusion is begun.

A final but important cardiac effect that lidocaine may occasionally produce is acceleration of the ventricular response of supraventricular tachyarrhythmias (especially atrial flutter or atrial fibrillation). This results from a quinidine-like action of this drug that may decrease AV nodal refractoriness in certain patients. Consequently, lidocaine should *never* be used indiscriminately as a diagnostic measure in patients with wide complex tachyarrhythmias, since the drug may aggravate the condition (that is, accelerate the ventricular response) if the rhythm turns out to be supraventricular (Marriott and Bieza, 1972; Hilleman et al, 1985).

LIDOCAINE ELIMINATION

Lidocaine is eliminated from the body principally by hepatic metabolism. The half-life of this elimination phase is proportional to hepatic blood flow, and under normal circumstances takes between 1 to 2 hours. Patients in shock or congestive heart failure in whom hepatic blood flow may be greatly diminished, would therefore be expected to have a prolonged elimination phase half-life—and be more susceptible to accumulation of drug and lidocaine toxicity. Other groups at particularly high risk of developing lidocaine toxicity include patients with liver disease, those taking drugs such as propranolol or cimetidine (that decrease hepatic clearance of lidocaine), the elderly (in whom cardiac output is less), and patients with low body weight *(Table 12E-2)*. In addition, the elimination phase half-life of lidocaine may increase in patients with AMI (due to altered protein-binding of lidocaine), and in those receiving prolonged ($\geq$24 hour) infusion of the drug. For this reason, it may be prudent to reduce the rate of the maintenance infusion in patients receiving lidocaine for more than 24 hours.

Table 12E-2

Factors Impairing Lidocaine Clearance
-Congestive heart failure
-AMI
-Shock
-Liver disease
-Drugs (i.e., propranolol, cimetidine)
-Older age
-Low body weight
-Prolonged infusion (i.e., >24 hours)

Cimetidine inhibits the hepatic metabolism of a number of drugs, including lidocaine, warfarin, theophylline, and diazepam. The mechanism by which this occurs is thought to result from the drug's avid binding to the *cytochrome P-450 system* involved in drug elimination (Zimmerman and Schenker, 1985). Failure to reduce the rate of lidocaine infusion for patients receiving cimetidine may precipitate lidocaine toxicity. Although other H-2 blockers currently in use (i.e., *ranitidine, famotidine, nizatidine*) act to reduce gastric acid production in much the same manner as cimetidine, they do not appear to bind to the cytochrome P-450 system to nearly the same degree. Significant clinical interactions between other H-2 blockers and lidocaine have not been reported, and use of these drugs is therefore preferable to cimetidine for patients with ventricular arrhythmias.

It is important to appreciate that abrupt cessation of an IV maintenance infusion of lidocaine will *not* immediately result in subtherapeutic blood levels. This point is well illustrated by Figure 12E-2, in which serum drug levels do not fall into the subtherapeutic range for nearly 2 hours *after* the maintenance infusion is discontinued. Thus, *there would seem to be no pharmacokinetic rationale for tapering patients off lidocaine infusions!* The 1- to 2-hour elimination phase half-life of the drug *automatically* ensures a tapering effect.

ADJUSTMENTS IN DOSING TO AVOID TOXICITY

What adjustments in dosing should be made for those patients at high risk of developing lidocaine toxicity? Consider the case of a 70 year old woman who is admitted to the hospital for pulmonary edema associated with AMI. She is 5 feet 2 inches tall, and weighs 110 pounds (50 kg). The decision is made to begin her on prophylactic lidocaine. After receiving the usual 1-mg/kg IV loading dose (in this case 50 mg), the patient rapidly becomes toxic on a maintenance infusion administered at the seemingly "standard" rate of 2 mg/min *(Figure 12E-8)*.

The point to emphasize in this clinical scenario is that a maintenance infusion at the "standard" rate of 2 mg/min may well be too high for an elderly individual of low body weight with AMI and significant congestive heart failure. In this particular case, the infusion was held for 4 hours (open arrowhead in Figure 12E-8). The drip was then restarted (arrow) at the lower infusion rate of 0.5 mg/min. In a patient such as this, an *infusion rate of as low as 0.5 mg/min may be more than adequate to maintain therapeutic serum concentrations of the drug.*

If this same 70 year old, 50-kg woman was admitted to the hospital with AMI but *without* congestive heart failure, slightly more lidocaine would probably be needed to achieve and maintain adequate blood levels. *Figure 12E-9* shows that this could be done by administering two 50 mg loading boluses and setting the IV infusion to run at 1 mg/min.

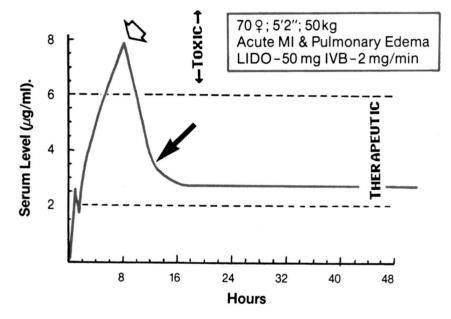

Figure 12E-8. Pharmacokinetic simulation of a 70-year-old woman (5 feet 2 inches, 50 kg) with AMI and pulmonary edema who receives 50-mg IV loading bolus of lidocaine and is begun on a maintenance infusion at 2 mg/min. The infusion is held after 8 hours (open arrowhead) when she becomes toxic. At 12 hours it is restarted (arrow) at the lower infusion rate of 0.5 mg/min.

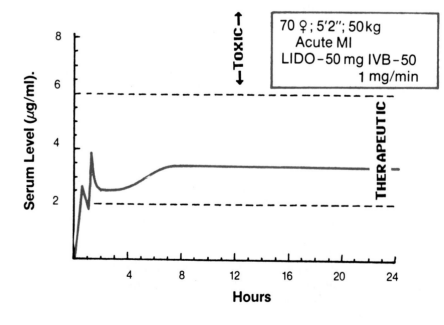

Figure 12E-9. Pharmacokinetic simulation for a 70-year-old woman (5 feet 2 inches, 50 kg) with AMI but *without* congestive heart failure. She is given two 50-mg IV loading boluses and then begun on an IV maintenance infusion at 1 mg/min.

Thus, the initial loading dose of lidocaine is fairly *independent* of patient variables other than body weight. A dose of 1 mg/kg (i.e., between 50-100 mg) is the usual amount recommended for this first bolus.

Many factors impair lidocaine clearance, however, and these factors must be taken into account if subsequent boluses are given and when determining the rate of the maintenance infusion (Table 12E-2). Failure to do so significantly increases the likelihood of developing lidocaine toxicity. Although 2 mg/min is the standard infusion rate recommended for most adults, lower rates (of 1 mg/min—or even 0.5 mg/min) may be advisable when lidocaine is administered to patients at high risk of developing toxicity.

PROPHYLACTIC USE OF LIDOCAINE

In the past it was thought that *"warning arrhythmias"* (5 or more PVCs per minute, 2 or more PVCs in a row, multiform PVCs, and the "R-on-T" phenomenon) regularly preceded the development of primary ventricular fibrillation in patients with AMI. Consequently, one would wait for the occurrence of such arrhythmias before initiating antiarrhythmic treatment in patients admitted with acute chest pain.

Today the concept of warning arrhythmias has been conclusively disproved. Ventricular fibrillation frequently occurs in AMI without warning arrhythmias. Sometimes it even occurs without any prior ectopic activity. Moreover, when warning arrhythmias do occur, they do not reliably predict which patients will subsequently develop ventricular fibrillation.

In view of the fact that more than 90% of patients with AMI have some ventricular ectopy, and 5% to 10% develop *primary* ventricular fibrillation,* it would seem reasonable to consider prophylactic use of antiarrhythmic therapy for patients with suspected infarction. Lidocaine has been the drug most commonly chosen for this purpose. It is easy to administer, is well tolerated by most patients, and effectively lowers the incidence of primary ventricular

---

*As discussed in Section B of this chapter, appreciation of the difference between *primary* and *secondary* forms of ventricular fibrillation is essential for understanding the goals and rationale for lidocaine *treatment* and *prophylaxis*. **Primary ventricular fibrillation** refers to the acute electrical instability that develops as a direct consequence of the infarction. It is most often seen within the first few hours of infarction, and is rare after 24 hours. In contrast, **secondary ventricular fibrillation** characteristically occurs several days after the onset of symptoms, and is usually associated with the development of cardiogenic shock. Lidocaine prophylaxis is aimed at preventing primary ventricular fibrillation. As might be expected, secondary ventricular fibrillation is generally resistant to any type of antiarrhythmic therapy.

fibrillation associated with AMI (MacMahon et al, 1988; Hine et al, 1989). Patients most likely to benefit from lidocaine prophylaxis are those seen soon (within the first few hours) after the onset of symptoms, especially if a high index of suspicion for AMI exists. This is because by far the greatest incidence of primary ventricular fibrillation associated with AMI occurs within the first few hours after the onset of infarction (ACC/AHA Task Force, 1990).

Lidocaine prophylaxis should *not* be used indiscriminately, however, since administration of this drug is associated with a 5% to 15% incidence of toxicity. The risk of lidocaine toxicity seems to be greatest for patients more than 70 years old (Goldman and Batsford, 1979; Lie et al, 1974). Since the risk of developing primary ventricular fibrillation is significantly less in this age group, elderly patients might reasonably be excluded from consideration for lidocaine prophylaxis. Also because primary ventricular fibrillation is rare after 24 hours, lidocaine prophylaxis is probably not warranted in patients who are initially seen after this period (ACC/AHA Task Force, 1990).

Unfortunately, the issue of whether to use prophylactic lidocaine for patients with suspected AMI remains controversial. As indicated earlier (in Section B of this chapter), meta-analysis of 14 randomized trials in the literature (involving more than 9,000 patients) failed to show a reduction in mortality in patients with suspected AMI who were routinely given prophylactic lidocaine (MacMahon et al, 1988). On the contrary, treatment of such patients with lidocaine appeared to slightly *increase* the risk of developing fatal asystole (from 0.2% to 0.4%) compared to patients with suspected AMI who were not given prophylactic lidocaine (Yusuf et al, 1988). We feel the jury is still out on this issue.

Despite the controversy, it may still be reasonable to consider lidocaine *prophylaxis* for the prevention of primary ventricular fibrillation in some selected patients with suspected AMI who:

1. Are less than 70 years of age.
2. Are seen soon after the onset of symptoms (especially if seen within the first 6 hours).
3. Are highly likely to be having AMI (i.e., who already demonstrate acute ECG changes.)

As indicated in Section B of this chapter, rather than endorsement of any particular policy, we feel it more important to *individualize* the decision of whether to use lidocaine, basing it on careful consideration of the pros and cons of such treatment, relevant pharmacokinetics of the drug (as discussed in this section), and the goals of therapy in the context of the clinical setting (as summarized in Table 12B-2).

Potential benefits of lidocaine prophylaxis are less for patients who are older (than 70), seen later in the course (after 12-24 hours of the onset of symptoms), and for whom the likelihood of AMI is less (i.e., history of atypical chest pain, absence of acute ECG changes). In addition, the potential risk of developing severe bradyarrhythmias (including advanced AV block or even asystole) is significantly greater in patients with pre-existing conduction disturbances. As a result, the overall risk-benefit ratio under any of these circumstances is unlikely to be favorable, and prophylactic use of lidocaine is probably *not* warranted.

The issue of whether to use lidocaine prophylaxis has almost become academic for patients receiving thrombolytic therapy. Because such individuals are at high risk of developing reperfusion arrhythmias, most clinicians tend to routinely administer lidocaine prophylactically in this setting. In addition, it is well to keep in mind that patients with suspected AMI who are treated with IV β-blockers probably *do not need* lidocaine prophylaxis (Conti, 1989).

> Lidocaine prophylaxis in an otherwise stable patient need *not* be continued beyond 12-24 hours. The risk of toxicity may be further minimized by limiting the number of loading boluses (to one, or at most two), and keeping the infusion rate at 2 mg/min. Use of lower infusion rates (of 0.5-1.0 mg/min) may be preferable when treating patients at especially high risk of developing lidocaine toxicity (i.e., the elderly, those with heart failure or liver disease, patients of lighter body weight).

LIDOCAINE TREATMENT IN AMI

In contrast to the uncertainties surrounding *prophylactic* use of lidocaine, most authorities still favor lidocaine *treatment* for patients with suspected AMI who manifest *new-onset* frequent and/or repetitive ventricular ectopy (ACC/AHA Task Force, 1990). It should be emphasized that not every PVC need be eliminated for lidocaine to exert a protective effect (in preventing primary ventricular fibrillation) in this setting. (See *Section B and Table 12B-2 in this chapter.*)

ANTIFIBRILLATORY EFFECT OF LIDOCAINE

A number of years ago, a point was made not to recommend lidocaine for treatment of ventricular fibrillation refractory to other measures out of concern that administration of the drug in this setting would be likely to abolish the only ventricular activity that was present and lead to asystole. For the most part, this concern has proved to be unfounded, although admittedly a slight increase in the incidence of asystole is associated with the use of lidocaine in this setting. Subsequently, the pendulum shifted and the recommendation was made to use lidocaine as an *antifibrillatory agent* for treatment of refractory ventricular fibrillation (White, 1984; AHA ACLS Text, 1986). Why was this done? How might lidocaine work to help in converting established ventricular fibrillation to a normal rhythm?

To answer this question, we must first consider the mechanisms that sustain ventricular tachycardia and fibrillation. The substrate for ventricular tachycardia is thought to be a fairly large reentry circuit that allows persistence of this tachyarrhythmia. In contrast, the wavefronts of depolarization for ventricular fibrillation are fragmented and follow circuitous paths. Seldom are such circuitous movements completed. Nevertheless, it appears that *reentry* is again the mechanism responsible for allowing the persistence of ventricular fibrillation, in this case prevailing throughout the ventricles in numerous small reentry circuits.

Lidocaine works by speeding conduction and prolonging refractoriness in ischemic zones. This may result in suppressing conduction along many of the fragmented wavefronts present with ventricular fibrillation. Subsequent electrical countershock might then facilitate removal of the remaining wavefronts that were sustaining ventricular fibrillation, and thus allow resumption of normal pacemaker function.

Thus, in addition to routine administration of lidocaine after conversion of ventricular fibrillation to sinus rhythm, the drug has also been recommended for use in treatment of refractory ventricular fibrillation in the hope that this antiarrhythmic agent might facilitate conversion to normal sinus rhythm with subsequent countershock.

> It should be noted that consensus is lacking regarding the overall net effect of lidocaine in the treatment of refractory ventricular fibrillation. Although its electrophysiologic effects may be beneficial in unifying conduction properties in the multiple small reentry circuits that are prevalent in this arrhythmia, this effect could be counterbalanced by an *increase* in energy requirements for defibrillation—as well as the small but real risk that administration of lidocaine may predispose to development of asystole (Wesley et al, 1991). Clearly, the jury is still out on this drug. . . .

Only time will determine the optimal role for lidocaine in the treatment of refractory ventricular fibrillation. At present, we still favor reserving its use for patients in persistent ventricular fibrillation that fails to respond to repeat countershock attempts. Once the patient is converted *out of* ventricular fibrillation, we favor its use as a *prophylactic* measure in the hope of preventing recurrence.

LIDOCAINE DOSING IN CARDIAC ARREST

Lidocaine pharmacokinetics during cardiac arrest are not very predictable. As a result, current guidelines suggest that only bolus therapy be used in this setting (AHA ACLS Text, 1986). In addition, due to markedly decreased clearance of the drug, it appears that less frequent administration of loading boluses is needed during this low-flow state (McDonald, 1985). Thus, *as little as one loading bolus* (1 mg/kg) *of lidocaine (or at most two boluses) is probably all that is required to maintain therapeutic levels of the drug during cardiac arrest.* Once the patient has been converted out of ventricular fibrillation, however, clearance of the drug markedly increases. Resumption of a normal dosing schedule (with rebolus and institution of a maintenance infusion) is then indicated.

> Practically speaking, it may be easier to continue the lidocaine maintenance infusion during the period of cardiopulmonary resuscitation. Doing so should *not* pose a significant risk of developing drug toxicity, since the amount of drug administered at an infusion rate of 2 mg/min during a 15 to 30 minute code will not exceed 30 to 60 mg. On the other hand, stopping (or never starting) the lidocaine infusion during the period of cardiac arrest makes it all too easy to forget to start (or restart) the infusion after conversion out of ventricular fibrillation, substantially increasing the risk of recurrence.

References

Adgey AAJ, Geddes JS, Webb SW, Allen JD, James RGG, Zaidi SA, Pantridge JF: Acute phase of myocardial infarction, *Lancet* 2:501-504, 1971.

American College of Cardiology/American Heart Association Task Force: Guidelines for the early management of patients with acute myocardial infarction, *Circulation* 82:664-707, 1990.

American Heart Association: Textbook of advanced cardiac life support, Dallas, 1987, The Association.

Barnaby PF, Barrett PA, Lvoff R: Routine prophylactic lidocaine in acute myocardial infarction, *Heart Lung* 12:362-366, 1983.

Church G, Biern RO: Intensive coronary care—a practical system for a small hospital without house staff, *N Engl J Med* 281:1155-1159, 1969.

Conti RC: Drug therapy of patients with acute myocardial infarction in the era of thrombolysis, *Mod Conc Cardiovasc Dis* 58:19-24, 1989.

Deglin SM, Deglin JM, Wurtzbacher J, Litton M, Rolfe C, McIntire C: Rapid serum lidocaine determination in the coronary care unit, *JAMA* 244:571-573, 1980.

El-Sherif N, Myerberg RJ, Scherlag BJ, Befeler B, Aranda JM, Castellanos A, Lazzara R: Electrocardiographic antecedents of primary ventricular fibrillation, *Br Heart J* 38:415-422, 1976.

Fuchs R, Scheidt S: Improved criteria for admission to cardiac care units, *JAMA* 246:2037-2041, 1981.

Goldman L, Batsford WF: Risk-benefit stratification as a guide to lidocaine prophylaxis of primary ventricular fibrillation in acute myocardial infarction: an analytic review, *Yale J Biol Med* 52:455-466, 1979.

Grauer K: Should lidocaine be routinely used in patients suspected of acute myocardial infarction? *J Fla Med Assoc* 69:377-379, 1982.

Harrison D: Should lidocaine be administered routinely to all patients after acute myocardial infarction? *Circulation* 58:581-584, 1978.

Hilleman DE, Mohiuddin SM, Destache CJ: Lidocaine-induced second-degree Mobitz II heart block, *Drug Intell Clin Pharm* 19:669-673, 1985.

Hine LK, Laird N, Hewitt P, Chalmers TC: Meta-analytic evidence against prophylactic use of lidocaine in acute myocardial infarction, *Arch Int Med* 149:2694-2698, 1989.

Koster RW, Dunning AJ: Intramuscular lidocaine for prevention of lethal arrhythmias in the prehospitalization phase of acute myocardial infarction, *N Engl J Med* 313:1105-1110, 1985.

Lie KI, Wellens JH, van Capelle FJ, Durrer D: Lidocaine in prevention of primary ventricular fibrillation, *N Engl J Med* 291:1324-1326, 1974.

Lopez LM, Mehta JL, Robinson JD, Roberts RJ: Optimal lidocaine dosing in patients with myocardial infarction, *Ther Drug Mon* 4:271-276, 1982.

Marriott JHL, Bieza CF: Alarming ventricular acceleration after lidocaine administration, *Chest* 61:682-683, 1972.

MacMahon S, Collins R, Peto R, Koster RW, Yusuf S: Effects of prophylactic lidocaine in suspected acute myocardial infarction: an overview of results from the randomized, controlled trials, *JAMA* 260:1910-1916, 1988.

McDonald JL: Serum lidocaine levels during cardiopulmonary resuscitation after intravenous and endotracheal administration, *Crit Care Med* 13:914-915, 1985.

Romhilt DW, Boomfield SS, Chou TC, Fowler NO: Unreliability of conventional electrocardiographic monitoring for arrhythmia detection in coronary care units, *Am J Cardiol* 31:457-461, 1973.

Stargel WW, Routledge PA: Lidocaine: therapeutic use and serum concentration monitoring. In Taylor WJ, Finn AL (eds): Individualizing drug therapy, New York, 1981, Gross, Townsend, Frank.

Wesley RC, Resh W, Zimmerman D: Reconsiderations of the routine and preferential use of lidocaine in the emergent treatment of ventricular arrhythmias, *Crit Care Med* 19:1439-1444, 1991.

White RD: Antifibrillatory drugs: the case for lidocaine and procainamide, *Ann Emerg Med* 13:802-804, 1984.

Wyman MG, Gore S: Lidocaine prophylaxis in myocardial infarction: a concept whose time has come, *Heart Lung* 12:358-361, 1983.

Wyman MG, Hammersmith L: Comprehensive treatment plan for prevention of primary ventricular fibrillation in acute myocardial infarction, *Am J Cardiol* 33:661-667, 1974.

Yusuf S, Wittes J, Friedman L: Treatments following myocardial infarction. In Overview of results of randomized clinical trials in heart disease, *JAMA* 260:2088-2093, 1988.

Zimmerman TW, Schenker S: A comparative evaluation of cimetidine and ranitidine, *Rational Drug Ther* 19:1-7, 1985.

SECTION F

AN ILLUSTRATIVE CASE STUDY

Mr. A is a 65 year old man who presented to the ED at **10:00 AM** with a chief complaint of severe chest pain. Mr. A has always been in good health. He does not take any medications, and had not seen a physician for years. He reports "fatigue" during the past week, and intermittent chest discomfort with exertion over the last 2 days.

YOU are asked to evaluate Mr. A, and to take over his care . . .

Mr. A has already received two sublingual nitroglycerin (NTG) in the ED, but is still complaining of severe chest pain. He has been placed on a telemetry monitor which shows normal sinus rhythm without ventricular ectopy. An IV line has been inserted, and D5W is running at KVO. Vital signs are normal (pulse = 75 beats/min; BP = 120/80 mm Hg). Physical examination is unrevealing (lung fields are clear; no murmurs, rubs or gallops are heard on cardiac auscultation; and there is no JVD, organomegaly or pedal edema).

Mr. A's initial 12-lead ECG (obtained at **10:20 AM**) is shown in *Figure 12F-1.*

PROBLEM   How would you interpret Mr. A's initial 12-lead ECG?

INTERPRETATION OF *FIGURE 12F-1* *Systematic evaluation* of Mr. A's initial 12-lead ECG reveals the following:

Normal sinus rhythm (at ≈80 beats/min), normal intervals (i.e., normal PR, QRS, and QT intervals), a normal QRS axis (of ≈ +45°), and no evidence of chamber enlargement.

There are tiny q waves in leads II and III. Although T waves are prominent and somewhat peaked in the inferior leads (i.e., "hyperacute" T waves), ST segments are only minimally elevated (at most 1 mm) in these leads. ST segments are slightly depressed in many of the remaining leads (i.e., "reciprocal" ST segment depression), and the T wave is frankly inverted in lead aVL.

In light of the clinical history, the overall picture is highly suggestive of an *acute ischemic syndrome.*

It is now **10:30 AM**. Mr. A is still complaining of severe chest pain. *What would you do at this point?*

Summarized History/Actions up to this point for the Case of Mr. A:

- **History of present illness**—"Fatigue" for 1 week; intermittent chest discomfort (with exertion) for 2 days

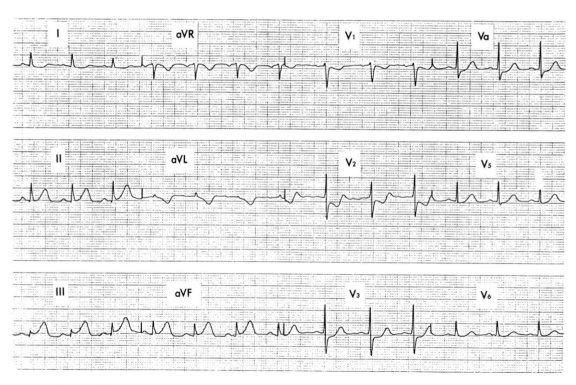

Figure 12F-1.   Mr. A's *initial 12-lead ECG*. The tracing was obtained 20 minutes after his arrival in the ED (i.e., at **10:20 AM**).

- **10:00 AM**—Arrival in ED—complaining of chest pain:
  —stable vital signs—unremarkable exam
  —sublingual NTG administered (× 2) without relief
  —IV line inserted (with D5W @ KVO)

- **Telemetry monitoring**—normal sinus rhythm without ventricular ectopy
- **10:20 AM**—Initial ECG obtained (Fig. 12F-1)
- **10:30 AM**—Severe chest pain persists. *YOU are asked to take over care.*

PROBLEM   **What *three* things would you do *first*?**
1.
2.
3.

ADDITIONAL PROBLEM: Reflect on the history obtained and the actions that had been taken up to this point. *Comment ???*

ANSWER   At the least, it appears that Mr. A is having some type of *acute ischemic syndrome* (new-onset anginal chest pain, preinfarction angina, and/or evolving AMI). Immediate actions that are indicated at this point include administration of:

1. **Aspirin** (160-325 mg PO)
2. **Oxygen** (by nasal cannula at 2-4 L/min)
3. More potent analgesia:
   a. **IV NTG** (beginning at an infusion rate of 10 μg/min, and gradually titrating the drip to 50-100 μg/min as needed).
       and/or
   b. **Morphine sulfate** (2-5 mg IV q5-30 min, as needed)

ASPIRIN

As emphasized in Section 12C, aspirin (ASA) is routinely recommended for *ALL* patients who present with new-onset chest pain of presumed ischemic etiology (provided there are no specific contraindications to the drug). Aspirin should be started *As Soon As Possible* (i.e., *"ASA—ASAP"*) *regardless* of whatever other interventions might be contemplated. *Aspirin should have been started BEFORE 10:30 AM in this case!*

OXYGEN

Oxygen is also recommended for all patients with suspected AMI *(Section 12B)*. One need not be concerned about the possibility of oxygen retention in this acute setting in which the patient is being so carefully monitored.

RELIEF OF CHEST PAIN

The chest pain of acute ischemic heart disease should be relieved as soon as possible. If this is not rapidly accomplished

with the use of sublingual NTG, more potent analgesia should be given. In patients who are not hypotensive or hypovolemic, our preference is to initiate an infusion of **IV nitroglycerin** as soon as we are convinced that the persistent chest pain is truly of ischemic etiology (*Table 12B-1 and Section 12B*).

Additional measures that may be considered for control of chest pain (*and* the anxiety component that so commonly accompanies such chest pain) include 2-5 mg IV incremental doses of **morphine sulfate** (Section 12B), and/or judicious use of **benzodiazepines** (Section 12B).

REFLECTION on the HISTORY OBTAINED/ACTIONS TAKEN up to this point: The history obtained in this case is notably lacking for information regarding the *onset of symptoms* that may be attributable to an acute event. Thus, Mr. A reports fatigue for 1 week and anginal chest pain for 2 days. *It is critically important to try to elucidate WHEN (the EXACT time) the severe and persistent chest pain that caused him to come to the hospital began*—as the *onset* of this symptom usually serves as the most reliable clinical indicator of the onset of AMI.

With respect to the evaluation and management of patients with suspected AMI, it is essential to remember that:

Time is muscle!

The "window of opportunity" for effective therapeutic intervention is extremely limited. In this particular case, *precious time was wasted.* Despite arrival of the patient in the ED at 10:00 AM, the initial ECG was not obtained until 10:20 AM, aspirin was not given until 10:30 AM, and severe chest pain was allowed to continue for 30 minutes with no more treatment than sublingual NTG. Moreover, consideration toward implementing additional therapeutic measures had not been addressed as of 10:30 AM. With *optimal* evaluation and management, *ALL of these actions/interventions would be accomplished (or at least considered) in far less time.*

PROBLEM   **What additional actions/therapeutic measures might be *considered* at this point?**

ANSWER   Actions/therapeutic measures to *consider* at this point might be classified as follows:

4. *Additional Medical Treatment*
   a. IV β-blockers
   b. Calcium channel blockers
   c. Prophylactic lidocaine
   d. Other drugs (i.e., magnesium sulfate)
5. *Attempted Reperfusion*
   a. Thrombolytic therapy (with IV streptokinase, rt-PA, APSAC, or other agent)
   b. Anticoagulation (with IV or subcutaneous heparin)

c. PTCA (as a *primary* procedure, *adjunct* to thrombolytic therapy, or as a "rescue" procedure)
6. *Laboratory Tests*

IV β-BLOCKERS

As emphasized in Section 12B, IV β-blockers effectively reduce mortality in patients with AMI, especially when administered within the first 3 to 6 hours of the onset of symptoms. Although patients with anterior AMI and signs of sympathetic overactivity (i.e., hypertension, tachycardia) are likely to benefit most from IV β-blockers, their use in AMI should *not* be restricted to such patients. In this case, since there are no obvious contraindications to the use of IV β-blockers for Mr. A (i.e., no history of bronchospasm, and no bradycardia, hypotension, or evidence of heart failure), they should be actively considered—*especially if his chest pain persists despite other analgesic measures (Tables 12B-4 and 12B-5).*

An additional benefit derived from using IV β-blocker therapy early in the course of AMI is that doing so appears to obviate any need for prophylactic lidocaine.

Strong consideration should be given to following IV β-blocker therapy with long-term oral β-blocker therapy as a secondary prevention measure.

CALCIUM CHANNEL BLOCKERS

Calcium channel blockers have *not* been shown to reduce mortality when administered early in the course of acute Q-wave infarction. As a result, they should *not* be a first-line intervention in the treatment of most patients with AMI—and, *we would probably NOT use them at this point in the case of Mr. A.* Calcium channel blockers may be helpful later in the course of AMI for treatment of persistent chest pain, and/or in follow-up treatment of patients with non-Q wave infarction. They are a drug of choice (with IV nitroglycerin and β-blockers) for treatment of unstable angina. Finally, they may be a helpful adjunct in selected patients when used *after* thrombolytic therapy to prevent post-reperfusion vasospasm that might otherwise lead to reocclusion of the IRA *(Section 12B and Table 12B-8).*

PROPHYLACTIC LIDOCAINE

Lidocaine is the antiarrhythmic agent of choice for *treatment* of new-onset ventricular ectopy associated with AMI. Up to this point in the case of Mr. A, however, there has been no evidence of ventricular ectopy—so that "treatment" per se is not necessary. Whether lidocaine should be used as a *prophylactic measure* for patients with *suspected* AMI who are not having ventricular ectopy (or who are only having rare PVCs without repetitive forms) remains controversial *(Sections 12B and 12E; Table 12B-2).* Because prophylactic administration of lidocaine has *not* been shown to reduce mortality, an increasing number of clinicians no longer use the drug for this indication.

Although our tendency has also been to use lidocaine less often than in the past, we still might *consider* antiarrhythmic prophylaxis in some selected patients with suspected AMI under the following circumstances:

1. When the patient is seen *soon* after the onset of symptoms (especially within the first 6 hours)
2. When the history and/or admission ECG *strongly suggest* that AMI is taking place
3. When the patient is *less* than 70 years of age

Two additional factors may facilitate the decision-making process:

4. Whether *thrombolytic therapy* is also used
5. Whether *IV β-blockers* are also used

Prophylactic administration of lidocaine is generally recommended for patients who receive thrombolytic therapy. This is because of the very high likelihood that "reperfusion arrhythmias" will occur with recanalization of the IRA. However, the antiarrhythmic effect of IV β-blockers may lessen (or even obviate) any need for antiarrhythmic prophylaxis. Thus, there is clearly more than one way to approach this case, and whether one decided to administer lidocaine would probably depend on a *combination* of factors.

If frequent and/or repetitive PVCs suddenly developed, *treatment* would certainly be indicated (but by definition, this would no longer constitute "prophylaxis"). On the other hand, if no PVCs developed, one might still *consider* the use of prophylactic lidocaine on the basis of the patient's age (*less* than 70), the suggestive history, and his abnormal initial ECG. Consensus on the use of prophylactic lidocaine is lacking, however, and an increasing number of clinicians would probably favor careful observation over antiarrhythmic prophylaxis in this situation. If the decision was made to use IV β-blockers, prophylactic lidocaine would probably not be needed—unless the decision was also made to use thrombolytic therapy, in which case the *addition* of lidocaine might further help to reduce the incidence and severity of reperfusion arrhythmias.

MAGNESIUM SULFATE

Although increasing use of magnesium in patients with AMI may be anticipated in the near future, routine administration of this drug (either prophylactically, or as specific treatment for ventricular ectopy) is not yet generally recommended. However, because serum magnesium levels are commonly reduced in the setting of AMI, it is probably worthwhile to routinely check the serum magnesium level in this setting—*especially in patients with frequent PVCs and/or in those predisposed to developing hypomagnesemia* (i.e., in patients with other electrolyte disorders, or in those who are taking diuretics, digitalis, or who have renal disease or a history of alcohol abuse). While the finding of a normal serum magnesium level does not rule out decreased body stores of this cation, a low serum level in the setting of AMI is a definite indication for magnesium replacement *(Section 12B; Chapter 14).* In the absence of ventricular ectopy and/or factors predisposing to hypomagnesemia, *we would not administer magnesium in this case unless Mr. A's serum level was low.*

Perhaps the biggest decision point in the case of Mr. A is the issue of thrombolytic therapy. Imagine the time is now **10:40 AM.**

PROBLEM   **If Mr. A's chest pain had begun suddenly at 6:40 AM (i.e., 4 hours ago), would he be a suitable candidate for the use of thrombolytic therapy? If so, *would he be likely to obtain substantial benefit from such treatment?*** (Base your answers on the history given in this case study, and on your interpretation of the initial 12-lead ECG shown in Figure 12F-1.)

ADDITIONAL PROBLEM: *Would it help clinically to repeat the ECG at this point?*

ANSWER   Mr. A is a suitable candidate for thrombolytic therapy because he satisfies *all of* the **Qualifying**

Criteria listed in *Table 12C-2:*

1. Age *less* than 75
2. History of new-onset (ischemic-sounding) chest pain that has not been relieved by nitroglycerin, and which began *less* than 6 hours ago
3. Acute ECG changes (with ≥1 mm of ST segment elevation in at least two contiguous leads)—*although admittedly these changes are fairly subtle*
4. No known contraindications to the use of thrombolytic therapy

However, based on his relatively late presentation and interpretation of his initial ECG, the *amount of benefit* that might be anticipated from using thrombolytic therapy is likely to be limited (Table 12A-2). That is, a full *4* hours have already passed since the onset of symptoms, the site of suspected infarction is *inferior,* and acute ST segment changes are minimal (i.e., *barely* 1 mm of ST segment elevation in the inferior leads with a relatively small amount of reciprocal ST segment depression). As a result, some clinicians might be less enthusiastic about using thrombolytic therapy in this case.

AMI is a *dynamic* and continually *evolving* process. As emphasized in Section 12A, the **initial ECG** will not always reveal the true nature and/or extent of this process for a number of reasons including:

- The possibility of a "lag time" (of several hours or longer) that may exist between the onset of symptoms and development of diagnostic ECG changes.
- The chance that the initial ECG was obtained at a time of *transition* (when ST segments have just returned to the baseline after the period of ST segment elevation, and just before the period of T wave inversion).
- The presence of a *competitive* condition (such as bundle branch block or ventricular hypertrophy with "strain") that may obscure diagnostic ECG findings.
- Infarction in an "electrically silent" area of the heart (such as the apex, right ventricle, or posterobasal portion of the left ventricle).

> Obtaining a **second (follow-up) ECG** *after a period of time* will occasionally provide invaluable insight that may help immensely in evaluation of the patient, and greatly facilitate management decisions.

The optimal "period of time" to wait before repeating the ECG is variable. It may be as short as several minutes (if the patient's condition has suddenly changed, or to evaluate the response to nitroglycerin)—or it may be several hours. Repeating the initial ECG may be especially helpful in determining whether (and to what extent) a patient is likely to benefit from thrombolytic therapy.

In the case of Mr. A, the clinical picture of persistent symptoms *despite* relatively little ST segment elevation on initial ECG—and the need to determine whether to initiate thrombolytic therapy—are reasons to consider repeating the ECG at this time.

PROBLEM   **Mr. A's follow-up (i.e., 10:45 AM) ECG is shown in *Figure 12F-2. Does it help you decide whether to initiate thrombolytic therapy?***

ANSWER   Despite an interval of only 25 minutes between tracings, considerable change has already occurred. In the inferior leads, Q waves have deepened, and ST segment elevation has definitely become more marked. Reciprocal ST segment depression has also become more prominent, especially in the anterior leads. In conjunction with the history, the overall picture is highly suggestive of AMI in evolution.

Compared to the initial 12-lead ECG (Figure 12F-1), the tracing shown in Figure 12F-2 suggests a higher likelihood of benefit from thrombolytic therapy *(See Table 12A-2).* Admittedly, the site of infarction is inferior, and a deep Q wave has now formed in lead III. However, the amount of ST segment elevation, as well as the amount of reciprocal ST segment depression are both significantly greater in this follow-up tracing. In particular, the presence of marked ST segment depression in the anterior leads, in association with ST segment elevation in the inferior leads suggests more extensive infarction (with possible posterior involvement) that would be more likely to benefit from reperfusion therapy *(See Section 12A).*

The decision is made to begin **thrombolytic therapy.*** Mr. A has already received **aspirin** (325 mg) and a dose of benzodiazepine (**diazepam**—5 mg PO). He is on a **nasal cannula** (at 2 L/min) and an **IV nitroglycerin infusion** (which has been gradually increased to its current rate of 80 μg/min). He is also started on an IV β-blocker (**metoprolol**—5 mg by IV bolus X 3) and *pro-phylactic* lidocaine (75 mg by IV bolus X 2, and a 2 mg/min IV infusion). As these actions/therapeutic measures are being accomplished, a number of laboratory tests are obtained.

PROBLEM   **Which laboratory tests would you order? Which test(s) would you not order? (Why?)**

6. *Laboratory Tests*
   a. **Blood/Urine Tests—?**
   b. **Arterial Blood Gases—?**
   c. **X-Ray Studies—?**
   d. **Echocardiogram—?**

ANSWER

BLOOD/URINE TESTS

We favor obtaining the following blood/urine tests on patients *admitted* to the hospital for suspected AMI:

- Routine tests (CBC, urinalysis, chemistry profile including serum electrolytes, BUN, creatinine, glucose, etc.).
- Serum magnesium (which is often not included in the standard chemistry profile)—*See Section 12B.*
- CK isoenzymes—obtained X 3 over the first 24 hours *(See Section 12A).*

---

*Refer to the **Addendum** at the end of this section for brief discussion of, *"Thrombolytic Therapy: Who Should Decide?"**

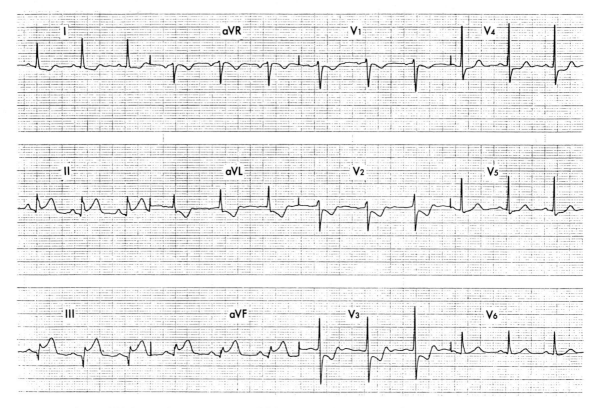

Figure 12F-2.   Follow-up 12-lead ECG obtained on Mr. A at **10:45 AM** (i.e., 25 minutes after his initial ECG was recorded). *Are you now more inclined to initiate thrombolytic therapy?*

- Bleeding parameters (including platelet count, fibrinogen level, pro time, and PTT)—if thrombolytic therapy is being contemplated.
- Blood type and hold (in the event excessive bleeding requiring transfusion develops).

Patients who receive thrombolytic therapy and/or IV heparin will need *serial monitoring* of selected bleeding parameters. Thus, the dosing and timing of IV heparin administration is usually adjusted to maintain a PTT value of 2 to 2.5 × the control value. Other parameters to monitor include serial hematocrits (for detection of occult bleeding), fibrinogen levels (to assess the degree of the systemic lytic state), and platelet counts (to guard against occult development of heparin-induced thrombocytopenia).

One test that we would *not* obtain in this case is LD isoenzymes, since the onset of Mr. A's severe chest pain was so acute. LD isoenzymes tend to be helpful diagnostically *only* when the onset of symptoms is one or more days earlier, because CK isoenzymes may have already returned to normal in such cases (See Section 12A).

ARTERIAL BLOOD GASES (ABGs)

Because of the increased risk of bleeding associated with the use of thrombolytic therapy, venipunctures should be kept to a minimum, and more invasive procedures avoided if at all possible. If a central line is required for optimal management, it should ideally be inserted *prior* to initiation of thrombolytic therapy.

ABG studies should be avoided if thrombolytic therapy is contemplated. Practically speaking, ABG analysis will rarely be essential for initial management of AMI.

X-RAY STUDIES

There are several reasons to routinely order a chest x-ray in patients with suspected AMI. These include:

- Obtaining a baseline.
- Making sure there are no "surprises" that might otherwise complicate or alter management (i.e., unsuspected pneumonia, pleural effusion, tumor, etc.).
- Ruling out pulmonary congestion/heart failure that may not have been evident from physical examination.
- Screening for potential contraindications to thrombolytic therapy—as may be suggested by widening of the aortic shadow (possible dissecting aneurysm) or a grossly enlarged, formless cardiac silhouette (possible pericardial effusion).

ECHOCARDIOGRAM

At this point in the process, *we would not obtain an echocardiogram.* Echocardiography is often invaluable as a noninvasive means for ruling out pericardial effusion, determining the etiology of valvular heart disease/congestive heart failure, and evaluating left ventricular function. However, an echocardiogram does *not* appear to be essential for optimal management in this case because:

- The site of AMI is *inferior* (and mural thrombus is rare with inferior infarction).
- No murmurs or rubs were heard on cardiac auscultation, and there is no other indication of valvular heart disease or pericarditis.
- There is no clinical evidence of heart failure.

Whether to routinely obtain an echocardiogram in the acute phase of a large, *anterior* AMI (as a screening test for mural thrombi) is another matter, and remains controversial.

It is now **11:15 AM.** Mr. A's chest pain has decreased, but is still moderately severe. Vital signs remain stable. Thrombolytic therapy is being infused.

PROBLEM   What is the most common complication associated with the use of thrombolytic therapy? *Anticipate how you would intervene if this complication developed.*

ANSWER   Bleeding is by far the most common complication of thrombolytic therapy. In most cases, bleeding complications are minor and related to the site of a vascular puncture (or other procedure). Firm *local pressure* (for *at least* 20 minutes) is often all that is needed.

As already emphasized, bleeding parameters must be closely monitored *regardless* of the agent used. Thrombolytic therapy should be STOPPED immediately if signs of significant bleeding occur (i.e., suspected intracranial bleeding, hematemesis, gross hematuria, retroperitoneal hemorrhage). Cryoprecipitate and/or fresh frozen plasma may be needed in such cases to replete clotting factors and fibrinogen; transfusion may be needed if bleeding is severe.

At **11:45 AM,** you are informed about a sudden change in the patient's rhythm. As a series of rhythm strips are recorded, Mr. A reports that the moderately severe chest pain he was having has dramatically decreased—*and that it virtually disappears as the last strip is recorded.*

PROBLEM   Review the following *serial* rhythm strips recorded on Mr. A between 11:45 AM and 11:50 AM *(Figures 12F-3, 12F-4, 12F-5, and 12F-6A).* How would you interpret these rhythms in light of the fact that they occurred almost *simultaneously* with resolution of his chest pain?

HINT: Your interpretation may be *greatly facilitated* by remembering five points:
1. That the rhythm strips were obtained *sequentially* from the *same* patient.
2. That the rhythm strips do *not* necessarily need to be interpreted sequentially!
3. That the patient was receiving thrombolytic therapy at the time, and that symptoms resolved as the last rhythm strip (Fig. 12F-6A) was recorded.
4. That attention to ST segments sometimes provides clues to rhythm analysis (and in this particular case also helps explains the resolution of Mr. A's symptoms).
5. That beats of different morphologies can "have children."

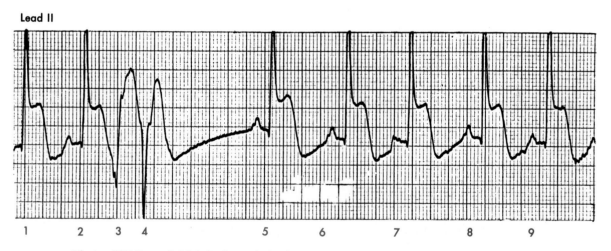

Lead II

Figure 12F-3.   Initial rhythm strip in the series—obtained from Mr. A at **11:45 AM.** Mr. A's chest pain is still moderately severe at this time.

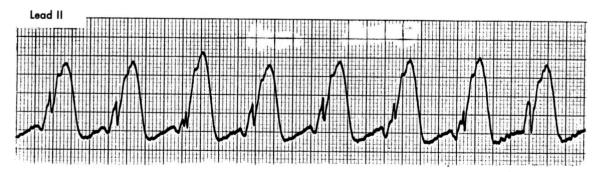

Lead II

Figure 12F-4.   Second rhythm strip in the series (recorded at **11:46 AM**)—demonstrating a sudden, dramatic change in QRS morphology.

Lead II

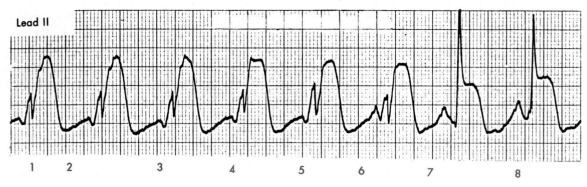

Figure 12F-5.   Third rhythm strip in the series (recorded at **11:47 AM**). Mr. A reports that his chest pain is "decreasing."

Lead II

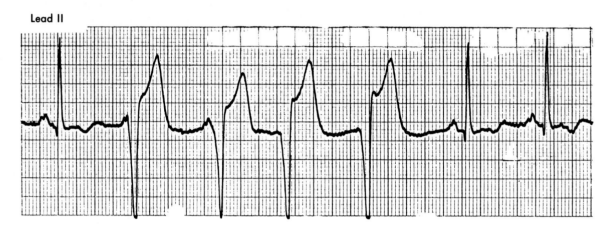

Figure 12F-6A.   Final rhythm strip in the series (recorded at **11:50 AM**). Mr. A's chest pain has virtually disappeared at this time.

ANSWER TO *FIGURES 12F-3, 12F-4, 12F-5, and 12F-6*/CLINICAL CORRELATION   As noted above, Mr. A is still having moderately severe chest pain at the time the initial rhythm strip in this series *(Figure 12F-3)* was recorded. Despite the irregularity in this rhythm, the underlying mechanism appears to be *sinus*, since an upright P wave with a constant (and normal) PR interval precedes most beats (i.e., beats #2, and #5-9) in this lead II monitoring lead. Thus, the underlying rhythm is *sinus arrhythmia*. Beats #3 and #4 are PVCs (and together they form a *ventricular couplet*).

> Although beat #4 does not appear to be very wide in this particular lead, its morphology is very different from the sinus-conducted beats in this tracing, and it is not preceded by a premature P wave. As a result, a ventricular etiology must be assumed until proved otherwise.
>
> At first glance, beat #3 appears to be *much wider* than beat #4. In reality, this is probably an illusion created by a combination of factors including a higher baseline and simultaneous occurrence of the downslope of the ST segment of beat #2 with the downslope of the S wave of the PVC. A post-ectopic pause follows the ventricular couplet.

An additional finding worthy of mention in *Figure 12F-3* relates to the ST segments. Although in general, ST segment analysis from a single monitoring lead is much less reliable than ST segment analysis from a complete 12-lead ECG, the amount and appearance of the ST segment elevation evident in this lead II is clearly consistent with the patient's evolving inferior AMI.

QRS morphology dramatically changes in *Figure 12F-4*. It isn't until beats #7 and #8 in *Figure 12F-5* that the QRS configuration of sinus-conducted beats returns. *Interpretation of these two rhythm strips will be easier if deferred until after evaluation of the arrhythmia shown in Figure 12F-6A.*

The initial beat in *Figure 12F-6A* is sinus conducted. It is followed by four predominantly negative complexes. These beats are presumably of ventricular etiology since they are widened and manifest a QRS morphology that differs markedly from that of the sinus conducted beats. Although the rate of this ventricular rhythm varies slightly, it clearly exceeds 40 beats/minute—and therefore represents an *accelerated* idioventricular rhythm (AIVR).

Two sinus-conducted beats end the tracing.

PROBLEM   **Is there evidence of *atrial activity* during the four-beat run of AIVR in *Figure 12F-6A?***

    HINT: Why might the QRS configuration of the first two ventricular beats in Figure 12F-6A (which seemingly manifest a small positive initial deflection) differ from the QRS configuration of the last two ventricular beats (which manifest a completely negative QS deflection)?

ANSWER   Use of calipers reveals that atrial activity remains regular throughout this tracing (arrows in *Figure 12F-6B*). Coincidental occurrence of P waves at the onset of beats #2 and #3 produces a "pseudo r wave," and accounts for the seemingly different QRS morphology of these beats compared to the totally negative (QS) deflections of beats #4 and #5. Arrows in *Figure 12F-6B* indicate that notching at the shoulder (onset) of the ST segment of beats #4 and #5 is also the result of atrial activity. Since none of these P waves have a chance to conduct, there is transient *AV dissociation*, which further supports our contention of a ventricular etiology for the four-beat run (beats #2 through #5).

Note that the dramatic ST segment elevation that had been present earlier has resolved for the sinus-conducted beats in *Figure 12F-6B* (i.e., beats #1, #6, and #7). In view of simultaneous clinical resolution of chest pain and the ventricular arrhythmias seen in these serial tracings, it is exceedingly likely that *reperfusion* of the IRA has occurred.

In addition to resolution of ST segment elevation, two subtle evolutionary changes are evident in the sinus conducted beats of Figure 12F-6B:

1. Slight deepening of the Q wave (compared to the q wave of sinus-conducted beats in Figures 12F-3 and 12F-5)
2. Beginning T wave inversion

It is important to emphasize that caution is always advised in interpreting morphologic/evolutionary changes from a single monitoring lead, and that confirmation (with a complete 12-lead ECG) will be needed to determine the clinical significance of such changes.

Clinical Indicators of Reperfusion

Because cardiac catheterization is not routinely recommended after administration of thrombolytic therapy for patients with AMI who otherwise appear to be doing well, *definitive* confirmation that the IRA has recanalized will usually not be possible. Nevertheless, assessment of three *clinical parameters* may be extremely helpful in predicting the likelihood of reperfusion. These parameters are:

1. Relief of chest pain.
2. Resolution of ST segment elevation.
3. Development of *reperfusion* arrhythmias.

Clinically, the specificity for predicting reperfusion approaches 100% if there is: (1) *complete* relief of chest pain; (2) *complete* resolution of ST segment elevation; and (3) development of *typical* reperfusion arrhythmias after administration of thrombolytic therapy (Kircher et al, 1987). Practically speaking, it is rare that all three of these parameters will be present and satisfied in their entirety. Specificity for clinical prediction of IRA patency is less when only one or two of these parameters are present, or if relief of chest pain or resolution of ST segment elevation is only partial (Califf et al, 1985; Kircher et al, 1987).

In contrast, recurrence of ST segment elevation after thrombolytic therapy—especially if associated with recurrence of chest pain—suggests reocclusion of the IRA (Kwon et al, 1991).

REPERFUSION ARRHYTHMIAS

The term **reperfusion arrhythmias** refers to those arrhythmias that develop with reestablishment of flow to the IRA. Although the precise mechanism responsible for this phenomenon is unclear, it may be that disparity in the conduction velocity and refractory period of ischemic myocardial cells leads to development of reentry pathways that form the substrate to sustain these arrhythmias. In this context, sudden reperfusion of ischemic tissue by oxygenated blood may then be the initiating stimulus.

Ventricular arrhythmias are commonly seen with reperfusion—especially late-occurring (i.e., *end-diastolic*) PVCs and AIVR (Gorgels et al, 1988).

Lead II

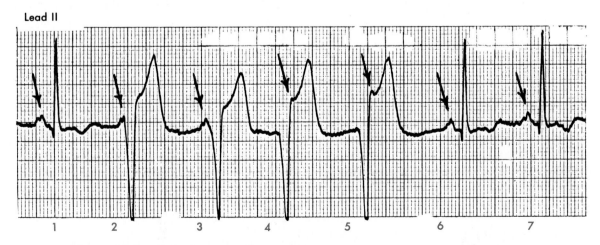

Figure 12F-6B.   Explanation of Figure '2F-6A. Arrows indicate that regular atrial activity continues throughout the tracing. Thus, there is transient *AV dissociation*, and beats #2 through #5 represent a short run of AIVR with a slightly irregular ventricular response.

Cercek et al (1987) studied the time course and characteristics of ventricular arrhythmias that develop in patients with AMI *after* administration of thrombolytic therapy. The findings of his study are insightful:

- Virtually 100% of patients developed PVCs during the first hour after reperfusion. PVCs were often extremely frequent (*exceeding* 1,000 PVCs/hour in a number of patients), and ventricular couplets were common. PVCs were especially frequent for the first 8 hours after reperfusion.
- *End-diastolic PVCs* (i.e., PVCs that have a relatively long coupling interval) were common with reperfusion. *This finding is in contrast to most other settings in which ventricular ectopy is seen where early-occurring PVCs are the rule.*
- *AIVR* (at a rate of between 50 to 120 beats/minute) occurred in 90% of patients. AIVR was especially likely to occur during the first hour after reperfusion. Many patients had multiple episodes of AIVR, which sometimes were *hundreds of beats* long! In addition, almost all patients had more than one morphologic form of AIVR.

  There were two general patterns of AIVR in the study. In one, the rhythm was usually initiated by a late-occurring (end-diastolic) PVC, the rate was relatively slow and regular, and the duration of the run tended to be long. Termination of the run was likely to result from gradual resumption of sinus rhythm (i.e., "recapture" of the ventricles by the sinus node).

  In contrast, the other pattern of AIVR typically began with an early-occurring PVC and was marked by a somewhat faster rate (i.e., between 100 to 120 beats/minute). Runs were more often irregular and of shorter duration (i.e., *less* than 10 beats long). This second pattern tended to end as abruptly as it began. *Neither type of AIVR degenerated to rapid ventricular tachycardia despite the fact that antiarrhythmic therapy was not used in the study.*
- **Fast ventricular tachycardia** (i.e., rate >125 beats/minute) occurred at least once in 85% of patients during the first 24 hours after reperfusion. In general, *fast ventricular tachycardia was much less common than AIVR.* Most runs of fast ventricular tachycardia were short (less than 15 beats long), and not accompanied by symptoms. *None of the runs of fast ventricular tachycardia deteriorated to ventricular fibrillation.*
- The frequency of ventricular arrhythmias dramatically decreased in virtually all patients after 24 hours. Although isolated PVCs were still commonly seen at the time of discharge from the hospital, ventricular couplets and fast ventricular tachycardia were rare. *None of the patients had AIVR on predischarge Holter monitoring.*

Thus, it appears that **reperfusion arrhythmias** are regularly seen within the first 8 hours after flow is restored to the IRA. End-diastolic PVCs and AIVR are especially common during this time. However, despite their frequent occurrence (and the occasional occurrence of fast ventricular tachycardia), *reperfusion arrhythmias tend to be relatively benign.*

A final phenomenon that is commonly associated with development of reperfusion arrhythmias is the frequent occurrence of **fusion beats.** This should not be unexpected considering the *end-diastolic* nature of these PVCs that are often delayed until the very last portion of the cardiac cycle (i.e., until *after* the P wave of the next beat). As a result, *fusion* of this next sinus-conducted impulse is likely to occur with the almost simultaneously-occurring discharge from the reperfused ventricular focus.

In a sense, AIVR may be thought of as a *series of late-occurring PVCs*—with each of these "late-occurring" PVCs being predisposed to developing some degree of fusion with the next sinus-conducted beat. Since runs of AIVR that occur in association with reperfusion are often extremely long (i.e., up to *hundreds of beats* in duration), multiple fusion morphologies may be seen. Unless the emergency care provider is aware of this phenomenon (and appreciates its usually *benign* consequences), the multitude of fusion morphologies seen with reperfusion could paint an alarming (and confusing) clinical picture.

PROBLEM   ***Return* to the series of rhythm strips recorded on Mr. A between 11:45 AM and 11:50 AM (Figures 12F-3 through 12F-6A). Considering the exceedingly high clinical likelihood that reperfusion of the IRA is occurring at this time:**

1. **How would you interpret the arrhythmia shown in Figures 12F-4 and 12F-5?**
2. **Should this arrhythmia be treated if the patient remains hemodynamically stable?**
3. **Now that infusion of thrombolytic therapy is complete (and reperfusion has presumably occurred), is there any additional medical therapy that should be started?**

ANSWER   As already noted, QRS morphology of the underlying rhythm changes between Figures 12F-3 and 12F-4. P waves appear to precede virtually all of the unusual-looking QRS complexes in Figures 12F-4 and 12F-5, although it is hard to determine the relationship (if any) of these P waves to the QRS. What *can* be said, is that the last two beats in Figure 12F-5 (beats #7 and #8) are clearly sinus-conducted. *What can also be said is* that a "marriage" between a normally conducted sinus beat and the negative (QS) deflection of Mr. A's ventricular beats (i.e., beats #3 and #4 in Figure 12F-3, and beats #2 through #5 in Figure 12F-6B) might produce a hybrid QRS morphology similar to that seen throughout Figure 12F-4, and for the first six beats of Figure 12F-5. Thus, the most likely explanation for the rhythm seen in Figures 12F-4 and 12F-5 is that there is *continual fusion* between the reperfusion arrhythmia (AIVR) and the patient's underlying (sinus) rhythm.

In this particular case, Mr. A has already been started on lidocaine. No additional antiarrhythmic treatment would be needed as long as he remains hemodynamically stable.

In general, AIVR (in which the rate of the ventricular rhythm is between 50 and 120 beats/minute) probably does not need to be treated, whereas rapid ventricular tachycardia (i.e., rate >125 beats/minute) should be suppressed. Discretion being the better part of valor, most clinicians tend to begin *prophylactic lidocaine* at the time they initiate thrombolytic therapy.

Finally, *anticoagulation* (with IV heparin) should be started at this time (and maintained for at least 24-72 hours) to minimize the chance that the IRA will reocclude *(See Section 12C)*.

Addendum

THROMBOLYTIC THERAPY: WHO SHOULD DECIDE?

Given the tremendous variation in AMI treatment regimens from one institution to the next, it is essential that some form of agreement be reached between members of the health care team at each location regarding the most appropriate protocol to follow at their particular institution for evaluation and management of patients who present with new-onset chest pain.

> Depending on the type and location of your practice, the *"initial contact"* person (designated as the one to assess the patient with new-onset chest pain for their suitability for thrombolytic therapy) may be an emergency care physician, primary care physician, cardiologist, or other member of the health care team. Considering the narrow "window of opportunity" for effective intervention, *expeditious evaluation is essential*. Ideally, **prior communication** between the group of "initial contact" health care providers and consulting cardiology team will have established who should be the one to decide/administer thrombolytic therapy, which thrombolytic agent to use (and in what dose), where in the hospital to begin thrombolytic therapy *(preferably in the ED!)*, and who should be called at the time of evaluation.

Practically speaking, the "initial contact" health care provider may be the most appropriate individual to initiate thrombolytic therapy in a *rural setting* where communication and/or cardiology consultation would necessitate significant delay in the institution of therapy. In contrast, in an *urban setting* (i.e., with help nearby) it may be easier to consult with the cardiologist on call after brief but careful review (of the relevant history, physical examination, and initial ECG) for *all* patients who potentially qualify as candidates for acute thrombolytic therapy. Decisions regarding the use of thrombolytic therapy can then be made based on your discussion with the consulting cardiologist.

References

Burney RE, Walsh D, Kaplan LR, Fraser S, Tung B, Overmyer J: Reperfusion arrhythmia: myth or reality? *Ann Emerg Med* 18:240-243, 1989.

Califf RM, O'Neill WW, Stack RS, Aronson L, Mark DB, Mantell S, George BS, Candela RJ, Kereiakes DJ, Abbottsmith C, Topol EJ, and the TAMI Study Group: Failure of simple clinical measurements to predict perfusion status after intraveanous thrombolysis, *Ann Int Med* 108:658-662, 1988.

Cercek B, Lew AS, Laramee P, Shah PK, Peter TC, Ganz W: Time course and characteristics of ventricular arrhythmias after reperfusion in acute myocardial infarction, *Am J Cardiol* 60:214-218, 1987.

Gorgels APM, Vos MA, Letsch IS, Vershuuren EA, Bar FWHM, Janssen JHA, Wellens HJJ: Usefulness of the accelerated idioventricular rhythm as a marker for myocardial necrosis and reperfusion during thrombolytic therapy in acute myocardial infarction, *Am J Cardiol* 61:231-235, 1988.

Kircher BJ, Topol EJ, O'Neill WW, Pitt B: Prediction of infarct coronary artery recanalization after intravenous thrombolytic therapy, *Am J Cardiol* 59:513-515, 1987.

Kwon K, Freedman SB, Wilcox I, Allman K, Madden A, Carter GS, Harris PJ: The unstable ST segment early after thrombolysis for acute infarction and its usefulness as a marker of recurrent coronary occlusion, *Am J Cardiol* 67:109-115, 1991.

CHAPTER 13

SPECIAL RESUSCITATION SITUATIONS

Special resuscitation situations are cardiopulmonary arrests or other life-threatening emergencies that require modification or ex- *tension of conventional life support techniques (AHA ACLS Text, 1986).*

SECTION A

DROWNING AND NEAR-DROWNING

Drowning is the third leading cause of accidental death, claiming between 5,000 and 10,000 lives each year in the United States (AHA ACLS Text, 1987; Pruessner, et al, 1988). It is second to motor vehicle accidents as the most common cause of accidental death in children and young adults, with as many as 40% to 50% of all drowning accidents occurring in *swimming pools* (O'Carroll et al, 1988). The incidence of near-drowning episodes is much more common than the incidence of drowning fatalities, although accurate determination is difficult due to significant underreporting. Near-drowning episodes may occur as many as 500(!) times more often than actual drowning (Orlowski, 1988). Many victims of near-drowning do not completely recover, and an estimated one third of all survivors are left with some degree of neurologic impairment from anoxic brain damage (Orlowski, 1988). Thus, the importance of this special resuscitation situation stems from the fact that many episodes are potentially preventable, and that the injury incurred may be reversible if appropriate treatment can be promptly instituted.

Definitions

Drowning is defined as *death* from suffocation by submersion in water (Modell, 1981). In contrast, use of the term **near-drowning** implies that the victim *survives* (at least temporarily) the episode of submersion.

Near-drowning episodes are most commonly **"wet,"** which means that the victim aspirates water into the lungs. Aspiration generally precipitates laryngospasm. This results in asphyxia and loss of consciousness. Glottic relaxation usually follows, leading to additional (and continued) aspiration of water into the lungs.

As many as 10% to 20% of episodes of near-drowning are **"dry"** and *not* accompanied by aspiration (Gonzalez-Rothi, 1987; Knopp, 1988). Laryngospasm in this instance is immediate, complete, and results in sustained glottic closure so that little or no fluid ever enters the lungs (Modell, et al, 1976).

Secondary drowning refers to a near-drowning episode in which death is *delayed* (minutes, hours, or days) after initial recovery. Death from secondary drowning most commonly results from ventricular fibrillation (in victims of cold-water submersion) or development of respiratory distress syndrome (Pruessner et al, 1988).

An important protective mechanism associated with cold-water immersion is the **diving reflex.** The reflex is especially well developed in certain sea-diving mammals (such as seals), allowing them to remain safely submerged for as long as 15 to 30 minutes at a time. Sudden, intense cold exposure results in apnea, severe bradycardia, peripheral vasoconstriction, and preferential shunting of blood to the heart and brain (Gonzalez-Rothi, 1987). Oxygen demand is thereby reduced, and oxygen utilization by vital organs is maximized. The same reflex may also occasionally be operative (albeit to a much lesser extent) in humans (especially children), and possibly accounts for case reports of survival with complete neurologic recovery despite prolonged submersion (Gooden, 1972; Knopp, 1988).

Less fortunate individuals sometimes respond to sudden cold-water exposure with an **immersion syndrome** in which cold precipitates arrhythmia-induced cardiac arrest (from ventricular fibrillation or asystole).

Pathophysiologic Changes

In theory, pathophysiologic changes associated with drowning or near-drowning depend on the type of fluid aspirated. **Freshwater** is *hypotonic.* Aspirated freshwater is therefore rapidly absorbed from alveoli into the pulmonary vasculature and the general circulation. This should result in an increase in overall blood volume and a reduction (by a dilutional effect) in the serum concentrations of most electrolytes.

In contrast, **saltwater** is extremely *hypertonic.* As a result, saltwater aspiration should be expected to osmotically draw off fluid from the vascular space into the alveoli. Overall blood volume should be reduced and serum concentrations of most electrolytes would be expected to increase.

The importance of electrolyte abnormalities in drowning and near-drowning is probably overemphasized in the literature. Practically speaking, most victims do not aspirate enough fluid to produce life-threatening alterations in blood volume or serum electrolyte concentrations (Modell et al, 1976; Knopp 1988; Pruessner et al, 1988). Instead, morbidity and mortality from drowning and near-drowning result from impaired gas exchange (hypoxemia) and direct pulmonary injury. Freshwater inactivates surfactant. This leads to widespread areas of microatelectasis (from collapse of alveoli). Because perfusion to these collapsed alveoli remains intact, significant pulmonary shunting (from the resultant ventilation-perfusion mismatch) is produced, leading to ever increasing degrees of hypoxemia.

The mechanism for lung injury with saltwater drowning may be somewhat different. Contact with saltwater during aspiration disrupts alveolar capillary membrane integrity. This allows plasma proteins and fluid to flood intraalveolar air spaces and results in pulmonary edema, severe hypoxemia, and adult respiratory distress syndrome (ARDS). Pulmonary insult may be further complicated if there are contaminants (such as mud, sand, sewage, or bacteria) in the water aspirated (Knopp, 1988).

Evaluation, Management, and Prognosis

Evaluation and management of victims of near-drowning is summarized in *Tables 13A-1, 13A-2,* and *13A-3*. In general, survival depends most on the extent of neurologic and pulmonary involvement. Prognosis is relatively good for victims of near-drowning who are alert at the time of arrival in the emergency department. In contrast, prognosis is extremely poor for patients who remain comatose following the episode, especially if CPR was required and spontaneous respiration does not resume (Modell, 1986; Gonzalez-Rothi, 1987; AHA ACLS Text, 1987). Although the precise mechanism for neurologic injury is unclear, it probably relates to a combination sequence of events including persistent hypoxemia and hypercapnia, resultant decreased cardiac output, impaired cerebral perfusion, tissue acidosis, diffuse neuronal damage, loss of cell membrane integrity, extracellular leakage of fluid, cerebral edema, and increased intracranial pressure (Gonzalez-Rothi, 1987).

Hyperventilation reduces cerebral blood flow, and may help in management by lowering ICP (intracranial pressure). ICP monitoring should be considered for patients with persistent coma. More aggressive measures (barbiturate coma, use of corticosteroids or osmotic diuretics, and induction of controlled hypothermia) have not been shown to be beneficial, could be detrimental, and are *not* recommended at this time unless there is documented evidence of sustained intracranial hypertension (Modell, 1986; Gonzalez-Rothi, 1987).

Table 13A-1

Physical Findings That Might Be Seen with Near-Drowning

Temperature

Hypothermia—if the victim was immersed in cold water

Fever—which may be neurogenic from central nervous system (CNS) injury or the result of secondary infection (especially pneumonia)

Cardiovascular System

Bradycardia—from the diving reflex

Peripheral vasoconstriction—from hypothermia or the stress-induced increase in circulatory catecholamines

Cardiac arrhythmias (including ventricular fibrillation or asystole)—from increased circulating catecholamines, the immersion syndrome, or as a direct result of hypoxemia

Hypotension—if the fluid aspirated was saltwater or high in contaminants, especially if the amount aspirated was extensive

Neurologic Findings

Altered level of consciousness—from hypoxemia, cardiac arrest, or the cerebral hypoperfusion, edema, and increased intracranial pressure that is commonly associated with near-drowning episodes during the initial 24 hours of recovery

Pulmonary System

Respiratory insufficiency—Presentation may vary greatly depending on the type and severity of the near-drowning episode, and the moment in the time course that the patient is observed. Patients may be asymptomatic, mildly tachypneic with only minimal pulmonary findings, or in severe respiratory distress with air hunger, pulmonary edema, and the full-blown syndrome of ARDS

Treatment of Pulmonary Complications

In patients who do not remain comatose following a near-drowning episode, survival is usually determined by the extent of the pulmonary complications. The potential range of these complications is highly variable. Pulmonary involvement may be minimal or pronounced on initial presentation. In the former case, development of pulmonary insufficiency may be insidious. It would therefore seem prudent to routinely observe victims of significant submersion (with close monitoring of oxygenation status and frequent follow-up chest x-ray studies) for at least 24 hours, even when symptoms and pulmonary findings are minimal or absent on initial examination.

Supplemental oxygen should be routinely provided for victims of near-drowning. Additional measures are needed for patients who remain hypoxemic (PaO_2 <55-60 mm Hg) despite adequate ($\geq$40%) inspired oxygen concen-

Table 13A-2

Laboratory Tests to Routinely Consider in Evaluation of Victims of Near-Drowning

ABGs—Acidosis is commonly present, which initially tends to be respiratory in nature (from hypoventilation). To this a metabolic component is often added (from development of lactic acidosis), especially if hypoxemia is persistent and severe.

Serum Electrolytes—Values can be highly variable, and should be checked frequently until they stabilize. Freshwater drowning may lower serum electrolyte values (from a hemodilutional effect), whereas saltwater drowning tends to raise them (from a hemoconcentrating effect). In most instances, however, the amount of water aspirated will not be enough to significantly alter serum values. Serum **magnesium, calcium,** and **phosphate** should nevertheless be checked along with the other standard electrolyte values.

BUN, Creatinine, and **Urinalysis**—Near-drowning may precipitate renal insufficiency and/or exacerbate preexisting renal disease. This may result in proteinuria, hematuria, oliguria (or even anuria), abnormal urine sediment, and elevated BUN and creatinine values.

Hematocrit—Hemoconcentration or hemodilution may occur if large amounts of salt or freshwater were aspirated.

Clotting Studies—The effects of near-drowning on clotting studies are variable. A **prothrombin time, partial thromboplastin time,** and **platelet count** should probably all be obtained as a baseline.

Chest X-Ray—Pulmonary findings vary greatly depending on the type and severity of the near-drowning episode, and the moment in the time course that the patient is observed. A baseline chest x-ray is essential, and serial films should be obtained thereafter at a frequency dictated by the patient's clinical course.

Other X-Ray Studies—Consideration should be given to obtaining a **C-spine** and/or other x-ray studies if there is the possibility that trauma may have caused (or contributed) to the near-drowning episode. C-spine injury is especially likely for victims of near-drowning associated with diving accidents, and should be strongly considered in victims who present in an unconscious state.

ECG and **Continuous Electrocardiographic Monitoring**—The stress of near-drowning and/or associated hypoxemia may precipitate acute myocardial infarction or a variety of cardiac arrhythmias, especially in patients with preexisting coronary artery disease.

Blood Alcohol Level—There is a definite association between increased blood alcohol levels and accidental drowning in adults (Calder and Clay, 1990). For the same reason, a **Toxicology Screen** might be obtained.

trations (Gonzalez-Rothi, 1987). *Positive airway pressure breathing* is essential in such cases to reverse the underlying pathophysiology (microatelectasis and/or alveolar flooding with pulmonary edema). Positive airway pressure may be delivered either by use of a pressurized CPAP (continuous positive airway pressure) mask or by endotracheal intubation and mechanical ventilation with PEEP (positive end-expiratory pressure) or CPAP.

Bacterial pneumonia may complicate pulmonary injury from near-drowning. However, diagnosis of superimposed infection may be extremely difficult if the baseline chest x-ray is already abnormal (as it so commonly is in victims of near-drowning). As a result, some clinicians have favored prophylactic use of broad spectrum antibiotic coverage for near-drowning victims, especially if submersion occurred in a stagnant lake, pond or canal where aspiration of contaminated water was likely (Gonzalez-Rothi, 1987). Other clinicians oppose this practice on the grounds that prophylactic antibiotics have never been shown to improve survival of near-drowning victims, and prophylactic treatment runs the risk of increasing susceptibility to antibiotic-resistant superinfection (Oakes et al, 1982). Reserving antibiotic treatment for patients with changing (evolving) infiltrates on chest x-ray, persistent fever, positive blood cultures, leukocytosis, and/or purulent secretions may

thus be the most prudent course of action (Gonzalez-Rothi, 1987; Knopp, 1988). Prophylactic use of corticosteroids has not been shown to be of benefit for victims of near-drowning, and is no longer recommended (Modell et al, 1976; Oakes et al, 1982; Modell, 1986).

References & Suggested Readings

Chapter 15: *Special resuscitation situations.* In Jaffe AS (ed): *Textbook of advanced cardiac life support,* Dallas, 1987, American Heart Association.

Calder RA, Clay CY: Drownings in Florida: 1977-1986, *J Fla Med Assoc* 77:679, 1990.

Gonzalez-Rothi RJ: Near drowning: consensus and controversies in pulmonary and cerebral resuscitation, *Heart Lung* 16:474, 1987.

Gooden BA: Drowning and the diving reflex in man; *Med J Aust* 2:583, 1972.

Knopp RK: *Near-Drowning.* In Rosen P (ed) *Emergency medicine: concepts and clinical practice,* St Louis, 1988, Mosby–Year Book.

Modell JH: Drown versus near-drown: a discussion of definitions, *Crit Care Med* 9:351, 1981 (editorial).

Modell JH: Treatment of near drowning: is there a role for H.Y.P.E.R. therapy? *Crit Care Med* 14:593, 1986.

Modell JH, Graves SA, Ketover A: Clinical course of 91 consecutive near-drowning victims, *Chest* 70:231, 1976.

Oakes DD, Scherk JP, Maloney JR, Charters AC: Prognosis and management of victims of near-drowning, *J Trauma* 22:544, 1982.

Table 13A-3

Management of the Victim of Near-Drowning

1. Assure an adequate airway. *Immobilize the C-spine if there is any possibility of cervical trauma and/or injury!*

2. Ventilate the patient who is not spontaneously breathing. *Rescue breathing may be curative.** Provide supplemental oxygen as indicated. Intubate if needed.†

3. Assess circulation. Take special pains (and time) to palpate for a pulse which may be difficult to feel because of vasoconstriction and/or reduced cardiac output. Assume ventricular fibrillation, asystole, or EMD if no pulse is found, and treat accordingly (with CPR, drugs, or defibrillation as needed).

4. Determine the patient's temperature:
   - Rule out *hypothermia* (especially for victims of cold-water submersion). If present, begin treatment. *(Consider the principles of management suggested in Table 13B-5 of Section B on Hypothermia).*
   - If fever is present, consider the possible causes (i.e., neurogenic, infection, etc.).
   - Try to maintain the patient's temperature as close to the euthermic range as possible, especially during the initial 24 hours of recovery (to minimize susceptibility to secondary neuronal damage).

5. Insert large bore intravenous line(s).

6. Consider obtaining laboratory tests, ABGs, ECG, and x-rays *(as suggested in Table 13A-2).*

7. Institute continuous ECG monitoring.

8. Insert Foley catheter (if patient not alert and spontaneously voiding) to monitor urine output.

9. Consider NG tube insertion (to decompress the stomach and minimize the chance of aspiration).

10. Treat pulmonary complications:
    - Observe (and monitor oxygenation) of victims of near-drowning for at least 24 hours, even if they are completely asymptomatic at the time they initially present.
    - Add *positive airway pressure breathing* if hypoxemia (PaO_2 <55-60 mm Hg) persists despite adequate inspired oxygen concentrations:
      - CPAP mask *or* endotracheal intubation (and mechanical ventilation) with PEEP or CPAP
      - Treat bronchospasm if present (with inhaled β-agonists or aminophylline)
      - Consider use of broad-spectrum antibiotic coverage prophylactically *(controversial!)* or if suggestive signs of superinfection develop (i.e., fever, purulent sputum, infiltrates on chest x-ray, leukocytosis, or positive blood cultures)

11. Assess neurologic function. Consider ICP monitoring and/or hyperventilation (to lower ICP) for victims of near-drowning who remain comatose.

---

*If unable to ventilate the patient, consider the possibility of particulate foreign matter obstruction of the airway. If such matter is visible (i.e., seaweed, sand), remove it. If not, consider the Heimlich maneuver (subdiaphragmatic abdominal thrusts). It is important to emphasize that the Heimlich maneuver is *not* recommended for initial management of near-drowning victims if there is no evidence of particulate matter airway obstruction. It has not been shown to remove aspirated fluid, and it may aggravate the situation by inducing vomiting and aspiration (Ornato, 1986; AHA ACLS Text, 1987; Orlowski, 1987).

†Protect the C-spine if cervical trauma and/or injury is a possibility!

O'Carroll PW, Alkon E, Weiss B: Drowning mortality in Los Angeles County, 1976 to 1984, *JAMA* 260:380, 1988.

Orlowski JP: Vomiting as a complication of the Heimlich maneuver, *JAMA* 258:512, 1988.

Orlowski JP: Drowning, near-drowning, and ice-water drowning, *JAMA* 260:390, 1988.

Ornato JP: The resuscitation of near-drowning victims, *JAMA* 256:75, 1986.

Pruessner HT, Zenner GO, Hansel NK: Management of the near-drowning victim, *Am Fam Physician* 37:251, 1988.

SECTION B

Hypothermia

Temperature is the most frequently forgotten vital sign in a code situation (Grauer, Green, Cavallaro, 1990). None of the 12 Emergency departments surveyed by Harris and Smith routinely recorded temperature during resuscitation efforts (Harris and Smith, 1988). Our 1990 national survey of 237 critical care nurses from across the country and 50 physician ACLS Affiliate Faculty for the state of Florida suggested a similar lack of attention to this vital sign (Grauer et al, 1990). Only 5% of nurses reported that temperature is routinely recorded at cardiac arrests in their institution, and 74% indicated they had *never* seen a temperature recorded at a cardiac arrest; only 4% of physician ACLS Affiliate Faculty routinely requested temperature be taken during cardiac arrest (Grauer et al, 1990). Considering the special considerations needed for management of hypothermic cardiac arrest, this omission may have profound clinical implications.

Cardiac arrest from hypothermia definitely occurs! It is seen not only in northern states during winter months, but also in southern states during warmer months (Kramer et al, 1989). We have even seen it occur in a hospitalized patient who was normothermic at the time of admission! In an even more extreme example of oversight, we are familiar with a case in which resuscitative efforts were terminated and a patient was declared "dead," only to later recover after dethawing from the warmth of the lamps that illuminated the Emergency Department (Personal Communication—Ellie Green).

Awareness of the settings in which hypothermia is most likely to occur can go a long way toward facilitating its diagnosis. Admittedly, recognition of hypothermia rarely poses a problem in the middle of winter when a patient with a long history of alcohol abuse is brought to the Emergency Department in an unresponsive state after being out on the street all night without shelter or adequate clothing. At other times and under less obvious conditions, however, the clinical presentation of hypothermia may be much more subtle. A study by Goldman et al in which unsuspected hypothermia was found at the time of hospital admission in more than 3% of elderly patients highlights how easy it is to overlook this disorder (Goldman et al, 1977).

For easy reference, we list the types of patients most likely to develop hypothermia in *Table 13B-1*. Often, several predisposing conditions are present at the same time (Kramer et al, 1989)—as in an elderly immobile patient with multisystem disease who may also be septic or the victim of a fall that resulted in a cerebral hemorrhage. It is easy to forget to check the temperature during the excitement of a cardiac arrest. Hypothermia will not be diagnosed as the cause of the arrest unless this is done.

Table 13B-1

Patients Especially Predisposed to Developing Hypothermia

- The elderly

- Young children and infants

- Victims of cold exposure (i.e., skiers, hikers, alcoholics)

- Patients with a history of alcohol abuse

- Inactive patients or those immobile for long periods of time

- Patients with certain endocrine disorders (i.e., hypothyroidism, adrenal insufficiency, hypopituitarism, diabetics with hypoglycemia or in diabetic ketoacidosis)

- Patients with anorexia nervosa

- Patients with certain CNS disorders (i.e., stroke, head injury, intracranial bleeding)

- Acutely ill patients with multisystem disease (especially if the patient is septic!)

- Victims of drug overdose (especially from medications such as phenothiazines, tricyclic antidepressants, or barbiturates)*

- Victims of major trauma (especially if they were resuscitated with large amounts of unwarmed blood or cold intravenous fluid)

*Use of these medications in *therapeutic doses* may predispose certain susceptible individuals to developing hypothermia.

Definition, Clinical Characteristics, and Management

Hypothermia is the state of subnormal temperature when the body is unable to generate sufficient heat to function efficiently (Maclean and Emslie-Smith, 1977). It is defined clinically as a core temperature below 35° C (Zell and Kurtz, 1985; AHA ACLS Text, 1987). Hypothermia is said to be *mild* when core temperature is between 33°-35° C, *moderate* when core temperature is between 28°-32° C, and *severe* when core temperature drops below 28° C (Danzyl, 1988). Although more severe degrees of hypothermia are associated with a poorer prognosis, complete recovery has been documented in a patient with an initial core temperature as low as 17° C (Reuler, 1978). As a result, *a patient with hypothermia should never be pronounced dead until he/she is "warm and dead."* Even the presence of body stiffness, cyanosis, fixed pupils, inaudible heart sounds, and the absence of visible respirations do not preclude the possibility of successful resuscitation (Gregory and Doolittle, 1973; Danzyl, 1988). Death from hypothermia can only be declared when resuscitation fails despite active rewarming (AHA ACLS Text, 1987).

An interesting study by Schaller et al (1990) suggests that *"some people are dead when they're cold and dead"* (Auerbach, 1990). In a small, retrospective study, victims of moderate to severe hypothermia (median rectal temperature of <30° C) were not able to be resuscitated despite effective rewarming (by cardiopulmonary bypass or peritoneal lavage) if serum potassium levels were markedly elevated (*at least* 6.8 mEq/L, with a median value of over 14 mEq/L!). In contrast, patients with a similar degree of hypothermia were uniformly resuscitated when serum potassium values at the time of presentation were not elevated.

Prolonged induced hypothermia typically *lowers* serum potassium as a result of a shift between intracellular and extracellular concentrations of this cation (Schaller et al, 1990). In contrast, end-organ tissue hypoxia and/or the autolytic condition of death raise serum potassium, and may explain the results of the above study (Auerbach, 1990). Admittedly, other potentially reversible causes of hyperkalemia (i.e., metabolic acidosis, drug effects, crush injury, rhabdomyolysis, renal failure, postsubmersion hemolysis) may *coexist* with hypothermia, and need to be actively considered in the evaluative process. Nevertheless, rapid determination of serum potassium may prove to be a helpful *prognostic indicator* for hypothermic patients who present comatose and in cardiopulmonary arrest. Obtaining a markedly elevated serum potassium value (i.e., >10 mEq/L) in this setting (in the absence of any potentially reversible cause of hyperkalemia) suggests that prolonged resuscitation may not be warranted.

The principal physiologic and clinical characteristics of the various stages of hypothermia are summarized in *Table 13B-2.* Laboratory tests to routinely consider in evaluation of hypothermic patients, and the abnormalities most likely encountered are suggested in *Table 13B-3.* General and specific principles of management are listed in *Tables 13B-4* and *13B-5.*

Table 13B-2

Physiologic and Clinical Characteristics of the Three Stages of Hypothermia
Mild Hypothermia (33-35° C = 91.4-95° F)
- Initial tachycardia, hyperventilation
- Peripheral vasoconstriction (to preserve core temperature)
- Shivering
- Increased reflexes
- Increased metabolic rate
- Altered mental status/impaired judgment
Moderate Hypothermia (28-32° C = 82.4-89.6° F)
- Bradycardia and other arrhythmias (i.e., atrial fibrillation, PVCs)
- Progressively decreased respiratory rate
- Shivering absent
- Decreased reflexes
- Decreased metabolic rate
- Mental stupor
Severe Hypothermia (<28° C = <82.4° F)
- Decreased heart tones
- Hypotension
- More serious arrhythmias (i.e., severe bradycardia, asystole, ventricular fibrillation susceptibility)
- Hypoventilation/development of major acid-base disturbances
- Absent reflexes
- Stupor/coma
Adapted from AHA ACLS Text, 1987; Danzyl, 1988; Grauer et al. 1990.

Table 13B-3

Laboratory Tests to Routinely Consider in Evaluation of Hypothermic Patients

ABGs—Acidosis is often present, which may be metabolic (from decreased tissue perfusion or increased lactate production) or respiratory (from hypoventilation).

Serum Electrolytes—Values are highly variable, and should be checked frequently. In addition to the effect of lowered temperature and fluid shifts on serum sodium, serum potassium* may be affected (increased or decreased) by changing acid-base status. Serum **magnesium, calcium,** and **phosphate** should also be checked.

BUN and Creatinine—Preexisting renal disease and/or acute insult (hypothermia-induced renal hypoperfusion) may result in elevated values. Rapid and unpredictable fluid shifts make it difficult to gauge volume status on the basis of BUN or hematocrit values. Renal failure may sometimes occur on rewarming.

Serum Glucose—Values are highly variable depending on preexisting glucose metabolism (i.e., presence of diabetes), severity of hypothermia (insulin release and activity are markedly reduced below 30° C), and duration of hypothermia (long-term cold exposure ultimately depletes glycogen stores). Because of the possibility of hypoglycemia, a **Dextrostix** should be immediately drawn, and an ampule of D50 given if the value is low.

Hematocrit—Hypothermia increases the hematocrit by an average of 2% for each 1° C drop in temperature. Altered fluid status and preexisting disease (i.e., anemia) are other contributing factors.

White Blood Cell (WBC) Count—Acute stress, dehydration, and/or infection may all elevate the WBC count. However, because sepsis is such a common (and often subtle) predisposing condition, all hypothermic patients should probably have **blood cultures** drawn, regardless of whether their initial WBC count is elevated.

Clotting Studies—Hypothermia may increase the tendency toward either enhanced coagulation or bleeding. Development of DIC (disseminated intravascular coagulation) has been reported. As a result, **prothrombin time, partial thromboplastin time, platelet count,** and a **fibrinogen level** should all be ordered.

Amylase—Although the mechanism is unclear, hyperamylasemia and clinical pancreatitis occur surprisingly often in association with hypothermia.

Toxicology Screen—Drug ingestion should be actively considered as an etiology of hypothermia.

Thyroid Profile and **Serum Cortisol**—Although uncommon, precipitating causes of hypothermia, hypothyroidism, and adrenal insufficiency should be ruled out.

Urinalysis (U/A) and **Urine Culture**—A U/A may provide useful baseline information on specific gravity (hydration status), sediment abnormalities (i.e., presence of protein, casts), bleeding tendency (if hematuria present), or infection (presence of WBCs, bacteria).

Chest X-Ray—Hypothermia patients are susceptible to a variety of pulmonary disorders including pneumonia (from cold exposure, hypoventilation, sepsis), heart failure (from fluid shifts, decreased contractility, shock), aspiration (from impaired mental status), and ARDS (from shock).

Other X-Ray Studies—Consideration should be given to obtaining a **flat plate** of the **abdomen** (looking for ileus, free air from unsuspected perforation) and a **C-spine** (to rule out unsuspected cervical trauma in patients who are unconscious).

ECG and **Continuous Electrocardiographic Monitoring**—Any cardiac arrhythmia may be seen with hypothermia, especially when temperature depression is severe. Myocardial infarction should be ruled out. In addition, electrocardiographic intervals (the PR, QRS, and QT interval) may all be prolonged, ST-T wave abnormalities may develop, and a J (Osborn) wave may be seen as a notching at the juncture of the QRS complex and ST segment. The common occurrence of artifact (from shivering or muscle rigidity) often makes interpretation of the ECG from a hypothermic patient difficult.

*As noted earlier, the finding of a markedly elevated serum potassium value (i.e., >10 mEq/L) in a patient who is comatose and in cardiopulmonary arrest is an extremely poor prognostic sign.
Adapted from AHA ACLS Text, 1987; Danzyl, 1988; Grauer et al 1990.

Table 13B-4

General Principles of Management of Hypothermia

1. Never discontinue resuscitation of a hypothermic patient until adequate rewarming (to ≥35° C) has occurred, or unless continued attempts would place rescuer in danger from cold exposure.

2. Strive to obtain as complete a history as possible (with special attention to causative or potentially correctable predisposing factors, such as those listed in Table 13B-1).

3. Prevent further heat loss.

4. Rewarm the patient as soon as is safely possible at a safe rate. Minimize manipulations. Assume severe hypothermia if the patient is unresponsive and shivering is absent.

5. Rewarm the "core" before the "shell."

Adapted from AHA ACLS Text, 1987; Danzyl, 1988; Grauer et al, 1990.

Table 13B-5

Specific Principles of Management of Hypothermia

1. Assure an adequate airway.

2. Ventilate the patient who is not spontaneously breathing. Intubate if needed.

3. Assess circulation. Take special pains (and time) to palpate for a pulse. Assume ventricular fibrillation, asystole, or EMD if no pulse is found, and treat accordingly (with CPR, drugs, or defibrillation as needed).

4. Prevent further heat loss (by transporting patient to shelter, gently removing wet clothing, applying blankets, etc.), but do not actively massage extremities (as this may suppress shivering, increase vasodilatation, and predispose to development of ventricular fibrillation). Be careful in moving the patient with severe hypothermia, as even minimal manipulation may induce refractory ventricular fibrillation.

5. Begin *active rewarming* of the patient while resuscitative efforts are continued.*

6. Insert a large-bore intravenous line.

7. Consider obtaining laboratory tests, ABGs, ECG, and x-rays (as suggested in Table 13B-3).

8. Institute continuous ECG monitoring.

9. Insert Foley catheter (to monitor urine output).

10. Consider NG tube insertion.

11. Treat potentially reversible causes of unresponsiveness:
    - Administer an ampule of D50 solution after drawing Dextrostix.
    - Administer Narcan if narcotic ingestion suspected.

12. Consider broad-spectrum antibiotic coverage (especially for infants or other patients who are likely to have a hypothermia-associated infection).

13. Provide supplemental oxygen (as indicated).

*Methods of **active rewarming** include **external** *rewarming* (i.e., by heated blankets) and **core** *rewarming* (i.e., inhalation of heated humidifed oxygen, administration of warmed IV fluids, warmed nasogastric or rectal irrigation—and in the most severe cases, peritoneal lavage and cardiopulmonary bypass).

Active external rewarming modalities should be applied only to the thorax so as to allow the extremities to remain at least partially vasoconstricted. Doing so minimizes the chance of developing *"rewarming shock"* (from vasodilatation of the peripheral vasculature with subsequent flooding of the central circulation with cold, lactate-containing peripheral blood). Active external rewarming should probably *not* be chosen as the sole rewarming technique, but should be combined with active core rewarming.

Adapted from AHA ACLS Text, 1987; Danzyl, 1988; Grauer et al, 1990.

Additional Special Considerations in Management of Hypothermia

In addition to the principles of management discussed in Tables 13B-4 and 13B-5, the following special considerations should also be borne in mind when attending to patients with hypothermia.

TAKING THE TEMPERATURE

Many standard thermometers are incapable of registering temperatures at the lower end of the scale. It is therefore essential to be sure the thermometer you are using records below 34° C.

PALPATING PULSES

Although reflex vasoconstriction is a beneficial physiologic adaptation that helps preserve body core temperature, it may make clinical detection of pulses and blood pressure more difficult (AHA ACLS Text, 1987). As a result, extra attention should be directed toward palpation of pulses *before* concluding that no pulse is present.

EXAMINING THE ABDOMEN

The abdominal examination of hypothermic patients is often unreliable (due to reduced or absent bowel sounds and the possibility of cold-induced rectus muscle rigidity). Extra caution is needed in evaluation.

SELECTING A SITE FOR INTRAVENOUS ACCESS

Adequate intravenous access is essential in resuscitation of the patient with severe hypothermia. Selection of an upper torso central site (subclavian or internal jugular line) is probably optimal (Curley and Irwin, 1986; Grauer et al, 1990). This is because the intense vasoconstriction that accompanies severe hypothermia often makes insertion of a peripheral intravenous catheter extremely difficult, as well as subjecting the limb to increased risk from traumatizing a frostbitten extremity. Even if a peripheral vein is successfully cannulized, intense vasoconstriction lessens the reliability of drug delivery. Pulmonary artery (Swan-Ganz) catheters should probably be avoided early on in the resuscitation process because of their potential to precipitate ventricular tachycardia or ventricular fibrillation if the tip of the catheter is inserted too far.

INTERPRETING ABGS

Because cold impairs buffering capacity and mobilization of organic acids, proper ABG interpretation is only possible if obtained values are corrected for temperature. For example, if a patient's temperature is 30° C, 0.10 pH units should be *added* to the pH obtained; 0.15 pH units should be *added* to the obtained pH if the patient's temperature is 27° C (Danzyl, 1988).

PERFORMING CARDIOPULMONARY RESUSCITATION

Cardiopulmonary resuscitation of the *severely* hypothermic patient differs from resuscitation of normothermic or mildly hypothermic individuals. Chest compression should be avoided if at all possible because of the tendency this manipulation has to induce refractory ventricular fibrillation when core temperature is greatly reduced, especially when it drops below 28° C (Danzyl, 1988). It is important to realize that chest compression will *not* necessarily be needed for bradycardia, even if heart rate is markedly reduced. Metabolic demands are dramatically decreased with severe hypothermia, and cardiac output may be adequate despite an extremely slow heart rate (Harris and Smith, 1988; Danzyl, 1988).

Although still indicated as treatment of ventricular fibrillation, *defibrillation is unlikely to be successful as long as core temperature remains below 28° C* (Zell and Kurtz, 1985; AHA ACLS Text, 1987). Similarly, emergency cardiac drugs are significantly less effective in the setting of severe hypothermia (AHA ACLS Text, 1987). Active rewarming must therefore accompany the resuscitative process if it is to be successful.

In addition to ventricular fibrillation, asystole, and EMD, non-lifethreatening atrial arrhythmias (especially atrial fibrillation) and AV block commonly occur in hypothermic patients. In general, these non-lifethreatening arrhythmias tend to spontaneously resolve on rewarming (Curley and Irwin, 1986). Because of uncertain efficacy of antiarrhythmic agents in the setting of severe hypothermia, drug treatment is probably best reserved for patients with lifethreatening arrhythmias.

Finally, if basic life support is required on a hypothermic patient, slower rates of ventilation and chest compression may be adequate (and perhaps even safer than rates recommended for normothermic resuscitation). Unfortunately, optimal rates and ratios for chest compression and ventilation with severe hypothermia are not universally agreed upon (Danzyl, 1988).

References and Suggested Readings

Chapter 15: *Special resuscitation situations*. In Jaffe AS (ed): *Textbook of advanced cardiac life support*, Dallas, 1987, American Heart Association.

Auerbach PS: Some people are dead when they're cold and dead, *JAMA* 264:1856, 1990 (editorial).

Curley FJ, Irwin RS: Disorders of temperature control: hypothermia (Part III), *J Inten Care Med* 1:270, 1986.

Danzyl DF: Chapter 38: Accidental hypothermia. In Rosen P (ed): *Emergency medicine: concepts and clinical practice*, St Louis, 1988, Mosby–Year Book.

Goldman A, Exton-Smith AN, Francis G, O'Brian A: A pilot study of low body temperatures of old people admitted to hospital, *J R Coll Physicians Lond* 11:291, 1977.

Grauer K, Green E, Cavallaro D: Less publicized aspects of cardiac arrest: a survey of caregivers at the bedside, *Fam Pract Recert* 12:32, 1990.

Gregory RT, Doolittle WH: Accidental hypothermia. Part II: clinical implications of experimental studies, *Alaska Med* 15:48, 1973.

Harris ML, Smith J: Temperature determination during CPR, *Ann Emerg Med* 17:296, 1988 (Letter).

Kramer MR, Vandijk J, Rosin AJ: Mortality in elderly patients with thermoregulatory failure, *Arch Intern Med* 149:1521, 1989.

Maclean D, Emslie-Smith D: *Accidental hypothermia*, Philadelphia, 1977, J B Lippincott.

Reuler JB: Hypothermia: pathophysiology, clinical settings, and management, Ann Intern Med 89:519, 1978.

Schaller MD, Fischer AP, Perret CH: Hyperkalemia: a prognostic factor during acute severe hypothermia, *JAMA* 264:1842, 1990.

Zell SC, Kurtz KJ: Severe exposure hypothermia: a resuscitation protocol, *Ann Emerg Med* 14:339, 1985.

SECTION C

HEAT ILLNESS

Normal individuals are able to maintain euthermia and dissipate environmental heat through the adaptive physiologic mechanisms of radiation, convection, and evaporization. Heat illness occurs when this ability is impaired. It encompasses a spectrum of disorders ranging from very mild to potentially life-threatening disturbances in temperature regulation. In this section we focus our attention on the most severe form of heat illness because of the special problem it may pose in resuscitation.

Definitions

Minor heat syndromes are common and characterized by the ability to maintain normal temperature regulation despite the heat-related disorder. **Heat cramps** is the mildest and most prevalent form. Cramps develop either during or following vigorous exertion in the heat. Individuals who are poorly conditioned or not well acclimated to the environment are particularly susceptible. The most-used muscle groups (especially the calves) are typically involved. The direct cause of spasm in these muscle groups is unclear, but is probably related to altered salt and fluid balance. Hypokalemia and hypocalcemia are surprisingly uncommon. Conservative measures (i.e., application of direct pressure or counterstretch to the affected muscle group), removal from the environment, and fluid replacement (either orally or intravenously) is generally curative within a short period of time.

Heat exhaustion is a more severe form of heat illness in which there may be nausea, vomiting, malaise, headache, tetany, and muscle cramps. Symptoms of cardiovascular compromise (such as tachycardia, orthostatic hypotension, and syncope) are sometimes also seen. Although there may be irritability and mild impairment of judgment, cerebral function is otherwise intact. Temperature is usually only mildly or moderately elevated, and rarely exceeds 39° C (102.2° F). Treatment includes rest in a cool environment, rehydration, and electrolyte replacement. Recovery is usually complete within 12 to 24 hours, and there are no long-lasting sequelae.

At the other end of the spectrum of heat illness disorders is **heat stroke,** which may be considered as an extreme form of heat exhaustion. Morbidity is much more severe with the full-blown syndrome of heat stroke, and mortality is reported at being between 10% and 80% (Callaham, 1988). Heat stroke is distinguished from heat exhaustion by the *loss of thermoregulatory control* and the more severe degree of neurologic impairment. Loss of thermoregulatory control results in dramatic temperature elevations to levels that may produce cellular and organ damage. Although no absolute temperature criterion exists for defining the

point that heat exhaustion becomes heat stroke, temperatures with this disorder almost always exceed 40° C (104° F), and often attain 41° to 42° C (105.8°-107.6° F) or more. We focus on this more severe form of heat illness in the rest of this section.

Pathophysiologic and Clinical Features of Heat Stroke

Associated with development of heat stroke is the risk of diffuse tissue injury. Tissue damage becomes increasingly likely at temperatures above 42° C, especially when the duration of exposure to the elevated temperature is extended (Callaham, 1988). Organ system damage is not always reversible. The most common pathologic findings associated with hyperthermic tissue injury are edema and hemorrhage. Specific organ involvement and resultant pathophysiologic changes that may occur are shown in *Table 13C-1*.

Clinical features of heat stroke are shown in *Table 13C-2*. There must be a *heat load*. This may be *environmental* (i.e., from elevated ambient temperatures, especially if associ-

Table 13C-1

Potential Organ System Damage from Hyperthermic Tissue Injury
Heart—myocardial injury and/or infarction (from subendocardial hemorrhage) and/or muscle fiber rupture)
Kidneys—Acute tubular necrosis (from diffuse hemorrhage, impaired renal perfusion, myoglobinuria, or rhabdomyolysis)
Liver—diffuse hepatocellular damage and deterioration
Gall Bladder—cholestasis with jaundice
Gastrointestinal Tract—diffuse hemorrhage
Skeletal Muscle—diffuse muscle fiber degeneration
Hematologic System—small vessel thrombi, impaired generation of clotting factors (from liver injury), disseminated intravascular coagulation
Central Nervous System—cerebral edema (from hemorrhage and/or degenerative neuronal changes)
Adapted from Callaham, 1988.

Table 13C-2

Predisposing Factors and Clinical Features of Heat Stroke

Exposure to a Heat Load—which may be environmental (elevated ambient temperatures, high humidity), and/or internally generated (severe physical exertion, fever from infection or other illness, neurogenic, medication-induced, etc.).

Predisposing Factors—In the presence of a heat load, development of heat stroke is most likely:
- in the very young, the very old, debilitated or poorly conditioned individuals
- in patients with dehydration, or congestive heart failure (decreased blood flow to the skin with resultant impaired ability to dissipate heat from the skin-air interface), or other debilitating illness
- in patients on medications that may interfere with temperature regulation (anticholinergics, tricyclic antidepressants, phenothiazines, MAO inhibitors, amphetamines, cocaine, alcohol), or which may depress cardiovascular function (β-blockers, sympatholytics)

Clinical Features

Temperature elevation—usually to at least 40° C (104° F), and often significantly higher.

Cutaneous vasodilation—as a physiologic response to temperature elevation to maximize heat loss at the skin-air interface.

Hyperventilation—which may be marked (with respiratory rates up to 60/minute) as a physiologic response to maximize heat loss.

Sinus tachycardia—which may be marked (with heart rates up to 150-180/minute) as a physiologic response to increase cardiac output and maximize heat loss through the dilated skin vasculature.

Hemodynamic response—may be varied. Cardiac output is initially increased as a result of significant shunting (of blood through dilated skin vessels) and compensatory sinus tachycardia (hyperdynamic circulation). New (functional) heart murmurs may be heard as a reflection of the increased cardiac output. Initially blood pressure remains stable or increases. Ultimately, if temperature remains elevated, compensatory mechanisms fail and the patient may develop high-output heart failure. Persistently elevated temperatures may produce cardiac injury, infarction, or a direct depressant effect on contractility. Blood pressure falls with the onset of cardiovascular decompensation.

Neurologic abnormalities—CNS dysfunction is an essential element of the diagnosis of heat stroke. The neurologic abnormalities most commonly seen include tremor, headache, dizziness, confusion, delirium, and ultimately seizures and coma.

---

ated with high humidity) or *internally generated* (from physical exertion, fever from infection or other illness, neurogenic, or medication-induced). Vigorous exercise generates a surprisingly large amount of heat. For example, marathoners typically develop and maintain body temperatures between 38° and 40° C (100.4° and 104° F) when they run (Simon, 1990). Were it not for their efficient thermoregulatory compensation, the heat generated from running would raise body temperatures to a much higher level. Instead, these well-acclimated and conditioned athletes maintain thermal homeostasis by dissipating heat through evaporation (of large amounts of sweat) and radiation (from cutaneous vasodilatation which increases skin temperature with respect to the ambient environment).

Heat stroke develops when thermoregulatory control is lost. This may occur in less well-conditioned athletes (with less efficient thermoregulatory function) or when thermoregulatory mechanisms are overwhelmed by excessive heat production, exceedingly high ambient temperatures or humidity, dehydration, or other predisposing factors shown in Table 13C-2.

Physiologic compensation (in the form of cutaneous vasodilatation, hyperventilation, and increased cardiac output with sinus tachycardia) is no longer adequate to prevent marked temperature elevation. Ultimately, compensatory mechanisms fail and the patient develops high-output heart failure. Alternatively, temperature elevation per se may produce a direct cardiac depressant effect or precipitate acute infarction, leading to cardiogenic shock. Cardiac arrest may follow.

An essential component of the diagnosis of heat stroke is neurologic dysfunction. Initially, patients become confused or disoriented. With persistent temperature elevation, this often progresses to delirium and ultimately coma and/or seizure activity.

The clinical characteristics of heat stroke vary depending on the type *(Table 13C-3)*. **Classic heat stroke** most commonly occurs during heat waves. Individuals affected tend to be at the extremes of life (the very young and the very old), and typically have one or more of the predisposing factors listed in Table 13C-2. Onset is gradual (over days), the degree of dehydration is usually severe, and sweating has usually ceased by the time these patients present for medical attention.

In contrast, **exertional heat stroke** is seen in young or middle-aged adults who are often active and otherwise healthy. Onset is usually much more abrupt, and is typically precipitated by a period of intense physical exertion under less than optimal conditions (excessively hot ambient temperatures or high humidity, poor physical conditioning). Because of the rapid onset, not enough time

Table 13C-3

	Classic Heat Stroke	**Exertional Heat Stroke**
	Clinical Characteristics of the Types of Heat Stroke	
Occurrence	Most common in the very young (especially infants) or the very old	Most common in young or middle-aged adults
Precipitating Factors	Significant heat load presented to individual who is unable to maintain adequate fluid intake and seek a cooler environment	Significant physical exertion (e.g., jogging, other sporting event) performed in excess and/or by an individual who is less than optimally conditioned or acclimated to the environment
Onset	Usually *gradual* (over a period of days)	Usually *very rapid* (over a period of hours)
Clinical Features:		
Hydration Status	Significant dehydration common by the time patient presents	Dehydration usually less severe (because rapid onset allows less time for severe dehydration to develop)
Sweating	Anhydrosis (cessation of sweating) common by the time patient is seen	Patient may still be sweating profusely (as a result of the lesser degree of dehydration) at the time of presentation

Adapted from Callaham, 1988.

may have passed for severe dehydration to develop, and the patient may still be sweating profusely when first seen.

Evaluation and Management

Laboratory tests to routinely consider in evaluation of patients suspected of heat stroke and the abnormalities most likely encountered are suggested in *Table 13C-4*. General and specific principles of management are listed in *Table 13C-5*. It is important to emphasize that regardless of the type of heat stroke (classic or exertional), this disorder constitutes a *true medical emergency* demanding prompt recognition and immediate treatment. Delay in temperature reduction—*even for a period of minutes*—may result in significant additional damage and increased risk of cardiac arrest. Tissue damage to multiple organ systems is a direct consequence of the height of temperature elevation and the *duration* of time that the patient is exposed (Bynum et al, 1978). As a result, a high index of suspicion for the diagnosis must always be maintained in any patient exposed to a "heat load" who presents with elevated temperature ($\geq 40°$ C $= 104°$ F) in association with clinical signs of severe CNS dysfunction (confusion, delirium, seizures, or coma), especially if other predisposing factors are present.

After attending to the ABCs, *immediate cooling* assumes top priority. In most cases, this will result in prompt resolution of symptoms (temperature reduction, improved mental status). Persistent temperature elevation and depressed consciousness despite application of adequate cooling measures should suggest the possibility of another cause for the altered consciousness and temperature elevation (meningitis, other serious infection with delirium from fever, seizures or stroke with neurogenic fever, thyroid storm, etc.). The laboratory tests listed in Table 13C-4 may help narrow the differential diagnosis.

The initial method selected for cooling depends on where the diagnosis of heat stroke is made, and the availability of various cooling measures. Clothing should be removed and the patient moved to a cool environment. In the field, significant body cooling may be accomplished by spraying the patient with water, followed by fanning the areas sprayed (if possible) to keep air circulating. Although a cooling mattress may suffice in less severe cases, continued use of *evaporative cooling* (directing moving air over the wet patient) after the patient arrives in the Emergency Department appears to provide the most efficient method for temperature reduction (Callaham, 1988). A "heat stroke gurney" with drains facilitates the process by providing a place to put the patient where ice packs can be easily

Table 13C-4

Laboratory Tests to Routinely Consider in Evaluation of Patients with Heat Stroke
ABGs—Metabolic acidosis is common with heat stroke as a result of anaerobic metabolism (especially in exertional heat stroke). Hyperventilation often develops as compensation (respiratory alkalosis). Hyperventilation per se is also a specific compensatory mechanism for dissipating body heat.
Serum Electrolytes—Values are highly variable, and should be checked frequently. In particular, *hypokalemia* (from hyperventilation and respiratory alkalosis) and *hyperkalemia* (from metabolic acidosis, muscle tissue breakdown) should be watched for. Profuse sweating and resultant dehydration may affect serum sodium concentration. Serum **magnesium, calcium,** and **phosphate** should also be checked.
Hematocrit—Hemoconcentration is a common reflection of the severe dehydration that is often seen in patients with heat stroke.
White Blood Cell (WBC) Count—Acute stress (from heat stroke), dehydration, and/or infection may all significantly elevate the WBC count. Should there be any doubt about the diagnosis of heat stroke, **blood cultures** should be drawn.
SGOT, LDH, and **CPK**—Enzyme values are often markedly elevated (sometimes in the tens of thousands) with heat stroke. Serum enzyme elevations may persist for 1-2 weeks, even with prompt cooling.
BUN and Creatinine—Preexisting renal disease and/or acute insult (hyperthermia-induced renal hypoperfusion, tissue damage, or rhabdomyolysis) may result in elevated values. Rapid and unpredictable fluid shifts make it difficult to gauge volume status on the basis of BUN or hematocrit values alone.
Thyroid Profile—Although uncommon, thyroid storm (thyrotoxicosis) may present an identical clinical picture as heat stroke and should therefore be included in the differential diagnosis.
Clotting Studies—Clotting abnormalities including disseminated intravascular coagulation (DIC) have been reported with heat stroke. A **prothrombin time, partial thromboplastin time,** and **platelet count** should all probably be ordered as a baseline.
Urinalysis (U/A) and **Urine Culture**—A U/A may provide useful baseline information on specific gravity (hydration status), sediment abnormalities (i.e., presence of protein, casts), bleeding tendency (if hematuria present), or infection (presence of WBCs, bacteria).
ECG and **Continuous Electrocardiographic Monitoring**—Almost any cardiac arrhythmia may be seen with hyperthermia, especially when temperature elevation is severe. A 12-lead ECG should be obtained to rule out acute infarction.
Chest X-Ray—A chest x-ray should be routinely obtained as a baseline, as well as to rule out heart failure and other causes of fever (pneumonia, aspiration).
Lumbar Puncture—Should be considered as part of the work-up for high fever and mental status alterations if the diagnosis of heat stroke is at all uncertain (i.e., if the patient doesn't promptly wake up and respond to cooling measures).

applied to the neck, groin, and axillae (which are areas of maximal heat transfer). At the same time, the skin is kept wet with tepid (*not* cold) water and the patient is actively fanned to favor evaporization. Alternatively the patient may be unclothed and suspended over a tub in a net while the skin is sprayed and active fanning is applied. *Iced gastric lavage* may be a helpful adjunct to evaporative cooling.

Active cooling measures should be continued until core temperature is lowered to between 38° and 39° C (100.4°-102.2° F). Cooling beyond this point may overshoot and result in development of hypothermia. Because the loss in thermoregulatory control may persist for a period of time, continued close observation is essential to guard against the possibility of *rebound hyperthermia* in the initial hours (and first few days) after active cooling is stopped.

The use of many cooling techniques remains controversial (Rubenstein, 1990). Ice water baths are no longer as enthusiastically recommended as they were in the past because the cutaneous vasoconstriction they produce ultimately slows the rate of cooling (Callaham, 1988; Danzyl, 1988). Ice-tub immersion may also be counterproductive

because it usually produces shivering which generates heat. Practically speaking, ice-tub immersion is unpleasant for the patient, difficult to administer (since it requires a large tub and a greater supply of ice than is usually available in most Emergency Departments), and potentially dangerous for acutely ill and unstable patients who require continuous electrocardiographic monitoring and may be intubated.

Other methods of cooling that are less commonly used include cold IV solutions (which are not nearly as effective as evaporative cooling techniques), ice water enemas (which are of limited benefit due to the relatively poor pelvic venous circulation), administration of cold air by positive pressure inhalation (which is cumbersome to set up and of limited efficacy), and peritoneal lavage with cooled dialysate (which is effective but requires time, skilled personnel, and is an invasive procedure).

Antipyretics (i.e., aspirin, acetaminophen) are generally ineffective in reducing the temperature of patients with heat stroke unless there is an additional underlying organic etiology for the elevated temperature. Antipyretics work

Table 13C-5

Suggested Approach to Management of Heat Stroke

1. Assure an adequate airway. Provide supplemental oxygen as needed.

2. Ventilate the patient who is not spontaneously breathing. Intubate if needed.

3. Assess circulation (pulse, blood pressure) and hemodynamic status. Consider invasive hemodynamic monitoring if pulmonary edema or hypotension is present.*

4. Insert a large bore intravenous line. Administer IV fluids according to individual patient needs (i.e., depending on whether the patient is volume depleted from dehydration, in high-output heart failure, etc.).

5. Verify the temperature. Consider use of a rectal thermister probe which can be left in place to continuously monitor the temperature.

6. Institute cooling measures:
   - Remove clothing.
   - Move patient to a cool environment.
   - Consider an *evaporative cooling* technique (keeping the skin wet with tepid water and directing moving air over the patient by fanning to facilitate evaporation).
   - Consider *iced gastric lavage.*
   - Avoid (if possible) cooling techniques that may induce cutaneous vasoconstriction (which retards cooling) or shivering† (which generates heat).
   - Consider antipyretics *if* an underlying organic etiology is suspected of contributing to the reason for temperature elevation.
   - Continue active cooling measures until core temperature is lowered to between 38°-39° C (100.4°-102.2° F). Then stop.
   - Continue close observation (and temperature monitoring) after active cooling is stopped to guard against *rebound hyperthermia.*

7. Consider obtaining laboratory tests, ABGs, ECG, and x-rays *(as suggested in Table 13C-4).*

8. Institute continuous ECG monitoring.

9. Insert Foley catheter (to monitor urine output) if patient not spontaneously voiding.

10. Consider NG tube insertion (prevention of emesis, iced gastric lavage).

11. Consider other possible causes of temperature elevation or unresponsiveness (meningitis, other serious infection, seizure or stroke with neurogenic fever, thyroid storm, etc.), and treat accordingly:
    - Administer an ampule of D50 solution after drawing Dextrostix.
    - Administer Narcan if narcotic ingestion suspected.

12. Promptly treat seizures if they occur (IV diazepam, phenytoin).

---

*Hypotension associated with heat stroke may be due to dehydration or high-output heart failure. *Invasive hemodynamic monitoring* is often needed for definitive diagnosis and to guide therapy.
†Shivering generates heat and should be suppressed if it develops. Consider use of **chlorpromazine** (10-25 mg IV at a rate of 1 mg/min) as needed for this purpose.

---

by correcting the thermoregulatory setpoint. The setpoint is not altered in heat stroke. Instead, the reason for temperature elevation with heat stroke is the loss in ability to adequately dissipate heat and maintain body temperature within normal limits (Callaham, 1988).

Neuroleptic Malignant Syndrome/Malignant Hyperthermia

Two less commonly encountered but extremely important hyperthermic syndromes to be aware of are **neuroleptic malignant syndrome (NMS)** and **malignant hyperthermia (MH).** Prompt recognition and early institution of specific treatment may be essential for survival *(Table 13C-6).*

The keys to distinguishing NMS and MH from heat stroke are the *clinical setting* and the presence of *muscle rigidity* and *hypertonicity.* The degree of temperature elevation and the nature of associated symptoms may be similar in all three disorders. However, muscle tone is generally not increased with heat stroke. Patients with heat stroke have a history of exposure to a *heat load.* Supportive treatment with rapid cooling usually results in resolution of symptoms. In contrast, exposure to *medication* (rather than heat load) precipitates most cases of NMS (phenothiazines, tricyclic antidepressants, or other neuroleptics) and MH (halogenated anesthetics, succinylcholine). Although appli-

Table 13C-6

Clinical Characteristics of Malignant Hyperthermia and Neuroleptic Malignant Syndrome Compared to Heat Stroke		
	Malignant Hyperthermia (MH)	**Neuroleptic Malignant Syndrome (NMS)**	**Heat Stroke**
Genetic Predisposition	Yes	No	No
Pathophysiology	Genetic defect results in abnormal sarcoplasmic release of calcium ion, which leads to increased myoplasmic calcium levels and a hypermetabolic state of muscle contraction with marked temperature elevation	May be related to depletion of available dopamine in the brain	Depends on type (classic vs exertional heat stroke, as described in Table 13C-3)
Precipitating Cause	Usually from inhalation of halogenated anesthetics and/or administration of the skeletal muscle relaxant succinylcholine Much less commonly precipitated by physical or emotional stress, or trauma	Recent use of a neuroleptic agent (phenothiazine, butyrophenone, thioxanthene, or lithium-neuroleptic or MAO inhibitor-tricyclic antidepressant combination)	See Table 13C-3
Onset	Sudden	Gradual over 1-3 days	Relatively sudden (exertional heat stroke) or gradual (classic heat stroke)
Muscle Rigidity & Hypertonicity	Yes!	Yes!	No
Mortality	≈60%	≈30%	Variable (10-80%)
Treatment	- Cooling measures - Supportive therapy - Dantrolene	- Cooling measures - Supportive therapy - Dantrolene - Bromocriptine	- Cooling measures - Supportive therapy

Adapted from Callaham, 1988; Danzyl, 1988.

cation of cooling measures and supportive therapy are helpful, symptoms generally will not reverse unless the offending agent is withdrawn and specific treatment with Dantrolene is given.

Dantrolene is a hydantoin derivative that acts directly on skeletal muscle to suppress release of calcium (Callaham, 1988). It therefore reverses the primary abnormality in these two hyperthermic syndromes. An initial dose of 2.5 mg/kg IV is given, which may be repeated up to a total of 10 mg/kg. This may be followed with 4 to 8 mg/kg of dantrolene given orally every 6 hours for up to 3 days.*

Another drug that may be useful in treatment of NMS is the dopamine agonist **bromocriptine** (2.5-10 mg PO every 8 hours).

---

*Calcium antagonists should be avoided while the patient is on dantrolene.

Thus, one should suspect either NMS or MH in patients who present with marked hyperthermia if:

- fever and associated symptoms persist despite adequate cooling measures
- there is an appropriate clinical setting (i.e., absence of heat load, exposure to a neuroleptic, halogenated anesthetic, or succinlylcholine)

In such cases, specific treatment with **dantrolene** is indicated, and prompt reversal of symptoms confirms the diagnosis.

References and Suggested Readings

Bynum GP, Panoolf KB, Schuette WH, Goldman RF, Lees DE, Whang-Peng J, Atkinson ER, Bull JM: Induced hyperthermia in sedated humans and the concept of critical thermal maximum, *Am J Physiol* 235:R228, 1978.

Callaham M: Chapter 39: *Heat illness*. In Rosen P (ed): *Emergency medicine: concepts and clinical practice*, St. Louis, 1988, Mosby–Year Book.

Danzyl DF: Hyperthermic syndromes, *Am Fam Physician* 37:157, 1988.

Rubenstein E: *Heatstroke*. In Rubenstein E, Federman DD (eds): *Scientific American medicine*, New York, 1990, Scientific American.

SECTION D

LIGHTNING

Lightning-related injuries occur much more commonly than is generally suspected by the medical community. An estimated 300 to 600 Americans die each year as a result of lightning strikes, and a much greater number are injured, sometimes with permanent disability (Cooper, 1988; Epperly and Stewart, 1989; Blount, 1990). It is likely that many more less severe injuries go unreported.

Historical reference to lightning dates back to ancient times. Greek mythology explained the phenomenon as an expression of the wrath of Zeus, aimed at striking down those who dared to defy him. Other cultures believed the ground struck by lightning was sacred and worthy of worship. A number of myths about the medical consequences of lightning have persisted to this day, including the following (Cooper, 1980, 1988):

1. Lightning strikes are always due to direct contact of the lightning flash with the victim.
2. Lightning strikes are uniformly fatal.
3. Lightning injuries are similar to other high-voltage injuries. They often turn the victim into a "crispy critter."
4. Victims of lightning strikes remain electrified. Bystanders should never touch (try to help) such victims because they may also become electrified.

Lightning is a complex electrical phenomenon that results from a transfer of energy from the negative charge of a thundercloud's lower surface to the relatively positive charge of the earth below. The normal insulating effect of air is lost during an electrical storm in which warm air has risen in a cold air system to set up conditions predisposing to tremendous potential differences in the charged particles contained within the electrical field. Up to 1 billion volts (and 200,000 amperes of current) may be generated by the resultant electrical discharge (Cooper, 1980, 1987, 1988).

The type and severity of injury from a lightning strike depend on the mechanism of energy transfer. Lightning injury may occur by direct strike, splash, ground current, contact, or blunt trauma.

As might be expected, *direct strike* produces the most severe lightning-related injury. Fortunately, this mechanism is not nearly as common as *splash* which occurs when lightning strikes an object (such as a tree, car, or building) and then jumps (i.e., *"splashes"*) through the air to another object (such as a nearby person) of lower electrical resistance. In most cases of lightning injury that occur outdoors, the skin will be wet (from the rainstorm). As a result, electrical resistance to current will be extremely low all

along the skin's surface, and current *(which tends to follow the path of least resistance)* will usually *flashover* the person's skin *without* significant penetration into deep tissues. This explains why flashover most commonly produces relatively superficial burns.

In contrast, the path of current with other high-voltage electrical injuries is much more likely to penetrate into deep tissues. This is because the skin will usually be dry with these other injuries. The electrical resistance of dry, intact skin may be more than 1,000 times greater than that of wet skin (Kunkle, 1988). Bone, nerve, muscle, and blood vessels all offer significantly less resistance than dry skin, so that current will be preferentially directed through these deeper structures rather than travel along the skin's surface.

As a direct consequence of extremely rapid passage along the skin surface of the tremendously high electrical current of lightning flashover, an interesting phenomenon may be seen. Moisture on the skin may vaporize. The effect of this instantaneous vaporization may generate enough force to rip clothes or shoes apart and partially unclad the victim. Despite this dramatic presentation, the fact that most of the electrical current fails to penetrate deeper structures is the major reason victims of lightning flashover usually sustain less severe injury than might otherwise be expected.

It should be noted that flashover may not occur if the victim is electrically grounded as may occur if shoes having metal cleats are worn or the person is standing in water. In this case, the path of current from a lightning strike is much more likely to pass through the body and cause more damage to deeper structures.

The other common mechanisms of lightning injury are ground current, contact, and blunt trauma. *Ground current* (or *step voltage*) occurs when lightning hits the ground and is then transferred to the victim. With *contact*, the victim is directly touching an object that makes up a part of the current pathway. Finally, *blunt trauma* may be sustained as a result of the tremendous force of shock waves generated by rapid cooling of superheated air.

Lightning strikes are fatal in approximately 20% to 30% of cases (Cooper, 1980; Blount, 1990). This means that most (i.e., 70-80%) victims survive. Unlike high-voltage electrical injuries that deliver a relatively prolonged alternating (AC) current discharge, a direct lightning strike releases a massive instantaneous direct current (DC) discharge. This tends to produce asystole from simultaneous depolarization of the entire myocardium. In the absence of underlying cardiac disease, the heart's inherent automaticity usually resumes normal function (i.e., normal sinus rhythm) within short order. In contrast, the longer-lasting AC discharge from high-voltage electrical injuries is much more likely to induce ventricular fibrillation.

Several important points about the cardiopulmonary sequelae of lightning strikes should be emphasized:

1. The major cause of mortality from lightning-related injuries is cardiopulmonary arrest (AHA Textbook on ACLS, 1987; Cooper, 1988). *Victims of lightning strikes who do not develop cardiopulmonary arrest almost always survive* (although they may sustain any of the other lightning-related injuries indicated in *Table 13D-1*).

2. In addition to cardiac arrest (from asystole), lightning also has a tendency to produce respiratory arrest from passage of current through the brainstem (which temporarily paralyzes the respiratory center). *The associated respiratory arrest often lasts longer than the period of ventricular standstill* (Cooper, 1988). This is an extremely important point to appreciate because rescue breathing (by either a lay-bystander or an emergency care provider) may be potentially life-saving. Failure to breathe for the patient until spontaneous ventilation resumes may result in hypoxia and cause *secondary* ventricular fibrillation that will then require

Table 13D-1

Potential Lightning-Related Injuries and Sequelae

HEENT
- Skull or cervical fractures *(which may result from violent displacement of the victim by the lightning strike)*
- Tympanic membrane rupture *(which is due to the mechanical effects of lightning's shock wave and is surprisingly common!)*
- Temporary sensorineural hearing loss
- Cataracts *(which are common and sometimes only develop months after the event)*, corneal lesions, uveitis, vitreous hemorrhage, hyphema, retinal detachment

Pulmonary
- Pulmonary contusion
- Respiratory arrest

Cardiac
- Myocardial ischemia or infarction
- Cardiac arrest *(which is most often due to asystole)**
- Cardiac arrhythmias *(virtually any arrhythmia may be seen)*

Abdomen
- Blunt abdominal injury *(rare)*†

Extremities
- Extremity fractures/dislocations
- Vascular ischemia/infarction *(which commonly manifests as transient mottling, blue discoloration, coolness and/or paresthesias of one or both lower extremities—and which is often due to vasospasm—usually clearing within several hours)*
- Permanent limb paresthesias or paralysis *(uncommon)*

Skin
- Burns *(which are most often superficial and which clinically may not appear for several hours)*

Neurologic
- Confusion
- Transient loss of consciousness
- Anterograde amnesia
- Intracranial hemorrhage
- Seizures

*This differs from the mechanism of cardiopulmonary arrest from high-voltage AC electrical injuries which are usually the result of ventricular fibrillation.
†Lightning-related injuries have not been associated with the intraabdominal catastrophes that may be seen with high-voltage electrical injuries (such as gallbladder necrosis, mesenteric thrombosis, etc.).
Adapted from Cooper, 1988.

electrical defibrillation for resuscitation to be successful.

3. If ventricular fibrillation does develop and defibrillation is needed, *success rates for resuscitation from lightning strikes tend to exceed those for cardiopulmonary arrest due to other causes* (even when a relatively long period of time has transpired since the onset of the arrest). This is because the basal metabolic rate may dramatically slow as a result of a lightning strike, delaying the onset of tissue degeneration and reducing the likelihood of anoxic injury. *Therefore, an attempt should always be made to resuscitate a victim of a lightning strike who has suffered cardiopulmonary arrest, even when the duration of the arrest is relatively prolonged* (Taussig, 1968; Peters, 1983; Moran and Thupari, 1986; Seward, 1987; Blount, 1990).

4. Lightning strikes often injure more than one person at a time. Because of the potential viability of victims of lightning-induced cardiopulmonary arrest and the rarity of death in those who survive the initial strike, the usual priorities on trauma should be reversed. *Treatment of the moving, moaning victim should therefore be deferred until after an attempt is made to resuscitate the apparently dead victim* (Taussig, 1968; Blount, 1990).

Management of Lightning-Related Injuries

The best treatment of lightning-related injuries is prevention. The period of highest risk in the United States is between the months from May to September, which encompass the thunderstorm season. Outdoor activities most commonly associated with lightning-related injury during a thunderstorm include jogging, camping, participation in water sports, working on construction, being in an open field, or seeking shelter under an isolated tree. Being indoors does *not* eliminate the risk of lightning-related injury. Seemingly harmless activities such as taking a bath, talking on the telephone, and working with electrical appliances are all potentially dangerous during an electrical storm. Specific preventive measures to minimize the risk of exposure and lightning-related injury are summarized in *Table 13D-2*.

Evaluation of the victim of a lightning strike should focus on assessment for the injuries most likely to occur *(Table 13D-1)*. As already emphasized, first priority should be directed toward treatment of unconscious or apparently dead victims. Immediate attention to the **ABC**s (**A**irway, **B**reathing, and **C**irculation) with application of ventilatory and/or circulatory support as needed (for apnea or asystole) is essential, and may be successful in reviving such patients even after a relatively long period of unresponsiveness.

Table 13D-2

Preventive Measures for Avoiding Lightning-Related Injury

1. Respect the Power of Electrical Storms

- Terminate outdoor activities such as jogging, recreational sports, and especially swimming!
- Do not wear metal helmets or metal-cleated shoes, and do not handle potentially conductive items such as umbrellas, kites, fishing rods, golf clubs, or rifles.
- Seek enclosed shelter (in a car or building) as soon as possible.
- Avoid standing under tall or *isolated* objects such as a tree *(which increases your chance of sideflash)* or in an open field.
- Spread out if in a group (to minimize the chance that all group members will be injured and unable to help each other).

2. Don't Believe the Myth that Lightning Never Strikes the Same Spot Twice

- Conditions that predispose an object to the original lightning strike (i.e., height of the object, degree of isolation, ability to conduct electricity) tend to remain in effect and thus predispose to additional lightning strikes in the same place.

3. Even If Indoors, Realize (and Respect) the Potential for Lightning-related Injury During an Electrical Storm

- Seemingly benign activities such as taking a bath, talking on the telephone, and working with electrical appliances are all potentially dangerous during an electrical storm.

Adapted from Epperly and Stewart, 1989.

Although victims who show signs of life after a lightning strike may still be seriously injured, they will almost always survive. This is why assessment of these patients can (should) be deferred until unresponsive victims are evaluated and an attempt has been made at resuscitation.

Additional evaluative measures to consider in patients with lightning-related injuries are suggested in *Table 13D-3*. Admission to the hospital for observation and/or treatment should be considered for those with cardiac signs or symptoms (chest pain, ECG changes, cardiac arrhythmias), neurologic abnormalities (persistently altered level of consciousness, seizures, focal neurologic deficits) or significant trauma. Victims with only momentary loss of consciousness or rapidly resolving confusion or amnesia can be safely discharged home in most cases with appropriate observation by family members. Similarly, minor burns, and most hearing and visual deficits can usually be followed on an ambulatory basis.

Table 13D-3

Evaluative Measures to Consider for Patients with Lightning-Related Injury

History:

- Mechanism of injury *(Direct strike? Splash? Trauma from being thrown to the ground by the lightning strike?)*
- Any witnesses to the event? *(Loss of consciousness?)*
- Previous medical history *(Preexisting cardiac disease?)*

Physical examination:

    Vital signs—Shock? Febrile/hypothermic?
    HEENT—Vision? Hearing/intact tympanic membranes? Signs of trauma to head or neck?
    Skin—Burns? Other signs of trauma/cyanosis?/mottling?
    Extremities—Peripheral pulses/sensorimotor function?
    Lungs—Respiratory rate/breath sounds?
    Heart—Rate/regularity of rhythm?
    Abdomen—Bowel sounds? Localized tenderness?
    Neurologic—Level of consciousness? Memory *(Antegrade/retrograde amnesia?)*

12-Lead ECG—ST-T wave abnormalities including transient ST segment elevation (which may or may not reflect accompanying myocardial necrosis) are common.

Continuous ECG Monitoring—Asystole from the lightning strike is usually short-lived (in patients without underlying cardiac disease). Various other arrhythmias may be seen, especially if the lightning strike produced myocardial necrosis.

X-Rays—C-spine, chest x-rays, and other films as appropriate should be strongly considered for victims suspected of having sustained significant trauma from the lightning strike.

Routine Laboratory Studies—CBC, SMAC-25, urinalysis.

Additional Laboratory Studies to Consider—Cardiac enzymes (if myocardial necrosis suspected), urine myoglobin (if appropriate).

References and Selected Readings

American Heart Association: *Special resuscitation situations*. In Jaffe A (ed): *Textbook of advanced cardiac life support*, Dallas, 1987, American Heart Association.

Blount BW: Lightning injuries, *Am Fam Physician* 42:405, 1990.

Cooper MA: Lightning injuries: prognostic signs for death, *Ann Emerg Med* 9:134, 1980.

Cooper MA: *Lightning injuries*. In Rosen P (ed): *Emergency medicine: concepts and clinical practice*, St Louis, 1988, Mosby–Year Book.

Cooper MA, Karkal SS: Enhancing recovery from electrical and lightning injuries, *Emerg Med Reports* 8:57, 1987.

Epperly TD, Stewart JR: The physical effects of lightning injury, *J Fam Pract* 29:267, 1989.

Kunkle RF: *Electrical injuries*. In Rosen P (ed): *Emergency medicine: concepts and clinical practice*, St Louis, 1988, Mosby–Year Book.

Moran KT, Thupari JN, Munster AM: Electric- and lightning-induced cardiac arrest reversed by prompt cardiopulmonary resuscitation, *JAMA* 255:2157, 1986, (letter).

Peters WJ: Lightning injury, *Can Med Assoc J* 128:148, 1983.

Seward P: Electrical injuries, *Emerg Med* 19:67, 1987.

Taussig HB: "Death" from lightning—and the possibility of living again, *Ann Intern Med* 68:1345, 1968.

SECTION E

ELECTRICAL INJURIES

Electrical injuries may be caused by such diverse sources of electrical energy as household appliances, car batteries, high-tension telephone lines, and lightning. A wide spectrum of injuries may be produced including relatively minor entry and exit skin burns; deeper, more severe charring burns; cataracts; fractures or dislocations; internal injury to a variety of organs; and fatal electrocution. Morbidity and mortality from electrical injuries is appreciable; 1,000 to 1,500 people die from such injuries in the United States each year (Kunkle, 1988).

The type and severity of any electrical injury is a function of many factors, including (Cooper, 1988):
1. Parameters of the electrical circuit (voltage, current, and resistance).
2. The type of current (direct or alternating) and the frequency of cycle.
3. The pathway of the current.
4. Duration of current application.
5. The site and surface area of current entry.

The current, voltage, and resistance of an electrical circuit are related according to **Ohm's Law** by the following equation:

$$V = IR$$

where **V** = voltage *(in volts)*, **I** = current *(in amperes)*, and **R** = resistance *(in Ohms)*

Thus for any given potential difference (voltage), current will vary inversely with electrical resistance. If resistance is high, the amount of current passing through the circuit will be low. Conversely, if resistance is low, a correspondingly greater amount of current will flow through the circuit.

In general, it is the amount of *current* passing through the circuit (and through the patient) rather than the voltage of the electrical source that determines the severity of injury. *According to Ohm's Law, current may thus be surprisingly low* (and the extent of injury minimal) *despite high voltage if electrical resistance is high.* By the same reasoning, current may be quite high (and the extent of injury severe) despite seemingly low voltage if electrical resistance is greatly reduced. Because the current and resistance of an electrical injury are rarely known, it is usually impossible to accurately predict the potential hazard from a particular electrical exposure.

Electrical injury is usually more severe following exposure to alternating (AC) current than to direct (DC) current. Even though passage of a DC current burst through the heart may depolarize the entire myocardium and produce asystole, the heart's inherent automaticity will usually resume spontaneous activity (i.e., normal sinus rhythm) shortly thereafter.

For practical purposes, a lightning strike can be thought of as a massive DC discharge. *(See Section D on Lightning Injuries.)* Despite extremely high current (of up to 200,000 amperes), the exceedingly short duration of this current (from 0.001 to 0.0001 second) may result in delivery of a total amount of energy that is less than that associated with other types of electrical injuries (Cooper, 1988). Factors most responsible for determining whether victims of a lightning strike survive are the presence of underlying cardiac disease (which may favor persistence of asystole) and the duration of the accompanying respiratory arrest.

In contrast, the alternating (AC) current commonly associated with other types of electrical injuries presents a repetitive stimulus of relatively long duration. Passage of AC current through the heart from such injuries usually causes ventricular fibrillation. Defibrillation will be required for successful resuscitation. Despite exposure to a much lower current load than occurs with lightning injury, the repetitive fibrillatory stimulus of an AC current promotes tetanic muscle contractions that may actually "freeze" the victim to the energy source for an extended period of time. The unfortunate result of this prolonged contact to an AC current source may be significant charring of tissue, severe internal injury, and a progressively increasing tendency to develop ventricular fibrillation. This differs from a DC current discharge that produces a single large muscle contraction which often jolts the victim with sufficient force to disconnect them from the energy source.

Human muscular tissue responds most actively to alternating current with a frequency range of between 40 to 150 cycles per second (cps). Household current alternates at 60 cps, which is well within this range, and accounts for the predisposition to tetanic muscular contraction and potential injury when current in the electrical circuit is of sufficient intensity (Kunkle, 1988). Exposure to AC current sources alternating at higher frequencies (i.e., greater than 150 cps) are generally less dangerous at any given current load because they are less likely to produce tetanic muscle contraction.

As alluded to above, the intensity of current is a critical factor in determining the response to contact with an electrical source. Exposure to low current intensity (in the range of 1 milliampere [= 1 mA] or less) is usually perceived as no more than a tingling sensation in the area of contact. Greater current intensities become increasingly unpleasant and ultimately painful. Although subject to interperson variability and dependent on cycle frequency, the *"let go current"* (beyond which involuntary tetanic muscle contractions make it impossible for the subject to release their grasp on the current source) is usually within the range of 5 to 30 mA (Kobernick, 1982; AHA ACLS Textbook, 1987). Exposure to higher currents (i.e., greater than 40 mA) may precipitate tetanic contraction of the diaphragm and intercostal muscles, causing respiration to cease until contact with the electrical source is terminated. With exposure to still higher currents (of 100 mA or greater), respiratory arrest may be prolonged (due to direct inhibition of central breathing centers), or ventricular fibrillation may be induced. Paradoxically, exposure to currents of greater than 10 A may actually lessen the likelihood of precipitating ventricular fibrillation. This is because higher currents tend to maintain the heart in a state of sustained contraction (AHA ACLS Textbook, 1987). In such cases of prolonged myocardial contraction, normal sinus rhythm will usually resume once the current is terminated.

Electrical injuries may result from exposure to energy sources of either *high-tension* (greater than 1,000 volts) or *low-tension* (less than 1,000 volts). Although the amount of electrical resistance in the circuit also influences current load (according to Ohm's Law), low-tension electrical sources (such as the 110 volt exposure of household current) are generally less likely than high-tension electrical sources to produce extensive tissue injury. However, low-tension electrical exposure is far from being benign, and significant tissue injury or death (from ventricular fibrillation or respiratory arrest) may still occur. Because of the much greater incidence of low-tension electrical exposure, overall mortality is approximately equal to that from high-tension electrical injuries (Kobernick, 1982).

The final factor determining the extent of damage from electrical injury is the pathway of current flow. For example, death is likely to occur if the current pathway includes the heart or brain, unless there is prompt resuscitation. Passage of current directly through the body produces damage to muscle, nerve, blood vessels, and other internal structures of low electrical resistance. This is in contrast to what happens with the "flashover" phenomenon of a lightning strike in which damage to internal structures is often minimal because current preferentially passes along the outer body surface without significant penetration through the skin.

Internal injury is not only produced by passage of electrical current per se through structures in its path, but also by the accompanying generation of heat *(thermal in-*

jury). In particular, the high resistance of bone to electric current results in actual heating of the bone which may then burn surrounding tissue. Any of the injuries indicated in *Table 13E-1* may result. Low resistance structures such as blood vessels and nerves are particularly susceptible to the thermal effects of electricity. Direct damage to vessel walls may be produced and/or severe arterial spasm precipitated. Vascular occlusion or thrombosis may result and ultimately lead to ischemic necrosis with loss of limb. Peripheral nerve injury can be due to either direct thermal exposure or vascular compromise. Renal failure may likewise result from direct thermal injury to the kidneys, or more commonly from release of large amounts of myoglobin into the vascular system secondary to extensive muscle necrosis.

It is important to appreciate that the extent of deep tissue damage with electrical injuries is often significantly greater than might be expected from the cutaneous appearance of entry and exit skin burns that are often surprisingly small. There may also be a delay of 24 to 48 hours before the full extent of this thermal injury becomes evident. Factors determining the size of an entry or exit wound are the skin resistance and extent of the site of contact with the electrical source. Larger wounds are generated by contact at a site of high skin resistance (such as a dry, calloused palm or sole), especially when the area of contact is small (allowing concentration of current flow through a small area). At the opposite extreme, no entry or exit wound at all may be seen in cases of bathtub electrocution because the area of contact is large (the entire skin surface) and the skin resistance is very low as a result of being wet (Kunkle, 1988).

Management of Electrical Injuries

Prolonged involuntary contact to an AC current source is painful, frightening, exhausting (from sustained tetanic muscle contraction), and potentially life-threatening (from induction of respiratory arrest, ventricular fibrillation, or severe internal injury). The first priority in management of electrical injuries must therefore be to separate the victim from the electrical source. *It is imperative never to touch the victim until the rescuer can be certain that current is no longer flowing!* If it is not possible to shut off the current, the victim may need to be separated from the electrical source by force using a nonconductive material such as rubber, rope, or wood (AHA ACLS Textbook, 1987). All "live" electrical sources should be removed from an accident scene.

Once the victim is freed from contact with the electrical source, evaluative and management measures are similar to those discussed in the previous section for lightning-related injuries *(Section 13D)*. Attention should first be directed toward treatment of unconscious or apparently dead

Table 13E-1

Potential Injuries from Electrical Exposure

Burns

- May only be superficial (flash or flame burns of the skin at the site of contact), but are commonly also deep (involving almost any internal organ) and thermal in nature (due to conversion of electrical energy into heat), especially following exposure to high-tension electrical sources).
- Lip commissure and mouth burns (especially common in children under 2 years of age from chewing through a lamp cord or sucking the end of an electrical outlet).

HEENT

- Cataracts *(which are common and sometimes only develop months after the event)*

Pulmonary

- Respiratory arrest *(which may result from tetanic contraction of the diaphragm or intercostal muscles, or from direct inhibition of the respiratory center)*

Cardiac

- Myocardial ischemia or infarction
- Cardiac arrest *(which is most often due to ventricular fibrillation)* *
- Cardiac arrhythmias *(virtually any arrhythmia may be seen)*

Abdomen

- Internal abdominal injury *(relatively uncommon)* **

Renal

- Renal failure *(from direct passage of current through the kidney or indirectly from myoglobinuria secondary to muscle necrosis)*

Musculoskeletal

- Fractures, dislocations, contusions, and sprains *(either as a direct result of tetanic muscle contraction, or indirectly from trauma caused by a fall or from the victim being forcibly thrown from the electrical source)*.
- Compartment syndromes (especially in victims of high-tension electrical exposure who demonstrate an entry or exit wound on the sole of the foot).

Vascular

- Ischemic necrosis of extremity vessels *(from direct thermal injury to the vessel wall with resultant vascular occlusion)*, sometimes leading to limb amputation.

Neurologic

- Seizures which may be immediate *(from anoxia or direct current passage through the brain)* or delayed in onset *(due to scar tissue formation)* for up to 2 years after the event.
- Neurologic deficit (C-spine injury should be assumed until proven otherwise for any victim who is unconscious and/or who may have sustained significant trauma)
- Impaired memory
- Headache
- Peripheral neuropathy *(which may be delayed in onset from perineural scarring)*

---

*This differs from the mechanism of cardiopulmonary arrest from lightning injuries, which is usually due to asystole.
**Intraabdominal involvement is relatively uncommon with electrical injuries, but paralytic ileus and potentially catastrophic injuries such as hemorrhagic necrosis of the gallbladder, intestinal perforation, and hepatic and pancreatic necrosis have been reported.
Adapted from Cooper and Karkal, 1987; Adams, 1988; Kunkle, 1988.

victims, since basic life support measures (such as rescue breathing) may occasionally be lifesaving, even after a seemingly prolonged period of unresponsiveness. Evaluative measures to consider for victims of significant electrical exposure include obtaining a 12-lead ECG and continuous ECG monitoring, x-ray studies (C-spine, chest, and extremity films) and laboratory tests (ABGs, CBC, SMAC, cardiac enzymes, blood type and cross, urinalysis, urine myoglobin, etc.) as appropriate. Those with cardiac signs or symptoms (chest pain, ECG changes, arrhythmias), neurologic abnormalities (altered level of consciousness, seizures, focal neurologic deficits), or significant trauma should be admitted to the hospital.

Two important differences between electrical and lightning-related injuries should be stressed. If cardiac arrest does occur with electrical injury, it is much more likely to be due to ventricular fibrillation. As a result, prompt defibrillation will almost always be needed if resuscitation of a victim of electrical injury is to be successful. This is in contrast to cardiac arrest from lightning-related injury in which asystole is most often the primary mechanism of the arrest, and for which basic life support (rescue breathing and external chest compression) may be all that are needed to sustain viability until spontaneous cardiac and respiratory function resume.

The other major difference to be aware of is that cutaneous involvement is much more likely to be deceptively small with electrical injury despite potentially deep penetration of current with significant internal injury. Should doubt exist about the true extent of injury, hospital admission with a period of observation is usually the wisest course of action. Additional management concerns for patients with high-voltage electrical injuries include adequate fluid replacement, correction of acidosis, and prevention of renal failure (from myoglobinuria) by maintenance of a high urine output (of 50-100 ml/hr). Extensive muscle necrosis predisposes to myoglobinuria and acidosis. Exudation and sequestration of large amounts of fluid is a common accompaniment of this deep tissue injury that is commonly seen with significant electrical exposure. Fluid loss is all too often underestimated, especially if volume replacement requirements are judged solely by the size of the surface wounds (Kunkle, 1988).

Last but not least, tetanus immunization status must be updated.

References and Suggested Readings

American Heart Association: *Special resuscitation situations.* In Jaffe A (ed): *Textbook of advanced cardiac life support*, Dallas, 1987, American Heart Association.

Adams SL: Electrical injuries (questions & answers), *JAMA* 260:2119, 1988.

Cooper MA, Karkal SS: Enhancing recovery from electrical and lightning injuries, *Emerg Med Reports* 8:57, 1987.

Cooper MA: *Lightning injuries.* In Rosen P (ed): *Emergency medicine: concepts and clinical practice*, St. Louis, 1988, Mosby–Year Book.

Kobernick M: Electrical injuries: pathophysiology and emergency management, *Ann Emerg Med* 11:633, 1982.

Kunkle RF: *Electrical injuries*, In Rosen P (ed): *Emergency medicine: concepts and clinical practice*, St. Louis, 1988, Mosby–Year Book.

SECTION F

COCAINE

Cocaine abuse is probably the major illicit drug problem in the United States today. The prevalence of use has increased more than fivefold over the past 15 years, and an estimated 30 million Americans tried the drug at least once in 1989 (Gawin and Ellinwood, 1988; Digregorio, 1990). The drug is *everywhere*—in big cities, smaller cities, and rural communities. To deny the potential presence of cocaine in *all* parts of the country is to ignore the scope of the problem.

> Medical professionals are not immune to cocaine addiction. Anonymous surveys suggest 15% to 20% of medical students have tried the drug, and as many as 5% indulge in regular (i.e., at least monthly) use (Schwartz et al, 1990). Considering the potentially lethal effects of acute intoxication, the ever-increasing prevalence of cocaine abuse poses a medical dilemma of epidemic proportions.

The Substance

Cocaine is an alkaloid derivative that can be isolated from the leaves of the *Erythroxylon* coca plant, a shrub indigenous to the mountain slopes of Central and South America. Therapeutically, the drug has long been favored for use in nasal procedures because of its efficacy and ease of application as a topical vasoconstrictor and local anesthetic. Medical concerns stem from the drug's potent CNS stimulatory action and potentially disastrous effects on the cardiovascular system.

Routes of Administration

Cocaine may be consumed via a number of routes of administration including oral ingestion, sublingual deposition, inhalation (i.e., smoking of freebase), snorting (intranasally), injection (either subcutaneously, intramuscularly, or intravenously), and absorption from vaginal or rectal mucosa.

The hydrochloride salt of cocaine is water-soluble, and this is the form of the drug used intravenously and intranasally. Heat degrades the salt, rendering it unsuitable for smoking. By a relatively simple process, however, cocaine *base* can be *freed* from the hydrochloride salt, leaving a stable, smokable compound known as *"freebase"* ("crack"). As opposed to other street forms of cocaine that are almost always diluted with adulterants, freebase is 95% to 100%

pure cocaine. Pulmonary absorption of smoked freebase is exceedingly efficient and rapid (occurring within seconds). The very high blood levels achieved from "crack" produce an intense euphoria. This leads to almost immediate gratification, which together with increasing street availability and decreased cost account for the exceedingly high addictive potential of freebase. Rapidly achieved and elevated drug concentrations as well as unpredictable drug absorption account for its high toxicity.

There are many similarities between cocaine reactions and drug reactions from other stimulants (such as amphetamines). One major difference is the significantly shorter duration of action of cocaine. Cardiovascular effects from cocaine begin within minutes of IV injection and usually subside by 20 to 30 minutes. As noted, effects from freebase smoking have an exceedingly rapid onset (within seconds). Duration of action is usually less than with IV injection. Compared to IV injection and inhalation, intranasal administration has a slower onset of action (requiring up to 20 minutes to achieve peak levels). Cardiovascular effects usually dissipate by 45 to 60 minutes.

Regardless of the route of administration, duration of action of the cocaine experience is relatively short compared to that experienced from use of other drugs. This in another important reason for cocaine's strong addiction potential. Users crave more drug sooner, and are more likely to fall into a pattern of binge use with frequent readministration. During binges, a cocaine user typically loses interest in all other daily functions including life pleasures and responsibilities. Drug is continuously administered until the user's supply is exhausted. Several days may then pass until the supply is renewed, and the cycle (i.e., the start of a new binge) then repeats itself.

Mechanism of Action

The mechanism of action for cocaine's cardiovascular and CNS effects involves catecholamine neurotransmitters. The drug specifically blocks reuptake of norepinephrine and dopamine at central and peripheral presynaptic nerve endings in the nervous system. This results in an increased concentration of these catecholamine neurotransmitters at post-synaptic nerve endings, leading to central and peripheral adrenergic stimulation. Heart rate and blood pressure are increased as a result of this sympathetic discharge. Traditionally, drugs that counteract sympathetic discharge (i.e., β-blockers) have been recommended for treatment of cardiovascular complications. Although the use of β-blockers for treatment of cocaine intoxication/overdose seems logical, a potential downside to such therapy has been suggested by recent studies that show β-blockade may lead to unopposed α-adrenergic stimulation and enhanced vasoconstriction. β-Blocker–induced coronary vasoconstriction causing ischemia may result (Nademanee et al, 1989). Catecholamine neurotransmitters are also mediators in the ascending reticular activating system and hypothalamus. Appreciation of the fact that these centers regulate control of alertness, sleep, appetite, sexual arousal, and emotional expression facilitates our understanding of the principal clinical manifestations of cocaine use and abuse.

Clinical Application

Emergency care providers are likely to encounter patients with a number of patterns of cocaine use and abuse. These include acute simple intoxication, acute overdose, acute toxic psychosis, chronic abuse, and withdrawal. The salient features facilitating recognition of each of these patterns appear in *Tables 13F-1* through *Table 13F-5*. Special considerations for evaluation and management of acute intoxication and overdose follow in *Tables 13F-6* and *13F-7*.

Table 13F-1

Signs and Symptoms of Acute Simple Cocaine Intoxication*

Cardiovascular Manifestations
- Hypertension
- Tachycardia *(although a short-lived bradycardia may initially be seen from a reflex vagal effect)*

Other Systemic Manifestations
- Increased respiratory rate and depth *(which is often followed by dyspnea)*
- Mydriasis *(from sympathetic activation)*
- Increased temperature *(from heat generated by intense muscle contraction)*
- Decreased appetite

Psychologic Manifestations
- Restlessness/inability to sit still
- Emotional lability/increased irritability
- Increased energy/lack of fatigue
- Euphoria *(marked by a profound sense of well being, enhanced self-confidence in one's physical and mental abilities, mood elation, and a magnified sense of pleasure)*

Neurologic Manifestations
- Nonintentional tremor
- Twitching of the small muscles of the face, fingers, and feet
- Hyperexcitability *(marked by generalized stimulation to sensory input)*

*Practically speaking, we define **Acute Simple Cocaine Intoxication** as a reaction to a relatively low dose of cocaine from which there are no serious medical complications.

Table 13F-2

Signs and Symptoms of Acute Cocaine Overdose*

Cardiovascular Manifestations
- Hypertension
- Tachycardia and other cardiac arrhythmias
- Chest pain/ischemia/coronary spasm/acute MI
- Cardiac arrest *(from cocaine-induced ventricular fibrillation)*

Other Systemic Manifestations
- Hyperglycemia/hypoglycemia
- Hyperthermia ("cocaine fever")
- Dyspnea/irregular respiratory pattern
- Respiratory depression and/or arrest *(especially if other sedative drugs were also ingested)*

Psychologic Manifestations
- Toxic psychosis *(see Table 13F-3 below)*

Neurologic Manifestations
- Agitation
- Confusion
- Mydriasis
- Cerebral vascular accident *(from stroke or cerebral hemorrhage)*
- Tremor and muscle twitching which may lead to seizures *(either single seizures or status epilepticus)*

*As opposed to simple intoxication, we define **Acute Cocaine Overdose** as a reaction to a larger (potentially lethal) dose of cocaine that is associated with more serious clinical manifestations.

Table 13F-3

Signs and Symptoms of Acute Toxic Psychosis*

- Marked agitation and restlessness
- Hyperexcitability *(to even minimal external stimuli)*
- General fearfulness
- General suspiciousness
- Delusions of persecution *(especially of being observed or pursued)*
- Altered behavioral traits, often with a tendency toward becoming violent
- Grandiose feelings
- Visual and/or tactile hallucinations *(i.e., "cocaine bugs" crawling on the skin)*

*We define **Acute Toxic Psychosis** as a combination of acute psychiatric findings that are most often associated with ingestion of either a single large dose of cocaine, or with long-term abuse of the drug. In the latter case, signs and symptoms may persist for days (or even weeks) after stopping the drug. Clinically, acute presentation may very much resemble the presentation of a patient with paranoid schizophrenia in crisis. As with schizophrenia, recent memory as well as orientation to time, place and person usually remain intact.

Table 13F-4

Signs and Symptoms of Chronic Cocaine Abuse*

Cardiovascular and Systemic Manifestations
- Chronic pupillary dilatation *(which may lead to visual disturbances such as photophobia or impaired focusing ability)*
- *Other cardiovascular and systemic signs and symptoms often become blunted with time!*

Behavioral Manifestations
- Chronic fatigue
- Restlessness
- Insomnia
- Difficulty concentrating *(with poor performance at school or work)*
- Decreased appetite *(which together with chronic overstimulation may lead to weight loss)*
- Toxic psychosis *(see Table 13F-3)*
- Increased tendency to violence (either as a direct effect of the drug and/or related to the tremendous amounts of money involved with sale and illegal distribution of cocaine)

Complications from Chronic Drug Use
- Venereal disease *(including syphilis, gonorrhea, and AIDS, especially with IV cocaine use)*
- Endocarditis *(especially with IV cocaine use)*
- Local skin infection
- Sinusitis/perforated nasal septum
- Tics and other motor disorders
- Myoglobinuric renal failure *(from cocaine binge-related immobility)*
- Seizures

*We define the state of **Chronic Cocaine Abuse** as the result of long-term repeated use of the drug. With time (and development of tolerance), the physical signs of acute intoxication listed in Table 13F-1 become blunted. Ultimately, they may not be present at all. Instead the presenting complaint of long-term cocaine use is likely to be a *complication* arising from chronic drug abuse. Assessment is made even more difficult by frequent occurrence of the pattern of *mixed drug abuse* that is seen when alcohol and/or other sedative drugs are also ingested in an attempt to counteract the overstimulation from repeated cocaine use.

Table 13F-5

Signs and Symptoms of Cocaine Withdrawal*

Acute Withdrawal ("Crash")
- Intense depression *(which may lead to suicide ideation)*
- Generalized fatigue *(and a strong desire for sleep)*
- Ravenous appetite
- Craving for additional cocaine *(that may eventually subside with adequate rest, nutrition, and continued abstinence)*

Later Withdrawal
- Mood lability *(often in association with underlying anxiety)*
- Depression *(that is generally less intense than that seen during "crash")*
- Anhedonia *(loss of pleasure)*
- Low energy level/listlessness
- Sleep disturbances
- Suspiciousness
- Persistent urge for cocaine (which may persist for *years* after abstinence—and which probably accounts for the very high relapse rate)

*We define **Withdrawal** as the complex of symptoms occurring after a period of cocaine use. Withdrawal typically has two phases: (1) An initial *"crash"* that begins within hours of stopping the drug, and which lasts hours to several days; and (2) a *Later Withdrawal Phase* that begins a number of days after the "crash," and which lasts for weeks to several months.

Table 13F-6

Principles of Management of an Acute *(Potentially Life-Threatening)* Cocaine Reaction*

1. Attend to the **ABCs** *(Assure an adequate airway; ventilate the patient who is not spontaneously breathing; intubate if needed; provide supplemental oxygen as indicated; assess circulation and verify adequate perfusion.)*
2. Insert a large bore intravenous line.
3. Consider inserting a Foley catheter *(if urine output monitoring needed and/or the patient is unresponsive)*
4. Institute continuous ECG monitoring:
   - Consider **lidocaine** or **propranolol** (or other IV β-blockers) for ventricular arrhythmias in need of treatment
   - Consider **propranolol** (or other IV β-blockers) for supraventricular arrhythmias in need of treatment
5. Consider gastric lavage, activated charcoal, and use of a cathartic agent *after* securing airway IF:
   - Cocaine was orally ingested
   - Suspicion of other orally ingested drug abuse exists
6. Treat potentially reversible complicating factors:
   - **D50W** *(after drawing Dextrostix)*
   - **Narcan** *(if narcotic abuse suspected)*
   - **Thiamine**—100 mg PO, IM, or IV *(if patient has a history of alcohol abuse)*
7. Obtain appropriate laboratory tests:
   - Standard blood work (CBC, chem profile with electrolytes and BUN/creatinine)
   - Urinalysis
   - ABGs
   - ECG
   - X-ray studies (chest x-ray and flat plate of the abdomen if indicated)
   - Drug screen (including alcohol level)
8. Watch for seizure activity:
   - Consider **valium** (which may be needed in high doses!) for acute seizures
   - Consider IV **dilantin** and appropriate work-up as indicated *(i.e., CT scan)* for other causes if seizure activity persists
9. After stabilization of potentially lifethreatening complications, minimize *(as much as possible)* external sensory stimuli that might aggravate the patient's reaction to cocaine.
   - Use of valium *(for its antianxiety effect)* and haldol *(for its antipsychotic effect)* is controversial. In particular, the use of haldol must be balanced against the fact that the drug may lower seizure threshold.

Special Assessment/Treatment Measures

- Be sure to check **temperature** *(to rule out hyperthermia, which commonly complicates acute cocaine reactions)*
- Consider performing **rectal** and **pelvic examinations,** as well as obtaining a **flat plate x-ray of the abdomen** (to rule out the possibility of "body packing"). *Rectal and pelvic examinations should be performed with care to avoid rupturing concealed packets of cocaine.*
- Carefully monitor cardiovascular and pulmonary status with:
  1. Frequent vital sign checks (of heart rate, blood pressure and respiratory rate)
  2. Continuous ECG monitoring (for arrhythmias)
  3. ABGs/oxygen saturation monitoring *(to assure adequate ventilation/oxygenation)*
- Consider treatment of severe hypertension with IV β-blockers, labetalol, or nitroprusside.
- Consider treatment of hypotension/shock with dopamine, isoproterenol, and/or IV fluid administration as indicated.

Specific Drug Therapy to Consider

Propranolol—0.5 to 1 mg by *slow* IV (over ≥ 1 minute) up to 5 mg total
Labetalol—20 mg IV as an initial bolus, followed by 20 to 80 mg IV increments q 10 minutes as needed (up to a maximum cumulative dose of 300 mg). The drug may also be given as an IV infusion at 2 mg/minute

---

*Although acute cocaine reactions can be extremely serious, emergency care providers may at least take some comfort from the fact that the acute reaction is usually self-limited (due to the short half-life of cocaine), and prognosis for survival is good if initial treatment effectively controls lifethreatening aspects of the reaction.

Table 13F-7

Selected Special Considerations

- An unfortunate consequence of the relatively *short duration of action* of cocaine reactions is that all too many patients never receive medical attention. Milder reactions tend to resolve spontaneously in the home, while more severe reactions that lead to cardiovascular collapse are often fatal before arrival at an emergency facility.

- Although early in the process of cocaine abuse the physical signs and symptoms of acute intoxication are quite characteristic (Table 13F-1), they often become blunted with chronic use and development of tolerance. As a result, it may be exceedingly difficult to recognize acute intoxication in a long-term, chronic abuser.

- Street cocaine is often diluted with adulterants such as amphetamine, caffeine, and phencyclidine (PCP). This explains why drug screens of cocaine users are often positive for multiple substances. Management is complicated because the adulterants may be concentrated enough to produce adverse effects of their own.

- The intense **euphoria** of acute intoxication usually lasts 15 to 90 minutes (depending on the amount of cocaine taken and the route of administration), and is the major factor leading the chronic abuser to the typical pattern of repeated use. Euphoria is usually followed by a longer state (lasting several hours) of anxiety, dysphoria and ultimately depression (which may be marked by crying spells and other strong feelings of negativity).

- "Drug hunger" for cocaine may last for *years*. The potential for relapse after a period of abstinence is so great that even *memories* associated with previous use may bring on an attack! An entirely new social network must therefore be developed for there to be any realistic chance of curing addiction.

- The *increased temperature* that is often seen with acute cocaine intoxication or overdose may be an extremely helpful differential sign for distinguishing this type of stimulant abuse from other acute psychologic reactions.

- Although it is common for respiratory rate to increase initially with acute cocaine overdose, it ultimately becomes depressed. Respiratory status must therefore be monitored closely to guard against respiratory arrest *(which otherwise is a frequent cause of death, especially if other sedative drugs were also taken.)*

- The intense α- and β-adrenergic stimulatory effects of cocaine may produce a number of potentially serious (lifethreatening) cardiovascular complications, including hypertensive urgency/emergency; coronary vasospasm/ischemia/infarction; cardiac arrhythmias; and cardiovascular collapse/shock.

    Cocaine overdose may precipitate acute myocardial infarction in young adults, even in the absence of preexisting coronary disease. *It is probably the major cause of acute myocardial infarction in adults under 30* (Tokarski et al, 1990; Goldfrank and Hoffman, 1991). As a result, an ECG should be routinely obtained in all cocaine abusers with any cardiac symptoms regardless of their age or previous health status.

- Be aware of the practice of **"body packing"** in which addicts/drug smugglers may conceal large amounts of cocaine in latex-covered packets that are swallowed or inserted into body cavities (i.e., vagina, rectum). Rupture of one or more of these packets (either spontaneously or through manipulation during attempted removal) may release enough of the drug to cause a rapidly lethal cocaine reaction. A flat plate x-ray of the abdomen is surprisingly sensitive in detecting "body packing."

- **Propranolol** has long been recommended for management of arrhythmias and hypertensive crisis associated with acute cocaine reactions.* However, caution is urged in patients with underlying coronary disease, especially if the possibility of acute ischemia or infarction exists. β-Blockade in this case may enhance sensitivity to unopposed α-adrenergic receptors which may provoke coronary vasospasm (aggravating ischemia) and/or exacerbate hypertension (Nademanee et al, 1989; Lange et al, 1990). Treatment with other antiarrhythmic agents, calcium channel blockers, nitrates, and/or labetalol may constitute a more appropriate (and safer) approach in such patients.

- **Labetalol** is a non-selective β-blocker with α-blocking and direct vasodilatory properties. The drug lowers blood pressure through reduction of peripheral vascular resistance. Adverse effects tend to be dose dependent, and may be related to α-adrenergic blockade (i.e., orthostatic hypotension, dizziness) and/or β-adrenergic blockade (i.e., bronchospasm, decreased contractility, etc.). Labetalol is an excellent agent for treatment of hypertensive urgency/emergency because of its rapid onset (in ≤5 minutes) and ease of administration (minute-to-minute drug titration is not necessary, as it is for nitroprusside). Duration of action is 3 to 6 hours. Labetalol may be a better choice for management of cocaine-associated hypertensive crisis because of its effect on both α- and β-adrenergic receptors.

*IV **esmolol** (administered as a 500 μg/kg loading dose over 1 minute, followed by a 50 to 200 μg/kg/min infusion) may be an alternative to IV propranolol. Attractive features of this drug are β-1 selectivity and its very short half-life of action. A drawback is its more complicated dosing protocol.

References and Suggested Readings

Digregorio GJ: Cocaine update: abuse and therapy, *Am Fam Physician* 41:247, 1990.

Garber MW, Flaherty D: Cocaine and sudden death, *Am Fam Physician* 36:227, 1987.

Gawin FH: Cocaine abuse and addiction, *J Fam Pract* 29:193, 1989.

Gawin FH, Ellinwood EH: Cocaine and other stimulants: actions, abuse and treatment, *N Engl J Med* 218:1173, 1988.

Gay GR: Clinical management of acute and chronic cocaine poisoning, *Ann Emerg Med* 11:562, 1982.

Goldfrank LR, Hoffman RS: The cardiovascular effects of cocaine, *Ann Emerg Med* 20:165, 1991.

Hankes L: Cocaine: today's drug, *J Fla Med Assoc* 7:235, 1984.

Kossowsky WA, Lyon AF, Chou S: Acute non-Q-wave cocaine related myocardial infarction, *Chest* 96:617, 1989.

Lange RA, Cigarroa RG, Flores ED, McBride W, Kim AS, Wells PJ, Bedotto JB, Danziger RS, Hillis LD: Potentiation of cocaine-induced coronary vasoconstriction by beta-adrenergic blockade, *Ann Intern Med* 112:897, 1990.

Levine SR, Welch KMA: Cocaine and stroke, *Curr Concepts Cerebrovascular Disease Stroke* 22:25, 1987.

McMullen MJ: Chapter 116: *Stimulants*. In Rosen P (ed): *Emergency medicine: concepts and clinical practice*, St Louis, 1988, Mosby–Year Book.

Medical Letter: Acute reactions to drugs of abuse, *Med Letter* 32:92, 1990.

Miller NS, Gold MS, Millman RL: Cocaine, *Am Fam Physician* 39:115, 1989.

Nademanee K, Gorelick DA, Josephson MA, Ryan MA, Wilkins JN, Robertson HA, Mody FV, Intarachot V: Myocardial ischemia during cocaine withdrawal, *Ann Intern Med* 111:876, 1989.

Schwartz RH, Lewis DC, Hoffmann NG, Kyriazi N: Cocaine and marijuana use by medical students before and during medical school, *Arch Intern Med* 150:883, 1990.

Tokarski GF, Paganussi P, Urbanski R, Carden D, Foreback C, Tomlanovich MC: An evaluation of cocaine-induced chest pain, *Ann Emerg Med* 19:1088, 1990.

SECTION G

TRICYCLIC ANTIDEPRESSANT OVERDOSE

The tricyclic antidepressants (TCAs) are one of the most commonly misused classes of medications. TCA overdose accounts for an estimated 15% of all hospital admissions for self-poisoning with a disproportionate share of intensive care unit admissions and mortality compared to other drug ingestions (Frommer et al, 1987; Ware, 1987).

The potential for overdose from TCAs is huge. In addition to being the pharmacologic agent of choice for treatment of major depression, TCAs are also commonly used to treat patients with chronic pain disorders, diabetic neuropathy, and fibromyositis. More than 25 million prescriptions are written each year in the United States for TCAs (Callaham, 1988).

Relevant Pharmacology

TCAs were introduced in the 1960s. These drugs form a group of closely related compounds that have in common a three-ring chemical structure (ergo the name "tri-cyclic"). Recent years have seen development of a number of newer *(second generation)* antidepressants. Despite a somewhat different chemical structure, overall pharmacologic properties and therapeutic effects of the second-generation drugs are similar to those of the original tricyclics. Consequently, we include them in this chapter's discussion of TCA overdose. We list the commonly used antidepressant agents in *Table 13G-1*, together with relevant clinical characteristics specific for each drug.

In therapeutic doses, TCAs are generally well absorbed from the gastrointestinal tract. In overdose, however, absorption is often delayed (by up to 12 hours) because the anticholinergic properties of the drug slow peristalsis and delay gastric emptying. Because of the high lipid solubility of these drugs, they have an exceedingly large volume of distribution (10-30 L/kg!). In addition, renal clearance is extremely low (i.e., <5%). As a result, treatment measures such as dialysis or forced diuresis are not effective in facilitating removal of drug from the bloodstream.* On the contrary, excessive volume infusion may predispose to fluid overload and pulmonary edema, a potentially lethal complication considering the tendency of TCAs to produce cardiovascular toxicity in overdose.

Serum drug concentrations (SDCs) reflect the total amount of circulating drug. This includes an inactive portion (i.e., drug bound to serum proteins) and the active portion ("free" or unbound drug). Because the percentage of total drug that is bound is so highly variable (demonstrating up to a ninefold difference among patients receiving the same dose), SDCs provide little useful clinical information in overdose other than to document that tricyclic ingestion has in fact occurred (Frommer et al, 1987; Callaham, 1988).

> Appreciation of how alteration in the degree of protein binding affects serum concentration of active drug becomes important in management of acute TCA overdose. **Alkalinization** *of serum pH increases protein binding.* This significantly lessens the potential for drug toxicity because it reduces the amount of available free drug (Frommer et al, 1987; Callaham, 1988).

Much attention is often devoted to assessing how much drug was ingested in a given overdose attempt. Although inquiry to the amount and type of medication kept in the home is recommended, trying to determine whether the patient could have ingested a "lethal dose" of TCAs is usually neither possible nor practical because:

1. the degree of protein binding exerts an important but unpredictable influence on the amount of free (active) drug
2. TCA ingestions are often mixed with other agents (especially alcohol and/or benzodiazepines), and this may significantly affect their potential toxicity (Kathol and Henn, 1983; Ware, 1987)
3. the history regarding the amount of drug ingested is often unreliable, and
4. there is high interpatient variability in the amount of drug that constitutes a lethal dose (Callaham, 1988).

Death has been reported following TCA ingestion of as little as 500 mg (which is no more than a handful of 100 mg pills). In contrast, other patients have survived following TCA ingestion of more than 10 gm (Turbiak, 1983; Ware, 1987).

Signs and Symptoms of TCA Overdose

Manifestations of TCA overdose primarily affect the neurologic and cardiovascular systems. In most cases of significant TCA ingestion, symptoms are seen within hours of taking the drug. Earliest manifestations include sinus tachycardia (the most frequent sign) and other an-

---

*The exception to this generality is amoxapine overdose, for which forced diuresis is recommended to prevent acute renal failure (Jennings et al, 1983; Ware, 1987).

Table 13G-1

Drug Class	Initial Dose (mg/day)	Therapeutic Dose (mg/day)	Anticholinergic Effect	Sedative Effect	Orthostatic Hypotension
Common Antidepressant Agents					
Tricyclics					
Amitriptyline (Elavil; Endep)	25-75 mg HS	50-300 mg	+ + + +	+ + +	+ +
Doxepin (Sinequan; Adapin)	25-75 mg HS	50-300 mg	+ +	+ + +	+ +
Imipramine (Tofranil; Janimine)	25-75 mg HS	50-300 mg	+ +	+ +	+ + +
Notriptyline (Aventyl; Pamelor)	25-50 mg HS	50-100 mg	+	+ +	+
Desipramine (Norpramin)	25-50 mg HS	75-300 mg	+	+	+
Protriptyline (Vivactil)	10-20 mg HS	20-60 mg	+ + +	+	+
Trimipramine (Surmontil)	50-75 mg HS	75-300 mg	+ +	+ + +	+ +
Second-Generation Antidepressant Agents					
Tetracyclics					
Maprotiline (Ludiomil)*	25 mg Tid	75-225 mg	+	+ +	+
Dibenzoxipine					
Amoxapine (Asendin)*	50 mg Tid	200-300 mg	+	+ +	+
Triazolopyridine					
Trazodone (Desyrel)**	50 mg Bid	200-600 mg	±	+ +	+ +
Fluoxetine (Prozac)***	20 mg Qd	10-80 mg	±	—	+
Unicyclic Aminoketone					
Bupropion (Wellbutrin)***	75 mg Tid	75-450 mg	+	—	—

*__Maprotiline__ and **Amoxapine**—appear to cause less cardiovascular toxicity in TCA overdose, but this effect is counterbalanced by an increased likelihood of seizures.
**__Trazodone__—appears to have almost negligible cardiovascular and CNS toxicity in TCA overdose. *(This feature may make this agent a drug of choice for depressed patients who appear to be at especially high risk of overdosing!)*
***__Fluoxetine__ and **Bupropion**—appear to have minimal cardiovascular toxicity in TCA overdose. The risk of seizures is relatively low, but these drugs should be used with caution in patients with a history of seizures.

ticholinergic effects of the drug. Thinking of the *"4 C's"* facilitates recall of the four most characteristic manifestations of severe ingestions: **c**oma, **c**onvulsions, **c**onduction defects, and depressed **c**ontractility. These and other signs and symptoms of TCA overdose are listed in *Table 13G-2*.

Management of TCA Overdose

Evaluative and management measures to consider for patients with acute TCA overdose are suggested in *Table 13G-3*. Unfortunately, there is no specific antidote, so that treatment of TCA overdose is largely supportive. Selected aspects of management are expanded upon and emphasized below.

GASTRIC LAVAGE/ACTIVATED CHARCOAL

Because excess anticholinergic activity may significantly delay gastric emptying, attempts at pill removal are recommended and may be effective for up to 12 hours following TCA overdose (Ware, 1987). Gastric lavage may be preferable to induction of emesis (with syrup of ipecac) for cases in which large amounts of drug were ingested. Sudden depression of mental status or seizures may occur at any time, which would greatly increase the risk of aspiration if ipecac was given. Another potential disadvantage of using ipecac is that its prolonged emetic effect may necessitate delaying instillation of activated charcoal.

Repeated doses of activated charcoal (and catharsis) are recommended for treatment of severe TCA overdose. In

Table 13G-2

Signs and Symptoms of TCA Overdose

Anticholinergic Signs and Symptoms
- Pupil dilatation (mydriasis) with blurred vision
- Dry mouth
- Fever
- Urinary retention
- Decreased peristalsis with delayed gastric emptying
- Anticholinergic psychosis (confusion, delirium, hallucinations)

Neurologic Signs and Symptoms
- Increased CNS irritability (agitation, hyperreflexia, myoclonus, seizures)
- Depressed level of consciousness (drowsiness, lethargy, and ultimately coma)

Cardiovascular Signs and Symptoms
- Sinus tachycardia (which is really an *anticholinergic* effect of the drug, unlike the other manifestations of cardiovascular toxicity that are listed here)
- Hypertension initially (from release of norepinephrine from presynaptic endplates); *ultimately hypotension* (from neurotransmittor catecholamine depletion, α-receptor blockade and/or direct cardiac depression)
- ECG abnormalities (ST segment and T wave abnormalities; right axis deviation; PR, QRS, and QT prolongation; and other conduction disturbances including bundle branch block or AV block)
- Cardiac arrhythmias (supraventricular and ventricular)
- Depressed myocardial contractility (aggravating hypotension and ultimately leading to heart failure and cardiovascular collapse)
- Cardiopulmonary arrest (from respiratory depression, cardiogenic shock, ventricular tachycardia or fibrillation, or torsade de pointes)

Adapted from Frommer et al, 1987.

Table 13G-3

Suggested Evaluative and Management Approach to Acute TCA Overdose

1. Attend first to the ABCs (establishment of an airway with respiratory and circulatory support as needed).
2. Establish IV access.
3. Place patient on continuous ECG monitoring.
4. Assess mental status.
   If patient comatose, administer **Narcan** and **Thiamine** (100 mg IM), followed by an ampule of D50W. Consider other possible etiologies for coma (i.e., cerebral hemorrhage, trauma, ingestion of other drugs, etc.), and initiate work-up as appropriate.
5. Perform a rapid, targeted physical exam (with special attention to cardiopulmonary function and detection of focal neurologic abnormalities).
6. Administer oxygen if consciousness impaired or hypoxia suspected.
7. Obtain 12-lead ECG, chest x-ray, ABGs, and other standard laboratory tests (CBC, SMAC, prothrombin time, urinalysis) to assess electrolyte balance, and renal and hepatic function.
8. Obtain toxicology screen (including alcohol level).
9. Place Foley catheter (if appropriate), and monitor urine output.
10. Pass nasogastric or preferably a large-bore (36 to 40 F) orogastric tube, and initiate gastric lavage. Follow with **activated charcoal** (50-100 g in a slurry) and **cathartic** (such as 300 ml of magnesium citrate). Repeat every 2 to 4 hours

Continued.

Table 13G-3—cont'd

to facilitate TCA elimination from the vascular compartment and reduce enterohepatic circulation of potentially active TCA metabolites.

11. Treat seizures:
    - **Diazepam** (Valium)—2-5 mg/min IV (up to 10 mg); May repeat 5-10 mg q10-30 minutes as needed

    or

    - **Ativan** (Lorazepam)—1-2 mg IV initially; May repeat 1-2 mg IV q 5-10 minutes as needed until desired effect. *(Unlike diazepam, loraze-pam is usually well absorbed and effective if given IM—which is a decided advantage if IV access is unavailable.)*
    - Consider **Phenytoin** (Dilantin) either as a therapeutic measure (if seizures have occurred) or *prophylactically* (even without seizures) in cases of significant TCA ingestion.
        Suggested dose of phenytoin = 10-15 mg/kg (up to 1,000 mg) slow IV loading (i.e., *not* faster than 50 mg/min), with careful ECG monitoring during administration.
    - Consider Physostigmine if other measures not successful.*

12. Consider serum **alkalinization** (by **sodium bicarbonate** administration and/or hyperventilation) to achieve an arterial pH of 7.45-7.55, especially if there is evidence of significant toxicity (depressed mental status, hypotension, arrhythmias).

13. Consider treatment of worrisome ventricular arrhythmias (i.e., frequent or repetitive PVCs, ventricular tachycardia):†
    - **Lidocaine—***Use standard dosing of this drug*
    - Other measures—**alkalinization,** phenytoin *(as above)*
    - Consideration of magnesium sulfate
    - Physostigmine*

14. Treat torsade de pointes *(see Section C in Chapter 16):*
    - **Magnesium Sulfate** (10% solution)—1-2 gm given IV over 1-2 minutes, and repeated 5-15 minutes later if no response
    - Overdrive pacing
    - Correction of hypokalemia (if present)
    - Serum **alkalinization**

15. Treat hypotension:
    - Volume expansion
    - Serum **alkalinization**
    - Vasopressors (dopamine or norepinephrine infusion)—although dopamine may be tried initially, norepinephrine will often be needed because TCA-induced hypotension is often resistant to dopamine‡
    - Dobutamine (for inotropic effect if myocardial depression severe)

16. Arrange for appropriate psychiatric evaluation and follow-up.

---

*Reserve **physostigmine** for treatment of life-threatening complications (ventricular tachyarrhythmias, hypotension, seizures, or severe anticholinergic psychosis) that have *not* responded to other therapy. If used, the dose is 1-2 mg IV (given *slowly* over 2 minutes), which may be repeated in 20-30 minutes. Alternatively, the drug may be administered IM (1-2 mg q 2 hours). Because of physostigmine's short duration of action, repeat doses are often needed to prevent recurrence of TCA toxicity.
†Type I antiarrhythmics (i.e., quinidine, procainamide), bretylium, and β-blockers are best avoided in treatment of patients with TCA overdose.
‡Epinephrine might best be avoided for treatment of severe shock associated with TCA overdose because its β-adrenergic stimulating effect may further exacerbate hypotension. *Norepinephrine is the pressor of choice for severe hypotension associated with significant TCA overdose.*
Adapted from Frommer et al, 1987; Ware, 1987.

---

addition to decreasing absorption, activated charcoal may also shorten the overall duration of TCA toxicity by blocking enterohepatic recirculation of the ingested drug and its potentially active metabolites (Ware, 1987). Unfortunately, rapid tissue binding and the large volume of distribution of TCAs limit the clinical usefulness of this therapeutic measure.

CARDIAC MONITORING AND CARDIOVASCULAR TOXICITY

Patients who develop severe cardiovascular toxicity from TCA overdose tend to do so within the first few hours following drug ingestion (Callaham 1985, 1988). Although orderly progression of cardiac changes (from sinus tachycardia—to right axis deviation and conduction disturbances—to sustained ventricular tachyarrhythmias and/or torsade de pointes) is typically described, this sequence of progression rarely holds true in clinical practice. In fact, evolution of signs and symptoms may at times may be so rapid that a patient can be alert one moment and comatose with a life-threatening cardiovascular complication the next (Callaham, 1985; Frommer et al, 1987).

In the past, an extended period of ECG monitoring (48-96 hours) was routinely recommended for patients with significant TCA ingestion. Recent studies suggest *extended monitoring (beyond 24 hours) is not necessary for patients who do not demonstrate clinical evidence of major toxicity during this time.* If adverse cardiovascular reactions are to occur, they are almost always seen within the first 24 hours following ingestion. It is exceedingly rare for de novo cardiac toxicity to develop in a patient who remains alert and has a normal ECG during this initial period of monitoring (Goldberg et al, 1985; Ware, 1987).

It is of interest that the best predictor of potentially lethal complications (from either seizures or arrhythmias) is QRS prolongation to ≥ 0.10 seconds (Goldberg et al, 1985; Frommer et al, 1987).* Despite being extremely common, sinus tachycardia is not a good indicator of serious cardiovascular toxicity. Isolated sinus tachycardia may result from a number of factors including the anticholinergic effect of TCA ingestion, simultaneous ingestion of other drugs (especially alcohol), dehydration, and anxiety generated by the hospital treatment itself. Hypotension is clearly associated with a poor prognosis, and often precedes cardiac arrest. Unfortunately, this sign usually occurs too late in the course for it to be helpful as a prognostic indicator.

VENTRICULAR ARRHYTHMIAS

The treatment of choice of worrisome ventricular arrhythmias associated with TCA overdose (frequent or repetitive PVCs, ventricular tachycardia) is lidocaine. Adjunctive measures include serum alkalinization and administration of phenytoin. Type I antiarrhythmics (i.e., quinidine, procainamide) are contraindicated because of their tendency to aggravate conduction disturbances (QRS widening and QT prolongation) and/or precipitate torsade de pointes. Bretylium is best avoided because its mechanism of action (sympathetic ganglionic blockade) may further exacerbate hypotension. β-Blockers should probably also be avoided because of their potentially deleterious effects on blood pressure and myocardial contractility.

---

*The only reservation about using this criterion is the necessity of knowing the patient's baseline QRS duration. A QRS duration of 0.10 seconds may be (at the upper limit of) normal for some patients. Others may have preexisting bundle branch block. Availability of a prior tracing (or at least obtaining a 12-lead ECG at the time the patient presents to the ED) is therefore essential for evaluating the significance of QRS widening.

TORSADE DE POINTES

Torsade de pointes is a special type of ventricular tachyarrhythmia in which the polarity of QRS complexes constantly changes. We discuss the entity in detail in Chapter 16. Key points to emphasize here are the importance of early recognition and appropriate treatment of the disorder.

QT interval prolongation predisposes to development of torsade de pointes. Patients with significant ingestion of TCAs should be carefully observed with continuous ECG monitoring for the initial 24 hours following overdose, especially when there are ECG abnormalities on the baseline tracing. Longer periods of monitoring may be needed for those with persistent QT prolongation or QRS widening. Efforts should be made to correct conduction system abnormalities (reduction of circulating TCAs by gastric lavage/activated charcoal, correction of hypokalemia which may further lengthen the QT interval, and consideration of phenytoin and/or serum alkalinization). Type I antiarrhythmic agents *must* be avoided. Optimal treatment of full-blown torsade de pointes consists of *magnesium sulfate* and *overdrive pacing* until the serum level of the offending TCA returns to normal (Tzivoni et al, 1984, 1988; Martinez, 1987).

HYPOTENSION/CARDIOVASCULAR COLLAPSE

Hypotension associated with TCA overdose may result from a combination of factors including neurotransmittor catecholamine depletion, α-adrenergic receptor blockade-induced vasodilatation, peripheral β-adrenergic receptor stimulation, and/or a direct myocardial depressant effect. Treatment consists of volume infusion, serum *alkalinization* (to a pH of 7.45-7.55), and use of pressor agents (if needed). Because TCAs block catecholamine uptake in both central and peripheral adrenergic receptors, direct α-adrenergic pressor agents such as *norepinephrine* may be preferable to indirect agents such as dopamine which rely on release of norepinephrine at receptor sites (Frommer et al, 1987; Teba et al, 1988). Epinephrine might best be avoided for treatment of severe shock associated with TCA overdose because its β-adrenergic receptor stimulating effect may further exacerbate hypotension. Finally, if myocardial depression is severe, addition of the positively inotropic agent dobutamine may prove useful.

Despite the potential severity and life-threatening nature of severe TCA cardiovascular toxicity, overdose victims who do not have preexisting cardiac disease may respond to prolonged attempts at resuscitation, even in the face of seemingly pre-terminal arrhythmias such as refractory ventricular fibrillation, EMD, or asystole (Callaham, 1985; Ware, 1987; Frommer et al, 1987). As a result, an attempt at vigorous resuscitation is almost always warranted, and resuscitative efforts should be continued until it becomes clear that such measures are futile.

USE OF PHENYTOIN (DILANTIN)

Dilantin is especially suited for treatment of patients with TCA overdose because it has both anticonvulsant and antiarrhythmic effects. Clinically, its antiarrhythmic effect is not as potent as that of other drugs used for this purpose. However, the drug may be unique from other antiarrhythmic agents in its ability to improve conduction defects, a particularly useful property in cases of severe TCA cardiovascular toxicity (Uhl, 1981; Boehnert and Lovejoy, 1985; Ware, 1987). Moreover, there are isolated case reports in which torsade de pointes refractory to other treatment measures responded only to IV phenytoin (Vukmir and Stein, 1991).

Prevention of seizures is especially important in cases of significant TCA ingestion. Repetitive seizure activity leads to acidosis. This decreases protein binding and results in higher free TCA levels, further exacerbating cardiovascular toxicity. The effect of intravenously administered benzodiazepines (diazepam or lorazepam) is short-lived. IV loading with phenytoin is therefore indicated if seizures persist. IV phenytoin must be administered *slowly* (not faster than 50 mg/minute) and under direct electrocardiographic monitoring to prevent complications (severe bradycardia, asystole, or respiratory arrest) that may occur if the drug is given too rapidly.

In an attempt to prevent the problems that may arise from repetitive seizure activity, some clinicians prefer to routinely *(prophylactically)* administer IV phenytoin as soon as possible to all patients with a history of significant TCA ingestion.

USE OF PHYSOSTIGMINE

Physostigmine is a reversible cholinesterase inhibitor that had been enthusiastically billed in the past as an "antidote" for TCA poisoning (Frommer et al, 1987). The high lipid-solubility of this drug allows it to easily cross the blood brain barrier and enter the CNS where it blocks degradation of acetylcholine. This accounts for the drug's ability to reverse the anticholinergic effects of TCA overdose. Unfortunately, numerous adverse effects have been associated with physostigmine administration including vomiting, bronchospasm, severe bradycardia (and even asystole), seizures, and death (Pentel and Peterson, 1980; Frommer et al, 1987; Ware, 1987). As a result, use of the drug is probably best restricted to patients with TCA overdose who manifest life-threatening complications (arrhyth-

mias, hypotension, seizures, or severe anticholinergic psychosis), and who have not responded to other therapy. Although physostigmine may rapidly reverse coma, it should *not* be used just to "wake the patient up."

Practically speaking, it is well to recognize that physostigmine is generally not very effective in the treatment of severe cardiac toxicity. This should not be surprising considering its mechanism of action (cholinergic activation) and the fact that other than sinus tachycardia, cardiac toxicity associated with TCA overdose is not related to the anticholinergic effect of these drugs.

References and Suggested Readings

Boehnert M, Lovejoy FH: The effect of phenytoin on cardiac conduction and ventricular arrhythmias in acute tricyclic antidepressant overdose, *Vet Hum Toxicol* 28:297, 1985 (abstract).

Callaham M (Chapter 110): Tricyclic antidepressant overdose. In Rosen P (ed): *Emergency medicine: concepts and clinical practice*, St Louis, 1988, Mosby–Year Book.

Callaham M, Kassel D: Epidemiology of fatal tricyclic antidepressant ingestion: implications for management, *Ann Emerg Med* 14:1, 1985.

Driggers DA, Deiss F, Steiner JF, Hudgings DW: Tricyclic antidepressant overdose, *J Fam Pract* 25:231, 1987.

Frommer DA, Kulig KW, Marx JA, Rumack B: Tricyclic antidepressant overdose: a review, *JAMA* 257:521, 1987.

Goldberg RJ, Capone RJ, Hunt JD: Cardiac complications following tricyclic antidepressant overdose: issues for monitoring policy, *JAMA* 254:1772, 1985.

Jennings AE, Levey AS, Harrington JT: Amoxapine-associated acute renal failure, *Arch Intern Med* 143:1525, 1983.

Kathol RG, Henn FA: Tricyclics: the most common agent used in potentially lethal overdose, *J Nerv Ment Dis* 171:250, 1983.

Martinez R: Torsades de pointes: atypical rhythm, atypical treatment, *Ann Emerg Med* 16:878, 1987.

Pentel P, Peterson CD: Asystole complicationg physostigmine treatment of tricyclic antidepressant overdose, *Ann Emerg Med* 9:588, 1980.

Preskorn SH, Othmer SC: Evaluation of bupropion hydrochloride: the first of a new class of atypical antidepressants, *Pharmacotherapy* 4:20, 1984.

Teba L, Schiebel F, Dedhia HV, Lazzell: Beneficial effect of norepinephrine in the treatment of circulatory shock caused by tricyclic antidepressant overdose, *Am J Emerg Med* 6:566, 1988.

Turbiak TT: Antidepressant overdose, *Ear Nose Throat J* 62:82, 1983.

Tzivoni D, Banai S, Schuger C, Benhorin J, Keren A, Gottlieb S, Stern S: Treatment of torsade de pointes with magnesium sulfate, *Circulation* 77:392, 1988.

Tzivoni D, Keren A, Cohen AM, Loebel H, Zahavi I, Chenzbraun A, Stern S: Magnesium therapy for torsades de pointes, *Am J Cardiol* 53:528, 1984.

Uhl JA: Phenytoin: the drug of choice in tricyclic antidepressant overdose? *Ann Emerg Med* 10:270, 1981.

Vukmir RB, Stein KL: Torsade de pointes: therapy with phenytoin, *Ann Emerg Med* 20:198, 1991.

Ware MR: Tricyclic antidepressant overdose: pharmacology and treatment, *South Med J* 80:1410, 1987.

SECTION H

CARDIOPULMONARY ARREST IN PREGNANCY

Cardiopulmonary arrest during pregnancy is a special resuscitation situation that is only rarely encountered by most emergency care providers who do not regularly participate in the care of pregnant women or neonates. Nevertheless, it is an extremely important situation to consider because of its unique features and the impact resuscitative measures may have in determining the outcome of both mother and fetus.

Although most pregnant women are relatively healthy and in the prime years of their life, this in not always the case. The child bearing age encompasses adolescence until early middle age. In the extreme, pregnancy has been reported in a 5 year old child (who delivered a healthy infant by caesarean section) and in a 63 year old woman (Cunningham et al, 1989). The risk from pregnancy is increased by many factors including underlying medical disease (diabetes mellitus, asthma, substance abuse, a seizure disorder, etc.), poor socioeconomic conditions, inadequate access to (or underutilization of) prenatal care, and pregnancy at an excessively young or older age. Medical complications of pregnancy include hemorrhage (from threatened abortion, ectopic pregnancy, placenta previa or abruptio, etc.); preeclampsia (hypertension, edema and proteinuria after the 20th week) and eclampsia (preeclampsia signs and symptoms plus seizures); pulmonary embolus; and overwhelming infection with septicemia. Patients with a high risk profile are more likely to develop these complications which may predispose them to cardiovascular compromise. Cardiopulmonary arrest can occur as a result. The risk of developing severe cardiovascular complications is greater in the presence of preexisting cardiac disease (i.e., congenital or valvular heart disease, history of cardiac arrhythmias) or with development of new cardiac disease (i.e., peripartum cardiomyopathy, acute myocardial infarction)—especially in older women with risk factors (smoking, hypertension, positive family history, etc.) who become pregnant. Cardiopulmonary arrest may also occur in otherwise healthy pregnant women who are unexpected victims of trauma, motor vehicle accidents, a lightning strike or electrical injury, envenomation, illicit drug abuse (i.e., cocaine overdose) and/or drug withdrawal, or an anaphylactic reaction.

A key factor to consider in the management of cardiopulmonary arrest during pregnancy is the potential viability of the fetus. Current guidelines emphasize the importance of determining if the length of gestation at the time of arrest is greater than **24 weeks.** Realistic chances for fetal survival increase significantly after this point in the pregnancy (AHA ACLS Textbook, 1987; Lee et al, 1986). If cardiopulmonary arrest occurs in a pregnant

woman *prior* to the 24th week of gestation, resuscitative efforts should be directed primarily toward saving the mother. After the 24th week, cardiopulmonary arrest in pregnancy should be thought of as a *double* arrest, and equal priority must be given to saving the fetus as well as the mother. Finally, an extra dimension has now been added to clinical (as well as ethical) management decisions because of our ability to maintain vital function in otherwise "brain dead" mothers for extended periods until a more propitious time for fetal delivery (Lee et al, 1986).

Management of Cardiopulmonary Arrest in Pregnancy

Many of the standard measures for management of cardiopulmonary arrest are unaltered by pregnancy. Thus attention must first be directed to assessment and control of the ABCs (airway, breathing, and circulation) with performance of basic life support as indicated. Ventricular fibrillation should be defibrillated at standard energy levels. Adequate oxygenation is especially important to the pregnant patient because of the increased metabolic demands of breast, uterine, placental, and fetal growth, and the tendency of hypoxia to even further reduce uteroplacental perfusion (Lee et al, 1986).

The major differences in cardiopulmonary resuscitation during pregnancy relate to the use of certain medications and positioning of the patient. Lidocaine may be used as indicated because standard doses of this medication do not appear to have an adverse effect on the fetus. In contrast, vasopressors (epinephrine, dopamine, and norepinephrine) may compromise the fetal circulation because the vasoconstriction they produce decreases blood flow through uteroplacental vessels (Lee et al, 1986; AHA ACLS Textbook, 1987; McAnulty et al, 1990). As a result, vasopressors should only be used with extreme caution, especially in cases when high priority is placed on fetal salvage. IV β-blockers and digoxin may precipitate uterine contractions. IV verapamil may further reduce maternal blood pressure and produce uterine atony. Bretylium may adversely affect uterine perfusion (Lee et al, 1986; McAnulty et al, 1990). Emergency thoracotomy with open chest cardiac massage may therefore be preferable to "desperate polypharmacy" for preserving uteroplacental blood flow and increasing cardiac output of the pregnant patient in cardiac arrest (Lee et al, 1986).

Normal cardiovascular physiologic changes during pregnancy are marked by progressive augmentation of cardiac output (of up to 50%) by the 20th week of gestation. This is accompanied by a fall in vascular resistance of uterine blood vessels with a resultant increase in uterine blood flow (Sullivan and Ramanathan, 1985; Lee et al, 1986). Cardiac output during pregnancy is extremely sensitive to changes in body position. Supine positioning of the pregnant patient may thus compromise blood flow by a gravitational effect of the pre-term uterus in which this organ compresses the iliac vessels, inferior vena cava, and abdominal aorta. Cardiac output may be reduced as much as 25% by this effect, and hypotension may result (Kerr, 1965; Lee et al, 1986; AHA ACLS Textbook, 1987).

In an attempt to optimize perfusion to vital organs during resuscitation, rotation of the pregnant patient slightly on her **left** side (by placing a wedge or pillow under the right abdominal flank and hip) is recommended. This should displace the gravid uterus to the left, improving venous return to the heart and arterial blood flow to the uterus (by minimizing the potentially adverse effect of gravity on uterine flow—Sullivan and Ramanathan, 1985; Lee et al, 1986; AHA ACLS Textbook, 1987). It is important *not* to fully rotate the patient to the left lateral decubitus position, however, because doing so would render external chest compression ineffective.

Our suggestions for integrating the standard protocol for treatment of cardiopulmonary resuscitation with special considerations relevant to the pregnant patient who arrests appear in *Table 13H-1*.

Table 13H-1

Suggested Approach to Evaluation and Management of Cardiopulmonary Arrest During Pregnancy

1. Assess the patient and control the ABCs:
   - Assure an adequate airway/provide supplemental oxygen.
   - Ventilate the patient who is not spontaneously breathing. Intubate if needed.
   - Assess circulation. Initiate external chest compression if the patient is pulseless.*

2. Rotate the patient toward her **left side** (by placing a pillow or wedge under the right abdominal flank and hip).

3. Determine the rhythm.

4. Defibrillate (with 200, 300, and then 360 joules) if the patient is in ventricular fibrillation.

5. Establish IV access.

6. Establish continuous ECG monitoring.

7. Rapidly obtain essential elements of the history:
   - Medical history of the mother?
   - Course of the pregnancy? *Is the cause of the arrest due to a complication of pregnancy?†*
   - Length of gestation? **Equal priority must be given to saving the fetus as well as the mother if the estimated length of gestation exceeds 24 weeks!**

8. Consider epinephrine (if indicated), realizing potentially adverse effects of this drug on the uteroplacental circulation.

9. Assure adequate volume status (as much as possible).

10. Consider evaluation of fetal viability (via external monitoring or real-time ultrasound) if patient has not responded after 5-10 minutes of resuscitation.

    Additional measures to consider if the fetus is viable and/or there has been no maternal response to resuscitation include emergency thoracotomy with open-chest cardiac massage (which may be much more effective than closed-chest cardiac massage in pregnant patients) and emergency caesarean section.

11. Consult appropriately (with obstetrics, neonatology, etc.) to help in the decision-making process.

*The recommended hand position on the sternum for performance of external chest compression is unchanged in pregnancy. (In contrast, relief of airway obstruction during later pregnancy should be attempted by application of chest thrusts instead of abdominal thrusts.)
†If the cause of the arrest is due to a complication of pregnancy (such as hemorrhage or eclampsia), specific treatment measures (such as blood replacement, surgery, magnesium sulfate, etc.) may be needed.
Adapted from AHA ACLS Textbooks, 1987.

Peripartum Cardiomyopathy

Peripartum cardiomyopathy is a rare but potentially devastating primary myocardial disease that we feel merits special mention as a possible cause of unexpected cardiopulmonary arrest in a previously healthy pregnant patient.

Peripartum cardiomyopathy is a distinct clinical entity characterized by development of congestive heart failure of undetermined etiology during the last month of pregnancy or within the first 5 postpartum months (Demakis and Rahimtoola, 1971). Recognition of the disorder may be difficult because of its insidious onset and the common occurrence of easy fatigability, dyspnea, chest pain, palpitations, and syncope in completely healthy pregnant women. Physical exam may be equally misleading because normal pregnant women also commonly manifest visible neck vein pulsations (that may be confused with jugular venous distension), pulmonary rales, heart murmurs, and a third heart sound (McAnulty et al, 1990). Clearly, a high index of suspicion must be maintained, as well as a low tolerance for obtaining diagnostic studies (such as echocardiography) in pregnant women with disproportionate symptoms (i.e., dyspnea on *minimal* activity or paroxysmal nocturnal dyspnea) if early diagnosis is to be made. Awareness of factors associated with an increased likelihood of developing this entity (i.e., multiparity, black race, maternal age over 30, pregnancy complicated by hypertension, and twins) may also be helpful (O'Dell et al, 1986; McAnulty, 1990).

Although the etiology of peripartum cardiomyopathy remains unclear, myocarditis (confirmed by percutaneous transvenous endomyocardial biopsy of the right ventricle) appears to be present in a majority of cases (Midei et al, 1990). The course and prognosis of the disorder is highly variable. Some patients demonstrate spontaneous improvement following delivery, especially in cases in which cardiomegaly rapidly resolves. Others respond to standard medical treatment for heart failure and/or immunosuppressive therapy (with azathioprine and corticosteroids). Immunosuppressive therapy is usually continued for 1 to 2 months, and then gradually tapered over a period of several additional months if the patient remains stable. Unfortunately, progressive deterioration of cardiac function despite intense medical and/or immunosuppressive therapy marks the course of a small but significant number of cases. Selected patients may become candidates for cardiac transplantation.

Patients with peripartum cardiomyopathy should be counseled regarding the likelihood of recurrence with subsequent pregnancies with substantial increased risk of maternal and fetal mortality (O'Dell et al, 1986; McAnulty, 1990).

References and Suggested Readings

American Heart Association: *Special resuscitation situations*. In Jaffe A (ed): *Textbook of advanced cardiac life support*, Dallas, 1987, American Heart Association.

Cunningham FG, MacDonald PC, Gant NF: *Maternal adaptations to pregnancy*. In *Williams obstetrics*, Norwalk, Conn, 1989, Appleton & Lange.

Demakis JG, Rahimtoola SH: Peripartum cardiomyopathy, *Circulation* 34:964, 1971.

Kerr MG: The mechanical effects of the gravid uterus in late pregnancy, *J Obstet Gynaecol Br Commonw* 72:513, 1965.

Lee RV, Rodgers BD, White LM, Harvey RC: Cardiopulmonary resuscitation of pregnant women, *Am J Med* 81:311, 1986.

McAnulty JH, Metcalfe J, Ueland K: *Heart disease and pregnancy*. In Hurst JW, Schlant RC (eds) *The heart: arteries and veins*, New York, 1990, McGraw-Hill.

Midei MG, DeMent SH, Feldman AM, Hutchins GM, Baughman KL: Peripartum myocarditis and cardiomyopathy, *Circulation* 81:922, 1990.

O'Dell ML, Ruth W, Gollub S, Gortney C: Peripartum cardiomyopathy, *J Fam Pract* 22:505, 1986.

Sullivan JM, Ramanathan KB: Management of medical problems in pregnancy: severe cardiac disease, *N Engl J Med* 313:304, 1985.

SECTION I

AIRPLANE EMERGENCIES

Among the least opportune times for a medical emergency to occur would seem to be in the middle of an airplane flight. Concern about such occurrences has been expressed since the inception of commercial air travel. Factors predisposing susceptible individuals to development of an in-flight medical emergency include the stress of air travel itself, relative hypoxia (despite pressurization of commercial aircraft), orthostasis (from arising after a prolonged period of sitting), disturbance of circadian rhythms (when flying across multiple time zones), exposure to cosmic radiation, and the ready availability of alcohol (Cottrell et al, 1989).* Individuals who are most at risk of developing an in-flight medical emergency are those who have one or more chronic medical illnesses. An estimated 5% of all air travelers have some type of underlying medical disease. A significant percentage of these individuals are completely disabled by their disease, and suffer from a condition that may be intensified by flying (Rodenberg, 1988). Given the prevalence of underlying disease among commercial air travelers and the multitude of predisposing factors, in-flight medical emergencies turn out to be surprisingly less common than one might anticipate.

Data on the Occurrence of In-Flight Medical Emergencies

In an attempt to document the prevalence and type of medical emergencies among commercial air travelers, Cummins and Schubach performed a 1-year prospective survey of all emergency calls excluding motor-vehicle injuries to the Seattle Tacoma International Airport (1989). Included in the survey were emergency calls for travelers, airport and airline employees and any other people at the airport who were attended to by physicians coincidentally on the scene (or on the flight) and/or the local two-tier EMS system.

During the period of study, a total of 14.4 million passengers flew on the 274,000 commercial flights. In-flight medical emergencies requiring emergency landing were exceedingly rare, occurring at a rate of 1 per 39,000 passengers (or once for every 753 flights). Moreover, retrospective analysis of these emergencies suggests that in most cases care of the patient could probably have been safely deferred for the 1 to 2 hours needed to complete the scheduled flight. Nevertheless, given the sheer numbers of Americans who fly each year (more than 500 million), a small (but definite) number of in-flight emergencies will continue to occur.

Results of the survey are insightful:

1. The most common emergency problems encountered were gastrointestinal (nausea, vomiting, diarrhea, and abdominal pain), shortness of breath (from asthma or COPD), chest pain, syncope (most often vasovagal in nature), or seizures.
2. Most (75%) emergency problems happened on the ground (in the airport, in the plane prior to takeoff, or after landing), rather than in flight. This probably reflects the enhanced stress travelers feel in the air terminal (obtaining tickets, rushing to make connections, unanticipated/annoying delays) compared to the rather "sedentary captivity experienced in flight."
3. Cardiac arrest was exceedingly uncommon. Only five cardiac arrests occurred during the year of the survey (of which none took place while the plane was actually in flight).

Flight attendants are not allowed to diagnose or administer medications in flight in the United States. As a result, commercial airlines depend on assistance from "good Samaritan" physicians in the event of an in-flight emergency. Other skilled health care providers (i.e., nurses, physician assistants, paramedics, etc.) should be encouraged to volunteer their services as well. Health care providers should be aware that the Federal Aviation Administration has mandated availability of a "doctors only" medical kit on all U.S. commercial aircraft (Cummins and Schubach, 1989; Dan, 1989). In the absence of a physician on board, non-physician providers may be allowed to use this kit at the discretion of the pilot. The contents of this kit are listed in *Table 13I-1*.

Practically speaking, epinephrine (1:1,000 dilution) may be the most important inclusion in the kit because its administration for an acute allergic reaction (such as anaphylaxis or angioedema from ingestion of peanuts or some other substance) is potentially lifesaving (Cottrell et al, 1989).

At the present time, there is little the emergency care provider can do to treat in-flight cardiopulmonary arrest. Left unresolved is the question of whether AEDs (automatic external defibrillators) should be regularly available on commercial aircraft.

The Effect of Altitude

Commercial aircraft usually fly at cruising altitudes between 28,000 to 43,000 feet. The partial pressure of any given gas progressively decreases as altitude increases. According to Boyle's Law, the concentration of oxygen mol-

---

*With the ban on smoking during commercial flights of less than 6 hours duration, exposure to environmental tobacco smoke is no longer a problem on domestic flights.

Table 13I-1

Contents of the "Doctors Only" Medical Kit*
- stethoscope
- sphygmomanometer
- oropharyngeal airways (3 sizes)
- selected medications (sublingual nitroglycerin, epinephrine [1:1,000 dilution], diphenhydramine, and 50% dextrose) with appropriate needles and syringes for administration**

*This "doctors only" medical kit is available on all U.S. commercial aircraft. In addition, high-flow oxygen is also regularly available.

**Addition of an inhaled β-adrenergic agonist to this list for use in acute bronchospastic conditions has been suggested (Cottrell et al, 1989). In an addition, an *aspirin* might be given if the emergency is suspected to be acute infarction.

ecules becomes progressively less as altitude increases. Thus, a patient with a PaO_2 of 98 at sea level will have a PaO_2 of approximately 70 mm Hg at 5,000 feet (Rodenberg, 1988). Although this drop in the partial pressure of oxygen is of little clinical significance in an otherwise healthy individual, it may have profound clinical consequences on a patient with compromised cardiopulmonary function.

Commercial aircraft are pressurized to compensate for the drop in pressure that occurs with increases in altitude. It is important to appreciate, however, that this pressurization does not restore the partial pressure of oxygen to the level that is present on the ground. Thus, a commercial aircraft flying at 35,000 feet will usually be pressurized to approximately 5,000 feet (AMA Commission on Emergency Medical Services, 1982). An aircraft flying at 41,000 feet may only be pressurized to 6,700 feet. In the example cited above, an individual who had a PaO_2 of 98 mm Hg at sea level would only have a PaO_2 of approximately 60

mm Hg at this latter altitude. In view of this, it is easy to understand how selected individuals with compromised cardiopulmonary function (i.e., patients with COPD, reactive airway disease, ischemic heart disease, cerebrovascular disease, etc.) may become hypoxic and develop symptoms during a routine commercial flight.

These relationships underscore the importance of administering *supplemental oxygen* as a primary treatment for air travelers who become hypoxic as a result of this altitude-induced depressurization. In addition, requesting the pilot to decrease the plane's altitude to 23,000 feet (a level at which the aircraft may be pressurized to sea level) will be extremely helpful in optimizing oxygenation until the plane arrives at its destination.

A recent study by Dillard et al (1991) sought to determine the frequency and outcome of airline travel among patients with COPD. Less than one third of the study group consulted with their physician prior to the flight. An increase in symptoms (compared to baseline) developed in 18% of the patients. Symptoms included dyspnea (especially among those patients who ambulated on board), wheezing, edema, and chest pain. Fortunately, no serious sequelae resulted, although several patients required administration of oxygen during the flight, and symptoms persisted for up to 48 hours *after* the flight in a few patients. Clearly, COPD patients should consider consulting their physician prior to flying, and be advised that they may develop symptoms in flight—and that they may benefit from administration of supplemental oxygen.

References and Suggested Readings

AMA Commission on Emergency Medical Services: Medical aspects of transportation aboard commercial aircraft, *JAMA* 247:1007, 1982.

Cottrell JJ, Callaghan JT, Kohn GM, Hensler EC, Rogers RM: In-flight medical emergencies: one year of experience with the enhanced medical kit, *JAMA* 262:1653, 1989.

Cummins RO, Schubach JA: Frequency and types of medical emergencies among commercial air travelers, *JAMA* 261:1295, 1989.

Dan BB: The accidental tourist: medical emergencies in the air, *JAMA* 261:1328, 1989.

Dillard TA, Beninati WA, Berg BW: Air travel in patients with chronic obstructive pulmonary disease, *Arch Intern Med* 151:1793, 1991.

Rodenberg H: Prevention of medical emergencies during air travel, *Am Fam Physician* 37:263, 1988.

SECTION J

TRAUMATIC CARDIAC ARREST

Cardiac arrest resulting from major trauma requires a number of special considerations in evaluation and management. Prognosis is generally much poorer than for non-traumatic cardiac arrest. *Priorities change.* Medical treatment of ventricular fibrillation will do little if the cause of this arrhythmia is a gunshot wound to the heart or an aortic tear from acceleration-deceleration forces of a motor vehicle accident. Practically speaking, survival is unlikely unless the cause of traumatic injury is identified and successfully treated (Cavallaro et al, 1988; Jorden and Barkin, 1988).

Special considerations in evaluation and management of traumatic cardiac arrest are listed in *Table 13J-1.* Admittedly, many of the resuscitative measures and interventions listed in this table extend beyond the scope of ACLS. Nevertheless, we feel it important to illustrate the type of prioritization necessary for successful management of traumatic cardiac arrest (American College of Surgeons, ATLS Course, 1989).

It is important to emphasize the concept of *"load and go"* in the approach to the victim of life-threatening trauma. In general, the amount one can (and should) do at the scene is limited (AHA ACLS Textbook, 1987; Cavallaro et al, 1988). The C-spine can be stabilized, the patient's level of consciousness rapidly assessed, the airway secured, and the adequacy of ventilation determined. If spontaneous ventilation is inadequate (or absent): (1) the patient may need to be intubated; and/or (2) there may be a potentially life-threatening pulmonary complication (such as tension pneumothorax) that needs to be immediately treated. Intravenous fluid resuscitation can be started for patients in shock. However, the most important determinant of the patient's prognosis is the time until definitive treatment (Cavallaro et al, 1988). As a result, transport to the nearest trauma care facility assumes highest priority (i.e., "load and go"). After initial stabilization measures, transport of the severely traumatized victim should not be held up for any reason, even to establish IV access. In contrast, when the pulseless condition is known to be of pure cardiac origin (in the certain absence of trauma), initiation of ACLS procedures (CPR, defibrillation, administration of epinephrine or lidocaine) is preferable in an attempt to stabilize the patient prior to transport.

References and Suggested Readings

Advanced Trauma Life Support Course for Physicians: Subcommittee on Advanced Trauma Life Support (ATLS) of the American College of Surgeons Committee on Trauma, 1989.

Cavallaro D, Mominee P, Michlin JP, Hillman J, Grauer K, Craver B: An algorithm for trauma victim assessment, *JEMS* 13:28, 1988.

Chapter 15: *Special resuscitation situations.* Jaffe AS (ed): In *Textbook of advanced cardiac life support,* Dallas, 1987, American Heart Association.

Jorden RC, Barkin RM: Chapter 8: *Multiple trauma.* In Rosen P (ed): *Emergency medicine: concepts and clinical practice,* St Louis, 1988, Mosby–Year Book.

Table 13J-1

Special Considerations in Evaluation and Management of Traumatic Cardiac Arrest

1. Stabilize the cervical spine:
   - Always assume a C-spine injury in a trauma patient until proved otherwise (especially in victims of blunt trauma).
   - Immediately immobilize the C-spine of all trauma victims.
   - Maintain C-spine stabilization until cervical injury can be ruled out with a cross-table lateral C-spine x-ray that demonstrates *all* 7 cervical vertebrae.

2. *Rapidly* assess the patient's level of consciousness:
   - Alert?
   - Responsive to verbal or painful stimuli?
   - Unresponsive?

3. *Rapidly* evaluate the **ABC's.** Institute life-saving treatment measures as needed.
   Airway
   - Assure an adequate airway. (Use the jaw-thrust maneuver *without* head tilt because of the high incidence of associated C-spine injuries.)
   Breathing
   - Ventilate the patient who is not spontaneously breathing.
   - Intubate if needed. *Nasotracheal* intubation is preferable for patients who are unresponsive but still breathing spontaneously because it may be accomplished without cervical manipulation.*

Continued.

Table 13J-1—cont'd

- Perform rapid chest exam to assess the adequacy of ventilatory exchange and to rule out major (life-threatening) injury. *Airway patency does not necessarily guarantee adequate ventilation.* Major chest injury must be identified early and promptly treated:
  - emergently decompress tension pneumothorax
  - immediately cover (with vasoline dressings sealed on three sides only) open chest wounds
  - stabilize flail chest with tape (*not* sand bags)

Circulation
- Assess circulation (pulse, capillary refill, blood pressure) and hemodynamic status. If no pulse is present, determine the cause (ventricular fibrillation, asystole, or EMD) and treat accordingly (with CPR, drugs, or defibrillation as needed).

4. Treat hemorrhagic/hypovolemic shock
- Identify external wounds that are actively bleeding; control visible hemorrhage by direct pressure.
- Replace lost volume with IV fluid (Ringer's lactate, normal saline, and/or whole blood—using type-specific blood if needed when cross-matched blood is not yet available).
- Consider use of pneumatic antishock (MAST) trousers as a temporizing measure to help in the management of shock.
- Consider autotransfusion (if available).
- Do *not* treat hemorrhagic/hypovolemic shock with pressor agents.

5. Prioritize further management:
- Realize that chances for survival from cardiac arrest that develops as a direct result of trauma hinge on rapid identification and immediate treatment of the precipitating cause.
- Direct physical assessment and laboratory evaluation at determining this cause. Potential precipitating causes of traumatic cardiac arrest to consider include:
  - tension or open pneumothorax
  - flail chest with pulmonary contusion
  - gunshot or other penetrating wound to chest or abdomen with resultant internal (exsanguinating) hemorrhage
  - pericardial tamponade
  - aortic rupture
  - severe neurologic injury (cerebral contusion, hemorrhage, spinal cord injury, etc.)
  - complete airway obstruction from facial trauma

- Delegate someone to obtain as much history as possible to help determine the mechanism of injury (i.e., speed of automobile, loss of consciousness, use of seat belts, collapsed steering wheel, etc.)

- Consider need for early invasive/surgical intervention for victims of traumatic cardiac arrest:
  - Open-chest resuscitation for exsanguinating hemorrhage (cross-clamping the aorta and performance of open-chest cardiac massage)
  - Emergency thoracotomy/surgery for penetrating chest wounds (i.e., repair of myocardial defects, aortic rupture)
  - Emergency exploratory surgery for blunt/penetrating abdominal trauma with significant internal hemorrhage
  - Emergency surgical airway intervention (i.e., cricothyroidotomy)

- Continually reevaluate the patient.

---

*For apneic patients, *orotracheal* intubation may be attempted with special attention directed at avoiding cervical manipulation if cervical spine injury has not been ruled out. Use of a second rescuer to exert *longitudinal* traction and stabilize the C-spine during intubation may help in this regard. *Cricothyroidotomy* may be needed for apneic patients when C-spine injuries are strongly suspected and/or for severe maxillofacial injuries and bleeding.

PART V

Beyond the Basics

CHAPTER 14

A COMPENDIUM OF ADDITIONAL DRUGS USED IN EMERGENCY CARDIAC CARE

Ken Grauer, MD
John Gums, Pharm D
Dan Cavallaro, REMT

SECTION A

AGENTS FOR SHOCK

Dobutamine (Dobutrex)

How Dispensed: 250 mg per 20-ml vial
Indication: Cardiogenic shock

DOSE AND ROUTE OF ADMINISTRATION

Mix 250 mg in 250 ml of D5W (1,000 μg/ml), and begin drip at 10 to 15 drops/min. This will infuse ≈2.5 μg/kg/min for a 60- to 80-kg patient. Titrate according to clinical effect. Usual range of infusion = 2.5 to 10 μg/kg/min.

COMMENTS

Dobutamine is a synthetic catecholamine with predominantly β-1-adrenergic receptor stimulating effects. At usual doses (below 10 μg/kg/min), the drug improves myocardial contractility with only a minimal effect on heart rate and peripheral vascular resistance. It commonly produces a degree of reflex *vasodilatation* in response to this increased contractility and improved cardiac output. As a result, it is important that the patient not be hypovolemic, or else hypotension may result.

Dobutamine is most useful for treatment of patients with cardiac failure who maintain a normal (or near normal) blood pressure, especially in the setting of acute myocardial infarction. For treatment of cardiac failure with hypotension, an agent such as dopamine (with its greater vasoconstrictor effect) is preferable. After blood pressure has been restored to the normotensive range, addition of dobutamine may produce a further increase in contractility (and in cardiac output).

For similar reasons, dopamine is likely to be much more effective than dobutamine for treatment of conditions such as septic shock in which systemic vascular resistance is low.

The effects of dobutamine are frequently confused with those of dopamine. These drugs differ in many ways. Dobutamine has no effect on dopaminergic receptors (in the renal or mesenteric vascular bed), and exerts a much lesser effect on the peripheral vasculature than does dopamine. If anything, use of dobutamine may result in mild *vasodilatation* (as a reflex response to the increase in contractility). In general, dobutamine is less arrhythmogenic than dopamine, and significant increases in heart rate usually are not seen unless high doses (>20 μg/kg/min) of the drug are used. Increases in cardiac output produced by dobutamine are generally the result of enhanced contractility (and therefore an increased stroke volume). This is in contrast to the increase in cardiac output produced by dopamine, which is more likely to reflect an increase in heart rate rather than a change in contractility.

Practically speaking, because dobutamine does not significantly increase blood pressure in most patients, the drug is *not* frequently used in the setting of cardiac arrest. In patients with spontaneous circulation, it is difficult clinically to titrate the dose of dobutamine because of its lack of effect on blood pressure—unless a Swan-Ganz catheter is in place.

Norepinephrine (Levophed)

How Dispensed: 1 mg/ml (4-ml vial)
Indications: Cardiogenic shock; hemodynamically significant hypotension (not due to hypovolemia)

DOSE AND ROUTE OF ADMINISTRATION

Mix 1 ampule (4 mg) in 250 ml of D5W (16 μg/ml), and begin drip at 10 drops/min (≈2-3 μg/min). Titrate according to clinical effect and adjust the infusion to the lowest rate that maintains desired hemodynamic response.

The half-life of norepinephrine is short (≈2 min), and pressor effects generally resolve within 1 to 2 minutes after discontinuing the infusion. The usual dose range of norepinephrine infusion for treatment of shock is between 4 and 20 μg/min (Ferguson and Abboud, 1990). Prognosis is poor for patients requiring prolonged high-dose (i.e., ≥30-40 μg/min) infusion of the drug.

COMMENTS

Norepinephrine is an endogenous catecholamine with both α- and β-receptor stimulating effects. It is an extremely potent vasoconstrictor (i.e., α-1 adrenergic stimulating effects predominate) that is used most often in the treatment of hypotension associated with reduced peripheral vascular resistance. *The drug should not be given to patients in shock from hypovolemia!*

The effects of norepinephrine on the heart are variable. Cardiac output may either increase or decrease, depending on circulating blood volume, peripheral vascular resistance, the state of the myocardium, and carotid baroreceptor reflex activity.

> Although the β-1 adrenergic effect of norepinephrine acts to increase cardiac contractility, this effect is often counterbalanced by the potent vasoconstrictor (α-adrenergic) action of the drug. The resultant increase in peripheral vascular resistance leads to an increase in afterload, which tends to limit any improvement in cardiac output. Myocardial oxygen consumption may also increase as a result of the increased afterload.
>
> Beneficial effects of norepinephrine infusion include an increase in blood pressure and improved myocardial perfusion (from the increase in aortic diastolic pressure it produces). However, renal, cerebral, hepatic, and skeletal muscle blood flow may all decrease as a result of significant regional vasoconstriction and shunting (Chatterjee, 1990). Other adverse effects associated with norepinephrine infusion include tachycardia and ventricular arrhythmias. Special care must be given to the IV site because skin sloughing is likely to occur if there is extravasation of the drug into surrounding tissues.

Because of the potentially deleterious effects of norepinephrine, use of this drug is usually reserved for patients in profound shock who have not responded to other vasoactive agents. The drug may be invaluable for treatment of shock in association with catecholamine depletion states such as severe tricyclic antidepressant overdose (*see Section 13G*).

> Use of norepinephrine may be combined with *low-dose* dopamine infusion (i.e., at a rate of 2-5 μg/kg/min) in an attempt to optimize hemodynamic parameters of patients in shock not due to hypovolemia. The rationale for this combination is to preserve renal perfusion and maintain urine output (with the dopaminergic effect of low-dose dopamine) while increasing systemic vascular resistance and blood pressure (by the α-1 adrenergic stimulating effect of norepinephrine).

Amrinone (Inocor)

How Dispensed: 5 mg/ml (20-ml vial = 100 mg)

Indications: Short-term treatment of severe congestive heart failure refractory to conventional therapy

DOSE AND ROUTE OF ADMINISTRATION

An initial 0.75 mg/kg IV loading dose is administered over 2 to 3 minutes, followed by an IV infusion of 5 to 10 μg/kg/min. Titrate according to clinical effect. An additional 0.75 mg/kg IV loading dose may be given (if needed) 30 minutes after the initial loading dose. The total daily dose should not exceed 10 mg/kg.

> Amrinone should not be added directly to dextrose-containing solutions because the combination may result in a loss of the drug's activity.

COMMENTS

Amrinone is a synthetic, nonglycoside, nonsympathomimetic (i.e., non-β-agonist) positive inotropic agent. The precise mechanism of action of the drug is unclear, but it may be related to selective phosphodiesterase inhibition with resultant increase in the level of myocardial cyclic AMP. Peak development of myocardial fiber tension, the maximal rate of tension development, and the maximal rate of relaxation all increase (Chatterjee, 1990). Clinically, this results in *enhanced cardiac contractility* (positive inotropic action) and *potent vasodilatation of both arterial and venous vascular beds*. Which of these effects predominate in any given individual will vary according to the dose used and the patient's pretreatment condition.

IV administration of amrinone may improve hemodynamic parameters and the cardiac performance of selected patients with severe heart failure that had been refractory to other therapy. Cardiac output and stroke volume generally increase, while filling pressures and systemic vascular resistance are reduced. Although ideally the net effect of the dual actions of IV amrinone result in improved hemodynamic status without significant alteration of baseline heart rate or blood pressure, careful monitoring and dose titration are essential to prevent development of excessive tachycardia and/or hypotension. The drug should never be abruptly discontinued.

Overall, despite the fact that IV amrinone is usually well tolerated, and that hemodynamic status may temporarily be improved, there is no evidence that long-term survival is increased. As a result, IV amrinone is approved only for short-term use in treatment of patients with severe congestive heart failure that has *not* responded to conventional therapy. Because of its relatively long half-life (of at least several hours), the drug is used less often in the acute care setting.

> The most common adverse effects associated with administration of IV amrinone are thrombocytopenia (≈2%), arrhythmias (≈3%), and hypotension (≈1%). Special caution is advised when the drug is used in the setting of acute myocardial infarction, particularly for patients who are hypotensive and/or not in heart failure. In such individuals, the potent venodilator action of the drug is much more likely to produce a hypotensive response.

Oral amrinone is not nearly as effective as the IV form of this drug. Due to a lack of sustained benefit with long-term therapy and an inordinately high incidence of side effects (gastrointestinal intolerance, headache, lightheadedness, thrombocytopenia, liver-function abnormalities, fever, and ventricular arrhythmias), oral amrinone is no longer being studied in clinical trials and is not available for general use. Evaluation of related compounds (i.e., milrinone and others) is still ongoing.

SECTION B:

AGENTS FOR HYPERTENSIVE CRISIS

Nitroglycerin

How Dispensed: Pharmacy dependent

Pharmacies vary greatly in the way they prepare IV nitroglycerin (dilutions may vary from 25-500 μg/ml) so that is *essential* to become familiar with the concentrations employed at one's particular institution.

Indications: Acute ischemic chest pain (angina pectoris, coronary spasm, acute myocardial infarction); complications of acute myocardial infarction (hypertension, left ventricular failure); limitation of infarct size (i.e., *prophylactic* use in the setting of AMI even in the absence of chest pain)

DOSE AND ROUTE OF ADMINISTRATION

Mix 50 mg in 250 ml of D5W (200 μg/ml), and begin drip at 3 drops/min (= 10 μg/min). Carefully titrate according to clinical response. Although there is no clearly defined upper dosage limit, it is usually best not to exceed 200 μg/min since adverse reactions (especially hypotension) are common at this higher dose range.

When nitroglycerin is used *prophylactically* (i.e., in an attempt to limit infarct size in patients who are no longer having chest pain), an infusion rate of between 25 to 100 μg/min is usually selected and empirically continued for 24 to 48 hours.

COMMENTS

The beneficial action of nitroglycerin in ischemic heart disease has been known for well over 100 years. Even today, the drug remains the first line of treatment for this disorder. Although multiple preparations of nitroglycerin are available, we limit our comments here to the intravenous form of administration.

The mechanism of action of nitroglycerin is multifactorial. The drug's most pronounced effect is to decrease venous tone. This produces a marked reduction in *preload*. Systemic vascular resistance is decreased (*afterload* reduction), although not nearly to the same extent as the reduction in preload. Nitroglycerin also increases coronary blood flow (by dilating epicardial coronary arteries) and dilates collateral vessels. Autoregulation of the normal vascular bed is preserved however, so that shunting of blood flow away from ischemic areas of myocardium (i.e., *coronary "steal"*) tends not to occur (Frishman, 1985).

IV nitroglycerin is the drug of choice for the treatment of severe chest pain and hypertension that complicate acute myocardial infarction. It is also extremely effective in treatment of congestive heart failure in this setting. Finally, prophylactic use of the drug (i.e., for patients with AMI who are not having chest pain) may limit infarct size and reduce mortality, especially if given early in the course to patients with moderate-to-large size infarction (Yusuf et al, 1988). Although close observation (and frequent blood pressure checks) in an intensive care unit is essential when using IV nitroglycerin, invasive hemodynamic monitoring will not be needed in many patients.

One should be particularly careful in using IV nitroglycerin when blood pressure is normal or slightly decreased (i.e., systolic blood pressure is in the range of 90-100 mm Hg), if left ventricular filling pressures are not elevated, and in the setting of acute right ventricular infarction. Under such circumstances the drug's vasodilatory and preload reducing effect may result in a net lowering of stroke volume and cardiac output and lead to hypotension and/or tachycardia.

Occasionally during nitroglycerin infusion paradoxical *bradycardia* will be seen in association with marked hypotension. If this occurs, the drug should be immediately stopped and the patient placed in Trendelenburg position. Administration of IV fluid and atropine are indicated if hypotension and bradycardia persist.

In general, IV nitroglycerin appears to be most effective when used in patients with significantly impaired left ventricular function. In such individuals the drug exerts a greater afterload-lowering effect, resulting in an increase in stroke volume and cardiac output (*see Section 12B for additional information on the use of IV nitroglycerin for patients with AMI*).

Sodium Nitroprusside (Nipride)

How Dispensed: 50 mg per 5-ml vial
Indications: Hypertensive crisis; treatment of complications of acute myocardial infarction (hypertension, left ventricular failure)

DOSE AND ROUTE OF ADMINISTRATION

Mix 50 mg in 250 ml of D5W (200 μg/ml), and begin drip at 3 drops/min (10 μg/min). This may be increased by 3 drops/min (10 μg/min) every 5 minutes.

- Usual range of infusion = 0.5 to 10 µg/kg/min
- Onset of action of the drug = within 1 to 2 minutes of starting the infusion; effects disappear within minutes of stopping the drip
- Hemodynamic monitoring and minute-to-minute titration of dose is essential when nitroprusside is used

COMMENTS

Nitroprusside is an extremely potent peripheral vasodilator of both the arterial and venous vascular beds. *It is the most effective agent currently available for treatment of hypertensive emergencies.* As such, it is indicated for treatment of hypertensive encephalopathy and severe hypertension associated with intracranial hemorrhage, acute head injury, dissecting aneurysm, catecholamine crisis, and perioperative complications. It may also be useful in the treatment of congestive heart failure, due to its ability to lower preload and afterload.

> Compared to IV nitroglycerin, nitroprusside is a far more potent antihypertensive agent due to the greater arterial vasodilation it produces. However, because nitroprusside is at least theoretically more likely to produce *coronary steal*, IV nitroglycerin is preferred by many for *initial* treatment of mild-to-moderate hypertension and congestive heart failure that complicate acute ischemic heart disease. Failure to respond to IV nitroglycerin is an indication to switch to IV nitroprusside. In contrast, IV nitroprusside may be preferable as initial therapy for assuring rapid afterload reduction in AMI patients who suddenly develop heart failure as the result of acute mitral regurgitation or ventricular septal rupture.

Potential problems associated with nitroprusside infusion include hypotension (from overaggressive use of the drug), headache, photodegradation of the solution (which is why the IV bottle should always be covered with aluminum foil), and *cyanide* or *thiocyanate toxicity.*

> Sodium nitroprusside is converted to cyanide by sulfhydrel groups in erythrocytes and tissue, and then to thiocyanate by metabolism in the liver. Fortunately, cyanide and thiocyanate toxicity are both extremely uncommon when the duration of nitroprusside infusion is limited and dosing recommendations are followed (Gifford, 1991).
> *Cyanide toxicity* typically manifests by clinical deterioration in association with progressive metabolic acidosis. It may be treated by infusion of sodium nitrite, followed by sodium thiosulfate.
> *Thiocyanate toxicity* is suggested by nausea, vomiting, headache, restlessness, tinnitus, blurred vision, depressed deep tendon reflexes, and a pinkish coloration of the skin. Ultimately, delirium or a toxic psychosis may develop. The risk of thiocyanate toxicity is greatest in heavy smokers and patients with renal insufficiency, especially when high doses of the drug are used for a prolonged period of time (i.e., for more than 48 hours). Clinical suspicion of toxicity is confirmed by a thiocyanate level in excess of 1.7 mmol/L. The condition reverses with discontinuation of the nitroprusside infusion.

> In summary, IV nitroprusside is the drug of choice for the acute treatment of most hypertensive emergencies. Use of this drug requires careful dose titration with moment-to-moment monitoring capability (and usually admission to an intensive care unit). Initial treatment of less severe blood pressure elevation in association with acute ischemic heart disease may be attempted with IV nitroglycerin, but there should be a low threshold for changing to IV nitroprusside if significant hypertension persists. Although sublingual nifedipine is an extremely effective agent for treatment of hypertensive urgency, it should *not* be used for acute blood pressure reduction in patients with potentially unstable conditions such as evolving infarction or stroke. Instead, the moment-to-moment titration capability of IV nitroprusside makes it the drug of choice in these situations.

Labetalol (Normodyne/ Trandate)

How Dispensed:
  For IV administration: 5 mg/ml
  For oral administration: 100-, 200-, and 300-mg scored tablets
Indications: Hypertensive urgency/emergency

DOSE AND ROUTE OF ADMINISTRATION

IV Dose: 20 mg IV as an initial "mini"-bolus, followed by incremental dosing in the amount of 20 to 80 mg IV q 10 minutes (up to a maximum cumulative dose of 300 mg).

> The reason for beginning with a relatively low dose (i.e., 20 mg) is to avoid the possibility of an excessive hypotensive response that may occasionally be seen if larger doses (of 50 mg or more) are given first. The full antihypertensive effect of the drug is usually observed within 5 to 10 minutes of an IV dose, which explains the suggested 10-minute interval for incremental dosing. As an alternative to repeated IV dosing, an **IV infusion** of labetalol (at a rate of 2 mg/min) may be used to sustain the antihypertensive effect.

Oral Dose: Begin with 100 to 200 mg PO Bid (up to a maximal dose of 1,200 to 2,400 mg/day).

COMMENTS

Labetalol is a *non-selective* β-adrenergic blocker with α-blocking and direct vasodilatory properties. As a result of these latter two effects, peripheral vascular resistance is reduced. This not only augments the antihypertensive action of the drug, but also minimizes the negative inotropic effect of the β-blocking component (i.e., by afterload reduction). The net result is that cardiac output is usually preserved.

It is of interest that the relative β- to α-blocking potency ratio of labetalol depends on the route of administration of the drug:

β : α = 3:1 for oral labetalol
β : α = 7:1 for IV labetalol

Thus, β-blockade contributes relatively more to the mechanism of action of the IV form of the drug than to the oral form. This point is clinically important because patients are often begun on long-term maintenance therapy with the oral form of the drug if the IV form has been successful. As suggested by the above relationship, clinical effects of the two preparations are *not* identical.

> Adverse effects of labetalol tend to be dose-dependent, and may be related to either α-adrenergic blockade (i.e., orthostatic hypotension, dizziness) and/or β-adrenergic blockade (i.e., bronchospasm, decreased contractility, etc.). Orthostatic hypotension may be minimized by keeping patients supine for 1 to 2 hours *after* the last IV dose—and then ambulating them cautiously (Wilson et al, 1983). As might be expected, adverse effects related to β-blockade are somewhat more likely to occur with the IV form of the drug.

IV labetalol is an extremely effective agent for the treatment of hypertensive urgency. With incremental IV dosing according to the above suggested protocol, safe and effective blood pressure reduction may be achieved in up to 90% of patients with this disorder (Wilson, et al, 1983).

> Advantages of IV labetalol are several. Administration of the drug does not necessarily require hospitalization in an intensive care unit and the moment-to-moment monitoring that is essential when IV nitroprusside is used. Moreover, the reflex tachycardia so commonly associated with administration of potent vasodilators (such as IV nitroprusside, IV nitroglycerin, or sublingual nifedipine) is *not* seen with IV labetalol (because of the β-blocking effect). This may make IV labetalol a safer agent for use in the treatment of patients with acute ischemic syndromes or suspected underlying coronary artery disease. Effective blood pressure lowering is seen with IV labetalol even in patients who are concurrently receiving β-blockers (Wilson, et al, 1983). Cerebral blood flow is generally preserved with the drug, so that IV labetalol can be used safely in patients with acute neurologic syndromes (Brott

and Reed, 1991). Overall patient tolerance of IV labetalol is good, and adverse effects are usually minimal when the drug is carefully titrated. Finally, an oral preparation of labetalol is available for long-term maintenance therapy, albeit with a slightly different hemodynamic profile (i.e., β:α potency ratio) than is seen for the IV form of the drug.*

Nifedipine (Procardia, Adalat)

How Dispensed: 10- and 20-mg capsules
Indications: Hypertensive urgency

DOSE AND ROUTE OF ADMINISTRATION

Sublingual administration: Split a 10-mg capsule longitudinally, and place the contents under the patient's tongue for several minutes. Alternatively a patient may be asked to chew a capsule with several puncture holes in it to express its contents. Having the patient swallow the remains of the capsule will provide a more sustained effect.

> Although the dose of sublingual nifedipine is sometimes repeated in 20 to 30 minutes if an adequate blood pressure response is not seen by this time, caution is advised. A delay in the onset of action of the initial dose could produce an excessive hypotensive response if additional doses are prematurely given.
>
> Blood pressure should be checked frequently (i.e., every few minutes) after sublingual nifedipine is first given, and less often thereafter. It should be noted that comparable blood pressure reduction is achieved with oral administration of the drug, albeit with a slightly delayed onset of action (of 30 to 60 min).

COMMENTS

Among the currently available calcium channel blocking agents, nifedipine exerts the most potent vasodilating effect on the peripheral vasculature. Thus, although all calcium channel blockers are effective in the long-term management of hypertension, nifedipine has been the agent most commonly selected for treatment of hypertensive urgency. When administered *sublingually* for this indication, blood pressure begins to fall within minutes, and usually remains depressed for one to several hours.

> Compared to other agents used to treat acute elevations in blood pressure, sublingual nifedipine offers the advantages of being easy to administer, well tolerated, and rapidly effective. Treatment may be initiated in the office or emergency de-

---

*Alternatively, Gonzalez et al (1991) have shown that *oral* labetalol (in a single dose of 200 mg) may effectively treat less severe blood pressure elevations *without* the need for additional doses within a 4-hour period.

partment *without* the need for continuous blood pressure monitoring that is essential when nitroprusside is used.

The key point to emphasize regarding the use of sublingual nifedipine relates to the indications for treatment. The drug should *not* be used to treat hypertensive emergencies in which moment-to-moment blood pressure control is essential (Grauer and Gums, 1992). Thus, other agents (i.e., IV nitroglycerin or nitroprusside) are preferable for treatment of hypertension in the setting of acute ischemic heart disease. The unpredictable blood pressure lowering effect of sublingual nifedipine in this setting may exacerbate ischemia and/or precipitate extension of an infarct (Gifford, 1991). Similarly, sublingual nifedipine should *not* be used to treat hypertension associated with an acute cerebrovascular accident (i.e., TIA, stroke-in-evolution) since excessive blood pressure reduction in this situation might worsen an already compromised cerebral circulation. Hospitalization in an intensive care unit and institution of IV nitroprusside constitute the treatment of choice for hypertensive emergencies associated with acute neurologic events.

In summary, sublingual nifedipine is a safe, effective agent to consider for treatment of acute blood pressure elevation when cardiac and/or neurologic complications are absent (i.e., *hypertensive urgency*). Other agents are preferable for treatment of hypertensive emergencies when moment-to-moment blood pressure control is essential.

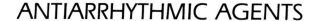

SECTION C

ANTIARRHYTHMIC AGENTS

Digoxin

How Dispensed:

For IV use: 0.25 mg/ml (2-ml ampule = 0.5 mg)

For oral use:

    Lanoxin—tablets of 0.125 mg, 0.25 mg, and 0.5 mg

    Lanoxicaps—capsule of 0.05 mg, 0.1 mg, and 0.2 mg

Indications: Limited in the acute care setting to atrial fibrillation/flutter with a rapid ventricular response (and perhaps PSVT as a 2nd or 3rd drug of choice after verapamil, adenosine, and/or IV esmolol).

Precautions: Digoxin should be used only with great caution (if at all) for treatment of MAT. The drug is *contraindicated* for treatment of rapid atrial fibrillation in patients with WPW (because digoxin may facilitate anterograde conduction over the accessory pathway and thus precipitate ventricular fibrillation).

> *Synchronized cardioversion* can usually be safely carried out in patients who have received therapeutic amounts of digoxin. However, because of the increase in myocardial excitability and decrease in fibrillatory threshold with digitalis excess, cardioversion is potentially dangerous *(and should be avoided if at all possible!)* when there is a chance of toxicity (Easterling and Tietze, 1989). If emergency cardioversion is necessary in such circumstances, it is particularly important to select the lowest amount of energy likely to be successful in converting the arrhythmia (Antman and Smith, 1986).

DOSE AND ROUTE OF ADMINISTRATION

IV Dose: For patients not previously digitalized, consider IV loading with an initial dose of 0.25 to 0.50 mg. This may be followed with 0.125- to 0.25 mg IV increments every 2 to 6 hours until a total of 0.75- to 1.50 mg has been given over the first 24 hours—that may then be followed the next day with the daily maintenance dose.

> The above schedule is suggested only as a rough guideline. It may need to be varied according to patient tolerance, the underlying medical condition, and the resultant ventricular response.
>
> The effects of IV digoxin occur much more rapidly than is generally appreciated. Onset of action may begin within 5 to 10 minutes! An initial peak of action is seen at about 30 to 60 minutes, with the maximum peak effect in about 4 to 6 hours.
>
> Digoxin is also effective when administered orally, albeit with a slightly delayed onset of action. The most commonly used preparation, lanoxin, has a bioavailability of 68%. Thus, when using this oral form of the drug, one would have to prescribe approximately one third *more* than the amount prescribed with the IV form to obtain the same effect. In contrast, bioavailability of the less commonly used Lanoxicaps is much

better (90-100%), and probably no correction at all need be made when switching from IV digoxin to this oral form.

Oral Maintenance Dose: ≈0.25 mg PO Qd (for most adults under 60 years of age who have normal renal function). Lower doses (i.e., 0.125 mg PO Qd or Qod) are recommended for older individuals and/or in those with renal impairment. *(Serum digoxin levels may help determine optimal dosing.)*

COMMENTS

Although frequently the source of controversy, digitalis has been a mainstay in the treatment of congestive heart failure ever since William Withering's first description of the foxglove in 1785.

> The drug has several actions. It increases the force and velocity of myocardial contraction (positive inotropic effect). When used in patients with congestive heart failure, heart size decreases and overall cardiac performance is improved. Digoxin also prolongs the refractory period of the AV node and, in so doing, helps to slow the ventricular response to most supraventricular tachyarrhythmias.

Despite these beneficial effects, *indications for the use of digoxin in the emergency care setting remain quite limited.* This is because the increase in cardiac contractility that the drug produces tends to be relatively modest (and is at least partially offset by an increase in myocardial oxygen consumption). Other medications (i.e., IV nitroglycerin, dobutamine, diuretics) are therefore preferable for treatment of congestive heart failure in the acute care setting. On the other hand, digoxin has long been favored as a drug of choice when supraventricular tachyarrhythmias (especially rapid atrial fibrillation) complicate acute myocardial infarction.

> It is important to appreciate that the principal mechanism by which digitalis slows the ventricular response to rapid atrial fibrillation is through an increase in vagal tone. As a result, even high doses of the drug will sometimes not be effective in controlling the heart rate of certain acutely ill patients for whom the tachyarrhythmia primarily reflects increased secretion of endogenous catecholamines (and/or patients receiving catecholamine infusion with agents such as epinephrine or dopamine). In these individuals the direct catecholamine inhibiting effect of *β-blockade* and/or the more direct AV nodal slowing action brought about by *IV verapamil* (or *IV diltiazem*) are much more likely to control the ventricular response to rapid atrial fibrillation than the vagotonic effect of digitalis (Falk and Leavitt, 1991).
>
> Alternatively, *combination therapy* (i.e., concomitant use of IV digoxin *and* IV verapamil) may produce a synergistic effect on heart rate control in the emergency setting. At the same time adverse effects can be minimized because lower doses of each agent can be used.

Digitalis Toxicity

The biggest potential drawback to the use of digitalis is the ever present risk of developing toxicity. The very narrow "therapeutic window" that exists between beneficial effects of the drug and toxicity makes it essential to carefully monitor patients on this medication. Clinically, one should be alert to the possibility of **digitalis toxicity** whenever any of the signs or symptoms shown in *Table 14C-1* occur in a patient taking digoxin.

Table 14C-1

Clinical Signs and Symptoms Suggestive of Digitalis Toxicity
• Nausea or vomiting • Disturbances in color vision (especially of red-green color perception, or seeing halos around light bulbs) • New-onset symptoms of psychosis • New-onset of nonspecific complaints of weakness, fatigue, or dizziness • Recent addition of drugs that may increase serum digoxin levels (i.e., quinidine, calcium channel blockers, amiodarone) • Recent worsening of renal failure • Development of certain cardiac arrhythmias suggestive of digitalis toxicity (i.e., frequent and/or multiform PVCs, ventricular tachycardia, atrial tachycardia with block, accelerated junctional rhythms, Wenckebach rhythms, atrial fibrillation with a slow or "regular" ventricular response).

Lower doses of digoxin are recommended for patients who may be especially susceptible to developing toxicity. Such individuals include patients with chronic obstructive pulmonary disease (who may be hypoxemic), patients with electrolyte disturbances (especially hypokalemia, hypomagnesemia, or hypercalcemia), the elderly, patients with renal impairment, hyperthyroidism, and/or in the setting of acute ischemia. It is well to remember that such individuals may sometimes manifest signs of toxicity at serum digoxin levels that are still within the "therapeutic range" (i.e., at serum digoxin levels between 1.2 and 2.0 ng/ml). Thus, *the diagnosis of digitalis toxicity is a clinical one that is not made exclusively on the basis of the serum digoxin level* (Grauer et al, 1982).

Treatment of *digitalis toxicity* consists of:

1. Withdrawing digoxin
2. Telemetry monitoring
3. Correcting electrolyte abnormalities (especially hypokalemia and hypomagnesemia)
4. Optimizing the patient's underlying medical condition (i.e., normalizing acid-base and volume status, correcting hypoxemia, treating ischemia, etc.)
5. Consideration of antiarrhythmic therapy (i.e., with lidocaine or phenytoin) as needed if worrisome ventricular arrhythmias develop
6. Consideration of digoxin antibody fragments (Digibind)

In many cases of digitalis toxicity, *little more than withdrawing the drug is needed*. Telemetry monitoring is advised if symptoms are associated with significant arrhythmias. It should be emphasized that the half-life of digoxin is commonly prolonged to 3 to 5 days in older individuals with impaired renal function. As a result, it may take several *days* (or even a week or more!) for markedly elevated levels in such patients to return to the normal range.

The pharmacokinetic elimination of digoxin is linear. This means that it takes approximately one half-life of the drug for the serum digoxin level to decrease by 50%. Thus, a patient with a 3-day half-life who presents with an initially toxic level of 4.0 ng/ml would require approximately 6 days (= two half-lives) for their serum digoxin level to return to 1.0 ng/ml (i.e., 3 days to decrease from 4.0 to 2.0 ng/ml, and an additional 3 days to decrease to 1.0 ng/ml).

Correction of electrolyte abnormalities is an important component of the treatment of digitalis toxicity. However, care should be taken *not* to administer IV potassium or magnesium too rapidly, since doing so may temporarily exacerbate cardiac arrhythmias (Antman and Smith, 1986).

Lidocaine (in standard doses) and/or phenytoin have been recommended as the antiarrhythmic agents of choice for digitalis-induced cardiac arrhythmias. **Phenytoin** is administered in 100-mg incremental doses by *slow* IV infusion (over a period of *at least* 5 minutes for every 100-mg dose!) until the arrhythmia is controlled, a total of 600 to 1,000 mg have been given, or phenytoin toxicity develops.

At the present time, the principal indication for administration of **digoxin antibody fragments** is for treatment of potentially life-threatening arrhythmias (i.e., sustained ventricular tachycardia, ventricular fibrillation, and/or severe bradyarrhythmias not responsive to atropine) that are the direct result of digitalis toxicity. (*Detailed discussion on recommendations for the use of digoxin antibody fragments follows below.*)

A Final Word on Digitalis: *A Drug Whose Time Has Gone?*

Recently, Falk and Leavitt (1991) have questioned whether digoxin should still be a drug of first choice for treatment of supraventricular tachyarrhythmias. As we have already noted, the principal mechanism by which digitalis slows AV conduction is an *indirect* one (through enhancement of vagal tone). One should therefore *expect* the drug to be *relatively ineffective* for treatment of conditions in which vagal tone is either withdrawn or overridden by excessive sympathetic stimulation.

Whereas digitalis may well provide adequate heart rate control for sedentary older patients with atrial fibrillation, it is much less likely to be effective in treating younger adults—especially if they are fairly active individuals (Klein and Kaplinsky, 1986; Falk and Leavitt, 1991). Similarly, in an acute care setting, catecholamine excess (from sympathetic stimulation) is likely to override the indirect vagotonic effects of the drug.

Two additional points should be stressed about the use of digoxin for treatment of atrial fibrillation:

1. In patients who are not in heart failure, the drug *by itself* appears to be *no more effective than placebo* for converting the arrhythmia to sinus rhythm.

   Many patients who present with new-onset rapid atrial fibrillation do not persist with this arrhythmia. Despite the common practice of acutely digitalizing such patients, conversion to sinus rhythm is most often a *spontaneous* event that is more likely attributable to correction of one or more underlying precipitating factors (such as hypoxemia, heart failure, ischemia, and/or electrolyte disturbance) than to antiarrhythmic properties of the drug (Falk et al, 1987).

2. The beneficial vagotonic effect of digoxin on the AV node may be *counteracted* by an adverse effect on atrial tissue.

   In addition to its effect on the AV node, digoxin exerts both a direct and indirect effect on atrial tissue. Whereas the former action results in slight prolongation of the atrial refractory period, the drug's indirect (vagotonic) effect usually predominates and acts in the opposite manner to *shorten* the atrial refractory period. As a result there is *increased* dispersion in atrial refractoriness (Falk and Leavitt, 1991). Under certain circumstances these physiologic changes may paradoxically *increase* susceptibility to development (or recurrence) of atrial fibrillation, as well as *increasing* the atrial (and therefore the ventricular) rate during such episodes (Rawles et al, 1990).

   Thus, having digoxin "on board" does not necessarily prevent recurrence of atrial fibrillation, nor does it protect against development of an excessively rapid ventricular response if such a recurrence occurs. On the contrary, most recurrent episodes of atrial fibrillation appear to be associated—at least initially—with a predominance of sympathetic tone—and might therefore be expected to respond poorly to digoxin (Rawles et al, 1990; Falk and Leavitt, 1991).

We definitely are *not* advocating abandonment of the use of digoxin for treatment of atrial fibrillation. The drug has withstood the test of time, and it clearly retains a place in the treatment regimen. What we are indicating, however, is that for patients with atrial fibrillation who are not in heart failure, other treatment modalities (i.e., use of β-blockers, verapamil, and/or diltiazem) may be preferable—especially for treatment of conditions in which sympathetic tone is likely to be increased. It is well to remember that digoxin is not a benign medication, and that *by itself,* the drug per se does not appear to facilitate conversion of atrial fibrillation or flutter to sinus rhythm compared to the effects of placebo.

In summary, digoxin can still be effectively used for the treatment of supraventricular tachyarrhythmias. However, it is no longer necessarily the drug of choice. If the decision is made to use digoxin, the possibility of less than optimal arrhythmia control should be kept in mind, and consideration given to alternative therapy if the desired clinical response is not achieved.

Digoxin Antibody Fragments (Digibind)

How Dispensed: Digoxin-immune Fab (Digibind) is a preparation of digoxin-specific antibody fragments obtained from immunized sheep. It is dispensed in vials:

> **1 vial of Digibind** (= 40 mg)
> **will bind ≈ 0.6 mg of digoxin**

Indications: Potentially life-threatening cardiac arrhythmias that are the direct result of digitalis toxicity (i.e., sustained ventricular tachycardia/fibrillation, severe bradyarrhythmias *not* responsive to atropine)

   There may be occasion to use Digibind as a *diagnostic tool* in selected patients with borderline serum digoxin levels (i.e., between 1.5- 2.0 ng/ml) when it is important to determine if a potentially life-threatening arrhythmia is a manifestation of digitalis toxicity. If the arrhythmia does not resolve with administration of a therapeutic dose of Digibind, one can conclude that the arrhythmia was not the result of digitalis toxicity.

DOSE AND ROUTE OF ADMINISTRATION

Digibind is administered IV over 15 to 30 minutes (ideally being infused through a 0.22-μm membrane filter). It may be given as a bolus if cardiac arrest is imminent. The dose will vary depending on the amount of digoxin that needs to be neutralized, but consideration of the following may help with empiric dosing (Medical Letter, 1986):

- An average dose of 10 vials has been used in clinical testing of digoxin overdose patients.
- For acute ingestion of a large *unknown* quantity of digoxin, an empiric dose of 20 vials (=800 mg) may be tried in adults or large children. Larger doses of Digibind may have a more rapid onset of action, but also carries the risk of causing a febrile reaction.
- A second empiric dose of Digibind may be administered several hours later (if needed).

It should be emphasized that once Digibind is administered, it will *no longer be possible* to follow the patient's serum digoxin level by the usual monitoring methods (i.e., serum digoxin levels increase markedly after administration of Digibind!). Elimination of antibody fragments may require up to 1 week (depending on renal function), so that if redigitalization is needed, it may be necessary to wait at least a week before restarting the drug!

- Much smaller doses of Digibind (on the order of 1 to 3 vials) are needed to treat digitalis toxicity arrhythmias that are not due to digoxin overdose (i.e., in association with serum digoxin levels of 2-4 ng/ml).

To Estimate the Dose of Digibind:

$$\underset{\text{(in \# of vials)}}{\text{Dose}} = \underset{\text{(in ng/ml)}}{\underset{\text{Level}}{\underset{\text{Digoxin}}{\text{Serum}}}} \times \underset{\text{(in kg)}}{\text{Bodyweight}} \div 100$$

Thus, to estimate the *neutralizing dose* for treatment of a 70-kg adult with a potentially life-threatening digitalis toxicity arrhythmia and an initial serum digoxin level = 4 ng/ml, *one should infuse 3 vials of Digibind IV over 30 minutes* (i.e., **4** ng/ml **×** **70** kg = 280 ÷ **100** = 2.8, or approximately **3 vials** of Digibind).

Clinically, the onset of action of Digibind begins within 15 to 30 minutes after completion of the infusion, with the maximal effect usually occurring within 3 to 4 hours. Duration of action is approximately 12 hours.

> Precautions to observe during (and after) administration of Digibind include telemetry monitoring for cardiac arrhythmias, frequent notation of vital signs (especially blood pressure and temperature recording), and frequent determination of serum potassium and magnesium values (with special attention directed at preventing hypokalemia). Because *therapeutic effects* of digoxin are also reversed by Digibind, it is important to realize that the drug may cause a recurrence of congestive heart failure and/or accelerate the ventricular response to atrial fibrillation.

COMMENTS

Up until recently, morbidity and mortality from massive digitalis overdose and/or severe digitalis toxicity arrhythmias had been alarmingly high. Development of digoxin-specific antibody fragments (Digibind) holds promise of significantly improving upon the results of conventional therapy for this potentially life-threatening condition.

> In a study by Antman et al (1990) of 150 patients with potentially life-threatening digitalis toxicity, use of Digibind resulted in resolution of all signs and symptoms of digitalis toxicity in 80% of study subjects. An additional 10% of patients improved, and only 10% failed to respond. After administration of Digibind infusion, the median time for an initial response was less than 20 minutes, with 75% of patients demonstrating evidence of a beneficial effect by 60 minutes. Less than 10% of patients developed an adverse event from Digibind (with hypokalemia and/or exacerbation of congestive heart failure being the most commonly reported side effects). There were no allergic reactions. Among those patients who experienced cardiac arrest as a manifestation of digitalis toxicity, more than 50% survived hospitalization. Thus, *a beneficial treatment response can be expected with the use of Digibind in more than 90% of cases of severe, life-threatening digitalis intoxication!*

Hyperkalemia is one finding that merits special mention. Development of this electrolyte abnormality is a poor prognostic sign in digitalis toxicity because it implies a more severe degree of impairment of the sodium-potassium-ATP pump mechanism. The result is leakage of potassium out of the cell membrane and into extracellular fluid. Early use of Digibind for patients with digitalis toxicity who develop hyperkalemia may improve prognosis.

> If severe, digitalis-induced hyperkalemia should be treated with D10/Insulin and/or Kayexalate. *Calcium should not be used (since this cation is contraindicated in digitalis toxicity)!* Special effort should be made not to overshoot correction of digitalis-induced hyperkalemia because hypokalemia may further aggravate the arrhythmias of digitalis toxicity.

Esmolol (Brevibloc)

How Dispensed: Ampules containing 10 mg/ml and 2.5 g/10 ml

Indications: Emergency treatment of supraventricular tachyarrhythmias (as an alternative agent to IV verapamil and/or adenosine); for selected patients with ventricular tachyarrhythmias, hypertensive urgency, and/or with acute myocardial infarction; treatment of peri-operative complications resulting from excessive sympathetic tone and/or β-blocker withdrawal.

Precautions: Similar to those for other β-blockers (i.e., caution in the presence of heart failure, tendency to bronchospasm, bradycardia, AV block, and following recent administration of IV verapamil). Compared to other β-blockers, however, the short duration of action of esmolol makes it less likely that these precautions will be problematic.

DOSE AND ROUTE OF ADMINISTRATION

Dosing recommendations for IV esmolol are somewhat complex and entail administration of an initial IV loading dose, initiation of an IV maintenance infusion, gradual upward titration of the maintenance infusion, and readministration of the loading dose before each incremental increase in the rate of the maintenance infusion (to ensure rapid achievement of each new steady-state level). The following protocol has been recommended (Medical Letter, 1987):

---

1. Administration of an **initial IV loading dose** (of 500 μg/kg to be administered over a 1-min period).
2. Initiation of an **IV maintenance infusion** at 50 μg/kg/min (to be continued over the next 4 min).
3. If steps **1** and **2** have not produced the desired

effect, **readministration** of the **loading dose** (i.e., 500 μg/kg over a 1-min period).

4. **Increasing** the rate of the maintenance infusion by 50 μg/kg/min (to a rate of 100 μg/kg/min).

5. **Repeating the process** (i.e., readministration of the loading dose, and incremental increase of the infusion rate to 150—and then to 200 μg/kg/min if needed).

Allow the maintenance infusion to continue for *at least* 4 minutes after each incremental increase in rate. If the desired clinical response is achieved during this time, the maintenance infusion may be continued at this rate. If not, readminister another loading dose (of 500 μg/kg over a 1-min period) and increase the rate of the maintenance infusion by an additional 50 μg/kg/minute.

After achieving control of the arrhythmia with IV esmolol, the patient may be switched over to alternative oral therapy (i.e., with digoxin, verapamil, and/or an oral β-blocker). To do this, the rate of the IV esmolol maintenance infusion may be reduced by 50% within 30 minutes after starting oral antiarrhythmic therapy. If the patient remains stable after receiving the second oral dose, the IV esmolol maintenance infusion may be discontinued an hour later (Frishman, et al, 1988).

Almost all patients who respond to the drug do so at maintenance infusion rates of between 50 to 150 μg/kg/minute. Infusion rates greater than 200 μg/kg/minute are generally not advised because additional clinical benefit is unlikely, and the risk of producing significant hypotension is unduly increased (Medical Letter, 1987; Frishman et al, 1988).

COMMENTS

Esmolol is a cardioselective β-adrenergic blocking agent with a rapid onset of action following IV administration and a short duration of action. Because its elimination phase half-life is *less* than 10 minutes, adverse effects are generally short-lived and pharmacologic effects will usually dissipate within 15 to 30 minutes of discontinuing the drug. This confers the drug with a decided advantage compared to other IV β-blocking agents such as propranolol and metoprolol which have a significantly longer duration of action (of several hours or more).

IV esmolol effectively slows the ventricular response to rapid atrial fibrillation/flutter, and it appears to be more effective than IV verapamil in converting these arrhythmias to sinus rhythm. The drug is also an effective alternative agent (to IV verapamil or adenosine) for treatment of reentry supraventricular tachyarrhythmias such as PSVT.

IV esmolol is generally safe to administer to patients with acute myocardial infarction, even in the presence of mild to moderate left ventricular dysfunction (Kirshenbaum et al, 1988). Because adverse effects are rapidly reversed, the drug may find a special role for use in this setting when it becomes important to determine whether a β-blocking agent can be tolerated (Kirshenbaum, 1989). The relative cardioselectivity of the drug makes esmolol less likely than other β-blockers to precipitate bronchospasm in potentially susceptible patients.

Practically speaking, two factors limit the use of esmolol: (1) a high incidence of hypotension; and (2) the complex nature of protocols for its administration.

Hypotension has been reported to occur in as many as 20% to 50% of patients who receive the drug (Medical Letter, 1987; Frishman et al, 1988). Because hypotension is generally a dose-related phenomenon, careful dose titration (and reduction in the rate of infusion of the drug if hypotension occurs) is essential. As is the case for other adverse effects, blood pressure almost always normalizes within 15 to 30 minutes of discontinuing the infusion.

In summary, esmolol is an exciting new cardioselective β-blocking agent that may become the treatment of choice for those situations in which it is desirable to administer a rapidly-acting β-blocker whose actions will reverse promptly if an adverse effect does occur. However, drawbacks of the drug (i.e., complex dosing regimen, high incidence of hypotension, need to avoid concomitant administration of IV verapamil) make it less likely that IV esmolol will establish a niche in the routine treatment of supraventricular tachyarrhythmias.

DILTIAZEM (Cardizem)

How Dispensed:
For IV use: 5.0 mg/ml (25 mg in a 5 ml vial; 50 mg in a 10 ml vial)
For oral use:
  Cardizem: tablets of 30, 60, 90, and 120 mg
  Cardizem SR: 60-, 90-, and 120-mg Sustained Release capsules
  Cardizem CD: 180-, 240-, and 300-mg capsules (for once daily dosing)

Indications: Supraventricular tachyarrhythmias (including PSVT, rapid atrial fibrillation, atrial flutter); acute ischemic heart disease (?).

Although experience to date is limited, use of IV diltiazem holds great promise of being beneficial for treatment of select patients with acute ischemic heart disease (Jaffe, 1992).

Precautions/Contraindications: In general, similar precautions are advised when using IV diltiazem as for the use of IV verapamil. Thus, caution is urged when considering use of the drug in patients with impaired left ventricular function (although the risk of precipitating or exacerbating heart failure does not appear to be as great as it is with administration of IV verapamil). Similarly, caution is urged when using IV diltiazem in patients with a history of sick sinus syndrome or conduction system disease (i.e., 2° or 3° AV block).

> Clinically, the most common adverse effect associated with IV use of diltiazem is hypotension. Fortunately, the overall incidence of this complication is low (*less* than 5%), and most cases are mild and transient enough so as not to require additional treatment. Nevertheless, special caution is urged when considering the use of IV diltiazem for treatment of supraventricular tachyarrhythmias associated with borderline blood pressure readings (i.e., with systolic pressures of 100 to 110 mm Hg or less).

Clinical situations in which *neither* IV diltiazem *nor* IV verapamil should be used include:

- treatment of a wide complex tachycardia of uncertain etiology (i.e., that could be ventricular tachycardia)
- treatment of patients with atrial fibrillation or flutter in the presence of an accessory pathway (i.e., WPW)
- treatment of patients who have just received an IV β-blocker

> Diltiazem is extensively metabolized by the liver and excreted by the kidneys. As a result, IV diltiazem should be used cautiously (and downward adjustment in dosing may be necessary) in patients with significant renal or hepatic impairment.

DOSE AND ROUTE OF ADMINISTRATION

IV Bolus Dosing: The *initial* recommended dose for IV use of diltiazem in an average-sized adult is administration of an **IV bolus** of approximately **20 mg** (i.e., 0.25 mg/kg) given over a 2-minute period. If this fails to produce the desired clinical response within 15 minutes, the dose may be increased with a *second* IV bolus of approximately **25 mg** (i.e., 0.35 mg/kg).

- Dosing for subsequent IV boluses should be individualized for each patient. Although some patients may respond to an IV bolus of as little as 15 mg, higher doses will be needed in most cases.
- Recall of recommendations for IV diltiazem dosing is facilitated by use of round numbers (i.e., use of 15, 20, or 25 mg for the amount of drug in an IV bolus). While round number approximations are appropriate for most patients, use of the *specific* milligram per killigram recommendations (i.e., **0.25 mg/kg** for the *initial* bolus— and **0.35 mg/kg** for the *second* bolus—based on **actual** *body weight*) is advised when treating patients who are either much lighter or heavier than "average."

Clinical effects from an IV bolus of diltiazem begin within 3 minutes of administration and usually peak by 7 minutes. Effects of the bolus last for approximately 1 to 3 hours (Ellenbogen et al, 1991).

IV infusion: For maintenance of antiarrhythmic effect (and continued rate control), an **IV infusion** of diltiazem is often started following bolus administration.

> Calculations for preparing an IV infusion of diltiazem may be simplified by incorporation of two modifications into the **"Rule of 250 ml"** (that was first presented in Section C of Chapter 2):
> 1. Use of **250 mg** (= the contents of *five* 50 mg vials—instead of the contents of one vial) as **"one unit"** of drug
> 2. Initiation of the infusion at a rate of **10 drops/min** (instead of 30 drops/min).

With the above two modifications in mind, an IV infusion of diltiazem may be prepared by mixing **1 "unit"** of drug (= **250 mg**) in **250 ml** of **diluent**.* Doing so results in a *concentration* of 1 mg/ml:

$$\boxed{\frac{1 \text{ unit of drug}}{250 \text{ ml}}} = \frac{250 \text{ mg}}{250 \text{ ml}} = \frac{1000 \text{ mg}}{1000 \text{ ml}} = \frac{1 \text{ mg}}{1 \text{ ml}}$$

The **recommended initial infusion rate** for IV diltiazem is **10 mg/hr** (= 10 mg/60 min). One should therefore set the rate of the IV infusion to deliver **1 mg of drug** (i.e., the contents of **1 ml**) every **6 minutes** in order to deliver 10 mg of drug/hour:

$$\boxed{\frac{10 \text{ mg}}{\text{hour}}} = \frac{10 \text{ mg}}{60 \text{ min}} = \frac{1 \text{ mg}}{6 \text{ min}} = \frac{1 \text{ ml}}{6 \text{ min}}$$

> Since **1 ml = 60 drops** for a **microdrip**, the *initial* rate of the IV infusion should be set to run at **10 drops/min** (to deliver 10 mg/hour):

$$\boxed{1 \text{ ml} = 60 \text{ drops} \text{ for a } \textbf{microdrip}}$$

$$\frac{1 \text{ ml}}{6 \text{ min}} \times \frac{60 \text{ drops}}{1 \text{ ml}} = \frac{60 \text{ drops}}{6 \text{ min}} = \boxed{\frac{10 \text{ drops}}{\text{min}}}$$

According to the above *concentration*, a rate of:
- 5 mg/hr = 5 drops/min
- **10 mg/hr = 10 drops/min**
- 15 mg/hr = 15 drops/min

> It should be noted that an infusion rate of 10 mg/hr (= 10 drops/min) may not be sufficient for some patients. In such cases the higher rate of infusion (i.e., 15 mg/hour = 15 drops/

*NOTE—As indicated above, *five* 10-ml vials of diltiazem are used for preparation of the IV infusion (50 mg of drug being contained in each 10-ml vial). This means that a **"unit"** of diltiazem (= 250 mg) will be contained within 50 ml of diluent (5 vials × 10 ml in each vial = 50 ml)—so that *only* **200 ml of D5W** will need to be added for preparation of the infusion to come up with the total 250 ml of diluent.

min) may be needed. In contrast, other patients may maintain an adequate therapeutic effect at an infusion rate as low as 5 mg/hour (= 5 drops/minute).* The capability of titrating the dose of drug delivered by IV infusion provides the distinct advantage of regulating whether control of heart rate will be "tighter" or "looser" (Ellenbogen, 1992).

COMMENTS

The recent approval of diltiazem for IV use is an exciting development with potentially far-reaching implications in our pharmacologic armamentarium. Although additional studies and clinical experience are clearly needed before definitive recommendations can be made, it appears that IV diltiazem may:

1. become an agent of choice for achieving and maintaining acute *rate control* of rapid atrial fibrillation and flutter
2. become an agent of choice for acute treatment of PSVT
3. be *preferable* to use of other IV antiarrhythmic agents (such as verapamil, digoxin, adenosine, and esmolol) for acute treatment of *certain* patients with supraventricular tachyarrhythmias.

Results from initial studies have been extremely encouraging:

A multicenter, double-blind, randomized, placebo-controlled trial by Salerno et al (1989) suggests that administration of IV diltiazem is *both* safe and effective in slowing the ventricular response of patients with rapid (i.e., average heart rate >120 beats/min) atrial fibrillation and atrial flutter. More than 90% of patients in their study responded with *at least* a 20% reduction in average heart rate to IV bolus treatment with diltiazem. Most patients responded to the *initial* IV bolus (of 0.25 mg/kg—or about 20 mg)—with the rest responding to a *second* IV bolus (of 0.35 mg/kg—or about 25 mg).

Adverse effects in the study were minimal. Less than 10% of patients developed hypotension (i.e., a systolic blood pressure of <90 mm Hg), and *none* required treatment for hypotension. Efficacy of the drug was rapidly achieved, and the *median* time until maximal heart rate control was *less* than 5 minutes!

A similar beneficial response to IV bolus administration with diltiazem was demonstrated in a study by Ellenbogen et al of patients with rapid atrial fibrillation or flutter (1991). In this trial, initiation of an IV infusion of diltiazem at a rate of between 10 to 15 mg/hour, and continuation of the infusion over the ensuing 24 hours was shown to maintain effective rate control during this period in more than 80% of study subjects (Ellenbogen et al, 1991).

Equally favorable results to administration of one or two boluses of IV diltiazem have been obtained in patients with PSVT. Thus, conversion of PSVT to normal sinus rhythm is

rapidly achieved (i.e., usually within 2 minutes of bolus administration) in approximately 85% to 90% of cases, with only a minimal incidence of adverse effects (Huycke et al, 1989).

COMPARISON OF IV DILTIAZEM WITH OTHER IV ANTIARRHYTHMIC AGENTS:

The number of IV antiarrhythmic agents available for acute treatment of supraventricular tachyarrhythmias continues to expand. Initial experience with **IV diltiazem** suggests that this drug may offer a number of advantages compared to other agents that are currently being used (Ellenbogen, 1992). We summarize these beneficial features of IV diltiazem as follows:

*Compared to **IV verapamil**:*
- The risk of exacerbating/precipitating heart failure appears to be less
- The risk of producing significant hypotension is less
- The degree of drug interaction with digoxin (with resultant increase in the serum digoxin level) is less
- An *approved* formulation of the drug is available for use as a *continuous IV infusion* for maintenance of the antiarrhythmic effect.*

*Compared to **IV digoxin**:*
- Onset of action is more rapid
- Rate control is more effective
- The chance of significant antiarrhythmic drug interaction is much less (compared to the high likelihood of significant drug interaction between digoxin and quinidine or verapamil)
- An *approved* formulation of the drug is available for use as a *continuous IV infusion* for maintenance of the antiarrhythmic effect
- The drug may also be beneficial for treatment of acute ischemic syndromes (whereas digoxin could exacerbate ischemia by increasing myocardial oxygen consumption)

*Compared to **IV esmolol**:*
- There is much greater facility in dosing
- Time until peak clinical effect in most patients is shorter (as a result of the much greater facility in dosing)
- Duration of action is longer (so that the need for continuation of the IV infusion is less)
- The incidence of hypotension is less
- Depression of left ventricular contractility is less

*Compared to **IV adenosine**:*
- There is wider clinical application (since adenosine is not useful in acute treatment of atrial fibrillation or flutter)
- Duration of action is longer (with consequent decreased chance of PSVT recurrence)
- An *approved* formulation of the drug is available for use as a *continuous IV infusion* for maintenance of the antiarrhythmic effect
- The drug may also be beneficial for treatment of acute ischemic syndromes (whereas adenosine could exacerbate ischemia by predisposing to deleterious redistribution of coronary flow)

---

*At the time of this writing, IV infusion rates of *greater* than 15 mg/hour have not been adequately studied (and are therefore *not* recommended). For similar reasons, continuation of an IV infusion of diltiazem for longer than 24 hours is generally not recommended.

---

*At the time of this writing, verapamil has not yet been approved for use as a continuous IV infusion.

Clinical Perspective

Many drugs are currently available for acute treatment of supraventricular tachyarrhythmias—each with its own unique set of clinical characteristics. Recent development of IV diltiazem adds yet another agent to our clinical armamentarium. While the drug will only rarely convert atrial fibrillation or flutter to sinus rhythm, it reliably slows the ventricular response to these tachyarrhythmias with a favorable side effect profile compared to other agents. In addition, IV diltiazem is almost equally effective as IV verapamil in converting PSVT to normal sinus rhythm. Although the role that this new drug will have in management of acute ischemic heart disease and hypertensive urgency remains to be determined, its potential clinical impact in the acute treatment of supraventricular tachyarrhythmias is exciting indeed.

SECTION D

MISCELLANEOUS DRUGS

Furosemide (Lasix)

How Dispensed: Ampules of 20 mg and 100 mg
Indications: Acute pulmonary edema, congestive heart failure, hypertensive emergencies, other edema states

DOSE AND ROUTE OF ADMINISTRATION

IV Dose: The usual initial dose for treatment of pulmonary edema is 40 to 80 mg IV. Incremental doubling of the dose is advised if there is no response within 30 to 60 minutes.

> Some patients who have never received furosemide before will be exquisitely sensitive to the effects of the drug. In such individuals, a 20-mg IV dose may be all that is needed to produce a brisk (and profound) diuresis. In contrast, much higher doses (up to 160 mg and more) may be needed in patients with poor renal function to achieve diuresis.
>
> An extremely useful clinical pearl to remember in patients resistant to high doses of furosemide is that addition of a low dose (2.5 to 5 mg PO) of **metolazone (Zaroxolyn)** may result in a therapeutic diuresis. The likely reason for this response is that metolazone acts at a different site in the nephron, and thus produces a synergistic effect when combined with furosemide. Addition/substitution of other diuretic agents such as 25 to 50 mg of **hydrochlorothiazide (HCTZ),** 1 to 2 mg of **bumetanide (Bumex),** and/or 50 mg of IV **ethacrynic acid (Edecrin)** may sometimes produce a similar beneficial response in patients resistant to high doses of furosemide.

PO Dose: *Not advised for acutely ill patients in need of an immediate diuretic effect.*

COMMENTS

Furosemide is a potent loop diuretic. As such it inhibits tubular resorption of sodium chloride in the ascending loop of Henle.

Following IV administration, diuresis begins within 5 to 15 minutes, peaks at 20 to 60 minutes, and continues for approximately 2 hours. It is important to emphasize, however that the initial therapeutic effect of IV furosemide in pulmonary edema stems *not* from this diuresis, but rather from the ability of the drug to rapidly reduce preload by increasing venous capacitance. This phenomenon explains why clinical improvement may occur with pulmonary edema *even before* diuresis begins!

> In patients who are not acutely ill, oral furosemide is well absorbed and works almost as effectively as the IV preparation. Diuresis following oral ingestion usually begins within 30 to 60 minutes, peaks by 1 to 2 hours, and continues for 4 to 8 hours. However, with acute heart failure (especially if there is a significant component of right-sided heart failure),

> intestinal absorption may be impaired due to edema of the gut. Oral furosemide (even in large doses!) may not be effective in this situation. As a result, *we routinely favor the use of IV furosemide for patients who are hospitalized with heart failure.*

Naloxone (Narcan)

How Dispensed: 0.4 mg/ml (1-ml ampules [= 0.4 mg] and 10-ml vials [= 4 mg])
Indications: *None* in the setting of cardiac arrest (unless narcotic overdose is suspected as a precipitating cause)

DOSE AND ROUTE OF ADMINISTRATION

For suspected narcotic overdose— 2 to 4 mg IV
For shock—???

COMMENTS

Among the most intriguing of concepts to be proposed is the idea that the narcotic antagonist naloxone might be beneficial in treatment of cardiac arrest.

> The theory is based on the properties of *endorphins*. These endogenous opiate-like substances are produced by the pituitary gland and released in the body in response to physiologic stress states. Because endorphins are known to lower peripheral vascular resistance and exert a myocardial depressant effect, it was thought that they might play a role in various shock states. By extension they could also be operative in cardiac arrest, since this condition has been viewed as "the ultimate shock state" (Rothstein et al, 1985).

If release of endorphins is at least partially responsible for the myocardial and peripheral vascular depression of cardiac arrest, might these effects not be reversed by administration of naloxone?

> Despite suggestive evidence from animal studies, clinical trials in humans have failed to demonstrate improved survival when patients in shock are treated with naloxone (Reynolds et al, 1980; Wilson, 1985; Benton, 1985). Most published reports on the use of naloxone in shock are retrospective case studies in which the drug had been used to treat patients with sepsis after conventional therapy had failed. Little prospective work has been done in the setting of cardiac arrest. Rothstein et al (1985) examined the effects of the drug after inducing ventricular fibrillation in mongrel dogs. Although naloxone was not found to be helpful in facilitating defibrillation, animals who developed EMD recovered after receiving the drug.
>
> At the present time, *there appears to be no indication for the use of naloxone in the setting of cardiac arrest* (unless narcotic overdose is suspected as a precipitating cause). One should be aware that the doses of naloxone used in the study by Rothstein et al (1985) were massive (5 mg/kg!).

Clearly, much more work would have to be done in a prospective manner on human subjects before it would be possible to make any recommendations regarding any potential use of this drug. Nevertheless, the idea that EMD might be treated by narcotic antagonism is fascinating indeed.

Corticosteroids

How Dispensed:

Methylprednisolone (Solu-Medrol): available in 40-mg, 125-mg, 500-mg, 1,000-mg, and 2,000-mg packages with diluent attached

Dexamethasone (Decadron): vials of 1 ml (4 mg), 5 ml (20 mg), and 25 ml (100 mg)

Indications: *None* in the setting of cardiac arrest (unless other potentially steroid-responsive conditions are felt to be present)

DOSE AND ROUTE OF ADMINISTRATION

IV Dose: Large doses (of up to 30 mg/kg of solumedrol) had been recommended in the past for treatment of shock.

COMMENTS

The question of whether high-dose corticosteroids should be administered to patients with conditions such as shock, aspiration pneumonia, adult respiratory distress syndrome (ARDS), and/or cerebral edema from anoxic brain insult, has always stirred great controversy. Although enthusiasm for the use of corticosteroids in these situations has dramatically decreased in recent years, full discussion of the subject clearly extends well beyond the scope of this book. However, the issue of whether corticosteroids should be considered for treatment of patients in a *pulseless idioventricular rhythm (PIVR)* is one that is pertinent to the interests of the emergency care provider managing cardiac arrest.

> The mechanism of action that has been postulated for corticosteroids is stabilization of myocardial membranes, an effect that might limit leakage of lysosomal enzymes and ischemic damage. Use of steroids might also facilitate release of ATP from myocardial mitochondria in a manner that could make ATP more available for the sodium/potassium pump, thus restoring membrane polarization and impulse conduction (Carden, 1984).

Clinically, enthusiasm for using corticosteroids stems from a report by White in 1976 that the drug was successful in resuscitating a small group of patients with PIVR. Although scattered additional reports in support of the use of corticosteroids followed (Paris et al, 1984), confirmatory studies demonstrating a beneficial treatment response to this form of therapy are lacking in recent years.

> Retrospective analysis of subjects responding to steroids in earlier studies suggests that other variables (such as septic shock and cerebral hematoma) may have accounted for some of the success in treatment. Only a minority of patients who responded appear to have actually arrested as a direct result of cardiac disease.

In summary, although a theoretical basis may exist for the use of corticosteroids in patients with PIVR, this has *not* been borne out by clinical studies in recent years. At the current time, *there is no indication for the use of corticosteroids in the setting of cardiopulmonary arrest.*

References

American Heart Association Subcommittee on Emergency Cardiac Care: Standards and guidelines for cardiopulmonary resuscitation (CPR) and emergency cardiac care (ECC), *JAMA* 255:2905-2992, 1986.

Antman EM, Wenger TL, Butler VP, Haber E, Smith TW: Treatment of 150 cases of life-threatening digitalis intoxication with digoxin-specific fab antibody fragments: final report of a multicenter study, *Circulation* 81:1744-1752, 1990.

Bernton EW: Naloxone and TRH in the treatment of shock and trauma: what future roles? *Ann Emerg Med* 14:729-735, 1985.

Brott T, Reed RL: Intensive care for acute stroke in the community hospital setting: the first 24 hours, *Cur Conc Cerebrovasc Dis* 24:1-5, 1989.

Carden DL: High-dose corticosteroids in the treatment of pulseless idioventricular rhythm, *Ann Emerg Med* 13:817-219, 1984.

Colucci WS, Wright RF, Braunwald E: New positive inotropic agents in the treatment of congestive heart failure: mechanisms of action and recent clinical developments, *N Engl J Med* 314:290-299, 349-358, 1986.

Denes P, Gabster A, Huang SK: Clinical, electrocardiographic and follow-up observations in patients having ventricular fibrillation during Holter monitoring, *Am J Cardiol* 48:9-16, 1981.

Easterling R, Tietze PE: Digitalis Toxicity, *J Am Bd Fam Prac* 2:49-54, 1989.

Ellenbogen KA, Dias VC, Plumb VJ, Heywood JT, Mirvis DM: A placebo-controlled trial of continuous intravenous diltiazem infusion for 24-hour heart rate control during atrial fibrillation and atrial flutter: a multicenter study, *J Am Coll Cardiol* 18:891-897, 1991.

Ellenbogen KA: Role of calcium antagonists for heart rate control in atrial fibrillation, *Am J Cardiol* 69:36B-40B, 1992.

Falk RH, Knowlton AA, Bernard SA, Gotlieb NE, Battinelli NJ: Digoxin for converting recent-onset atrial fibrillation to sinus rhythm: a randomized, double-blind trial, *Ann Int Med* 106:503-506, 1987.

Falk RH, Leavitt JI: Digoxin for atrial fibrillation: a drug whose time has gone? *Ann Int Med* 114:573-575, 1991.

Ferguson RK, Vlasses PH: Hypertensive emergencies and urgencies, *JAMA* 255:1607-1613, 1986.

Flaherty JT: Parenteral nitroglycerin: clinical usefulness and limitations. In Conti CR (ed): Cardiac drug therapy, cardiovascular clinics, Philadelphia, 1984, FA Davis.

Frishman WH: Pharmacology of the nitrates in angina pectoris, *Am J Cardiol* 56:81-131, 1985.

Frishman WH, Murthy VS, Strom JA: Ultra-short-acting β-adrenergic blockers 72:359-372, 1988.

Genton R, Jaffe A: Management of congestive heart failure in patients with acute myocardial infarction, *JAMA* 256:2556-2560, 1986.

Gifford RW: Management of hypertensive crises, *JAMA* 266:829-835, 1991.

Gonzalez ER, Peterson MA, Racht EM, Ornato JP, Due DL: Dose-response evaluation of oral labetalol in patients presenting to the emergency department with accelerated hypertension, *Ann Emerg Med* 20:333-338, 1991.

Grauer K, Curry RW, Robinson JD: Prediction of serum concentrations of digoxin in a family practice center, *J Fam Prac* 15:1081-1086, 1982.

Grauer K, Gums J: Oral antihypertensive agent, *J Fam Prac* 34:397, 1992, (letter).

Huycke EC, Sung RJ, Dias VC, Milstein S, Hariman RJ, Platia EV, and the Multicenter Diltiazem PSVT Study Group: Intravenous diltiazem for termination of reentrant supraventricular tachycardia: a placebo-controlled, randomized, double-blind, multicenter study, *J Am Coll Cardiol* 13:538-544, 1989.

Jaffe AS: Use of intravenous diltiazem in patients with acute coronary artery disease, *Am J Cardiol* 69:25B-29B, 1992.

Kirshenbaum JM, Kloner RF, McGowan N, Antman EM: Use of an ultrashort-acting beta-receptor blocker (esmolol) in patients with acute myocardial ischemia and relative contraindications to beta-blockade therapy, *J Am Coll Cardiol* 12:773-780, 1988.

Kirshenbaum JM: Non-thrombolytic intervention in acute myocardial infarction, *Am J Cardiol* 64:25B-28B, 1989.

Klein HO, Kaplinsky E: Digitalis and verapamil in atrial fibrillation and flutter: is verapamil now the preferred agent? *Drugs* 31:185-197, 1986.

Medical Letter: Intravenous amrinone for congestive heart failure, *Med Lett Drugs Ther* 26:104-105, 1984.

Medical Letter: Digoxin antibody fragments for digitalis toxicity, *Med Lett Drugs Ther* 28:87-88, 1986.

Medical Letter: Esmolol: a short-acting IV beta blocker, *Med Lett Drugs Ther* 29:57-78, 1987.

Paris PM, Stewart RD, Deggler F: Prehospital use of dexamethasone in pulseless idioventricular rhythm, *Ann Emerg Med* 13:1008-1010, 1984.

Platia EV, Michelson EL, Porterfield JK, Das G: Esmolol versus verapamil in the acute treatment of atrial fibrillation or atrial flutter, *Am J Cardiol* 63:925-929, 1989.

Rajfer SI, Anton AH, Rossen JD, Goldberg LI: Beneficial hemodynamic effects of oral levodopa in heart failure: relation to the generation of dopamine, *N Engl J Med* 310:1357-1362, 1984.

Rawles JM, Metcalfe MJ, Jennings K: Time of occurrence, duration, and ventricular rate of paroxysmal atrial fibrillation: the effect of digoxin, *Br Heart J* 63:225-227, 1990.

Reynolds DG, Gurll NJ, Yargish T, Lechner RB, Faden AI, Holaday JW: Blockade of opiate receptors with naloxone improves survival and cardiac performance in canine endotoxic shock, *Circ Shock* 7:39-48, 1980.

Rothstein RJ, Niemann JT, Rennie CJ, Suddath WO, Rosborough JP: Use of naloxone during cardiac arrest and CPR: potential adjunct for postcountershock electrical-mechanical dissociation, *Ann Emerg Med* 14:198-203, 1985.

Salerno DM, Dias VC, Kleiger RE, Tschida VH, Sung RJ, Sami M, Giorgi LV, and the Diltiazem-Atrial Fibrillation/Flutter Study Group: Efficacy and safety of intravenous diltiazem for treatment of atrial fibrillation and atrial flutter, *Am J Cardiol* 63:1046-1051, 1989.

White BC: Pulseless idioventricular rhythm during CPR: an indication for massive intravenous bolus glucocorticoids, *JACEP* 5:449-454, 1976.

Wilson RF: Science and shock: a clinical perspective, *Ann Emerg Med* 14:714-723, 1985.

Wilson DJ, Wallin JD, Vlachakis ND, Freis ED, Vidt DG, Michelson EL, Langford HG, Flamenbaum W, Poland MP: Intravenous labetalol in the treatment of severe hypertension and hyptensive emergencies, *Am J Med* 75:95-102, 1983.

Young GP: Calcium channel blockers in emergency medicine, *Ann Emerg Med* 13:712-722, 1984.

CHAPTER 15

DIFFERENTIATION OF PVCs FROM ABERRANCY

BASIC PRINCIPLES

One of the most difficult problems confronting those involved in emergency cardiac care is the differentiation of PVCs from aberrantly conducted beats. The issue is *not* merely academic. Whereas ventricular arrhythmias may be potentially life-threatening if not adequately controlled, supraventricular beats that conduct aberrantly are most often benign and can usually be safely observed without treatment.

How can one distinguish between PVCs and aberrancy?

Is this differentiation reliable? *Are there ways to make it more reliable?*

PROBLEM **Consider the rhythms shown in *Figures 15A-1* and *15A-2*, taken from two patients admitted for acute myocardial infarction. *Should one (or both) of these patients be treated for ventricular ectopy?***

(HINT: *At least one of these patients does not need to be treated.*)

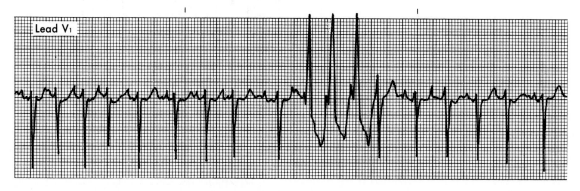

Figure 15A-1.   Should this patient be treated for ventricular ectopy?

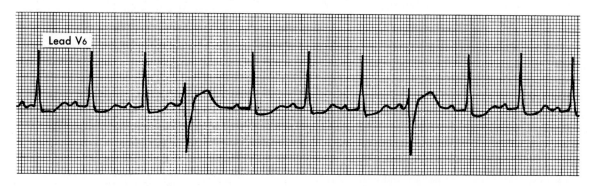

Figure 15A-2.   Should this patient be treated for ventricular ectopy?

Although we'd like you to *write down* your response to this question *now*, we intentionally defer discussing our answer until the end of this section (on page 505).

The purpose of this chapter is to suggest guidelines for helping to distinguish between abnormal-appearing *(anomalous)* QRS complexes that are ventricular in origin (PVCs), and those that are supraventricular but conducted with aberration. *The guidelines work most of the time.* It is important to appreciate, however, that occasionally anomalous beats will defy even our most earnest attempt at differentiation. In such cases, correlation of the arrhythmia to the clinical situation at hand becomes critical. For example, the treatment of choice for a hemodynamically significant tachyarrhythmia is synchronized cardioversion *regardless* of whether the arrhythmia is supraventricular or ventricular in nature.

We emphasize that the burden of proof must always lie with demonstrating that an anomalous QRS complex is aberrant, *rather than the other way around.* Thus,

> *A beat must be judged as "guilty" (a PVC) until proven innocent!!!*

Application of the basic principles presented in this chapter (and frequent use of a pair of calipers) should greatly facilitate your ability (and make you much more comfortable) in exercising this judgement. Brief description of the key rules for diagnosing aberration follows. Numerous examples will illustrate our points along the way.

Basic Rules for Differentiating PVCs from Aberrancy

Although there are many rules for diagnosing aberration, the three most helpful findings in our experience are the presence of the following:

i. A ***"typical" right-bundle branch block (RBBB) pattern*** when the anomalous complex is viewed in a *right-sided* monitoring lead (*either* lead V_1 or MCL$_1$).

ii. A **similar initial deflection** (with similar direction *and* slope) of the anomalous and normally conducted beats.

iii. A ***premature*** *P wave* preceding the anomalous beat.

All three of these features are demonstrated in the short rhythm strip shown in *Figure 15A-3* in which beat #4 is

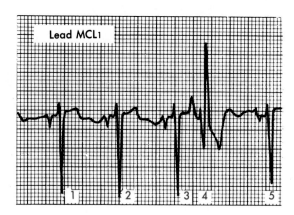

Figure 15A-3. Beat #4 manifests three of the most characteristic features of aberration: a typical RBBB (rSR′) pattern in this right-sided lead, a similar initial deflection to the normally conducted beats, and a *premature* P wave.

conducted with aberration. Although this beat looks markedly different from the others, it manifests a *typical* RBBB pattern (rSR′ configuration in this right-sided lead), and its initial QRS deflection is in the same upward direction (with the same slope) as the normally conducted beats. Inspection of the T wave immediately preceding beat #4 reveals extra peaking (compared to the normal T waves) due to a premature P wave.

THE "TYPICAL" RBBB PATTERN

The system for QRS nomenclature denotes the first negative deflection of the QRS complex as a Q wave, the first positive deflection as an R wave, and the first negative deflection *after* the R wave as an S wave. Not every QRS complex will have a Q wave, R wave, and S wave. Sometimes there may be two positive deflections, in which case the second positive deflection receives a *prime* (′) notation. Larger deflections (greater than 3 little boxes, or so) are denoted by capital letters, whereas smaller deflections are designated by lower case letters.

If we apply this system for QRS nomenclature to the complexes in Fig. 15A-3, it can be seen that beats #1 to #3, and #5 all demonstrate an rS configuration (small initial positive [r wave] deflection and deep negative [S wave] deflection). The aberrantly conducted beat (#4) manifests an rSR′ configuration (small initial positive [r wave] deflection, fairly deep negative [S] deflection, and a second [terminal] tall positive [R′ wave] deflection).

It is particularly important to note that for an RBBB pattern to be "typical," the *second* positive deflection of the QRS complex (the R′) must be *taller* than the initial positive deflection. That is, the QRS complex has a **taller right rabbit ear.** This is the case for both of the examples shown in *Figure 15A-4A.*

Although the amplitude of the negative deflection may be either small or large, for the RBBB to be "typical" the S wave (or s wave) *must descend back to the baseline!* Note that this is the case for both examples shown in Fig. 15A-4A.

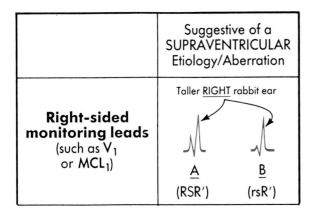

	Suggestive of a SUPRAVENTRICULAR Etiology/Aberration
Right-sided monitoring leads (such as V₁ or MCL₁)	Taller <u>RIGHT</u> rabbit ear <u>A</u> <u>B</u> (RSR′) (rsR′)

Figure 15A-4A. Appearance of a **typical RBBB pattern** in a *right-sided* lead. **A)** RSR′ configuration. **B)** rsR′ configuration. Note that for both **A** and **B,** the second positive deflection (the R′) is taller than the initial positive deflection (i.e., there is a **taller right rabbit ear**). Note also that the negative deflection in both cases (S wave in **A** and s wave in **B**) descends back to the baseline.

	Suggestive of a VENTRICULAR Etiology
Right-sided monitoring leads (such as V₁, or MCL₁)	Taller <u>LEFT</u> rabbit ear <u>F</u> <u>G</u> <u>H</u>

Figure 15A-4B. QRS configurations with a **taller left rabbit ear** in lead V₁ or MCL₁. **F)** RR′ configuration. **G)** "R-slur-prime configuration." **H)** QR configuration. Each of these configurations strongly suggests ventricular ectopy.

When the *left* rabbit ear is taller (i.e., when the initial positive deflection is taller than the second [R′] positive deflection), ventricular ectopy is strongly suggested (Example **F** in *Figure 15A-4B)*. Ventricular ectopy is also suggested by an "R-slur-prime" configuration (Example **G**) in which there is no distinct terminal (R′) positive deflection, and by the presence of a Q wave *prior* to the initial positive deflection (Example **H**). *In all three of these cases, the initial positive deflection predominates* (i.e., there is a **taller left rabbit ear**) and ventricular ectopy is strongly favored.

Unfortunately, QRS morphology in lead V₁ or MCL₁ is of *no assistance* in the differentiation between ventricular ectopy and aberration when an *intermediate* pattern is seen *(Figure 15A-4C)*. Thus, despite the fact that the right rabbit ear is taller for Examples **C, D,** and **E** in this figure, the QRS configuration is *not* that of a typical RBBB pattern. As a result, nothing can be said from the appearance of the QRS complex in this lead about the likelihood of aberrant conduction.

Specifically, the reason QRS configuration does not qualify as "typical" for RBBB (in a right-sided lead) in the middle panel of Figure 15A-4C is the lack of an initial distinct positive deflection in **D,** the presence of a Q wave in **E,** and failure of the negative deflection to descend back to the baseline in **C.**

EXPLANATION OF THE RULES FOR RECOGNIZING ABERRATION

The reason aberrant beats most often conduct with a **RBBB pattern** is that the refractory period of the right bundle branch tends to be longer than that of the left bundle branch. As a result, a premature supraventricular impulse (PAC or PJC) arriving at the ventricles is much more likely to find the right bundle branch still in a refractory state *(Figure 15A-5)*.

As suggested above, for persons with an otherwise normal heart, the overwhelming majority of aberrantly conducted

	Suggestive of a SUPRAVENTRICULAR Etiology/Aberration	Of NO HELP in Differentiation	Suggestive of a VENTRICULAR Etiology
Right-sided monitoring leads (such as V₁ or MCL₁)	Taller <u>RIGHT</u> rabbit ear <u>A</u> <u>B</u>	Taller <u>RIGHT</u> rabbit ear <u>C</u> <u>D</u> <u>E</u>	Taller <u>LEFT</u> rabbit ear <u>F</u> <u>G</u> <u>H</u>

Figure 15A-4C. Comparison of QRS morphology with an **intermediate pattern** in lead V₁ or MCL₁ with the QRS appearance shown previously in Fig. 15A-4A (that was suggestive of aberration) and 15A-4B (that was suggestive of a ventricular etiology). **C)** RR′ configuration (with a taller right rabbit ear). **D)** Monophasic R wave. **E)** QR configuration (with a taller right rabbit ear). None of these intermediate patterns are of any assistance in differentiation between ventricular ectopy and aberration.

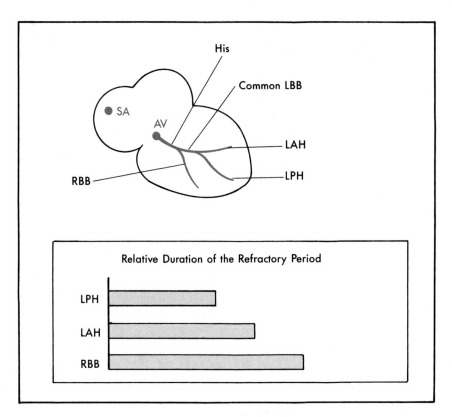

Figure 15A-5.   Explanation for the frequency of RBBB aberration. In persons with an otherwise normal heart, the RBB tends to have a longer refractory period. As a result, a premature supraventricular impulse (PAC or PJC) arriving at the ventricles is much more likely to find the RBB still in a refractory state and conduct with a pattern of RBBB aberration. The same is *not* necessarily true for patients with underlying heart disease *(see text).*

SA—sinoatrial node. AV—atrioventricular node. His—bundle of His. RBB—right bundle branch. Common LBB—common left bundle branch. LPH—left posterior hemibranch. LAH—left anterior hemibranch.

complexes manifest a RBBB pattern (with or without an accompanying hemiblock). Only a minority demonstrate a pure LBBB or isolated hemiblock pattern. Although the RBBB pattern of aberration is still the predominant one in the diseased heart, the *other forms become relatively more important.* Thus, there may be LBBB aberration, a bifascicular block pattern of aberration (RBBB and left anterior or posterior hemiblock), or isolated left anterior or posterior hemiblock aberration. Discussion of morphology characteristics for recognition of each of these different forms of aberration extends beyond the scope of this book.

The ***initial deflection*** of aberrant beats frequently is similar to that of the normally conducted beats, since the initial portion of the conduction pathway is usually unaffected. Thus, the wave of depolarization is conducted normally until it encounters that part of the conduction system that is still refractory. Statistically one might imagine a 50% chance exists for any ventricular ectopic beat to manifest a similar direction for its initial deflection to that of the normally conducted beats. A beat can be directed in only one of two ways (up or down). Consequently, detection of a similarly directed initial deflection supports the diagnosis of aberration, but *in no way* rules out the possibility that the anomalous beat could be a PVC (that by chance has a similarly directed initial deflection). On the other hand, finding that the direction of the initial deflection of an anomalous beat is *opposite* to the initial QRS vector of the normally conducted beats favors ventricular ectopy.

The usefulness of the similar initial deflection criterion applies *only* to aberrant beats that conduct with a *pure* RBBB pattern. This is because the initial vector of conduction may be significantly altered if either a LBBB or mixed pattern of aberration (RBBB and left anterior or posterior hemiblock) is present.

In addition to a similar *direction*, the initial deflection of the beat in question should also manifest a similar *shape* and *slope* for this criterion to be a reliable indicator of a supraventricular etiology.

Perhaps the most convincing finding in favor of aberration is the third feature we listed—identification of a **premature P wave** in the T wave preceding the anomalous QRS complex. This premature P wave is often not nearly as obvious as it is in Fig. 15A-3, and close scrutiny of the preceding T wave with careful comparison to the appearance of a normal T wave may be needed to detect it.

> The key to determining whether a premature P wave is hidden in the preceding T wave is to first establish what a "normal T wave" looks like. This is *not* always easy to do, especially during cardiac arrest or with acutely ill patients who so commonly manifest movement artifact on the electrocardiographic tracing. For example, note that the "normal T waves" of beats #1 and #2 in Fig. 15A-3 are not exactly the same. Although this slight difference is most likely the result of artifact (since the R-R interval for these two beats does not change), it is easy to imagine how the J point notching seen at the takeoff of the ST segment of beat #2 might be misinterpreted as a partially hidden premature P wave. Fortunately in this example, the peaking of the T wave preceding beat #4 is so dramatic that there is little question of the existence of a premature P wave.

It should be emphasized that *none* **of the signs for differentiating between aberration and ventricular ectopy are perfect.** Exceptions abound, and one often has to weigh one factor against another in making a judgement about the nature of conduction for any given case. *Frequently the result is a probability statement rather than a definite determination.* Occasionally, no matter how diligent one's efforts are (or how expert one's arrhythmia interpretation abilities may be), it will be absolutely impossible from the surface electrocardiogram to determine whether aberrancy or ventricular ectopy is present. *A major purpose of this chapter is to help in the recognition of such cases.* It is perfectly acceptable (and in our opinion preferable) to indicate *"anomalous complex(es) of unknown etiology"* as an interpretation instead of hazarding a wild guess. Fortunately, most of the time enough clues *will* be present to allow reliable differentiation between PVCs and aberrancy.

Therefore, when confronted with an anomalous (abnormal-appearing) QRS complex (or a run of anomalous beats), application of the principles suggested in this chapter should allow you to determine that the beat(s) in question is (are):

  i. Likely to be of ventricular etiology (a PVC or ventricular tachycardia)
  ii. Likely to be supraventricular (and conducted with aberration)

OR

  iii. Not allow you to make any determination from the information provided.

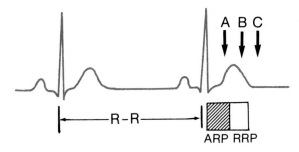

Figure 15A-6. Conduction of premature impulses A, B, and C. Premature impulse A arrives earliest during the ARP (absolute refractory period). It is "blocked" (not conducted to the ventricles). Premature impulse B arrives during the RRP (relative refractory period). It is conducted with aberration. Premature impulse C occurs after completion of the refractory period, and is conducted normally.

THE RELATIVE REFRACTORY PERIOD

Supraventricular impulses arriving at the AV node may or may not be conducted to the ventricles. If the process of repolarization is complete and the conduction system has fully recovered, the impulse will be conducted normally. This would be the case for premature impulse C in *Figure 15A-6* (or for any supraventricular impulse occurring *later* in the cycle than impulse C).

If on the other hand, the premature impulse occurs very *early* during repolarization, it may find the ventricles unable to conduct the stimulus. This situation is represented by premature impulse A in Fig. 15A-6, which occurs during the *absolute refractory period (ARP)*. As a result, conduction is "blocked." Premature impulse B occurs at an intermediate point during the *relative refractory period (RRP)*. It is this impulse that conducts *aberrantly* since it finds a portion of the conduction system still in a refractory state.

PROBLEM **Examine** *Figure 15A-7.* **Is beat #10 a PVC?** *Why does this beat look different than beat #6?* **How can you explain the pause after beat #2?**

ANSWER TO FIGURE 15A-7 The underlying rhythm in this figure is sinus. Premature atrial contractions (PACs) notch the T waves of beats #2, #5, and #9. The PAC that occurs *earliest* (A in Fig. 15A-7) is *blocked*. This premature impulse has the shortest *coupling* interval (0.27 second—as measured here from the onset of the R wave until the onset of the premature P wave) and corresponds to premature impulse A in Figure 15A-6 (which occurs during the ARP). Beats #6 and #10 in Figure 15A-7 are *aberrantly* conducted, with the latter complex manifesting a greater degree of aberrancy. This is because premature impulse B occurs at an earlier point (it has the shorter coupling interval of 0.29 second) when the conduction system is more refractory (corresponding to premature impulse B in Fig. 15A-6). Premature impulse C has the longest coupling interval (of 0.33 second), and probably occurs late in the RRP. As a result beat #6 is conducted

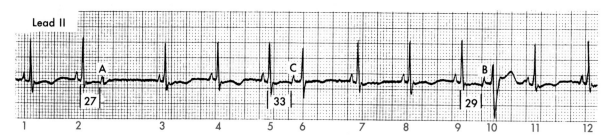

Figure 15A-7. *Can you explain the events that follow the premature P waves (PACs) labeled* **A, B,** *and* **C** *in this tracing?*

with only a minimal degree of aberrancy. Were this PAC to occur any later, it would most likely fall beyond the refractory period and be conducted normally.

In contrast to the situation shown in Fig. 15A-7, *all* of the anomalous QRS complexes in *Figure 15A-8A* (beats #2, #4, #5, #8, #10, and #12) occur at a relatively later point in the cycle. One would not anticipate aberrant conduction for any of these beats, since they occur well after the T wave (at a time when one would expect the conduction system to have fully recovered). A key point to emphasize whenever contemplating the diagnosis of aberrancy is the need to determine whether a *reason* exists for the altered conduction. Relatively short coupling intervals explain the aberrant conduction of beats #6 and #10 in Fig. 15A-7. Anomalous beats with long coupling intervals (such as those seen in Fig. 15A-8A) don't have any "reason" to conduct aberrantly, and therefore are much more likely to be PVCs.

Several additional points may be brought out by analyzing Fig. 15A-8A. Note that beat #8 in this figure is *preceded* by a P wave. *If a P wave precedes this beat, why isn't it aberrant???*

The answer is simply that the P wave preceding beat #8 is *not* premature. *Instead it occurs precisely on time!*. The fact that this QRS complex *is* preceded by a P wave actually provides strong supportive evidence that beat #8 *must* be a PVC. The normal PR interval in this tracing for each of the sinus-conducted beats (beats #1, #6, #7, #9, #11, and #13) is 0.14 second. Because the PR interval preceding beat #8 is signif-icantly *shorter* than this, something else *(other than a sinus-conducted complex)* must be occurring *before* this atrial impulse can stimulate the ventricles—namely, a PVC.

PROBLEM   **Why do you suppose that beat #8 in Fig. 15A-8A looks so different from all of the other PVCs in this tracing?**

(HINT: Feel free to refer back to Fig. 3B-25 in explaining your answer.)

ANSWER TO FIGURE 15A-8A   The reason the appearance of beat #8 differs from that of the other PVCs in this tracing is that it represents *fusion* of a supraventricular (sinus-conducted) impulse with a PVC. That is, the P wave preceding beat #8 is only able to conduct partially through the ventricles until (somewhere in its path) it meets the wave of depolarization emanating from the PVC *(Figure 15A-8B)*. The result (a *fusion* beat) manifests characteristics of both impulses (i.e., if beats #7 and #10 were to "have children," *one of the offspring might look like beat #8*).

As discussed in Section B of Chapter 3 (in our explanation of Figs. 3B-21 through 3B-25), fusion beats are not seen all that often, but when they do occur they provide overwhelming support in favor of ventricular ectopy.

PROBLEM   **Apply what we have covered up to this point to work through the example shown in *Figure 15A-9,* taken from a patient in a bigeminal rhythm. There are two abnormal-looking complexes present (beats #2 and #6). *Are these beats PVCs, or are they aberrantly conducted?***

ANSWER TO FIGURE 15A-9   Beats #2 and #6 manifest the three most characteristic features of aberrancy:

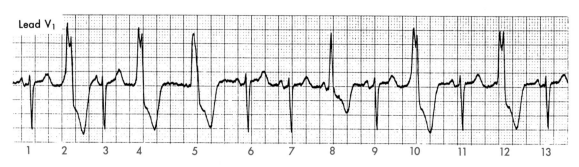

Figure 15A-8A.

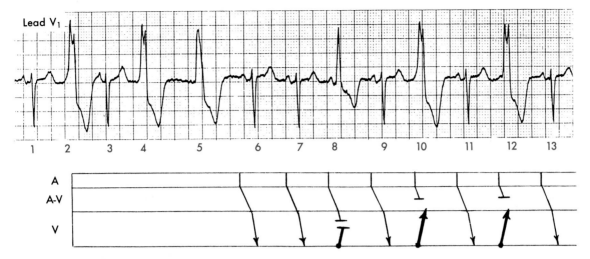

Figure 15A-8B. Laddergram illustrating the reason for the short PR interval of beat #8 in Fig. 15A-8A. This complex is a *fusion* beat, which explains why its morphology is intermediate between that of a PVC and that of the normally conducted sinus beats.

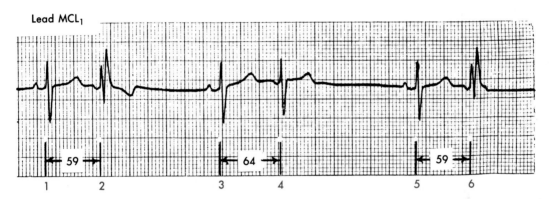

Figure 15A-9. Bigeminal rhythm. *Are beats #2 and #6 PVCs or aberrantly conducted?*

- a RBBB pattern in a right-sided monitoring lead
- an initial deflection similar to that of the normally conducted beats
- a *premature* P wave (which in this case is a tiny negative deflection with a short PR interval seen just before the onset of the QRS complex)

We can therefore say with relative certainty that beats #2 and #6 are premature supraventricular impulses— probably premature junctional contractions (PJCs) that conduct aberrantly.

PROBLEM **Why does beat #4 in Fig. 15A-9 conduct normally?**

ANSWER Beat #4 conducts normally because it has a longer coupling interval than the aberrantly conducted beats. That is, the coupling interval of beats #1-2 and #5-6 is 0.59 second. It is slightly longer than this (0.64 second) for beats #3-4.

Beat #4 occurs at a time when the ventricles have recovered the ability to conduct (corresponding to premature impulse C in Fig. 15A-6). In contrast, beats #2 and #6 occur during the RRP. They correspond to the situation that was seen for pre-

mature impulse B in Fig. 15A-6, and are therefore conducted to the ventricles with aberration.

Note that there is a *reason* for the aberrant conduction seen in Fig. 15A-9. That is, the premature beats that are conducted with aberration (beats #2 and #6) have a shorter coupling interval than the premature beat that conducts normally (beat #4).

This type of analysis in which one carefully examines coupling intervals to assist in determining if aberration is present is known as **cycle-sequence comparison.** Although the method is far from being foolproof, it often works and can be extremely helpful in explaining why certain beats in a rhythm strip conduct normally while others are conducted with aberration. Use of cycle-sequence comparison in conjunction with the morphologic features described above provides *incontrovertible evidence* that beats #2 and #6 in Fig. 15A-9 are not PVCs!

THE ASHMAN PHENOMENON

In addition to the coupling interval, another important determinant of aberrancy is the duration of the R-R interval that *precedes* the anomalous beat in question. This concept is explained in *Figure 15A-10A.*

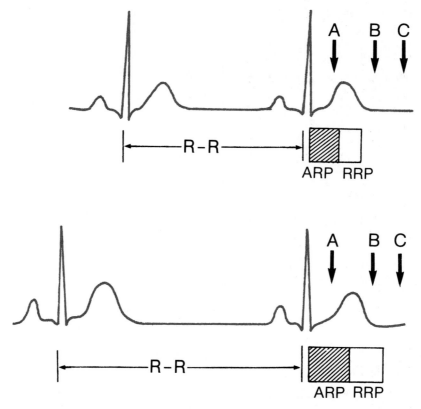

Figure 15A-10A. Explanation of the Ashman phenomenon. The duration of the refractory period is directly proportional to the length of the *preceding* R-R interval *(see text)*.

As previously discussed, premature impulses occurring during the ARP are blocked, whereas those that occur after repolarization is complete are conducted normally. Premature impulses occurring during the RRP conduct with aberration. Thus in the upper panel of Figure 15A-10A, premature impulse A will be blocked, while B and C will be conducted normally.

Whether a premature impulse will fall within the RRP (and conduct with aberration) will also be determined by the length of the R-R interval *preceding* the anomalous best. **The duration of the refractory period is directly proportional to the length of the preceding R-R interval.** When the heart rate is slowed (as it is in the lower panel of Fig. 15A-10A), *both* the ARP and the RRP are prolonged.

If we now consider the timing of the premature impulses in Fig. 15A-10A, it can be seen that impulse A in the lower panel of the figure will be blocked (since it still occurs in the ARP) and impulse C will be conducted normally (since it still occurs *after* the refractory period is over). However, premature impulse B (which previously occurred *after* the completion of repolarization), will now occur *during* the RRP, and will therefore be conducted with aberrancy. This cycle-sequence manipulation is known as the **Ashman phenomenon.** Fortunately, the rather complex explanation of this phenomenon can be synthesized into a much more easily remembered format:

> *"The funniest-looking (i.e., most aberrant) beat is most likely to follow the longest pause."*

PROBLEM   **Use the Ashman phenomenon to explain why beat #12 in Figure *15A-10B* conducts aberrantly, whereas other beats in this tracing with comparable (or even shorter) coupling intervals do not.**

ANSWER TO FIGURE 15A-10B   The underlying rhythm in Fig. 15A-10B is sinus. There are multiple PACs (beats #3, #5, #7, #8, #10, #12, and #13—*at least*). The "funniest-looking beat" is #12. It follows the longest pause (the R-R interval between beats #10-11). Cycle-sequence comparison and reference to Fig. 15A-10A (i.e., the Ashman phenomenon) explain why this beat is conducted with aberration, while beats #5, #7, #8 (which have comparable coupling intervals) and beat #13 (which has an even *shorter* coupling interval) are not.

Utilization of the Ashman phenomenon may be extremely helpful diagnostically when it is applied to understanding the appearance of beats in arrhythmias obtained from patients who are in sinus rhythm. However, one should be aware that the Ashman phenomenon is of uncertain value with atrial

Lead MCL1

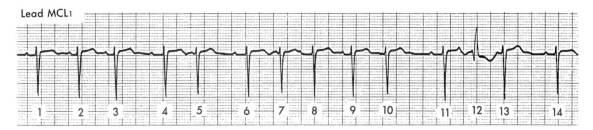

Figure 15A-10B. Illustration of the Ashman phenomenon. Beat #12 is conducted with aberration, while other beats with comparable (or even shorter) coupling intervals are not.

fibrillation. This is because the length of the R-R interval in atrial fibrillation is continually influenced by another phenomenon known as *concealed conduction** in which the variable penetration of atrial impulses through the AV node affects conduction in a way that the preceding R-R interval no longer accurately reflects the duration of the subsequent refractory period.

COMPENSATORY PAUSES

A frequently cited diagnostic criterion for ventricular ectopy is the finding of a full *compensatory pause*. In adults, PVCs usually do not conduct retrograde to the atria. Consequently, the sinoatrial (SA) node most often continues to discharge at its previous rate *unaffected* by ventricular ectopic activity. The P wave that follows the PVC

---

*The term **concealed** **conduction** refers to an advanced concept in which the occurrence of an electrophysiologic event can only be recognized *by its effect on the subsequent beat or cycle*. For example, retrograde conduction of a PVC to the AV node may prolong the PR interval of the subsequent sinus beat without leaving a trace of evidence that this is happening on the surface electrocardiogram! *(You will NOT need to know about concealed conduction to successfully complete the ACLS arrhythmia test.)*

(P′ in the left panel of *Figure 15A-11)* occurs precisely on time, and the pause containing the PVC is exactly *twice* the duration of the normal sinus cycle (58 + 92 = 150 = 75 × 2).

In contrast, a PAC is conducted throughout (and therefore depolarizes) the rest of the atria (including the SA node). As a result, a PAC *resets* the sinus cycle. Consequently, the pause containing a PAC would not be expected to equal twice the duration of the sinus cycle (44 + 98 = 142 ≠ 75 × 2 in the right panel of Fig. 15A-11).

Determining whether or not a full compensatory pause exists may be an additional helpful point in differentiating PVCs from aberrantly conducted beats. However, *caution must be advised!* PVCs sometimes *do* conduct retrograde to the atria, in which case they will reset the sinus cycle. Furthermore, a PAC can arise from a site in one of the atria that *by chance* lies at a distance such that the time required to depolarize the atria and reset the SA node *coincidentally* equals twice the normal R-R interval. Consequently, *PVCs do not always demonstrate a full compensatory pause, whereas PACs may occasionally do so.* One therefore cannot depend on the presence or absence of a full compensatory pause as a definitive diagnostic criterion. Instead this information should be used in the context of the

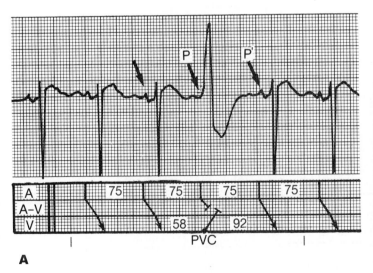

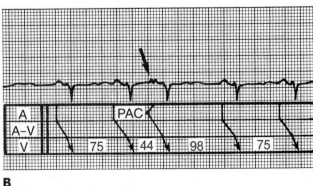

A   B

Figure 15A-11. **A)** Full compensatory pause. The pause containing the PVC is exactly twice the duration of the normal sinus cycle. **B)** Non-compensatory pause. The pause containing a PAC is usually not fully compensatory because the PAC resets the sinus cycle.

other characteristics of the abnormal beat in arriving at a decision about its likely etiology.

QRS Morphology

Analysis of QRS morphology may be among the most useful aids for differentiating between PVCs and aberrancy. As discussed earlier, the finding of a *typical* RBBB pattern (rSR′ with taller *right* rabbit ear) in a right-sided monitoring lead strongly suggests aberrancy. Thus in the example shown in *Figure 15A-12*, taken from a patient in atrial flutter, beats #4, #5, #6, and #9 are much more likely to be aberrantly conducted than ventricular ectopic beats. Each of these complexes manifests an rSR′ configuration with a *taller right rabbit ear* (the R′ of each complex is *taller* than the initial r).

In contrast, the rabbit ear for beat #6 in *Figure 15A-13* is taller on the *left*. This strongly suggests that the beat is a PVC.

Analysis of QRS morphology is especially helpful in evaluating the etiology of anomalous complexes when the underlying rhythm is not a sinus mechanism. This is because the "premature P wave" criterion may no longer be operative in such cases. QRS morphology then becomes the key determinant for assessing the likely etiology of the beat in question. This point is well illustrated in Figs. 15A-12 and 15A-13 (in which the underlying rhythm is atrial flutter and atrial fibrillation, respectively). In the former case, the finding of the typical RBBB morphology pattern for the anomalous complexes (in conjunction with the similar initial deflection) allows us to say with *at least* 90% accuracy that these beats are aberrantly conducted (Marriott and Conover, 1983). We emphasize that *this statement cannot be made with 100% accuracy*. Nevertheless, an accuracy of at least 90% for predicting the etiology of anomalous beats provides extremely nice odds that should help greatly in making clinical management decisions.

In contrast, the appearance of beat #6 in Fig. 15A-13 provides almost incontrovertible evidence that this com-

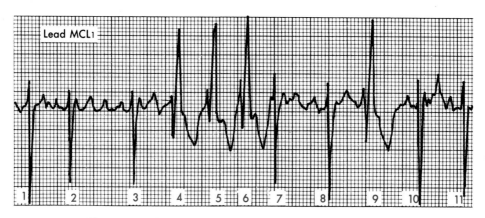

Figure 15A-12. Beats #4-6 and #9 manifest the typical RBBB (rSR′) pattern that is strongly suggestive of aberrant conduction. The underlying rhythm is atrial flutter.

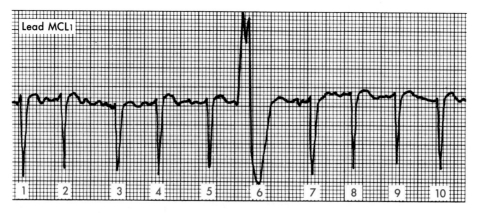

Figure 15A-13. The underlying rhythm is atrial fibrillation. Morphologic characteristics of beat #6 (marked widening, bizarre shape, oppositely directed initial deflection, and taller *left* rabbit ear) overwhelmingly favor a ventricular etiology.

plex must be a PVC. In addition to manifesting a taller *left* rabbit ear, beat #6 is markedly widened, bizarre in shape, and has an oppositely directed initial deflection.

WHEN THE ANOMALOUS COMPLEX IS *UPRIGHT* IN V₁ OR MCL₁

We have already emphasized the key morphologic features that suggest aberrant conduction when the QRS complex of the beat in question is *upright* in a *right*-sided lead (Fig. 15A-4C). We now incorporate this information with additional diagnostic features that may be detected from examination of QRS morphology in *left*-sided leads *(Figure 15A-14)*.

Left-sided monitoring leads are often neglected in morphologic evaluation of anomalous complexes. This is unfortunate since they may sometimes provide the *only* clues to the diagnosis. The most commonly used (and most helpful) left-sided leads are V_6 and MCL_6. (Similar information can usually also be derived from examination of left-sided leads I and V_5).

In our experience, the most easily remembered (and most helpful) left-sided morphologic clue is the finding of a *totally negative* (or almost totally negative) complex in lead V_6 or MCL_6 (Example **L** or **M** in Fig. 15A-14). When present, this finding is strongly suggestive of ventricular ectopy (*especially* if the complex in V_6 or MCL_6 is *entirely* negative).

Conceptually, this clue makes sense. The heart is a left-sided structure. As a result, electrical activity arising from the process of ventricular depolarization should be oriented toward the left (i.e., toward the heart). Even in the presence of a conduction defect (such as bundle branch block), at least *some* electrical activity should still be oriented toward the left. Thus, the finding of a *totally negative* QRS complex in a left-sided lead (**M** in the figure) strongly suggests a different site of origin for this electrical activity—as would be the case from a ventricular ectopic beat.

If instead of being totally negative, a small r wave precedes the deep S wave (**L** in Fig. 15A-14), the finding is still suggestive of ventricular ectopy, although it is somewhat less diagnostic since certain conduction defects (such as left anterior hemiblock) may also produce a similar morphology for the QRS complex in lead V_6 or MCL_6.

The finding of a QRS complex with an R wave of significant amplitude in a left-sided lead (regardless of whether the R wave is associated with a deep S wave) is of absolutely no diagnostic assistance (**K** in Fig. 15A-14).

A particularly interesting morphologic finding is the triphasic (qRS) pattern (**I**). Occurrence of this pattern in a left-sided monitoring lead represents the *reciprocal* of an rSR′ configuration in a right-sided monitoring lead. Because it is extremely unusual for a PVC to manifest a *small q wave* in a left-sided monitoring lead, the finding of a triphasic (qRS) pattern in lead V_6 or MCL_6 strongly favors aberration. Unfortunately, this pattern is only rarely seen. Instead, a much more common accompaniment of the typical RBBB morphology pattern of aberration is the finding of a *terminal wide S wave* in left-sided leads (**J**).

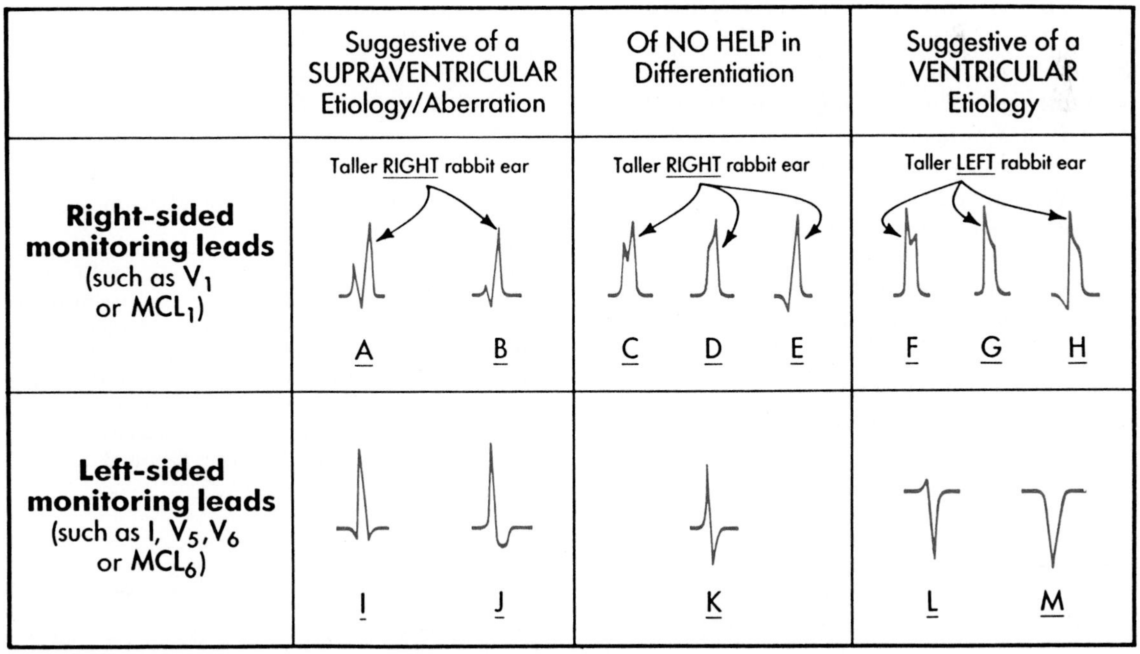

	Suggestive of a SUPRAVENTRICULAR Etiology/Aberration	Of NO HELP in Differentiation	Suggestive of a VENTRICULAR Etiology
Right-sided monitoring leads (such as V₁ or MCL₁)	Taller RIGHT rabbit ear A B	Taller RIGHT rabbit ear C D E	Taller LEFT rabbit ear F G H
Left-sided monitoring leads (such as I, V₅, V₆ or MCL₆)	I J	K	L M

Figure 15A-14. Utilization of morphologic clues for determining the etiology of anomalous beats **when the QRS complex is upright** in a right-sided lead. The finding of a typical RBBB pattern (example **A** or **B** above) in leads V₁ or MCL₁ strongly favors a supraventricular etiology or aberration. In contrast, the finding of a taller *left* rabbit ear in these leads, or of a predominantly or totally negative QRS complex in *left-sided* leads (example **L** or **M** above) strongly suggests a ventricular etiology.

For those who are less accustomed to seeking out morphologic clues in their diagnostic approach, memorization of the multiple patterns depicted in Fig. 15A-14 may seem somewhat cumbersome, to say the least. This need *not* be the case:

i. *There is no need to memorize.* Feel free to copy this Fig. 15A-14 and refer to it as often as needed in your clinical practice setting.

ii. The key patterns to remember from the figure are **A** (which should facilitate recall of **B**) and **M** (which should facilitate recall of **L**).

Simply stated, the key points to remember about patterns **A, B, L,** and **M** from Fig. 15A-14 are:

—**the finding of a *typical RBBB pattern*** (with a taller *right* rabbit ear) **in a *right*-sided lead strongly suggests aberration**

—**the finding of a *totally negative*** (or almost totally negative) **complex in a *left*-sided lead strongly suggests ventricular ectopy.**

WHEN THE ANOMALOUS COMPLEX IS *NEGATIVE* IN V₁ OR MCL₁

PVCs originate more often from the *left* ventricle than from the right. This is logical, since the left ventricle in adults is so much larger, thicker, and more likely to become ischemic than the right ventricle. In general, PVCs of left ventricular orgin *tend* to manifest a predominant R wave in right-sided monitoring leads. Because they arise from the left, their depolarization wavefront will be seen by right-sided leads as *approaching*—resulting in an upright QRS complex in lead V₁ or MCL₁. **This is why a majority of PVCs manifest an upright QRS complex in a right-sided monitoring lead** (*i.e., left ventricular PVCs are more common than right ventricular PVCs*). This is also why attention to the morphologic features reviewed in Fig. 15A-14 is so helpful in differentiating between PVCs and aberrantly conducted beats.

Although PVCs that originate from the *right* ventricle are less common than left ventricular PVCs, their diagnosis is often more problematic. *The morphologic clues suggested in Table 15A-14 for right-sided leads are simply not applicable.*

In general, right ventricular PVCs manifest a predominantly *negative* QRS complex in right-sided monitoring leads. That is, since they arise from the *right*, their depolarization wavefront is seen by right-sided monitoring leads as moving *away* (i.e., toward the left)—resulting in a predominantly negative QRS complex in lead V₁ or MCL₁. *The problem with right ventricular PVCs from a diagnostic standpoint is that their appearance may be very similar to that of the normally conducted beats.**

PROBLEM   **Consider the rhythm strip shown in *Figure 15A-15. Are beats #3 and #12 PVCs, or are they supraventricular impulses that are aberrantly conducted?***

ANSWER TO FIGURE 15A-15   The underlying rhythm is sinus. Because of a resemblance in the waveform of the anomalous and the sinus-conducted beats (both types of complexes manifest an rS morphology), and a similarly directed (upward) initial deflection, one might be tempted to diagnose beats #3 and #12 as supraventricular with aberrant conduction. Several factors weigh against this.

First, the setting is *not* ideal for aberrancy, since these beats are not particularly premature (they occur well after the termination of the preceding T wave). Moreover, they are relatively wide (0.14 second), are not preceded by a premature P wave, and occur in the middle of a full compensatory pause. Although these beats do manifest a similarly directed initial deflection, this finding has its greatest use when there is an RBBB pattern of aberration (which is *not* the case here). Taken together (and in the absence of any compelling reasons for aberrancy), these factors

---

*Reference to PVCs as being either of right or left ventricular origin is helpful in understanding (and remembering) the morphologic appearance of the two basic types of anomalous complexes. As indicated above, **left ventricular PVCs** tend to be upright in right-sided leads (V₁ or MCL₁), whereas the less commonly occurring **right ventricular PVCs** tend to be predominantly negative in these leads. It is important to emphasize that *this classification is purely for convenience, and that the origin of PVCs cannot always be reliably predicted by their morphologic appearance.*

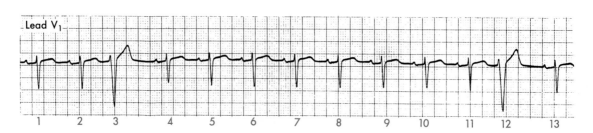

Figure 15A-15.   Are beats #3 and #12 PVCs or aberrantly conducted?

suggest that beats #3 and #12 are probably PVCs. A *right ventricular* etiology is suggested because the QRS complex is predominantly negative in this right-sided lead.

> An additional subtle clue is present on this tracing. Careful inspection of the initial deflection of each PVC reveals that it is slightly *broader* than the r wave of the normally conducted beats. It is distinctly unusual for an aberrantly conducted complex to alter the initial deflection of the r wave in a right-sided lead in this manner.

Although morphologic clues to the etiology of anomalous complexes that are predominantly negative in lead V_1 or MCL_1 are often quite subtle, they may nevertheless prove to be exceedingly useful in diagnosis. For example, the finding of a "fat" initial r wave in a right-sided lead strongly suggests ventricular ectopy. This is illustrated by the complex labeled **P** in *Figure 15A-16* (and corresponds to the morphology of beats #3 and #12 in Fig. 15A-15). The finding of a slurred (or delayed) downward initial deflection in a right-sided lead is also suggestive of ventricular ectopy (example **Q** in Fig. 15A-16).

In contrast, beats of *supraventricular* etiology that manifest an initial r wave in lead V_1 or MCL_1 are more likely to have a *very narrow* initial deflection **(N)**. In addition, the downslope of the S wave in this lead is more likely to be rapid **(O)**, although a slower (delayed) downslope does not rule out a supraventricular etiology (Kindwall et al, 1988).

> Recall of the implications of a slurred or delayed downward deflection in lead V_1 or MCL_1 (pattern **Q**) might be facilitated by conceptualizing the likely process of depolarization when it originates from a ventricular site (i.e., from a PVC)—*unorganized* and *delayed* by travel through unspecialized ventricular myocardial cells. In contrast, a premature supraventricular impulse conducted with LBBB aberration would seem more likely to manifest a neat, rapid downslope (with or without a slender initial r wave—patterns **N** or **O,** respectively)

due to the more organized initial component of depolarization (during which time the impulse is transmitted over the unblocked portion of the conduction system).

Admittedly, reliability of the criterion regarding the rapidity of the downslope of the S wave in lead V_1 or MCL_1 is far from perfect. Nevertheless, the following can be said:

 i. ***The finding of a "fat" initial r wave in a right-sided lead** (pattern **P** in Fig. 15A-16) **strongly suggests ventricular ectopy.***

 ii. ***The finding of a very rapid** (almost vertical) **downslope to the S wave in a right-sided lead** (pattern **O**) **is most consistent with a supraventricular etiology and aberration.***

PROBLEM   **Apply what we have covered up to now to the arrhythmia shown in *Figure 15A-17.* Do beats #7-9 represent a salvo (3 PVCs in a row), or are they premature supraventricular beats that are conducted with aberration? *Do morphologic characteristics of the 3 anomalous beats support your conclusions?***

ANSWER TO FIGURE 15A-17   The underlying rhythm is sinus tachycardia at a rate of 105 beats/minute. This is interrupted by a 3-beat run of anomalous complexes (beats #7-9). Careful inspection of the T wave preceding beat #7 reveals definite notching that is not seen in any other T wave. This notching must be the result of

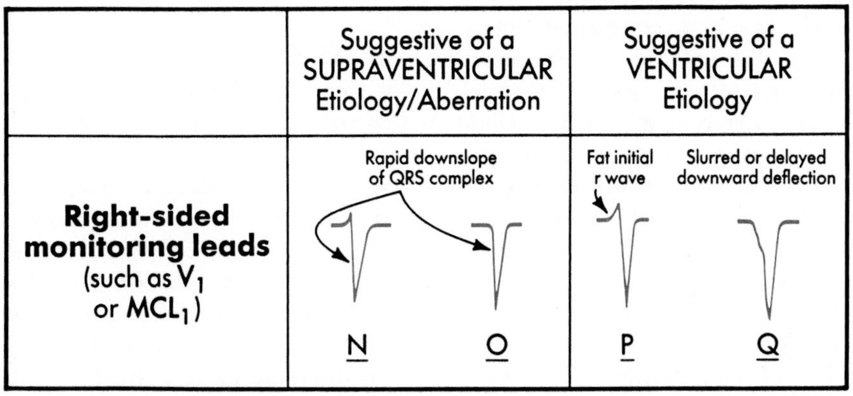

	Suggestive of a SUPRAVENTRICULAR Etiology/Aberration		Suggestive of a VENTRICULAR Etiology	
Right-sided monitoring leads (such as V_1 or MCL_1)	Rapid downslope of QRS complex		Fat initial r wave	Slurred or delayed downward deflection
	N	O	P	Q

Figure 15A-16.   Morphologic clues for determining the etiology of anomalous beats **when the QRS complex is negative** *in a right-sided lead.* The finding of a fat initial r wave or a slurred (or delayed) downward initial deflection strongly suggests ventricular ectopy. In contrast, the finding of a narrow initial r wave deflection and/or a rapid downslope of the S wave is more consistent with a supraventricular etiology.

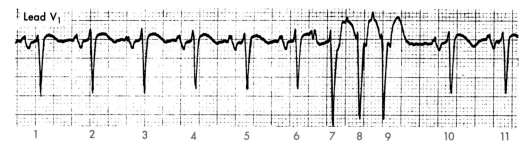

Figure 15A-17.   Are beats #7-9 PVCs or aberrantly conducted?

a *premature P wave*, and strongly suggests that beats #7-9 are *aberrantly conducted* supraventricular beats.

Morphologic analysis supports this conclusion. Note that the anomalous beats are predominantly *negative* in this right-sided V_1 monitoring lead. Reference to Fig. 15A-16 suggests the anomalous beats most closely resemble pattern **N** in this figure (slender initial r wave; very rapid, almost vertically downsloping S wave). Beats #7-9 in this figure are conducted with a pattern of *LBBB aberration*.

PROBLEM   ***Do you see evidence of additional atrial activity during this 3 beat run of anomalous complexes?* (If so, does this finding help in assessing the etiology of the anomalous complexes?)**

ANSWER   Close inspection of the T wave of beats #7 and #8 also reveals notching (at the peak of these T waves). *This reflects atrial activity.* Note that there is no notching (and presumably no atrial activity) in the T wave of beat #9.

Clinically, detection of these P waves does *not* solidify determination of the etiology of the three anomalous complexes in this tracing. Moreover, it is hard to be sure from this short rhythm strip alone if these P waves reflect anterograde (i.e., forward) or retrograde atrial activity. The former might result if the notching represented PACs, whereas the latter could result from either the retrograde atrial activity of a reentry circuit with PSVT (in which failure of atrial conduction after beat #9 might account for the termination of the run), or retrograde atrial conduction from PVCs. It should be emphasized that our purpose in drawing attention to these P waves is *not* to debate their role in this arrhythmia, but merely to point out that *evidence of atrial activity can often be found when (and if) carefully looked for!* Detection of hidden atrial activity such as this may sometimes provide an invaluable clue to uncovering the mechanism of the arrhythmia.

USE OF LEFT-SIDED LEADS IN MORPHOLOGIC ASSESSMENT

We have previously suggested how analysis of *left-sided leads* can help in determining the etiology of anomalous

beats when the QRS complex is upright in a right-sided lead (Fig. 15A-14). Inspection of left-sided leads may prove equally helpful in morphologic assessment when the anomalous complex is negative in lead V_1 or MCL_1. In either case, the finding of a totally negative (or almost totally negative) complex in a left-sided monitoring lead is strongly suggestive of ventricular ectopy. Thus, the same morphologic patterns presented previously in Fig. 15A-14 for the appearance of the anomalous beat in a left-sided lead (complexes **L** and **M**) are equally valid indicators of a probable ventricular etiology *regardless of whether the anomalous complex is upright or not in lead V_1 or MCL_1.*

Conceptually, since the heart is a left-sided structure, one might expect supraventricular complexes to have *at least some* of their electrical activity oriented toward the left. Thus, **the finding of predominant (or total) negativity in a left-sided lead** (*similar to complexes L and M in Fig. 15A-14*) **is a strongly suggestive clue to the presence of ventricular ectopy.**

QRS DURATION

Return for a moment to Fig. 15A-13. As previously discussed, morphologic characteristics alone (bizarre shape, taller *left* rabbit ear, *oppositely* directed initial deflection) are more than enough to suggest that beat #6 is a PVC. In addition to these morphologic clues, note that the duration of the QRS complex of beat #6 is *at least* 0.16 second. **QRS duration exceeding 0.14 second favors the diagnosis of ventricular ectopy.** Relatively narrow QRS complexes (of ≤0.11 second, as for beats #7-9 in Fig. 15A-17) are more likely to be due to aberrancy.

A word of caution is in order. The appearance of a PVC may vary markedly, depending on which lead is used to monitor the patient. Thus a premature beat that looks to be narrow (supraventricular) in one lead may appear much wider and more bizarre (suggesting ventricular ectopy) when viewed from another perspective.

This point is made abundantly clear in *Figure 15A-18*, which shows the simultaneous recording of a rhythm strip from leads

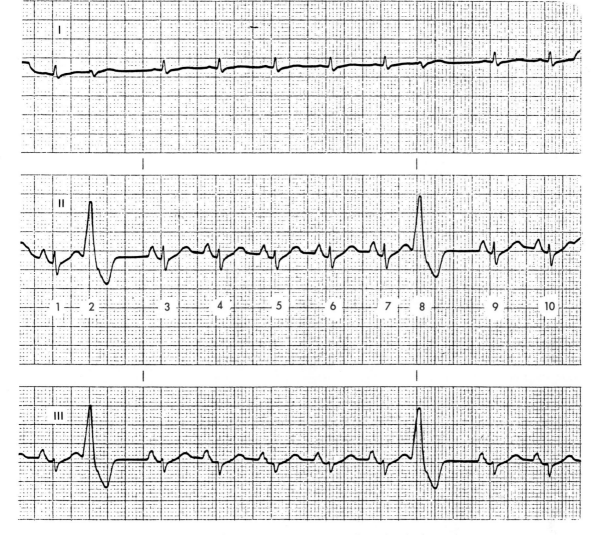

Figure 15A-18. Simultaneous recording of a rhythm strip from leads I, II, and III. Beats #2 and #8 are PVCs, despite the deceptively narrow appearance of these beats in lead I.

I, II, and III. Beats #2 and #8 in leads II and III are obviously much wider than the normally conducted beats in these leads. One would have little difficulty in recognizing these beats as PVCs. However, the same beats look surprisingly narrow when viewed from lead I. *If lead I was the only monitoring lead available, it would not be at all apparent that beats #2 and #8 were PVCs!*

The importance of examining an anomalous complex in more than one monitoring lead is further emphasized by *Figure 15A-19*, taken from a patient who is in ventricular bigeminy. Arrows indicate the PVCs in each lead. Note that ectopic morphology varies greatly. One certainly would have no difficulty identifying the PVCs in leads I, III, aVR, aVL, V₁, and V₆. The QRS is bizarre in shape and significantly wider than the normally conducted beats in each of these leads.

Identification of the bigeminal beats as PVCs is not nearly as apparent from inspection of leads II, aVF, V₂,

and V₃. In particular for leads V₂ and V₃, the normally (sinus) conducted QRS complexes are of much greater amplitude than the beats that follow them, and might be mistaken for PVCs if one did not see a preceding P wave. Furthermore notching in the T wave of the normally conducted beats in leads V₃ through V₆ simulates a premature P wave and adds another potential source of confusion.

Because the anomalous complexes in this example do not manifest a pure RBBB pattern, attention to the direction of the initial deflection is less helpful in differentiation. It can be seen that in some leads the initial deflection of anomalous beats is similarly directed as for the normally conducted beats, whereas it is oppositely directed in other leads. Even when similarly directed, however, the *slope* (shape and angle of incline) is often quite different, suggesting a different focus of origin (i.e., suggesting that one beat is supraventricular and the other is not).

The reason the QRS complex of PVCs appears deceptively narrow in leads II, V₂, and V₃ in Fig. 15A-19, is

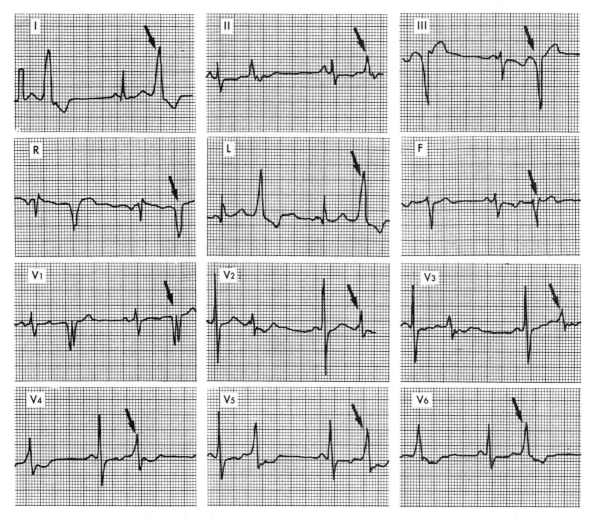

Figure 15A-19. 12-lead ECG from a patient in ventricular bigeminy. Arrows indicate the PVCs in each lead.

that a portion of the QRS lies on the baseline. This is the same phenomenon that produced a deceptively narrow QRS complex for beats #2 and #8 in Figure 15A-18. The moral is clear: ***the more leads available for analysis of anomalous beats, the more accurate our assessment will be.***

RECOGNITION OF ABERRANCY IN ATRIAL FIBRILLATION

Differentiation of PVCs from aberrancy is especially difficult in the setting of atrial fibrillation. The reason is twofold. First, because of the loss of organized atrial activity, P waves are no longer evident on the ECG. Consequently, the important differentiating feature of identifying a premature P wave is lost.

Second, the Ashman phenomenon is of uncertain validity in the presence of atrial fibrillation, since the length of the R-R interval is constantly being influenced by con-

cealed conduction. Fortunately, the *irregularity* of the atrial fibrillation itself provides an important clue.

PROBLEM **Examine the abnormal beats in *Figures 15A-20* and *15A-21*, taken from two patients who are completely asymptomatic. Is ventricular ectopy likely to be present in one or both of these tracings?**

ANSWER TO FIGURE 15A-20 The run of seven anomalous (abnormally wide) beats toward the end of this rhythm strip at least initially suggests a run of ventricular tachycardia. However, note that the rhythm remains irregularly irregular throughout the entire strip *irrespective of the width of the QRS complex*. *Ventricular tachycardia tends to be a fairly regular rhythm*, although admittedly at times there may be some variation to its regularity. The gross irregularity in this case persists, and is more than one usually expects to see with ventricular tachycardia. This suggests that the run of anomalous beats may well be the result of atrial fibrillation with aberrant conduction.

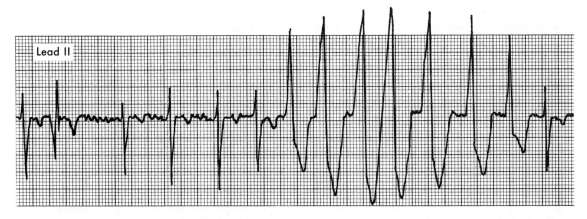

Figure 15A-20.   The underlying rhythm is atrial fibrillation.
Are the anomalous beats likely to be PVCs or aberrantly conducted?

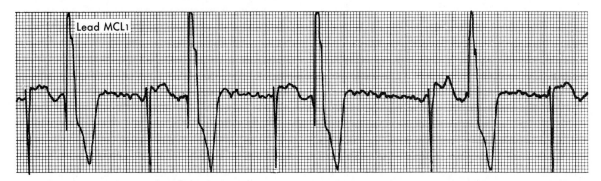

Figure 15A-21.   The underlying rhythm is atrial fibrillation.
Are the anomalous beats likely to be PVCs or aberrantly conducted?

Analysis of QRS morphology is not helpful in the differentiation of PVCs from aberrancy in a standard lead II as was used here. Only right-sided leads (V_1 or MCL_1) or left-sided leads (such as V_5, V_6, or MCL_6) are helpful in morphologic assessment.

It is important to emphasize that one cannot be sure from the rhythm strip shown in Fig. 15A-20 alone of the etiology of these anomalous beats. More information (i.e., additional monitoring leads) is needed. The patient in this case remained asymptomatic and demonstrated wide complexes with a typical aberrant morphology when switched to a right-sided monitoring lead.

ANSWER TO FIGURE 15A-21

Atrial fibrillation is again evident from the lack of P waves and the erratic baseline. A wide and bizarre QRS complex occurs every other beat. However, note that although the underlying rhythm is irregularly irregular, the coupling interval of each bigeminal beat is *fixed*. This strongly suggests that the anomalous beats are PVCs.

If the anomalous complexes were supraventricular impulses conducted with aberration, one would certainly expect them to occur with the same irregular irregularity as the underlying rhythm. In contrast, PVCs that have a similar appearance probably arise from the same ectopic focus. Because the most common mechanism of ventricular ectopy is *reentry* (through a well-defined circuit of myocardial cells), uniform PVCs tend to have a relatively constant coupling interval. Thus, *in the presence of atrial fibrillation, the finding of anomalous beats with a fixed coupling interval is suggestive of a ventricular etiology.*

Other factors strongly favor a ventricular etiology for the anomalous beats in this tracing. These include marked QRS widening (of at least 0.15 second), a QR-"slur" configuration of the QRS complex with a *taller left rabbit ear* in this right-sided lead, and an initial deflection that is *oppositely directed* (i.e., negative) to the small positive r wave of the normally conducted beats.

PROBLEM

As a conclusion to this section, RETURN to the question we posed at the start on page 489 regarding whether ventricular ectopy is present in *Figures 15A-1* and *15A-2*. Feel free to refer to Fig. 15A-14 in formulating your answer.

ANSWER

The underlying rhythm in Fig. 15A-1 is multifocal atrial tachycardia (MAT) with an irregularly irregular rhythm, but manifesting well-defined (albeit different) P waves in front of most QRS complexes.* Three

---

*Recognition and full discussion of MAT is covered in detail in Section A of Chapter 16.

anomalous complexes appear in the middle of the tracing. Application of the principles discussed in this section allow us to say with a high degree of certainty that these beats are supraventricular and conducted with aberration:

i. The anomalous beats manifest a typical RBBB pattern in this right-sided monitoring lead (similar to pattern **B** in Fig. 15A-14).
ii. Anomalous beats have an almost identical initial deflection (similarly directed *and* of similar slope) as the normally conducted beats.
iii. A *premature* P wave initiates the run (identified as a definite notching in the T wave immediately preceding the first anomalous beat).
iv. The Ashman phenomenon is present (i.e., the first abnormal-appearing beat follows the longest pause).

A final subtle point should be made about QRS morphology. Occasionally when there is a run of anomalous beats, QRS morphology may vary slightly from beat to beat. This is the case in Fig. 15A-1. *The key complex to focus on is the first anomalous beat in a run.* In Fig. 15A-1, the first anomalous beat manifests a classic rsR′ pattern (with an s wave that descends to the baseline and a *taller right rabbit ear),* and strongly suggests aberrant conduction.

In contrast, the two anomalous complexes in Fig. 15A-2 are PVCs. Although the initial deflection of these beats is similarly directed to that of the normally conducted beats, the initial *slope* appears to be somewhat different (i.e., slower rising). Moreover these beats are significantly widened, and P waves can be seen to walk right through the tracing, resulting in a perfectly compensatory pause. The P wave that precedes the second anomalous beat is *not* a PAC (that conducts aberrantly) since this P wave is *not* premature. On the contrary, the fact that the PR interval preceding this second anomalous complex is so much shorter than the PR interval of the sinus conducted beats is strong evidence that something else must have happened (i.e., a PVC) *before* this P wave was able to conduct to the ventricles.

Morphologic assessment of the two anomalous beats in this tracing is not extremely helpful. Although the rS pattern of these beats in this left-sided lead is consistent with a ventricular etiology, little can be said with certainty because of the amplitude of the r wave (which is *at least* 6 mm tall). A ventricular etiology is *only* suggested when the anomalous complex in a left-sided lead is totally negative or *almost totally negative*— which is not the case here.

By now it should be apparent that analysis of anomalous complexes is an art. Definite differentiation between ventricular ectopy and aberration is not always possible, and one is often left rendering a relative probability statement as an answer. We view this differentiation as a challenge. The principal tools needed for evaluation of anomalous complexes have all been introduced. Practice makes perfect. Numerous practice tracings in their clinical context await in the next section. *Are you up to the challenge?*

SECTION B

A *CHALLENGE* IN DIAGNOSIS: PVCS OR ABERRANCY?

This section will offer you a chance to test your mettle! In it we have included a host of challenging rhythm strips that illustrate the principles covered in the first section of this chapter. Many of these rhythms are **not** easy to interpret (and admittedly **we** still are not sure about the answers to some of them!). However, of much more importance than a yes or no answer— aberrant or not aberrant—is the rationale employed for arriving at your conclusion. Appropriate management decisions (whether to treat, and if so how) can then be based on the patient's underlying diagnosis and clinical condition. Hemodynamic status permitting, more information (additional leads, reference to previous tracings,

response to a vagal maneuver, etc.) may then be obtained if needed.

While completing this exercise you may find it impossible at times to be sure of *the answer*. To try and become comfortable at recognizing those times, it may be helpful to formulate your responses in terms of the *relative certainty* you have about a particular diagnosis (i.e., definite PVC, probable PVC, probable aberrantly conducted beat, or *cannot tell*).

Feel free to refer back to Fig. 15A-14 (on page 499) and 15A-16 (on page 501) as often as you like regarding questions on QRS morphology. As an additional aid to the task, we have consolidated in *Table 15B-1* the key non-

Table 15B-1

Non-Morphologic Diagnostic Features for Differentiating Between Ventricular Ectopy and Aberration			
+++ = Strongly favoring; ++ = moderately favoring; + = slightly favoring.			
Diagnostic Feature	**Relevant Leads**	**Favors Aberrancy**	**Favors Ventricular Ectopy**
• **QRS Duration**	Most leads	**+** (If ≤0.11 second)	**+** (If ≥0.14 second)
• **Initial Deflection**	Most leads	**++** (If similarly directed *and* of similar slope*)	**++** (If oppositely directed)
• **Preceding P wave**	Any leads	**+++** (If the preceding P wave is *premature*)	**+** (For the absence of any preceding P wave) **+++** (For the presence of a preceding P wave that is *not* premature)
• **Compensatory Pause**	Any leads	**+** (If absent)	**+** (If present)
• **AV Dissociation** (relatively uncommon)	Any leads		**+++** (If present)
• **Fusion Beats** (relatively uncommon)	Any leads		**+++** (If present)
• **Capture Beats** (very uncommon)	Any leads		**+++** (If present)
• **QRS Concordance** (very uncommon)	All of the precordial leads (V$_{1-6}$)		**+++** (If present)
*The finding of a similar initial deflection is less helpful diagnostically when there is a hemiblock or LBBB pattern of aberration.			

morphologic diagnostic features to keep in mind during the process of differentiation between ventricular ectopy and aberration.

You're now on your own . . . .

PROBLEM   *FIGURE 15B-1: PVCs or aberrant?*

ANSWER TO FIGURE 15B-1   The underlying rhythm is sinus. Beats #3, #11, and #12 are all *aberrantly* conducted. Each manifests a typical RBBB pattern (rSR′ with a taller right rabbit ear in this right-sided monitoring lead) in which the initial deflection closely resembles that of the normally conducted beats. A *premature* P wave is clearly seen to precede beat #3 (producing an obvious peak in the T wave of beat #2) and beat #11 (producing a subtle but definite notch in the T wave of beat #10).

> Beat #7 is also aberrantly conducted. Although it looks different than the other aberrantly conducted beats (it lacks a tall R′ component), it nevertheless manifests an rSr′ configuration with a similar initial deflection, and is preceded by a premature P wave (that notches the T wave of beat #6). The reason beat #7 is not quite as wide as the other anomalous beats that conduct with a pattern of complete RBBB aberration (and the reason beat #7 lacks a tall R′ component) is that beat #7 is conducted with a pattern of *incomplete* RBBB aberration.

Our degree of confidence in diagnosing aberration in this example?—almost 100%!

PROBLEM   **Beat #4 in *Figure 15B-2A* manifests an rsR′ pattern and is preceded by a P wave. *Is this beat also aberrant?***

ANSWER TO FIGURE 15B-2A   No! Note that the rhythm strip shown in Fig. 15B-2A was obtained from a lead II monitoring lead. Morphologic appearance is of absolutely *no* diagnostic assistance when assessed from a lead II. It is *only* of use when assessed from right-sided monitoring leads (V_1 or MCL_1) or left-sided leads (such as V_5, V_6, or MCL_6).

Although a P wave does precede the anomalous beat in Figure 15B-2A, this P wave is *not* premature! *Figure 15B-2B* demonstrates that this P wave occurs precisely on time. The fact that the PR interval preceding beat #4 is so much shorter than the normal PR interval (which is 0.24 second in this rhythm strip) provides incontrovertible evidence that *something* else must have occurred *before* the normal atrial impulse was able to conduct—and for practical purposes *proves* that beat #4 is a PVC.

In many institutions lead II remains the most commonly used monitoring lead. Although this is often the best lead for assessing atrial activity (and it offers the additional

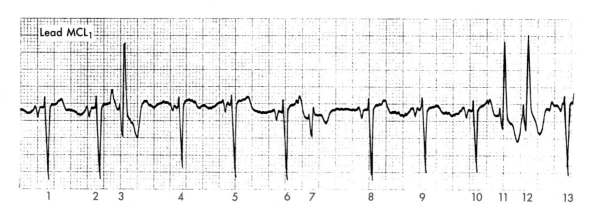

Figure 15B-1.   *PVCs or aberrant?*

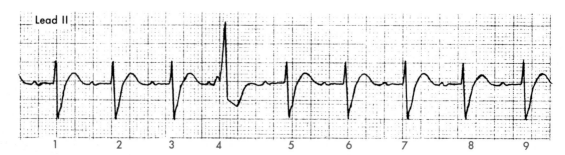

Figure 15B-2A.   Beat #4 manifests an rsR′ configuration and is preceded by a P wave. *Is it aberrant?*

advantage of facilitating recognition of LAHB), analysis of lead II is of no diagnostic assistance in the morphologic assessment of anomalous beats. If doubt exists about the etiology of such beats, switching to a right- and/or left-sided monitoring lead may hold the key to the answer.

> The question may have arisen in your mind about the possibility of beat #4 in Fig. 15B-2A being a premature *junctional* contraction (PJC) instead of a PVC. If this were the case, we would still be left with having to explain why this PJC looks so different from the normally conducted beats. Granted—its different appearance could be due to aberration (the likelihood of which is impossible to assess from this lead II monitoring lead). However, beat #4 occurs so *late* in the cycle (i.e., well *after* the T wave), that there is no reason to expect it to conduct with aberrancy. Thus, although one cannot absolutely rule out the possibility of beat #4 being an aberrantly conducted PJC, the odds of this are remote (less than 1%). Practically speaking, it makes sense to routinely assume a ventricular etiology whenever one sees a premature anomalous complex without preceding *premature* atrial activity *unless there is strong morphologic evidence to the contrary.*

to 95% certainty. The reason beats #4 and #7 also differ from the normally conducted beats is that they are also aberrant (they manifest a pattern of *incomplete* RBBB aberration).

> Note the long-short sequence that precedes *each* of the aberrant beats. This is the Ashman phenomenon *("funniest-looking beat" follows the longest pause).* Although the Ashman phenomenon is not as reliable in the setting of atrial fibrillation (due to the unpredictable effect of *concealed conduction* resulting from partial penetration of numerous atrial impulses bombarding the AV node), it appears to be operative in this example. Cycle-sequence comparison may then explain why beat #17 does not conduct with aberration. Although also preceded by a relatively long R-R interval (the R-R interval between beats #15-16), the coupling interval of this complex (the distance between beats #16-17) is ever so slightly *greater* than the coupling interval of the beats that conduct aberrantly.
>
> While cycle-sequence comparison may not be as reliable in the presence of atrial fibrillation (because of concealed conduction), it appears to offer supportive evidence in this case in favor of aberrant conduction for beats #4, #7, and #13.

PROBLEM   *FIGURE 15B-3: PVC or aberrant?*

ANSWER TO FIGURE 15B-3   The underlying rhythm in this tracing is atrial fibrillation. This eliminates looking for a "premature P wave" as a criterion for differentiating between PVCs and aberrancy. However, the morphology of beat #13 is so typical of *aberrancy* (perfect rSR′ pattern with identical initial deflection) that one should feel comfortable making this diagnosis with 90%

PROBLEM   *FIGURE 15B-4: PVC or aberrant?*

ANSWER TO FIGURE 15B-4   Beat #4 is *definitely* a PVC. It is wide, bizarre, and morphologically very suggestive of a PVC (monophasic R wave in this right-sided lead with, if anything, a taller *left* rabbit ear—most similar to pattern **G** in Fig. 15A-14). Confirmation of this impression is forthcoming from the P wave that precedes this beat—it is *not* premature, and the PR interval is *too*

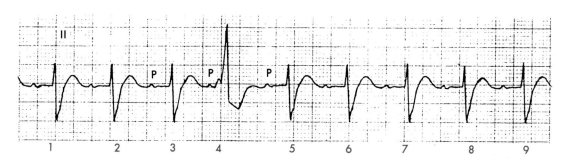

Figure 15B-2B.   The P wave preceding the anomalous complex (beat #4) is *not* premature but occurs precisely on time.

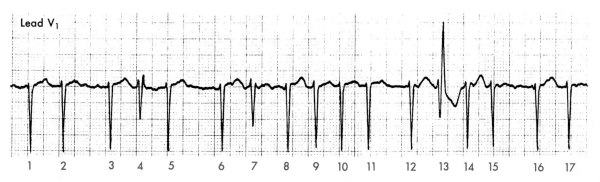

Figure 15B-3.   Is beat #13 a PVC or aberrant? *How certain are you of your answer?*

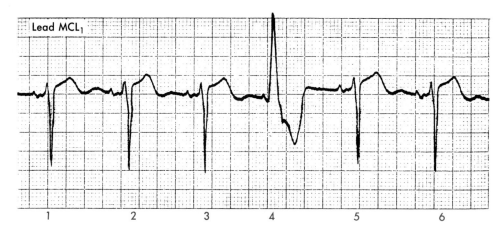

Figure 15B-4. Is beat #4 a PVC or aberrant? *How certain are you of your answer?*

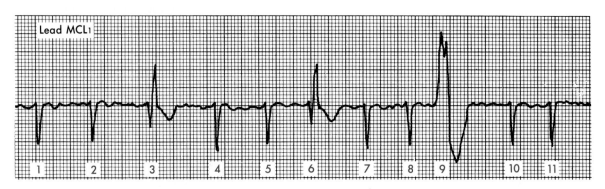

Figure 15B-5. Are beats #3, #6, and #9 PVCs or aberrant? *How certain are you of your answer?*

short to conduct. Thus, something must have occurred (i.e., a PVC) before this atrial impulse was able to conduct to the ventricles. Also in support of beat #4 being a PVC is the *lack of a reason for aberrancy.* Beat #4 occurs so late in the cycle that conditions needed for aberrant conduction (i.e., occurrence of a premature impulse during the relative refractory period) would not be expected to exist.

> In some circles, beat #4 is termed an **end-diastolic PVC.** The reason we like this terminology is that it verbally describes the relative position of the PVC in relation to the cardiac cycle—late, at a point that probably corresponds to the end of diastole.* Clinically, end-diastolic PVCs are commonly seen as a reperfusion arrhythmia in patients with acute myocardial infarction following successful thrombolytic therapy or angioplasty.

---

*It should be emphasized that systole and diastole are *mechanical* events, whereas ventricular depolarization and repolarization are *electrical* events. Nevertheless, we can approximate the period of **ventricular systole** as the interval between the QRS complex (onset of ventricular depolarization) and the end of the T wave (end of ventricular repolarization)—and the period of **ventricular diastole** as the interval from the end of the T wave until the next QRS complex. From this description it should be apparent why late-occurring PVCs (such as beat #4 in Fig. 15B-4) may be referred to as "end-diastolic" PVCs.

PROBLEM **FIGURE 15B-5: Are beats #3, #6, and #9 PVCs or aberrant? *How certain are you of your answer?***

ANSWER TO FIGURE 15B-5 The underlying rhythm is atrial fibrillation. Beat #9 is *definitely* a PVC— it is very wide, bizarre, and manifests an ectopic morphology (taller *left* rabbit ear in this right-sided lead— most similar to pattern **F** in Fig. 15A-14).

It is more difficult to be certain about the etiology of beats #3 and #6. Although each manifests a morphology suggestive of aberrancy (rSR' pattern with a taller *right* rabbit ear and similar initial deflection), confirmatory evidence is lacking because the presence of atrial fibrillation precludes identification of a premature P wave. Against the diagnosis of aberration is the *absence of a reason for aberration* for beat #3—it occurs so *late* in the cycle at a time when ventricular repolarization should long be over. Aberration would seem more plausible for a beat like #11, as it has a much shorter coupling interval. *We therefore hedge on our interpretation here,* pending more information (i.e., additional rhythm strips).

A diagnosis of aberrancy is always made more confidently if a "reason" exists for aberrant conduction to occur. Thus in

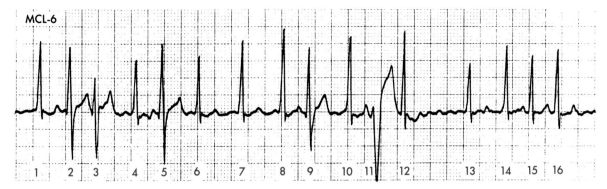

Figure 15B-6. Atrial fibrillation with anomalous complexes. *PVCs, aberrant, or both?*

the previous example of atrial fibrillation reviewed (Fig. 15B-3), each of the anomalous beats (#4, #7 and #13) had relatively short coupling intervals—and a reason to be aberrant. This is definitely not the case for beat #3 in Figure 15B-5. Because the morphologic appearance of beats #3 and #6 in this tracing is so similar, it is likely that both beats share the same etiology. However, we feel it impossible to be sure from this rhythm strip alone whether these beats are PVCs or aberrantly conducted.

PROBLEM   *FIGURE 15B-6: PVCs, aberrant, or both?*

ANSWER TO FIGURE 15B-6   Once again the underlying rhythm is atrial fibrillation, this time with a fairly rapid ventricular response. The normally conducted complexes have an Rs configuration. Beats #2, #3, #5, and #9 are in all probability *aberrant*—they are fairly narrow (≤0.11 second) and manifest a qRS configuration in this *left-sided* lead (comparable to pattern **I** in Fig. 15A-14, and which is the *reciprocal* of an rSR′ configuration in a right-sided lead). In addition, there is a *reason* for these beats to conduct aberrantly—they all have relatively short coupling intervals compared to those beats that conduct normally.

Although beat #11 also has a relatively short coupling interval, it is unlike the other aberrantly conducted beats in this tracing. This beat is wider and manifests a different morphology (it has an rS configuration that most resembles pattern **L** in Fig. 15A-14). Because of its morphology, and for lack of evidence in favor of aberrancy, one has to work on the assumption that beat #11 is a PVC (*"guilty until proved innocent!"*).

> It is of interest to note that R wave amplitude of the "normally" conducted beats varies throughout this tracing. The reason and clinical significance of this finding (if any) is not clear.

Clinically, the most important point to make about the tracing shown in Fig. 15B-6 is the need to **identify and treat the primary disorder.** The principal problem in this example is *not* whether beat #11 is a PVC or an aberrantly conducted supraventricular impulse. Instead, the *principal problem* is the primary disorder, which in this case is the underlying rhythm (i.e., *atrial fibrillation with a fairly rapid ventricular response)*. If this can be treated (and the rate of atrial fibrillation controlled and/or the rhythm converted to normal sinus rhythm), it is likely that the anomalous beats will disappear *regardless* of their etiology. That is, treatment of rapid atrial fibrillation should correct those conditions that predispose to aberrant conduction (short coupling intervals with enhanced likelihood that impulses will fall within the relative refractory period). Treatment should also correct those conditions that predispose to ventricular ectopy (i.e., ischemia from impaired blood flow resulting from the loss of atrial kick and reduced diastolic filling time). Thus medical treatment (with digitalis or antiarrhythmic agents such as quinidine) and/or institution of therapeutic measures to correct any predisposing causes of the arrhythmia (i.e., improved oxygenation, normalization of serum electrolytes) is likely to be much more effective than presumptive treatment with lidocaine.

PROBLEM   *FIGURE 15B-7:* **The initial deflection of the three anomalous beats in this tracing (beats #3, #6, and #9) is *opposite* that of the normally conducted beats.** ***Does this prove that these beats are PVCs?***

ANSWER TO FIGURE 15B-7   No! Despite the fact that the initial deflection of beats #3, #6, and #9 is oppositely directed to that of the sinus beats (and despite the rS configuration of beat #3 in this left-sided lead), there is incontrovertible evidence on this tracing that beats #3, #6, and #9 are all *aberrantly* conducted. First, note that the QRS complex of these beats is *not* significantly widened. Of even greater importance is the fact that *each* of these beats is preceded by a *premature* P wave (that noticeably peaks the T wave preceding it). Finally, *cycle-sequence comparison* provides a perfect explanation for why beat #9 should conduct with a greater degree of aberrancy than beat #6, and why beat #3 is the most aberrant of all (the premature P wave occurs *earliest* after beat #2,

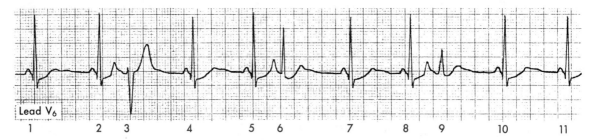

Figure 15B-7. The initial deflection of premature beats #3, #6, and #9 is *oppositely* directed to that of the normally conducted beats. *Does this prove that these beats are PVCs?*

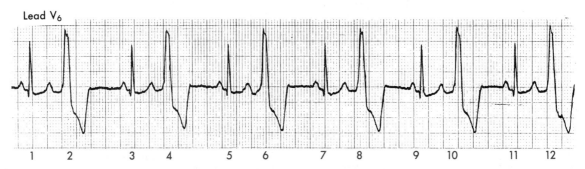

Figure 15B-8A. *PVCs or aberrant?* (Are premature P waves hiding in the T waves that precede each of the anomalous beats?)

and *latest* after beat #6). Thus the rhythm in this tracing is *atrial trigeminy* (i.e., sinus rhythm with a PAC occurring every *third* beat) in which PACs are conducted with varying degrees of aberration (depending on the length of their coupling interval).

> The reason the initial deflection of the anomalous beats in this tracing is oppositely directed to that of the normally conducted beats is that the aberrant conduction is with a hemiblock pattern. This reinforces the point we emphasized at the beginning of the chapter—**none of the rules for determining aberration are perfect.** Instead, one has to gather all available information, integrate it, correlate it clinically, and come up with a *best-educated guess* about the etiology of the arrhythmia.

PROBLEM   *FIGURE 15B-8A:* **Every other beat in this tracing is abnormal.** *Are the anomalous beats PVCs or aberrant?* **(Are premature P waves hiding in the T waves that precede each of the anomalous beats?)**

ANSWER TO FIGURE 15B-8A   Unfortunately, there is no way to tell for sure if a premature P wave is buried in the T wave that precedes each of the anomalous complexes (i.e., the T wave of beats #1, #3, #5, #7, #9, and #11). This is because one *never* sees two sinus beats in a row. Since a beat is "guilty until proven innocent," the even-numbered beats must be assumed to be ventricular since they are wide, bizarre in shape, and manifest an oppositely directed initial deflection. In addition, there are really no compelling reasons for aberrancy.

Figure 15B-8B was recorded from the same patient a little later. Now that two sinus beats occur in a row, we can compare the T wave preceding each of the anomalous beats with the appearance of a "normal" T wave. Even with close scrutiny, there is no definite deformity suggestive of premature atrial activity. Thus, Figure 15B-8A represents ventricular *bigeminy*, and Fig. 15B-8B ventricular *trigeminy* (i.e., every *third* beat is a PVC).

If you were satisfied with the above explanation for the arrhythmias shown in Figs. 15B-8A and 15B-8B, *read no further!* If, on the other hand, you were bothered by the slight variation in T wave morphology in Figure 15B-8A, read on . . . .

> Admittedly, T wave (and ST segment) morphology *does* change slightly from beat to beat in Fig. 15B-8A. Complicating matters even more is the slight variation in the R-R interval between some of the sinus-conducted beats (i.e., the R-R interval between beats #1-3, #3-5, and #9-11), suggesting that the underlying rhythm is sinus arrhythmia. Again, one is left with the fact that two normal sinus-conducted beats *never* occur in a row, anomalous beats are wide, bizarre in shape, and manifest an oppositely directed initial deflection, and the need to presume that an anomalous beat is "guilty" (i.e., a PVC) until *proved* innocent. Thus, despite the possibility that the slight variation in T wave morphology could be the result of hidden premature atrial activity, in the absence of firm proof to the contrary, the anomalous beats in this tracing must be assumed ventricular in etiology. Support of this assumption is provided by the follow-up tracing shown in Fig. 15B-8B, in which ST segment and T wave morphology is more consistent and fails to suggest even a hint of hidden premature atrial activity.

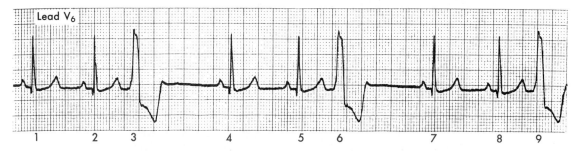

Figure 15B-8B.   Subsequent tracing recorded from the patient who was in a bigeminal rhythm in Fig. 15B-8A. *Are beats #3, #6, and #9 PVCs or aberrantly conducted?*

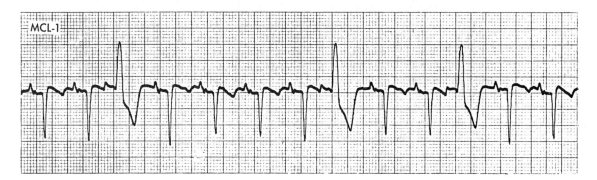

Figure 15B-9.   Lead MCL₁ rhythm strip obtained from a patient with acute myocardial infarction. *Should the anomalous beats be treated with lidocaine?*

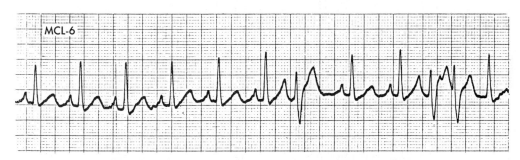

Figure 15B-10A.   Lead MCL₆ rhythm strip obtained from a patient with acute myocardial infarction. *Should the anomalous beats be treated with lidocaine?*

PROBLEM   *Figures 15B-9 and 15B-10A were* **taken from a patient having an acute myocardial infarction. Based on the anomalous beats seen in these (and numerous other) rhythm strips, the patient was treated with lidocaine.** *Do you agree?*

ANSWERS TO FIGURES 15B-9 AND 15B-10A

The underlying rhythm in Fig. 15B-9 is sinus tachycardia at a rate of 105 beats/minute. Unfortunately, morphologic analysis of the anomalous beats in this tracing is not of much assistance in diagnosis, since the initial r wave is absent. Anomalous beats manifest an "intermediate" pattern with a qR configuration that most closely resembles complex **E** in Fig. 15A-14. The reason the initial positive

deflection (r wave) is missing may be as a result of the acute infarction. However, because the normally conducted sinus beats *also* lack an initial r wave, a typical RBBB pattern might not occur even if aberration was present. Therefore, no conclusions can be drawn based on morphologic assessment of the anomalous beats in this lead.

On the other hand, *premature* atrial activity is *definitely* present, and this provides ample evidence to interpret the arrhythmia. Careful inspection of the T waves of normally conducted beats, and comparison with the T waves preceding each of the anomalous beats reveals the distinct notching of a "telltale PAC" in front of the latter. The finding of a PAC in front of *each* of the anomalous beats is strongly in favor of aberrancy.

This conclusion is further supported by extra peaking of the T waves that precede *each* of the anomalous beats in the MCL$_6$ lead rhythm strip (Fig. 15B-10A). Coincidence would not produce an abnormality *only* in the T waves that directly precede each of the anomalous beats in these two tracings.

> Morphologic assessment of the QRS complex in lead MCL$_6$ (Fig. 15B-10A) suggests an intermediate (RS) pattern (similar to complex **K** in Fig. 15A-14) that by itself does not help in differentiation. However, note that anomalous beats in this rhythm strip are not markedly widened, and that their initial deflection (direction *and* slope) is virtually *identical* to that of the normally conducted beats—factors consistent with a supraventricular etiology. In the context of the premature atrial activity described above, a strong case is made for aberrant conduction.

Figure 15B-10B was recorded a little later from this same patient. Arrows highlight extra peaking of the T waves (corresponding to hidden PACs) that precede beats #3 and #7. A third arrow precedes beat #9 and points out another, even more clearly identified premature P wave that notches the terminal portion of the T wave of beat #8.

PROBLEM   **In view of the fact that beats #3 and #7 are conducted with aberration in Fig. 15B-10B, why does the premature P wave preceding beat #9 conduct normally?**

ANSWER TO FIGURE 15B-10B

Cycle-sequence comparison explains why beat #9 conducts normally in this tracing. The premature P waves preceding beats #3 and #7 clearly occur *earlier* (i.e., have *shorter* coupling intervals) than the PAC that follows beat #8. As a result, this last P wave is most likely to occur at a later point in the refractory period at a time when normal conduction is possible.

> The importance of differentiating between PVCs and aberrantly conducted beats in the setting of acute myocardial infarction is obvious—the former often require treatment (usually with lidocaine) while the latter do not. Treatment of aberrantly conducted PACs with lidocaine is not only unnecessary, but it may sometimes be harmful, as we will see momentarily.
> A helpful point to keep in mind is that the occurrence of frequent premature supraventricular impulses (PACs or PJCs) may be a subtle clinical sign of incipient heart failure.

Figure 15B-11 shows what happened to this patient shortly after the lidocaine was given.

The beginning of Fig. 15B-11 is similar to Fig. 15B-9: sinus tachycardia at a rate of 105 beats/minute. Midway

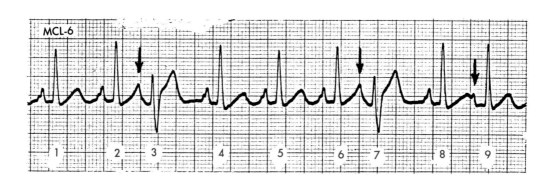

Figure 15B-10B.   Subsequent MCL$_6$ lead recording from this same patient with acute myocardial infarction. Arrows highlight premature P waves preceding beats #3, #7, and #9. *Why does the PAC preceding beat #9 conduct normally?*

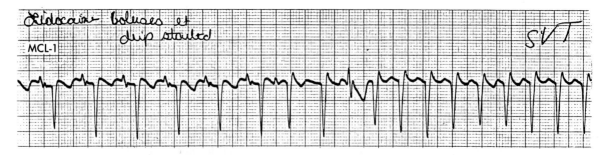

Figure 15B-11.   Rhythm strip obtained from this patient with acute myocardial infarction shortly after lidocaine was administered. *What happened?*

through the rhythm strip, a PAC occurs (the premature P wave notching the preceding T wave), and this sets off a run of supraventricular tachycardia (SVT). Although not a common response, **lidocaine may occasionally accelerate supraventricular rhythms!**

Treatment with lidocaine is *not* benign, and the drug should never be given as a "therapeutic trial." In addition to an incidence of adverse reactions that approaches 15%, lidocaine occasionally exerts a slight vagolytic effect that may *accelerate* the rate of the supraventricular rhythm (especially in patients with atrial fibrillation). Thus, the supraventricular tachycardia produced in this case was totally *iatrogenic* (i.e., the patient should *never* have received lidocaine), since strong evidence suggesting aberrancy was present on other rhythm strips (Figs. 15B-9, 15B-10A, and 15B-10B).

Full discussion of the types of supraventricular tachycardia will follow in Section A of Chapter 16. As a result, we defer discussion of the probable mechanism involved in Fig. 15B-11 until then. For now, we'd simply like to draw attention to the fact that evidence of atrial activity *during* the run of SVT is present in Figure 15B-11. *Do you see it?*

The normally conducted sinus beats in the beginning of this tracing manifest a QS (all negative) configuration. In contrast, the initial PAC, and each of the complexes during the run of SVT manifest a terminal positive deflection (i.e., they have a Qr configuration). This small, positive terminal deflection that has been added to the QRS complex represents *retrograde* atrial activity, and results from the reentry mechanism sustaining the SVT. As we will see in Section A of Chapter 16, *evidence of atrial activity can often be found during reentry supraventricular tachyarrhythmias if carefully looked for.*

PROBLEM   *FIGURE 15B-12: PVCs or aberrant?*

ANSWER TO FIGURE 15B-12   It is hard to be sure if the underlying rhythm is sinus with very frequent PACs or multifocal atrial tachycardia. In any event, P waves abound. A premature P wave notches the T wave preceding the first anomalous beat. The two anomalous beats are not greatly widened (they are ≤0.11 second), they have a similarly directed (upward) initial deflection to the normally conducted beats, and they manifest a typical RBBB pattern in this right-sided monitoring lead (comparable to complex **B** in Fig. 15A-14). Finally, the Ashman phenomenon is present (with the first anomalous

complex occurring with a short coupling interval after a relatively long pause). *Level of confidence in diagnosing aberrancy?*—almost 100%!

This tracing illustrates a subtle point made earlier regarding morphology—namely, that *the key complex to focus on for morphologic assessment during a series of anomalous beats is the initial complex in the run.* Thus, the first anomalous beat in Fig. 15B-12 manifests the typical rSR′ pattern of RBBB aberration, whereas the negative deflection (S wave) of the second anomalous complex is much less distinct, and by itself would be much less suggestive of aberration.

The saying, ***"Birds of a feather . . . . "*** holds equally true for arrhythmias as in life. Multiple PACs are evident on the tracing shown in Fig. 15B-12. Other than the two beats in question, there is not even the slightest hint of ventricular ectopy elsewhere. Considering the multitude of PACs present in the underlying rhythm, it would seem much more likely statistically for the two anomalous beats on this tracing to also be PACs (that conduct aberrantly), than to postulate sudden development of ventricular ectopy.

PROBLEM   *FIGURE 15B-13A: PVCs or aberrant?*

ANSWER TO FIGURE 15B-13A   Obviously PVCs (ventricular trigeminy). The anomalous beats are markedly widened, bizarre in shape, and are not preceded by a premature P wave. A full compensatory pause is present (i.e., the pause containing the anomalous beat is exactly twice the normal R-R interval). Finally, it appears that the sinus-conducted beats manifest a tiny q wave (initial negative deflection) that differs from the initial positive deflection of the wide beats.

Even if you have reservations about the existence of a small, initial negative deflection (q wave) for the sinus-conducted beats, it is clear that the *slope* (rate of incline) of the R wave of each anomalous beat is different (slower rising) than the

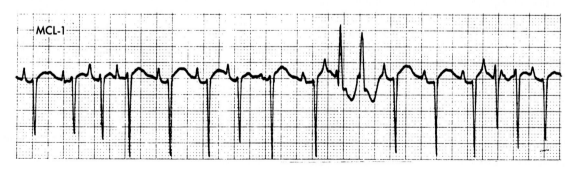

Figure 15B-12.   *PVCs or aberrant?*

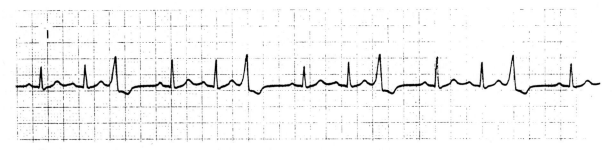

Figure 15B-13A. *PVCs or aberrant?*

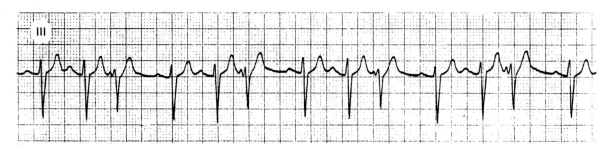

Figure 15B-13B. *PVCs or aberrant?*

almost vertical slope of the R wave of the sinus-conducted beats.

Level of confidence in diagnosing ventricular ectopy?—almost 100%!

___

PROBLEM *FIGURE 15B-13B: PVCs or aberrant?*

ANSWER TO FIGURE 15B-13B   The anomalous beats in this tracing appear to be aberrantly conducted. They look very much like the sinus-conducted beats, they do not appear to be wide, their initial deflection is similarly directed, and they seem to be preceded by a premature P wave.

Alas, this is a trick tracing!!! *Can you figure out why?*

More leads are better than one! At times the appearance of a beat in one particular monitoring lead may be extremely deceptive of its true appearance. Nowhere is this more true than for Fig. 15B-13B. For all the world from inspection of Fig. 15B-13B, each of the early beats (every third beat) seems to be narrow, similar in shape to the normally conducted beats, and preceded by a premature P wave.

Figure 15B-13C shows that this is *not* the case! Instead, the **timeline** drawn on this simultaneously recorded rhythm strip indicates that the small, pointed, positive deflections that were thought to be premature P waves in Fig. 15B-13B (lower panel of Fig. 15B-13C) are actually part of the QRS complex. Thus the anomalous beats in this tracing *are* wide, and are *not* preceded by a premature P wave.

Note in Fig. 15B-13C that the top panel displays the simultaneous recording of a lead I monitoring lead. This is the same rhythm strip we just saw in Fig. 15B-13A, and for which it was clear that the anomalous beats were PVCs. **More leads are better than one**—*and the anomalous beats in Fig. 15A-13B are all PVCs!*

___

PROBLEM *FIGURE 15B-14: Why do beats #5 and #9 in this tracing look different?*

ANSWER TO FIGURE 15B-14   Beats #5 and #9 look different than the normally conducted beats because they are PVCs (probably with some degree of *fusion*). The principal clue lies in the atrial rate, which remains *constant* throughout the rhythm strip. Thus a regular sinus P wave can be seen to slur the upstroke of the QRS complex of the anomalous beats. Since the PR interval in front of these beats (beats #5 and #9) is too short to conduct, an impulse (a PVC) must be arising from below.

> The anomalous beats in this tracing provide another example of *end-diastolic PVCs* (i.e., they occur toward the end of the R-R interval, which corresponds to the end of diastole). As might be imagined, this type of ventricular ectopy commonly produces fusion beats.
>
> Note how similar beats #5 and #9 are to the sinus-conducted beats. This is a common occurrence with right ventricular PVCs.

___

PROBLEM *FIGURE 15B-15: What is the rhythm? What are the different-looking beats?*

ANSWER TO FIGURE 15B-15   The underlying rhythm is irregularly irregular without definite P waves in

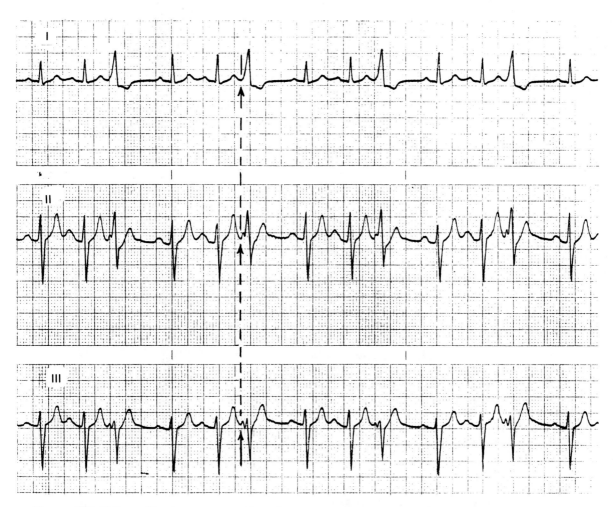

Figure 15B-13C. Simultaneous recording of the rhythm strips shown in Figs. 15B-13A and 15B-13B. The **timeline** shows that the small, pointed positive deflections that simulate a premature P wave in lead III (lower panel) are actually part of the QRS complex. *The anomalous beats are PVCs!*

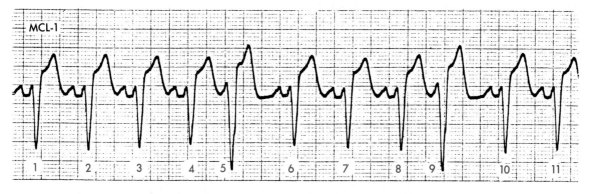

Figure 15B-14. *Why do beats #5 and #9 look different?*

this lead II monitoring lead. This is atrial fibrillation with a moderately rapid ventricular response. There are two types of "different-looking" beats in this tracing: negative complexes with a QS configuration (beats #3, #4, and #22), and biphasic complexes with an RS configuration (beats #6-9).

Beats #3, #4, and #22 are probably PVCs. They are wide, bizarre in appearance, and have a very different initial deflection from the normally conducted beats. In contrast, beats #6-9 are much more likely to be supraventricular impulses conducted with *aberration*. These complexes are not significantly widened and their initial de-

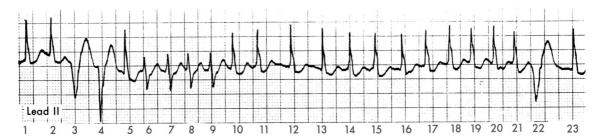

Figure 15B-15.   *What are the different-looking beats?*

flection is virtually identical (in direction *and* slope) to that of the normally conducted beats. Moreover, this run maintains the same rapid and irregular *cadence* as the underlying atrial fibrillation (i.e., it begins abruptly with beat #6, and ends equally abruptly with nary a pause before beat #10).

> Note that there is a *short **post-ectopic pause*** following beat #22. Interruption of the underlying cadence of atrial fibrillation by a short pause is a common finding associated with ventricular ectopy. Although the principle is similar to that which produces the "full" compensatory pause discussed in Section A of this chapter (concealed *retrograde* conduction from the PVC delaying or preventing antegrade conduction of the next supraventricular impulse), the inherent irregularity of atrial fibrillation understandably prevents determination of what constitutes "full" compensation.
>
> It is important to emphasize that *not* all PVCs that occur with atrial fibrillation are followed by a "post-ectopic pause" (beat #4 in this tracing is not!), and that the heart rate may by chance transiently slow down at times following aberrant conduction of a supraventricular impulse. Nevertheless, awareness of the phenomenon of a *post-ectopic pause* may sometimes prove very useful in the differential diagnosis of anomalous complexes that occur during atrial fibrillation.

PROBLEM   *FIGURE 15B-16A:* **The patient whose rhythm is shown in this tracing was hemodynamically stable.** *Should this run of anomalous beats be treated as a run of ventricular tachycardia (i.e., with lidocaine)?*

ANSWER TO FIGURE 15B-16A   The underlying rhythm is again atrial fibrillation (irregularly irregular rhythm, no definite P waves). Although one might be

tempted to call beats #3-8 a run of ventricular tachycardia, several factors argue against this conclusion. Morphologic assessment of the anomalous complexes is most in favor of aberration. Granted, a "neat" rsR′ configuration (with a distinct initial positive r wave deflection and s wave return to the baseline) is hard to make out. Nevertheless, we feel a RBBB pattern (similar to complex **B** in Fig. 15A-14) is probably present for the anomalous complexes in Fig. 15B-16A, at least for the initial beats in each run (beats #3 and #10). Moreover, the anomalous complexes do not appear to be significantly widened, and they once again do not disturb the rapid and irregular cadence of the patient's underlying atrial fibrillation (i.e., a slight but definite irregular irregularity persists throughout the run of anomalous beats). Statistically, when a series of irregularly occurring anomalous beats complicates rapid atrial fibrillation, it is much more likely to reflect aberrant conduction than ventricular ectopy. In this particular case, the run ends as abruptly as it begins, and there is no postectopic pause after beat #8 or #10. Taken together, the sum of these factors strongly favors *aberration* as the cause of the anomalous beats. Rather than an empiric trial of lidocaine, one might do better to try and control the ventricular response with medication such as digoxin and/or verapamil.

It is important to emphasize that at this point in the diagnostic process, *it is hard to be certain* of the etiology of the arrhythmia shown in Fig. 15B-16A. Despite the balance of evidence in favor of aberrancy, ventricular tachycardia *cannot* be completely ruled out. However, as was the case for the rhythm we discussed earlier in Fig. 15B-6, the

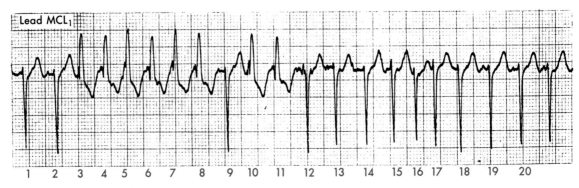

Figure 15B-16A.   *Should this run of anomalous beats be treated with lidocaine?*

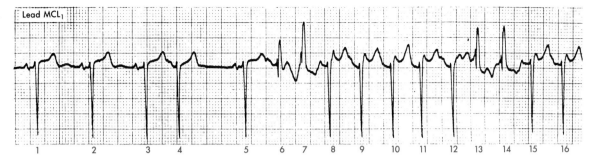

Figure 15B-16B.   Follow-up tracing to Fig. 15B-16A, obtained a short while after administration of IV digoxin. *Does this follow-up tracing support your previous assumption that the anomalous beats in Fig. 15B-16A were aberrantly conducted?*

principal clinical concern for this hemodynamically stable patient has to be **identification and treatment of the primary disorder** *rather* than definitive diagnosis of the anomalous beats. Since the "primary disorder" is atrial fibrillation with a *rapid* ventricular response, achievement of heart rate control and/or conversion to normal sinus rhythm is the principal therapeutic goal. Attaining this goal is likely to result in correction of those conditions causing the anomalous beats *regardless* of their etiology.

> A word of caution is again warranted regarding the use of the medications lidocaine and verapamil for treatment of anomalous complexes that occur in association with rapid atrial fibrillation. Lidocaine is not without side effects. It is important to appreciate that on occasion this drug may exert a vagolytic effect and actually *accelerate* the ventricular response of a supraventricular tachycardia (especially atrial fibrillation). IV verapamil is an excellent agent to use for treatment of supraventricular tachyarrhythmias, but its vasodilatory and negative inotropic effects may become extremely problematic if blood pressure is borderline or low, and/or the run of anomalous beats turns out to be sustained ventricular tachycardia.

The patient in this particular case was not given lidocaine, but was started on IV digoxin. A short while after receiving a second 0.25-mg IV dose of this drug, the rhythm shown in *Figure 15B-16B* was observed.

PROBLEM   **Does this new rhythm (shown in Fig. 15B-16B) support your previous assumption that the anomalous beats in Fig. 15B-16A were aberrantly conducted?**

ANSWER TO FIGURE 15B-16B   Sinus rhythm is temporarily restored (beats #1, #2, #3, and #5), but the rhythm then reverts back to atrial fibrillation. Beat #4 is clearly a PAC—the complex conducts normally, and a premature P wave distorts the preceding T wave. Similarly, a premature P wave produces a notch in the T wave preceding beat #6. Note that the morphology of beats #6, #7, #13, and #14 in Fig. 15B-16B is identical to that of beats #3-8, and #10 and #11 of Fig. 15B-16A. In the context of Fig. 15B-16B, the premature P wave that precedes beat #6, in conjunction with the similar initial deflection to the normally conducted beats and RBBB pat-

tern, establish *beyond doubt* that beat #6 is aberrantly conducted. It follows that *all of the other similar-appearing beats in this figure and in Fig. 15B-16A must also be aberrant.* Sometimes definitive diagnosis of an arrhythmia will only be possible *retrospectively.* Such is the case here, since we could not be 100% sure that the anomalous beats seen in Fig. 15B-16A were aberrantly conducted until after we had seen the follow-up tracing shown in Fig. 15B-16B.

PROBLEM   **There is one more finding in favor of aberrant conduction for beat #6 in Fig. 15B-16B. What is it?**

[HINT: Why might the first "funny-looking beat" in this tracing (beat #6) follow the longest pause (the R-R interval between beats #4-5)?]

ANSWER   Cycle-sequence comparison in the form of the Ashman phenomenon explains why beat #6 is conducted aberrantly in this tracing, while beat #4 is not. The premature P waves that notch the T waves of beats #3 and #5 occur at approximately similar points in the cardiac cycle. However, the longer pause (R-R interval) preceding beat #5 results in prolongation of the subsequent refractory period, and accounts for the aberration of beat #6.

You are now informed that a run of anomalous beats manifesting yet another QRS configuration has just occurred (beats #13-16 in *Figure 15B-17*).

PROBLEM   **Considering development of this new wide complex tachycardia (beats #13-16 in Fig. 15B-17), *should you give the lidocaine now?***

ANSWER TO FIGURE 15B-17   Although the presence of atrial fibrillation again precludes searching for telltale premature P waves, several other features suggest that beats #13-16 in this follow-up tracing are *also* aberrantly conducted, this time with an LBBB pattern of aberration. Note that the underlying irregular irregularity persists throughout the entire rhythm strip irrespective of the change in QRS morphology. Moreover, the run of

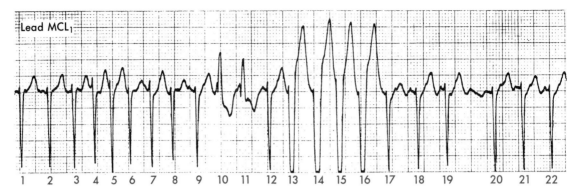

Figure 15B-17. Follow-up tracing of Fig. 15B-16B demonstrating a run of anomalous beats that manifest yet another QRS configuration (beats #13-16). *Should you give the lidocaine now?*

anomalous beats ends as abruptly as it begins without any post-ectopic pause, and the QRS complex during the run is *not* greatly prolonged (0.11 second). Finally, QRS morphology of the anomalous beats during the run is consistent with the pattern of LBBB aberration (similar to complex **N** in Fig. 15A-16) in which a slender initial positive deflection (r wave) is followed by an extremely rapid (almost vertical) descending S wave.

> Pure LBBB aberration is much *less* common than RBBB aberration. Moreover, supraventricular impulses that conduct with pure LBBB aberration are often much harder to recognize than those conducting with RBBB aberration because of a much greater resemblance to ventricular ectopic beats. The morphologic characteristics illustrated in Fig. 15A-16 provide some help in differentiating between right ventricular ectopy and LBBB aberration. Additional help may be forthcoming from appreciation of the fact that RBBB and LBBB aberration may *alternate* in the same patient. This phenomenon of **alternating RBBB and LBBB aberration should be especially suspected when runs of anomalous complexes are separated by a single normally conducted beat.** This is the case in Fig. 15B-17 in which RBBB aberration (beats #10 and #11) and LBBB aberration (beats #13-16) are separated by a single, normally conducted beat (#12).

Clinically, in the context of a hemodynamically stable patient having runs of beats that are *definitely* aberrant (the anomalous beats with RBBB configuration), it would seem reasonable to assume with a high degree of probability

that beats #13-16 in Figure 15B-17 also are aberrant. Additional administration of IV digoxin succeeded in controlling the ventricular response. Ultimately the patient converted to sinus rhythm, and no further anomalous beats were seen.

PROBLEM *Figure 15B-18: Aberrancy or ventricular tachycardia?*

ANSWER TO FIGURE 15B-18 *Ventricular tachycardia!* The QRS complex during the tachycardia becomes wide and looks very different from the normally conducted beats. Morphologically, the first few anomalous beats in this tracing most resemble complex **G** in Fig. 15A-14 (with, if anything, a taller *left* rabbit ear), and strongly suggest ventricular ectopy. A post-ectopic pause follows the seven-beat run. There is absolutely no reason to suspect aberrancy in this tracing; ventricular tachycardia *must* be assumed, *and the patient treated accordingly.*

PROBLEM *Figure 15B-19A: Ventricular tachycardia?*

ANSWER TO FIGURE 15B-19A Following three sinus-conducted beats, a long run of anomalous beats occurs. The QRS complex during the run is wide and looks

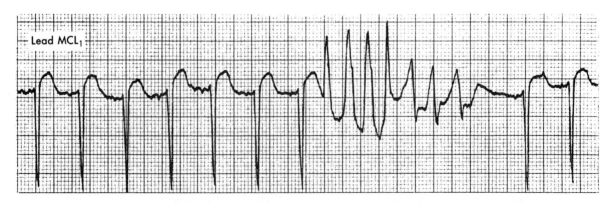

Figure 15B-18. *Aberrancy or ventricular tachycardia?*

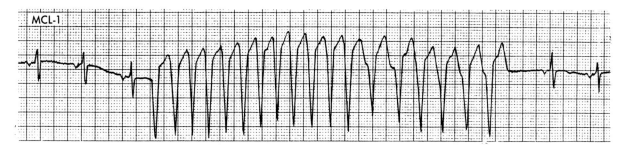

Figure 15B-19A.   *Ventricular tachycardia?*

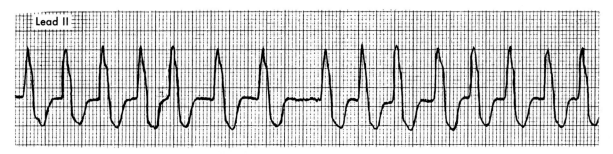

Figure 15B-19B.   The QRS complex is definitely widened.
Is this ventricular tachycardia?

very different from the normally conducted beats (most resembling complex **Q** in Fig. 15A-16). A postectopic pause follows the last beat of the run. Once again, ventricular tachycardia must be assumed, and the patient treated accordingly.

> In general, ventricular tachycardia tends to be a fairly *regular* rhythm. At times, however, it may exhibit either a **"warm-up"** or **"cool-down"** phenomenon. In the former, ventricular tachycardia starts off at a slower rate and then gradually accelerates (i.e., *"warms up"*) until it attains its eventual rate. In contrast, with a "cool-down" phenomenon, the rhythm starts off *faster* and then slows down to its eventual rate. The run of ventricular tachycardia seen in Fig. 15B-19A illustrates a "cool down" phenomenon in which the first few beats are decidedly faster than the heart rate toward the end of the run.

PROBLEM   *FIGURE 15B-19B:* **The QRS complex is definitely widened in this tracing.** *Is this ventricular tachycardia?*

ANSWER TO FIGURE 15B-19B   Probably not! Despite the fact that the QRS complex is obviously widened, the underlying rhythm is grossly irregular. Continual variation in the R-R interval from beat to beat, and the absence of atrial activity in this lead II monitoring lead suggest that the rhythm is atrial fibrillation.

PROBLEM   **If the rhythm in Figure 15B-19B is supraventricular (atrial fibrillation), how do you explain the QRS widening?** *What would be needed to prove your explanation?*

ANSWER   The most likely explanation for the QRS widening seen in Figure 15B-19B is to postulate the pres-

ence of a *pre-existing* bundle branch block. Access to a previous 12-lead ECG on this patient would be invaluable in confirming this impression.

> Unfortunately, morphologic assessment of the QRS complex in Fig. 15B-19B is of absolutely no assistance because the rhythm was recorded from lead II.

Compare the "rhythmicity" of the arrhythmia shown in Fig. 15B-19B with that of the run of anomalous beats in Fig. 15B-19A. Both rhythms are irregularly irregular. However, there is the suggestion of a *pattern* in Fig. 15B-19A (extremely rapid and fairly regular initial portion, followed by a fairly regular, slower terminal portion). In contrast, there is absolutely no pattern to the irregularity of the rhythm shown in Fig. 15B-19B. This is why we strongly suspect atrial fibrillation in this latter case, although admittedly this diagnosis *cannot* be made with 100% certainty *without* confirmatory evidence of preexistent QRS widening.

PROBLEM   *FIGURE 15B-20:* **Do beats #5 to #15 represent a run of ventricular tachycardia?**

ANSWER TO FIGURE 15B-20   The underlying rhythm in this tracing is sinus tachycardia at a heart rate of 105 beats/minute. This is interrupted by a long run of anomalous beats (#5-15). Note that a premature P wave initiates the run (notching the T wave preceding beat #5). The QRS complex during the run is not markedly prolonged (<0.11 second), and the morphology is consistent with a pattern of LBBB aberration (slender initial r wave, and extremely rapid downsloping S wave—similar to com-

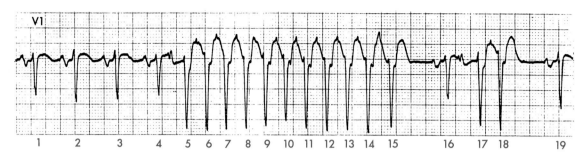

Figure 15B-20. *Ventricular tachycardia?*

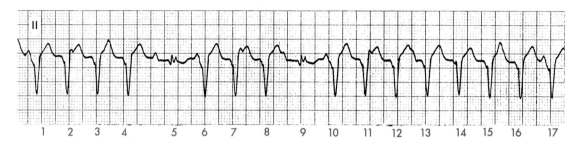

Figure 15B-21A. *Ventricular tachycardia?*

plex **N** in Fig. 15A-16). A premature P wave is also seen to notch the T wave preceding beat #17 (which together with beat #18 is conducted with a similar morphologic pattern as beats #5-15). Consideration of the *combination* of these factors strongly suggests that the anomalous run of beats in Fig. 15B-20 is the result of aberrant conduction (and *not* ventricular tachycardia)!

> It is of interest (but of unknown significance) that P waves *can* be seen to notch the apex of the T wave during the run of anomalous beats. This probably reflects retrograde atrial activity resulting from the reentry mechanism of the supraventricular tachycardia. No P wave is seen to notch the last T wave in the run (the T wave of beat #15—or the T wave of beat #18), suggesting a role for this retrograde atrial activity in sustaining the tachycardia. However, because ventricular tachycardia may also occasionally exhibit retrograde 1:1 conduction, the finding of P waves within the T waves of the anomalous beats during the run *by itself* is of little diagnostic assistance.

PROBLEM   *FIGURE   15B-21A:*   Ventricular tachycardia?

ANSWER TO FIGURE 15B-21A   The basic rhythm is composed of QS complexes that are 0.12 second in duration and regular at a rate of 135 beats/min. Two "unusual-looking" complexes (beats #5 and #9) interrupt this underlying rhythm. The first of these (beat #5) is preceded by a P wave that appears to be conducting, albeit with 1° AV block. Scanning the rest of the tracing for signs of atrial activity, notching and peaking at various points of the QRS complex in many beats is evident. *Setting one's calipers* to the interval defined by the P wave preceding beat #5 and the positive deflection that occurs just before beat #6, atrial activity can be *"marched out"* across the

rhythm strip (arrows in *Figure 15B-21B*). Because this atrial activity is for the most part *unrelated* to the QRS complex, there is *AV dissociation* in which the negative complexes (with a QS configuration) represent runs of ventricular tachycardia that are interrupted by *sinus capture beats* (beats #5 and #9). The q waves of these sinus-conducted beats and the 1° AV block are each manifestations of this patient's acute inferior myocardial infarction.

> The finding of **AV dissociation** during a wide complex tachycardia is an extremely useful diagnostic feature for identifying the tachyarrhythmia as being of ventricular origin. Although theoretically possible for a wide complex tachycardia to manifest AV dissociation as the result of aberrant conduction from an accelerated junctional focus, this is exceedingly rare. Unfortunately, persistent AV dissociation as demonstrated in Fig. 15B-21B is only seen in a minority of cases of ventricular tachycardia. It is most likely to occur in those cases in which the rate of the ventricular tachycardia is relatively slow—which are the cases that generally cause the least diagnostic difficulty.
>
> The finding of **sinus capture beats** is of similar diagnostic utility as AV dissociation. Unfortunately, this finding is even more uncommon than AV dissociation, and is also most likely to occur in cases when the rate of ventricular tachycardia is relatively slow (See Table 15B-1).

PROBLEM   *FIGURE 15B-22: Ventricular tachycardia?* **(The patient is hemodynamically stable.)**

ANSWER TO FIGURE 15B-22   The underlying rhythm appears to be atrial fibrillation with a rapid ventricular response (irregularly irregular rhythm with coarse undulations of the baseline, but no definite P waves). Beat #5 begins a run of a wide complex tachycardia. Morphologic assessment is complicated by uncertainty in knowing whether or not an initial positive deflection (r wave) com-

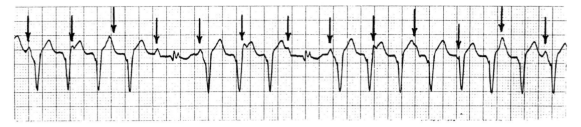

Figure 15B-21B.   Arrows indicate the presence of *regular* atrial activity throughout the rhythm shown in Fig. 15B-21A. Since most P waves are unrelated to the QRS complex, there is AV dissociation.

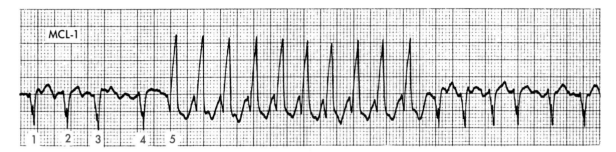

Figure 15B-22.   *Ventricular tachycardia?*

prises the first part of the anomalous complexes. If so, the anomalous beats would have an rSR′ configuration with a taller right rabbit ear in this right-sided lead (similar to complex **B** in Fig. 15A-14), which would strongly favor aberrant conduction. On the other hand, if the QR pattern of beat #5 (similar to complex **E** in Fig. 15A-14) represents the true configuration of the anomalous beats, morphologic assessment would be of little assistance in differentiation between ventricular ectopy and aberration.

> Other somewhat conflicting findings are present on the tracing. A long-short sequence (Ashman phenomenon) precedes the run, but this finding is decidedly less reliable in the setting of atrial fibrillation. The string of anomalous beats begins and ends *abruptly* (i.e., there is no post-ectopic pause), and careful measurement of the R-R interval *during* the run reveals an ever-so-slight irregularity of the rhythm. Although these findings are consistent with a supraventricular etiology, they in no way rule out ventricular tachycardia (which is usually a regular rhythm, but which may manifest some irregularity). Finally, the clinical finding that the patient was hemodynamically stable during the tachycardia is not helpful in differentiation.

Considering the above discussion, we favor *aberrant conduction* as the etiology of the anomalous beats in Fig. 15B-22, but *fully acknowledge the impossibility of knowing for sure*

from this one monitoring strip alone. So admittedly, our bets are hedged pending additional information. Obtaining a 12-lead ECG and/or comparison with previous rhythm strips done on this patient might clarify the issue. In the meantime, treatment of the primary underlying disorder (rapid atrial fibrillation) should be undertaken, and the patient closely observed until such time as the arrhythmia resolves or definitive diagnosis becomes possible.

PROBLEM   *FIGURE   15B-23A: Ventricular tachycardia?* **How certain are you of your diagnosis?**

ANSWER TO FIGURE 15B-23A   The initial portion of the tracing demonstrates sinus tachycardia at a rate of 105 beats/min as the underlying rhythm. This is interrupted by a wide complex tachycardia of different morphology (with, if anything, a taller *left* rabbit ear—most closely resembling complex **G** in Fig. 15A-14). *Ventricular tachycardia* must be assumed until proven otherwise.

Further support in favor of ventricular tachycardia as the etiology of the run of anomalous beats is provided by *Fig. 15B-23B*, in which arrows demonstrate AV dissociation during the first two beats of the run. Note also the

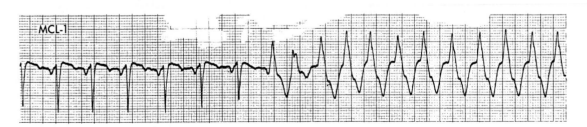

Figure 15B-23A.   *Ventricular tachycardia?* How certain are you of your diagnosis?

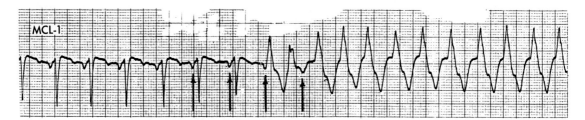

Figure 15B-23B. Sinus tachycardia is interrupted by a wide complex tachycardia. Morphologic assessment of anomalous beats (taller *left* rabbit ear in this right-sided lead) and the presence of AV dissociation strongly suggest ventricular tachycardia.

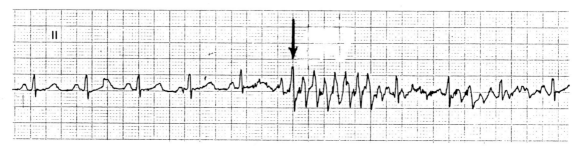

Figure 15B-24A. *Ventricular tachycardia or supraventricular tachycardia?*

relatively late onset of the wide complex tachycardia at a point in the cardiac cycle when aberrant conduction would *not* be expected.

Degree of certainty in the diagnosis of ventricular tachycardia?—virtually 100%!

PROBLEM *FIGURE 15B-24A: Ventricular tachycardia or supraventricular tachycadia?*

ANSWER TO FIGURE 15B-24A   Neither. Although the arrow in Fig. 15B-24A suggests the onset of a tachyarrhythmia, the heart rate during this short burst of anomalous complexes is *well over* 300 beats/min—much too fast to represent a real rhythm. *Fig. 15B-24B* (which demonstrates the simultaneous recording from lead V₅) is revealing.

It can be seen from lead V₅ of Figure 15B-24B that the normal QRS complex is *unaffected* by the disturbance in the baseline, and regular complexes continue to occur at a rate of 85 beats/min. This confirms *artifact* as the cause of the baseline disturbance (and of the pseudotachycardia) in lead II. This patient began seizing as the result of a hypoglycemic reaction at the point indicated by the arrow.

Artifact should be suspected whenever the electrocardiographic appearance of an arrhythmia is inconsistent with physiologic principles (i.e., a rate of 400-450 beats/min as shown in Fig. 15B-24A is *too fast* to be a real rhythm). Suspicion of artifact is supported by irregularities in the baseline, and may

often be confirmed by simultaneous lead recordings (as shown in Fig. 15B-24B) and/or clinical correlation (observation of the patient to see whether they are responsive, trembling, seizing, etc.).

PROBLEM *FIGURE 15B-25A: Ventricular tachycardia?* How certain are you of your diagnosis?

ANSWER TO FIGURE 15B-25A   Although small-amplitude undulations in the baseline make it somewhat hard to tell, the underlying rhythm appears to be sinus tachycardia at a rate of 135 beats/min. This is interrupted by an anomalous couplet, an additional normally conducted beat, and then a long run of an anomalous tachycardia. QRS morphology during the run differs greatly from that of the sinus conducted beats, and *of itself* suggests ventricular tachycardia. Close analysis of the R-R baseline between the two beats of the couplet provides confirmation *(Figure 15B-25B)*.

Solid arrows mark the sinus P waves in Fig. 15B-25B and indicate that AV dissociation is present for the anomalous couplet! The broken arrows indicate notching of the ST segment of beat #7 and of subsequent beats in the anomalous run. This is most likely due to *retrograde* conduction to the atria during the ventricular tachycardia.

Degree of certainty in the diagnosis of ventricular tachycardia?—virtually 100%.

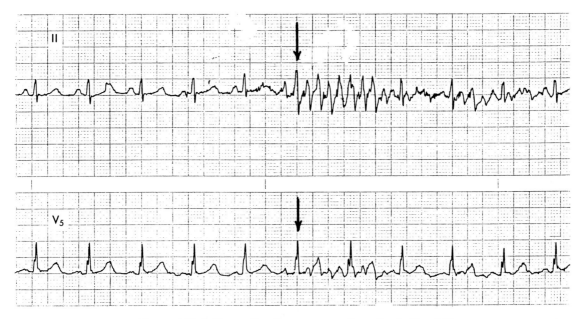

Figure 15B-24B.   Simultaneous recording of leads II and V₅ demonstrating that the normal QRS complex in lead V₅ is unaffected by the pseudotachycardia in lead II.

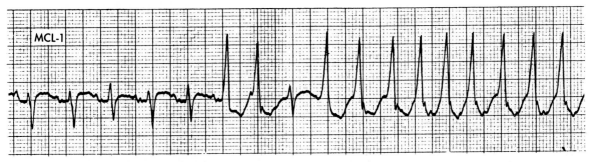

Figure 15B-25A.   *Ventricular tachycardia?* How certain are you of your diagnosis?

PROBLEM   *FIGURE 15B-26: How do you explain the QRS widening in this tracing?*

ANSWER TO FIGURE 15B-26   No atrial activity is evident in this 12-lead tracing, and the rhythm is irregularly irregular. This suggests atrial fibrillation as the underlying rhythm (in this case with a fairly rapid ventricular response). QRS widening would then be the result of preexisting RBBB and left anterior hemiblock.

Morphologic assessment of the QRS complex in leads V₁ and V₆ is consistent with a supraventricular etiology, although admittedly the QR pattern in lead V₁ and RS pattern in V₆ could *also* be the result of ventricular tachycardia. However, the degree of irregularity in the lead V₁ rhythm strip at the bottom of the tracing is more than one would usually expect with ventricular tachycardia, and is much more consistent with atrial fibrillation. Availability of a prior ECG with a similar pattern of QRS widening would be invaluable in confirming the impression of atrial fibrillation with preexisting bundle branch block.

PROBLEM   The patient whose rhythm is shown in *Figure 15B-27A* was treated with verapamil for presumed PSVT. *Would you have done the same?* (The patient was alert and hemodynamically stable at the time the tracing was recorded.)

ANSWER TO FIGURE 15B-27A   All one can say from Fig. 15B-27A is that there is a regular tachyarrhythmia at a rate of 170 beats/minute. Although the QRS complex in this one monitoring lead does not appear to be widened, a portion of it could conceivably lie on the baseline. Analysis of QRS morphology is not of much as-

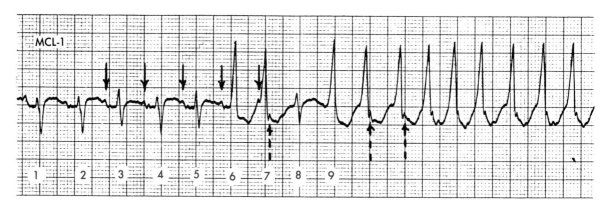

Figure 15B-25B.   Close analysis of the R-R baseline between the two beats of the anomalous couplet (beats #6-7) demonstrates AV dissociation (solid arrows). Broken arrows most likely reflect *retrograde* atrial conduction during the run of anomalous tachycardia.

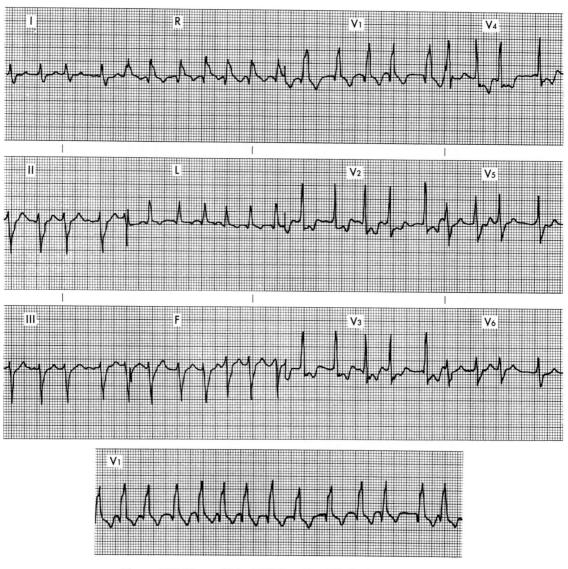

Figure 15B-26.   12-lead ECG and lead V₁ rhythm strip demonstrating an irregular wide complex tachycardia. *How do you explain the QRS widening?*

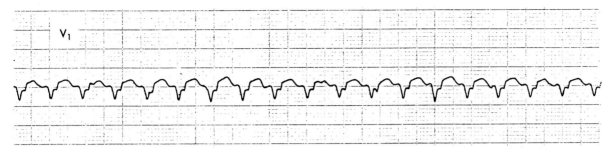

Figure 15B-27A. Lead V₁ rhythm strip. This hemodynamically stable patient was treated with verapamil. *Would you have done the same?*

sistance since it is hard to determine which of the four patterns shown in Fig. 15A-16 most closely resembles the QRS complex in this tracing.

Very subtle, tiny amplitude deflections are intermittently seen at various points of the cardiac cycle (for example, notching the early portion of the T wave of the 3ʳᵈ and 10ᵗʰ beats). Unfortunately, the relationship of these deflections (if any) to the QRS complex is unclear, and the clinical significance of this finding (retrograde atrial conduction? AV dissociation? artifact?) is open to conjecture.

PROBLEM **FIGURE 15B-27B is the 12-lead ECG of this patient. *Does it alter your opinion in any way?* (Does the fact that the patient was *alert* and *hemodynamically stable* at the time the tracing was recorded have any bearing on your answer?)**

ANSWER TO FIGURE 15B-27B Figure 15B-27B is the 12-lead ECG of a patient in *sustained ventricular tachycardia!* Normal atrial activity is absent, the QRS complex is markedly widened (in virtually all leads *except* V₁), and

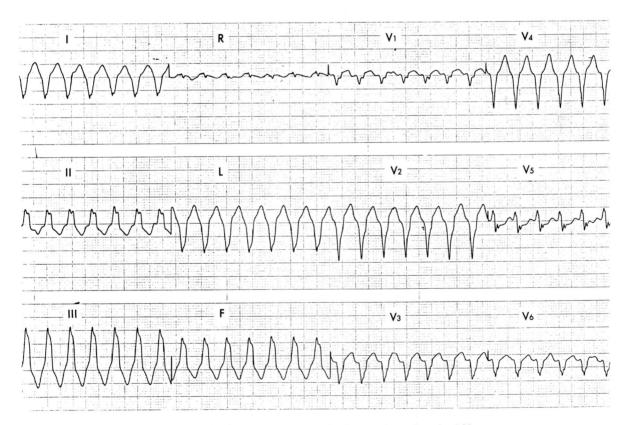

Figure 15B-27B. 12-lead ECG of the patient whose lead V₁ rhythm strip was shown in Fig. 15B-27A. *Does this alter your interpretation of the rhythm shown in Fig. 15B-27A?* (Does the fact that the patient was alert and hemodynamically stable have any bearing on your answer?)

Table 15B-2

Key Clinical Points in the Diagnosis of Ventricular Tachycardia

1. The width of the QRS complex may appear *deceptively narrow* if only one monitoring lead is used to view the arrhythmia.

2. Whenever doubt exists about the etiology of a tachyarrhythmia (in a patient who is hemodynamically stable), *immediately* obtain a 12-lead tracing *if at all possible!*

3. Once established that the QRS complex is wide, remember the *differential diagnosis* for a **regular wide complex tachycardia** in the absence of well-defined atrial activity:

    i. Ventricular tachycardia
    ii. VENTRICULAR TACHYCARDIA
    iii. **VENTRICULAR TACHYCARDIA**
    iv. Supraventricular tachycardia (SVT) with aberration
    v. SVT with preexisting bundle branch block

    Ventricular tachycardia *MUST* always be assumed until proven otherwise.

4. Hemodynamic status is *not* a reliable indicator of the etiology of an arrhythmia. Patients may remain alert for minutes, hours, or even *days* and maintain a normal (or even elevated) blood pressure *despite* the presence (and persistance) of ventricular tachycardia.

5. Verapamil should *never* be administered as a diagnostic/therapeutic "trial" in patients with a wide complex tachycardia of unknown etiology.

6. Assessment of QRS morphology (as suggested in Figs. 15A-14 and 15A-16), and attention to the nonmorphologic features included in Table 15B-1 may be extremely helpful in determining the probable etiology of a tachyarrhythmia.

7. Availability of prior 12-lead ECGs and/or rhythm strips on the patient may prove invaluable (as *comparison* tracings) by revealing the true configuration of normally conducted and/or ventricular ectopic beats.

8. Follow-up 12-lead ECGs and/or rhythm strips obtained on the patient *after* conversion to normal sinus rhythm may prove equally invaluable and sometimes allow definitive diagnosis of the tachyarrhythmia to be made *in retrospect*.

9. Ventricular tachycardia is a much more common cause of a wide complex tachycardia of unknown etiology than SVT with either aberration or preexisting bundle branch block—especially in older patients who have underlying heart disease.

10. *Always assume ventricular tachycardia until proven otherwise.*

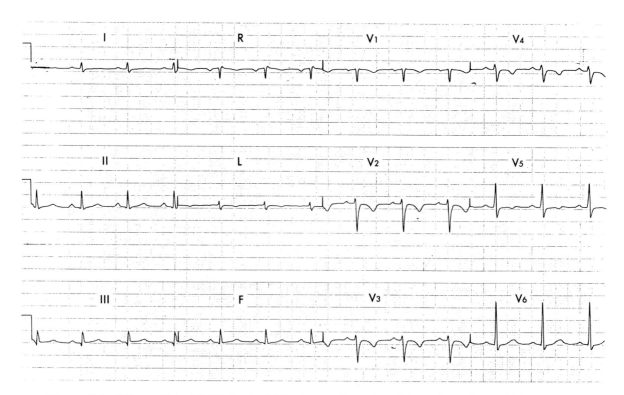

Figure 15B-27C.   12-lead ECG obtained following cardioversion of the patient whose initial tracing was shown in Fig. 15B-27B.

morphologic clues strongly suggestive of the diagnosis are present (i.e., almost totally negative complex in lead V_6, bizarre frontal plane axis).

This case illustrates a number of key points about the diagnosis of ventricular tachycardia. For clarity, we summarize these points in *Table 15B-2*. Interestingly, the patient remained alert and hemodynamically stable for more than 20 minutes *despite* persistence of the tachyarrhythmia. PSVT was initially diagnosed from an MCL_1 monitoring lead (in which the arrhythmia looked very similar to the tracing shown in Fig. 15B-27A). As a result, he was given IV verapamil. Shortly thereafter, his blood pressure dropped and he almost decompensated. Fortunately, the correct diagnosis was finally realized (from the 12-lead ECG shown in Fig. 15B-27B), and the patient was cardioverted. His 12-lead ECG following synchronized cardioversion is shown in *Figure 15B-27C*.

Verapamil should *never* be administered indiscriminately as a diagnostic/therapeutic "trial" to a patient with a regular wide complex tachycardia of unknown etiology. Although the drug may well convert the rhythm if it is supraventricular (SVT with either aberration or preexisting bundle branch block), potentially disastrous consequences are likely if this is not the case (Stewart, 1986; Buxton et al, 1987; Levitt, 1988). That is, if the tachyarrhythmia turns out to be ventricular, there is a significant chance that the vasodilatory and negative inotropic effect of this calcium channel blocking agent will precipitate acute decompensation (i.e., ventricular fibrillation).

The ***postconversion tracing*** of this patient is insightful and confirms beyond doubt that the rhythm in Fig. 15B-27B was ventricular tachycardia. With the return of normal sinus P waves, it is clear that the "true" QRS complex is narrow, upright in lead V_6 (as it should be), and the frontal plane axis is normal. In addition, symmetric T wave inversion in leads V_1 through V_5 suggest ischemia, which may have contributed to (and/or been the result of) the episode of ventricular tachycardia.

PROBLEM   *FIGURE 15B-28: Ventricular tachycardia?* **(The patient is alert and hemodynamically stable.)**

ANSWER TO FIGURE 15B-28   There is a regular, wide complex tachycardia at a rate of 155 beats/min. Atrial activity is absent. Although morphologic assessment of the QRS complex in lead V_1 is of little help (the slurred monophasic R wave of this complex lacks a definitive "rabbit ear"), the almost totally negative rS complex in lead V_6, in conjunction with the **bizarre** (markedly leftward) **frontal plane** axis strongly suggest *ventricular tachycardia* as the diagnosis. The patient's stable hemodynamic status should *not* alter this impression. *Ventricular tachycardia must be assumed (and the patient treated accordingly) until proven otherwise.*

PROBLEM   *FIGURE 15B-29A:* **This 12-lead ECG was obtained from a patient known to have complete LBBB. In view of this history, it was felt that the ECG shown here (Fig. 15B-29A) represented sinus tachycardia with preexisting LBBB.** *Do you agree?*

ANSWER TO FIGURE 15B-29A   A regular, wide complex tachycardia at a rate of 125 beats/min is seen on this tracing. Definite atrial activity is absent. Although the

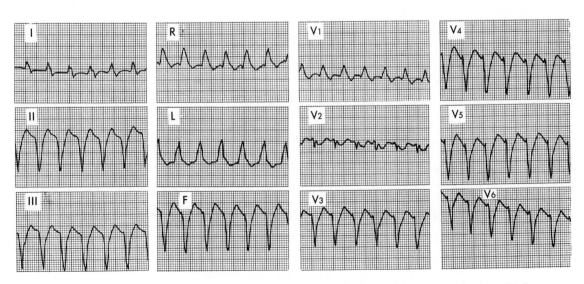

Figure 15B-28.   *Ventricular tachycardia?* (The patient is alert and hemodynamically stable.)

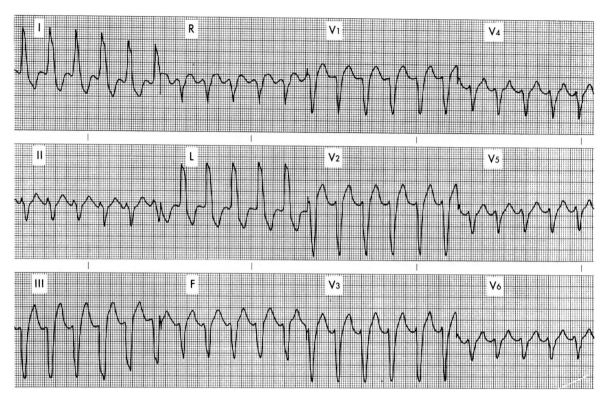

Figure 15B-29A. 12-lead ECG from a patient known to have complete LBBB. With this history in mind, *is there any cause for concern?*

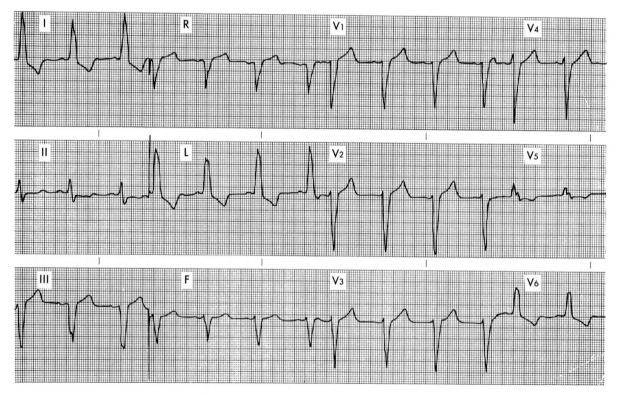

Figure 15B-29B. Follow-up 12-lead ECG obtained after cardioversion of the patient whose initial tracing was shown in Fig. 15B-29A.

ECG superficially resembles LBBB, QRS morphology in the precordial leads is *not* typical for this conduction disturbance for two reasons:

   i. The QRS complex is predominantly negative in lead V_6.

   ii. There is **concordance** (*global negativity* in this case) of the *direction* of QRS complexes in the precordial leads.

These findings strongly suggest that the patient is in *ventricular tachycardia*. This patient remained in ventricular tachycardia for *more than a day* before it was finally realized that his wide complex tachycardia was not the result of an old LBBB. Following synchronized cardioversion, the ECG shown in *Figure 15B-29B* was obtained.

Note that resumption of sinus rhythm in Fig. 15B-29B is marked by the return of normal atrial activity (i.e., an upright P wave in lead II) and the more "usual" morphologic pattern of LBBB in which a monophasic (upright) R wave is seen in *all* lateral leads.

> QRS concordance is one of the less commonly occurring non-morphologic diagnostic signs that may occasionally prove extremely helpful in differentiating between ventricular tachycardia and SVT (with either aberration or preexisting bundle branch block). As we indicated in Table 15B-1 at the beginning of this section, the finding of **QRS concordance** (with *either* global positivity *or* global negativity of QRS complexes in *all* six precordial leads) is virtually diagnostic of ventricular tachycardia. Awareness of this finding (and awareness of the fact that lead V_6 will almost always manifest a significant amount of positivity) could (should) have alerted the health care team much sooner that the patient in Fig. 15B-29A was in sustained ventricular tachycardia.

> ### Ventricular Tachycardia—*Almost a "Telephone Diagnosis"*
>
> REMEMBER—*Ventricular tachycardia* is by far the most common cause of a regular wide complex tachycardia—*regardless* of whether the patient is awake or not—and *regardless* of whether the patient has been in the rhythm for minutes, hours, or longer (Steinman et al, 1989). Statistically, in an adult (middle-aged or older) who has a history of documented cardiac disease (angina pectoris, prior myocardial infarction, and/or heart failure), the chance of a regular wide complex tachycardia of unknown etiology being ventricular tachycardia approaches 90% (Baerman et al, 1987; Akhtar et al, 1988; Steinman et al, 1989)—*so much so*—that one could almost make a **"telephone diagnosis."** That is, if you are told that an adult with a history of underlying heart disease presents in a hemodynamically stable, regular wide complex tachycardia of unknown etiology— you could guess (*sight unseen!*) that the patient was in ventricular tachycardia (i.e., make a "telephone diagnosis")—and be correct approximately 90% of the time!

The key principles for distinguishing between ventricular ectopy/tachycardia and aberrancy have been covered. Figs. 15A-14 and 15A-16A, Tables 15B-1 and 15B-2 remain as readily available reference material. *Mastery is attainable with continued practice.**

For those with an interest (and a true love of the topic), we have added a final section on aberrancy (Section C) with a few final pearls, and a few final challenge tracings.

---

*Use of a **12-lead ECG** is an invaluable part of the diagnostic process that can't be overemphasized. For *hemodynamically stable* patients who present with a wide complex tachycardia, obtaining a 12-lead ECG allows:

   1. Use of **morphologic criteria** (as discussed for leads V_1 and V_6)

   2. Optimal opportunity for finding P waves/AV dissociation (**"12 leads are better than one"**)

   3. Determination of mean QRS **axis** in the frontal plane (with VT being strongly suggested by the finding of either *marked* left or right axis deviation)

   4. Simultaneous lead comparison (for clarification of QRS width/appearance)

   5. Documentation (for later comparison) of the patient's rhythm *during* the tachycardia, **and**

   6. **A moment for you to reflect** (i.e., "stall") while you ponder the diagnostic possibilities (*and during which you may be blessed by spontaneous conversion to sinus rhythm*).

SECTION C

PVCS vs ABERRANCY: A FINAL CONCEPT & A FEW FINAL CHALLENGES

If you have followed the contents of Sections A and B in this chapter, this final section should be fun. A word of forewarning: *Many of these tracings contain much more than initially meets the eye!*

   i. *How many of the subtle findings can you identify?*
   ii. How *sure* are you of whether the anomalous complexes are ventricular or aberrantly conducted?

We suggest you reserve sufficient time to *carefully* go over each arrhythmia and *write out* your diagnosis (as well as the *degree of certainty* you have in this diagnosis) *before* looking at our answers. We begin with a final concept . . . .

PROBLEM   ***FIGURE 15C-1:* Do beats #3-18 in this rhythm strip represent a run of ventricular tachycardia?**

ANSWER TO FIGURE 15C-1   If one did not see the beginning and end of this run, it would be exceedingly difficult to rule out ventricular tachycardia because the QRS complex is wide and definite atrial activity is not seen between beats #4-18. Fortunately, readily detectable P waves (with a normal PR interval) precede beats #1, #2, #3, and #19. Thus Fig. 15C-1 begins and ends with

normal sinus rhythm, and the reason for the QRS widening is a preexisting bundle branch block. Since the QRS morphology during the run is very similar to its morphology during the sinus conducted beats, the tachyarrhythmia that begins with beat #3 is most likely to be *supraventricular* (although ideally we would like to see additional leads to be sure). The irregularity of the tachyarrhythmia (beats #4-18) suggests that this run most likely represents an episode of *paroxysmal atrial fibrillation.*

PROBLEM   **A short while following treatment with digoxin, the ECG shown in *Figure 15C-2A* was recorded from this patient. *What has happened?* Has the reason for the QRS widening in Fig. 15C-1 become more evident?**

ANSWER TO FIGURE 15C-2A   Digoxin has succeeded in converting the patient to normal sinus rhythm (with the exception of beat #5, which is either a PAC or a PJC). Of particular interest is the fact that the QRS complex is wide for beats #2-5, but of *normal duration* for beats #1 and #6-9!

Fig. 15C-2A illustrates the phenomenon known as **rate-dependent** *bundle branch block (BBB).* Under certain con-

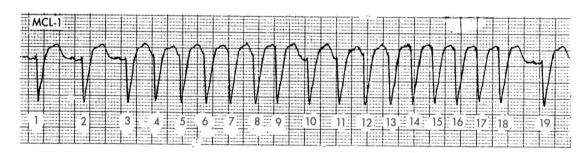

Figure 15C-1.   *Do beats #3-18 represent a run of ventricular tachycardia?*

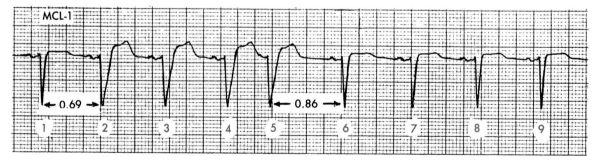

Figure 15C-2A.   Follow-up tracing to Fig. 15C-1 obtained after this patient was treated with digoxin.

ditions the refractory period (RP) of one of the bundle branches may become pathologically prolonged. If the heart rate then accelerates to a point where the cycle length (the R-R interval between two successive beats) *becomes less* than the RP of the diseased bundle branch, a rate-dependent BBB will develop and persist until the heart rate slows down enough for normal conduction to occur.

Thus for the case shown in Figure 15C-2A, a left bundle branch block (LBBB) pattern of aberrancy develops with beat #2 because of cycle length shortening between beats #1-2 (which demonstrate an R-R interval of 0.69 second). Normal conduction does not resume until beat #6. The pause following premature beat #5 allows the extra time needed for the left bundle branch to recover and conduct normally. Retrospectively in the context of Fig. 15C-2A, the QRS widening in Fig. 15C-1 may simply be the result of the cycle length shortening that is maintained throughout this rhythm strip.

That rate-dependent BBB does *not* always come and go at some precise cycle length is evident from Fig. 15C-2A, since normal conduction persists for beats #6-9 *despite* the fact that the R-R interval of these last few beats is as short as it was when the LBBB aberration developed at the beginning of the rhythm strip.

Although rate-dependent BBB is not a common form of aberration, the importance of recognizing it is obvious from inspection of *Figure 15C-2B*, recorded a little later from this same patient. Without knowledge of this patient's tendency to conduct with LBBB aberration at faster rates, it would be all too easy to misdiagnose beats #4-6 and #9-11 in Fig. 15C-2B as salvos of ventricular tachycardia.

Although admittedly, assessment of QRS morphology when anomalous beats are negative in lead V_1 is far from perfect, the very slender initial r wave, and almost vertically descending S wave of beats #4-6 and #9-11 in Figure 15C-2B is at least consistent with a supraventricular etiology (most closely resembling pattern **N** in Fig. 15A-16).

PROBLEM   *FIGURE 15C-3:* Interpret the arrhythmia. *Can you explain why QRS morphology changes throughout the rhythm strip?*

(HINT: What happens to the *cycling length* throughout the rhythm strip?)

Before formulating your answer for this arrhythmia (and the other arrhythmias to follow), it may be helpful to keep in mind the following principle:

The easiest diagnostic approach to complex arrhythmias is to:
  i. First determine the *underlying rhythm* (if there is one)
              and
  ii. Interpret those parts of the tracing that are *easiest* to interpret
                    before
  iii. Interpreting the *more difficult* part

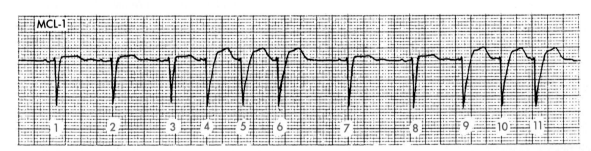

Figure 15C-2B.   Rhythm strip obtained later from this same patient. Without knowledge of this patient's tendency to conduct with LBBB aberration, it would be easy to misdiagnose beats #4-6 and #9-11 as salvos of ventricular tachycardia.

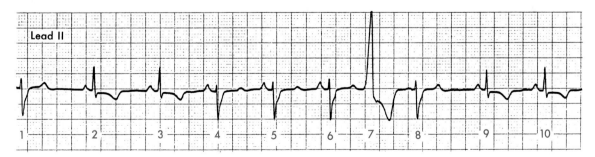

Figure 15C-3.   *Why does QRS morphology change throughout this rhythm strip?*

ANSWER TO FIGURE 15C-3   The *underlying rhythm* is sinus, as beats #2 and #3 are narrow and preceded by an upright P wave with a constant (and normal) PR interval in this lead II monitoring lead.

The *easiest* beat to interpret is #7—which is obviously a PVC. It is wide, bizarre in shape, and dramatically different in configuration from *all* other beats in the tracing.

> The small amplitude upright deflection preceding beat #7 is *not* a P wave. Instead, it is simply the T wave of beat #6.

The *more difficult* aspect of the tracing to interpret is the reason for the change in QRS morphology for beats #4-6 and #8. Although QRS morphology changes (from an Rs complex for beats #2 and #3, to an rS complex for beats #4-6 and #8) each beat continues to be preceded by a similar-appearing P wave with the same PR interval. This suggests that a normal sinus mechanism is still operative. Taking the HINT given above provides the answer: *cycle length shortens after beat #3!* Thus, beats #4-6 exhibit a *rate-related* conduction defect (in this case, aberrant conduction with a LAHB configuration).

> It is not clear what beat #8 is. No definite P wave precedes it, suggesting it is either a junctional beat or a sinus-conducted beat whose preceding P wave is buried in the T wave of the PVC, and for which retrograde concealed conduction from the PVC greatly prolonged the PR interval. This beat is clearly the *most difficult* part of the tracing to interpret. What *can* be said is that regardless of its etiology, the short coupling interval preceding it (the R-R interval between beats #7-8) explains why it too conducts with LAHB aberration.

Note that normal conduction resumes with beat #9 as the rate slows (i.e., the cycle length increases) toward the end of the rhythm strip.

> A final subtle (but important) finding on this tracing is the change in T wave morphology. During normal conduction (i.e., for beats #2, #3, #9, and #10), the T wave is symmetrically inverted in this inferior lead, suggesting *ischemia*. T wave inversion is *masked* for those sinus beats that conduct with LAHB aberration!

PROBLEM   ***FIGURE 15C-4A: PVC or PAC conducted with aberration?***

ANSWER TO FIGURE 15C-4A   This tracing is a good example of the difficulty that may be encountered

when the QRS complex of normally conducted beats is wide. Here the underlying rhythm is sinus with bundle branch block. The 5th beat occurs early. It is definitely different, and almost looks "more normal" than the other sinus-conducted beats. However, despite its relatively benign appearance, there is ample evidence on the tracing that this 5th beat is a PVC.

Confirmation of the ventricular ectopic origin of this beat is forthcoming from *Figure 15C-4B*, which demonstrates simultaneous recording of leads V_1, II, and V_6. It is clear from inspection of leads II and V_6 that the QRS complex is significantly widened and dramatically different in configuration from the normally conducted beats. Arrows in the upper panel (V_1 lead) of Fig. 15C-4B demonstrate persistence of regular atrial activity *throughout* the rhythm strip. Thus, the P wave preceding the 5th beat is *not* premature. Instead, it manifests a PR interval that is clearly *too short* to conduct, virtually proving its ventricular etiology.

The presence of preexisting bundle branch block often complicates the process of differentiating between ventricular ectopy and aberration. Despite resemblance of the 5th beat in Fig. 15C-4A to the normally conducted beats, the first key clue to its true etiology lies in the fact that even in the V_1 monitoring lead, this beat *is different*. The second key clue is that the atrial rate remains regular, so that the P wave preceding the 5th beat is *not* premature (and manifests a PR interval too short to conduct). Once additional leads are obtained (i.e., the simultaneous lead recording shown in Fig. 15C-4B) the case can be closed.

> Note that although QRS morphology of the 5th beat manifests an RS pattern with a fat initial R wave in a right-sided lead (similar to complex **P** in Fig. 15A-16), caution must be advised against depending on morphologic clues in the presence of preexisting QRS widening.

PROBLEM   ***FIGURE 15C-5: PVCs? Aberrant? Some of each?***

ANSWER TO FIGURE 15C-5   The underlying rhythm is sinus tachycardia at 135-140 beats/min. There are three "unusual" beats—#3, #10, and #15. Beat #15 is definitely a PVC. It is markedly widened and very different in configuration than the normally conducted beats.

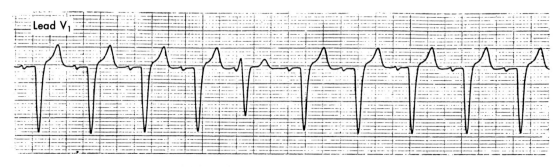

Figure 15C-4A.   *PVC or PAC conducted with aberration?*

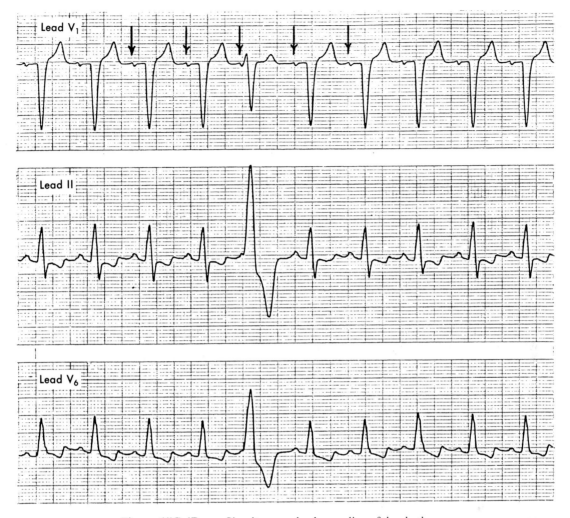

Figure 15C-4B. Simultaneous lead recording of the rhythm strip shown in Fig. 15C-4A. Arrows in the V₁ lead demonstrate regularity of the atrial rhythm. Despite the relatively benign appearance of the 5th beat in this lead, leads II and V₆ demonstrate how different this beat actually is compared to the normally conducted beats.

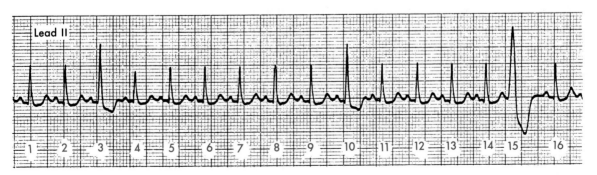

Figure 15C-5. *Are beats #3, #10, and #15 PVCs or aberrantly conducted PACs?*

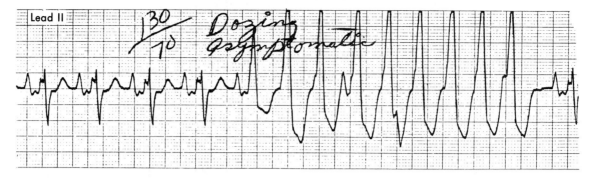

Figure 15C-6A.   Do the anomalous beats represent a run of ventricular tachycardia or SVT with aberrant conduction? *How certain are you of your diagnosis?*

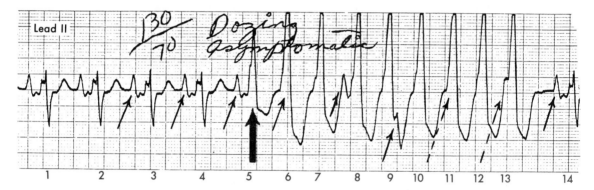

Figure 15C-6B.   Slanted slender arrows indicate persistence of regular atrial activity throughout the rhythm strip. Beat #5 (heavy solid arrow) is a fusion beat.

Close inspection suggests that the normally conducted beats begin with an ever so small negative initial deflection (a "micro q" wave). If so, the initial positive deflection of the PVC (which manifests a monophasic R wave configuration) is *oppositely* directed to that of the normally conducted beats. However, even if you question the existence of an initial negative deflection for the normally conducted beats, assessment of the initial deflection is still suggestive of ventricular ectopy because its *slope* is different (slower rising) for the PVC!

Beats #3 and #10 appear to be very similar in morphology to the normally conducted beats, but they are taller. Imagining a "marriage" between beats #14 and #15, the "children" might well be expected to look like beats #3 and #10. Comparison of T wave morphology between the PVC and the normally conducted beats provides further support that beats #3 and #10 represent an intermediate form and are **fusion beats.** The fact that the PR interval preceding each of these fusion beats is so close to the normal PR interval explains why beats #3 and #10 look more "normal" than ectopic.

PROBLEM   *FIGURE 15C-6A:* **Ventricular tachycardia? or a run of SVT with aberrant conduction?** *How certain are you of your diagnosis?*

ANSWER TO FIGURE 15C-6A   The first four beats are sinus at a rate of about 80 beats/min. As indi-

cated on the rhythm strip, the patient is hemodynamically stable (with a blood pressure of 130/70 mm Hg) and is "dozing" and "asymptomatic." No matter. The run of anomalous beats is *definitely* ventricular tachycardia!

Reasons for our certainty in making this diagnosis are evident on *Figure 15C-6B*. The slender, slanted arrows demonstrate persistence of regular atrial activity throughout the rhythm strip. Thus, there is *AV dissociation* since atrial activity is unrelated to anomalous beats #6-13. Anomalous beats are significantly widened, bizarre in shape, and very different in appearance from the normally conducted beats. Although they manifest a similarly *directed* initial deflection, the *shape* of this initial deflection is otherwise different than the notched initial deflection of the normally conducted beats. Finally, beat #5 (highlighted by the heavy solid arrow) is a fusion beat (the product of a "marriage" between beats #4 and #6). The combination of these factors overwhelmingly incriminates ventricular tachycardia as the etiology of the arrhythmia. Following a brief (post-ectopic) pause, normal sinus rhythm resumes with beat #14.

PROBLEM   *FIGURE 15C-7A:* **Interpret the arrhythmia. Are the anomalous beats PVCs or aberrant?** *How certain are you of your diagnosis?*

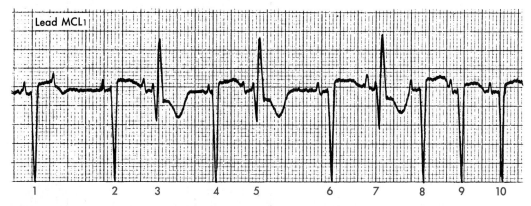

Figure 15C-7A.   Are the anomalous beats (i.e., #3, #5, and #7) PVCs or aberrant? *How certain are you of your answer?*

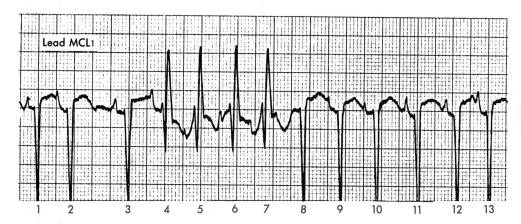

Figure 15C-7B.   Rhythm recorded a short while later from the same patient presented in Fig. 15C-7A. Should the run of anomalous beats (#4-7) be treated with lidocaine?

ANSWER TO FIGURE 15C-7A   A lot is happening. The underlying rhythm appears to be sinus, as suggested by beats #1, #2, #6, and #8. The rhythm is also irregular and marked by a brief pause (between beats #1 and #2), several anomalous beats (#3, #5, and #7), and a short run of tachycardia (beats #8-10). A single, underlying "theme" can explain *all* of these abnormalities!

Note first that the T wave of beat #1 is "spiked." This spike represents a PAC. Because this PAC occurs so early in the repolarization process, it is "blocked" (which explains the brief pause between beats #1 and #2).

The T waves of beats #2, #4, and #6 are also spiked. Each of these spikes is again the result of a PAC. Because they occur at a later point in the repolarization process (i.e., the coupling interval of each of these PACs is *longer* than the coupling interval of the first PAC that was blocked), each of these PACs *is* conducted, but with aberration. Thus beats #3, #5, and #7 each manifest the typical rSR' pattern of RBBB aberration in this right-sided lead. The PR interval preceding beat #4 measures only 0.07 second, which is significantly less than the PR interval of the sinus conducted beats. This supraventricular beat either arises from the AV node or from elsewhere in the atrium.

It is impossible to tell for sure from Fig. 15C-7A what the underlying sinus rate is. As a result, it is impossible to know if beats #9 and #10 are also PACs (that are conducted normally), or if they reflect an underlying sinus tachycardia. Regardless, it is safe to say that the underlying rhythm here is sinus, and that there are very frequent PACs—some of which are blocked, and others which are conducted with aberration. *Our degree of confidence in this diagnosis?*—virtually 100%!

PROBLEM   **A short while later, the rhythm shown in *Figure 15C-7B* was observed in this patient. Should this run of anomalous beats be treated with lidocaine? *How certain are you of your answer?***

ANSWER TO FIGURE 15C-7B   No! The underlying rhythm is sinus tachycardia. P wave morphology during the normally conducted beats does change slightly from beat to beat, suggesting that they may be PACs (and/or MAT). The run of anomalous beats is *definitely* supraventricular in origin with aberrant conduction. We know this (with 100% certainty) because QRS morphology is identical to that of the anomalous beats in Fig. 15C-7A (it manifests a typical rSR' pattern), the run is preceded by a premature P wave (which notches the T wave of beat

#3), and the Ashman phenomenon is present (the first "funny-looking" beat follows the longest pause). Not only would lidocaine *not* be helpful (since this drug is ineffective for SVT), but it might make matters worse because of its potential to further accelerate supraventricular rhythms.

PROBLEM   *FIGURE 15C-8: Are beats #2 and #4 PVCs or aberrant? Is there evidence of atrial activity associated with these beats?*

ANSWER TO FIGURE 15C-8   Beats #2 and #4 are *almost certainly* PVCs. Although they superficially resemble the normally conducted complexes in this tracing, these beats are definitely widened, and *not* preceded by a premature P wave. Moreover, despite their predominant negativity, close scrutiny reveals an initial deflection that is both oppositely directed *and* different in shape than that of the sinus-conducted complexes. That is, the initial deflection of beats #2 and #4 is downward (negative) and slightly rounded (most like that of complex **Q** in Fig. 15A-16), whereas the sinus conducted beats manifest a tiny initial positive (r wave) deflection with an almost vertically descending S wave.

Atrial activity *is* associated with each of these PVCs. It manifests as a notching in the T wave of beats #2 and #4, and probably reflects *retrograde* conduction from the PVC back to the atria.

> This is an excellent example of how closely right ventricular PVCs may resemble the normally conducted beats. Special attention focused on characteristics of the initial deflection is often essential to detect subtle differences in morphologic appearance between right ventricular PVCs and normally conducted beats.

PROBLEM   *FIGURE 15C-9A: The arrows in lead II of this 12-lead ECG indicate normal (upright) atrial activity, and prove that the rhythm is supraventricular Or do they???*

HINT (actually, a *"red herring"*): *Is there evidence of atrial activity elsewhere on this tracing?*

ANSWER TO FIGURE 15C-9A   If you interpreted the upright deflections highlighted by the arrows in lead II as normal (sinus conducted) atrial activity:

  i. You may be afflicted with the *"P preoccupation"* syndrome, and/or . . . .
  ii. You forgot the differential diagnosis of a regular, wide complex tachycardia.

The advantage of three-channel ECG machines is their ability to display the simultaneous recording of three leads at a time. Admittedly, if *only* lead II was viewed in Fig. 15C-9A, the small upright deflections highlighted by the arrows might well be mistaken for normal sinus P waves. *Figure 15C-9B* demonstrates that this is definitely *not* the case. Timelines in this tracing indicate that these small initial positive deflections in lead II are actually a part of the QRS complex (and *not* P waves!). Similarly, the "pseudoatrial activity" in leads aVF and V**6** of Fig. 15C-9A are also part of the QRS complex.

> The **P-Preoccupation Syndrome** is an *acquired* syndrome associated with a state of mind in which the affected individual—when faced with an arrhythmia—becomes obsessed with placement of undue emphasis on the pursuit and identification of P waves where there are none—and once "found" (or *thinking* that P waves have been found), attributes undue diagnostic value to them *(adapted from personal communication with Dr. HJL Marriott)*. The beauty of simultaneous lead recordings such as the one shown in Fig. 15C-9B is that unclaimed undulations in the ECG baseline can be assessed in other leads to determine if they are real or just artifactual (and if they are real, what their significance is likely to be).

Returning to the 12-lead ECG shown in Fig. 15C-9A, the first step in evaluation should be recognition of the presence of a **regular, wide complex tachycardia** *without* definite atrial activity. The differential diagnosis includes five entities—*the first three of which are:*

  i. Ventricular tachycardia
  ii. VENTRICULAR TACHYCARDIA
  iii. **VENTRICULAR TACHYCARDIA**

The diagnosis of ventricular tachycardia is overwhelmingly supported by marked QRS widening (to at least 0.16

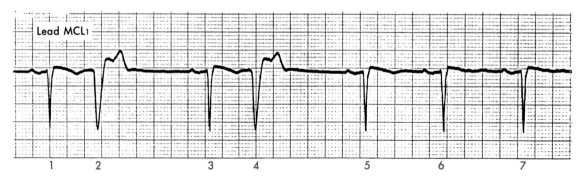

Figure 15C-8.   *Are beats #2 and #4 PVCs or aberrant?*

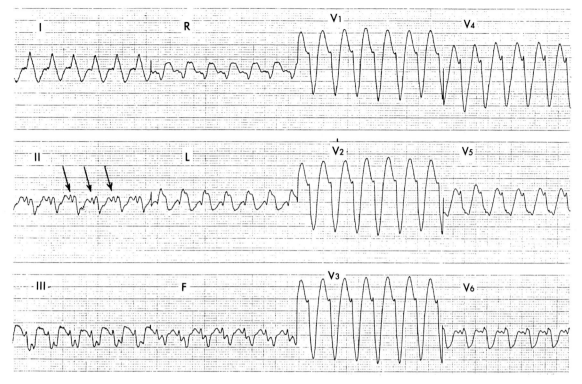

Figure 15C-9A. 12-lead ECG from a patient in a wide complex tachycardia. The arrows in lead II indicate normal (sinus conducted) atrial activity. *Or do they?*

second), an unusual (markedly leftward) frontal plane axis, QRS morphology (delayed descent of the S wave in lead V_1 and predominant negativity in lead V_6), and QRS concordance *(global negativity)* in the precordial leads.

PROBLEM **The patient whose 12-lead ECG is shown in *Figure 15C-10* is a 60-year-old woman who was admitted for severe, new-onset chest pain. At the time this tracing was recorded, she was alert, and had a blood pressure of 100/70 mm Hg. *What is the rhythm?* Clinically, what is going on with the patient?**

(HINT: *What are the arrows pointing to?*)

ANSWER TO FIGURE 15C-10 The overall rhythm is rapid (about 150 beats/min) and appears to be fairly regular, although QRS morphology is somewhat variable. The underlying (i.e., predominant) rhythm is characterized by a widened QRS complex without definite evidence of atrial activity. Thus, there is a regular, wide complex tachycardia—which once again means that *ventricular tachycardia must be assumed until proven otherwise.* Definitive evidence in favor of this presumption is present on this 12-lead tracing, and includes the unusual (markedly leftward) frontal plane axis of the widened beats, their QRS morphology (fat initial r wave in lead V_1, total negativity in lead V_6), QRS concordance of the widened beats *(global negativity)* in the precordial leads, fusion beats, and

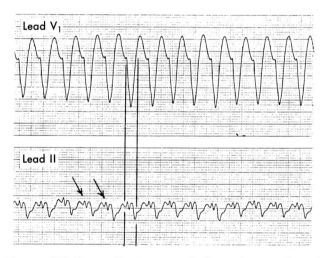

Figure 15C-9B. Simultaneous rhythm strip recording of leads V_1 and II from Fig. 15C-9A. Timelines indicate that the initial positive deflections in lead II (highlighted by the arrows) are *not* P waves, but instead make up the initial portion of the QRS complex.

one more sign that we have not yet discussed—**capture beats** (see Table 15B-1).

The importance of AV dissociation as a diagnostic clue to the presence of ventricular tachycardia has already been emphasized. Occasionally, if the timing of atrial activity is just right, some of the regularly occurring P waves may arrive at the AV node at precisely the moment when it is no longer

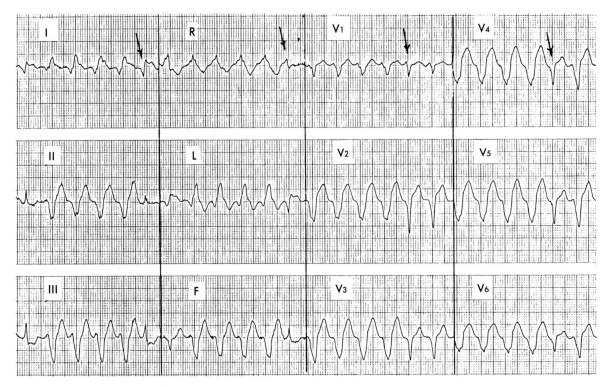

Figure 15C-10.   12-lead ECG from a 60-year-old woman complaining of new-onset chest pain. *What is the rhythm?* What are the arrows pointing to?

refractory from the retrograde conduction of the ventricular tachycardia. If this occurs, atrial impulses may "slip through" and be conducted to (i.e., "*capture*") the ventricles, producing normal (narrow) QRS complexes. These sinus conducted beats that are able to slip through and interrupt the run of an anomalous tachycardia are known as *capture beats*, and their presence virtually *proves* that the anomalous tachycardia is ventricular in origin.

The capture beats in Fig. 15C-10 are the narrow complexes denoted by the arrows. Although exceedingly subtle, the P waves producing the capture beats in leads I and V₁ appear to be present and hiding (notching) the terminal portion of the preceding T wave.

> It is almost impossible to evaluate the 12-lead ECG of a patient in sustained ventricular tachycardia for evidence of ischemia or acute infarction. However, because capture beats are *normally conducted complexes*, analysis of these beats may provide an invaluable clue to the occurrence of clinical events. Thus in Fig. 15C-10, the capture beats (arrows in leads I, aVR, V₁, and V₄—as well as the simultaneously occurring beats in the leads below) reveal that this patient is in the process of evolving an acute anterolateral infarction. Deep, wide Q waves and ST segment elevation is seen in the capture beats of leads I and aVL, with reciprocal ST segment depression being seen in the capture beats of the inferior leads. Furthermore, a QS complex with accompanying ST segment elevation is seen in the capture beats of leads V₂ through V₆. The last beat in this 12-lead ECG (i.e., the beat that appears *after* the arrow in lead V₄) is a *fusion beat* since it manifests an intermediate morphology between that of the sinus beat and the PVCs in this lead.

PROBLEM   *FIGURE 15C-11: Ventricular tachycardia?* **or SVT with aberration?**

ANSWER TO FIGURE 15C-11   The rhythm is a regular, wide complex tachycardia at a rate of about 200 beats/minute. Although there is periodic notching in the ST segment of certain leads and undulations in the baseline (especially in lead V₂), there is no definite atrial activity. The frontal plane axis is in "no man's land" (negative QRS complex in *both* leads I and aVF). QRS morphology in lead V₁ (which manifests an rR′ configuration similar to complex **C** in Fig. 15A-14) is not helpful in diagnosis. However, the almost totally negative rS configuration in lead V₆ (similar to **L** in Fig. 15A-14) is consistent with the other findings on this tracing (lack of atrial activity, indeterminate frontal plane axis, no compelling "reason" for aberration), and *very strongly* suggests that the rhythm is ventricular tachycardia.

PROBLEM   *FIGURE 15C-12: Ventricular tachycardia?* **or SVT with aberration?**

ANSWER TO FIGURE 15C-12   Once again, the rhythm is a regular, wide complex tachycardia. The heart rate is approximately 170 beats/minute. There is no definite evidence of atrial activity. The frontal plane axis is rightward, but not markedly so. Assessment of QRS morphology not only demonstrates a typical RBBB pattern

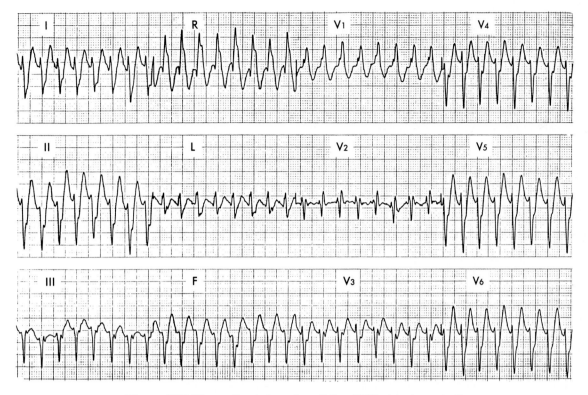

Figure 15C-11.   *Ventricular tachycardia?* or SVT with aberration?

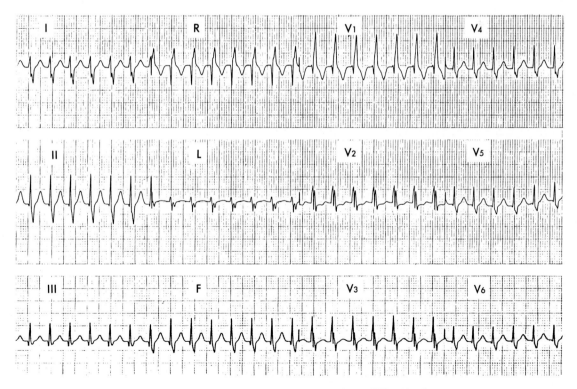

Figure 15C-12.   *Ventricular tachycardia?* or SVT with aberration?

(rSR' configuration with taller right rabbit ear) in lead V_1, but *also* demonstrates the *reciprocal* of this pattern in lead V_6 (i.e., a qRS configuration in this left-sided lead that closely resembles complex **I** in Fig. 15A-14). Thus, despite the need to always assume ventricular tachycardia until proven otherwise, morphologic features are so typical of RBBB aberration in this case that one should suspect a *supraventricular* etiology for this arrhythmia. *Our level of confidence in this diagnosis?*—about 90%!

PROBLEM **How would you proceed *clinically* at this point?**

ANSWER The answer depends on a number of factors. Clinically, the *most important* parameter to assess is the patient's hemodynamic status. If there were signs of hemodynamic instability (i.e., hypotension, depressed consciousness, chest pain, shortness of breath, etc.), *immediate synchronized cardioversion* would be indicated *regardless* of the etiology of the tachyarrhythmia.

Although hemodynamic stability would *in no way* rule out the *possibility* of ventricular tachycardia, it would at least allow time for more complete evaluation and/or a trial of medical therapy. *Search of the patient's chart for prior 12-lead tracings and/or rhythm strips may prove invaluable.* If documentation of pre-existing bundle branch block or definite aberrant conduction (with the *same* RBBB configuration) could be found, the diagnosis of a *supraventricular* tachycardia would be solidified.

Therapeutically, one might ask the patient to cough ("cough version"), try a vagal maneuver, treat with verapamil or adenosine (depending on your level of comfort that the tachycardia is supraventricular), or treat with IV procainamide (which may be effective for either VT or SVT)—all the while being ready to cardiovert *at any moment* should the patient suddenly become hemodynamically unstable.

PROBLEM *FIGURE 15C-13: Ventricular tachycardia? or SVT with aberration?*

ANSWER TO FIGURE 15C-13 There is a regular, wide complex tachycardia. The frontal plane axis is normal. Morphologic analysis of the QRS complex in lead V_1 (which manifests a monophasic R wave similar to pattern **D** in Fig. 15A-14) is of no diagnostic assistance. Although the RS complex in lead V_6 (similar to **J**) is consistent with a supraventricular etiology, it in no way rules out ventricular tachycardia.

Assessment of atrial activity poses a special problem in itself. It is hard to be sure from this 12-lead tracing if the upright deflections occurring between QRS complexes in lead II represent normal sinus P waves (in which case the rhythm would be sinus tachycardia with bundle branch block), the terminal portion of the T wave, or the combination of the T wave and P wave. A factor against the diagnosis of sinus tachycardia is the absence of any sign of atrial activity in most other leads. In particular, P waves

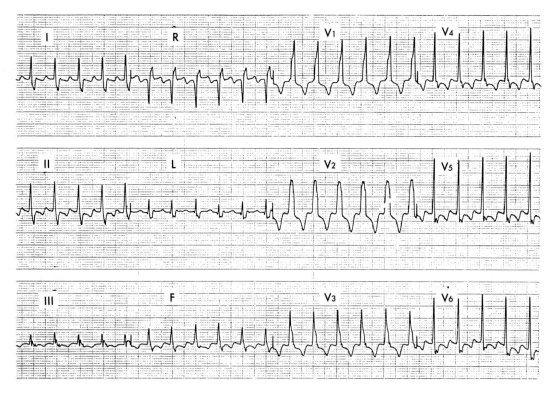

Figure 15C-13. *Ventricular tachycardia? or SVT with aberration?*

are almost always easily seen in leads V_1 and V_2. In this tracing, however, all that is seen in these leads is a deeply inverted T wave. The fact that the QT interval is so clearly prolonged in leads V_1-V_3 suggests that rather than a P wave, the upright deflections between QRS complexes in lead II make up the terminal portion of the T waves in that lead. **Bottom line—** *We don't know if P waves are present in Fig. 15C-13, and we really are not sure what the rhythm is!*

PROBLEM   **How would you proceed *clinically* at this point?**

ANSWER   In many respects, our clinical approach to this arrhythmia is similar to that suggested in our answer to Figure 15C-12:

   i. Assess the patient's hemodynamic status to determine if there is a need for *immediate* intervention (i.e., cardioversion).

   ii. If the patient is hemodynamically stable, try to obtain more information. Additional rhythm strips and/or different monitoring leads may help to determine if atrial activity is present. Comparison with previously obtained 12-lead ECGs might reveal whether QRS widening is new (and likely to be ventricular tachycardia), or whether the patient had preexisting bundle branch block.

   iii. Be aware of the diagnostic possibilities:
    —ventricular tachycardia
    —sinus tachycardia (with either bundle branch block or aberration)
    —atrial flutter (with either bundle branch block or aberration)
    —PSVT (with either bundle branch block or aberration)

   iv. Consider the therapeutic options. These might include an attempt at cough version, application of a vagal maneuver, or medical treatment with IV procainamide—all the while being ready to cardiovert *at any moment* should the patient suddenly become hemodynamically unstable. Because of a greater degree of diagnostic uncertainty (i.e., a greater possibility of ventricular tachycardia), treatment with either verapamil or adenosine would be less advisable in this case than for the patient whose rhythm was shown in Fig. 15C-12.

ACTUAL PATIENT COURSE: Review of this patient's chart revealed numerous old ECGs demonstrating sinus rhythm with RBBB conduction (of identical morphology to that shown in Fig. 15C-13)—proving a *supraventricular* etiology for the arrhythmia. As a result, a trial of IV verapamil was deemed safe—and resulted in prompt conversion to normal sinus rhythm. Alternatively—and perhaps preferentially—adenosine could have been used instead. The point to emphasize from this example, however, is that *definitive diagnosis was NOT possible from examination of the arrhythmia shown in Fig. 15C-13 alone!*

PROBLEM   ***FIGURE 15C-14A:* Ventricular tachycardia, SVT with aberration, *or neither???* (With what degree of certainty would you make this diagnosis?)**

ANSWER TO FIGURE 15C-14A   There is a regular, wide complex tachycardia at a rate of about 110 beats/minute. Bizarre (indeterminate) frontal plane axis, marked QRS widening (to at least 0.14 second), and morphologic assessment (total negativity in lead V_6) all strongly favor a ventricular etiology. Analysis of atrial activity settles the issue. Despite the absence of sinus-con-

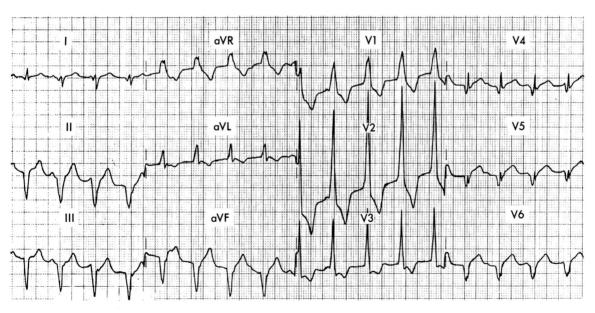

Figure 15C-14A.   Ventricular tachycardia, SVT with aberration, *or neither???*

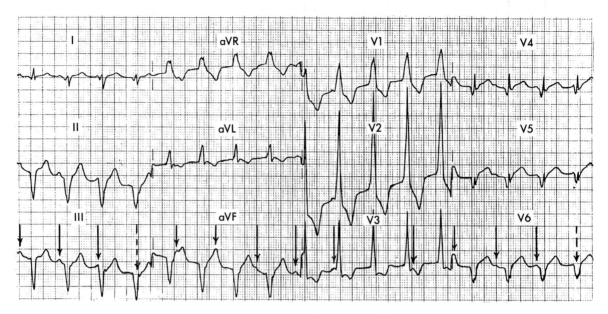

Figure 15C-14B.   Use of calipers to evaluate the rhythm shown in Fig. 15C-14A reveals regular atrial activity (arrows) at a rate of about 85 beats/minute. P waves are totally unrelated to the QRS complex (i.e., complete AV dissociation is present).

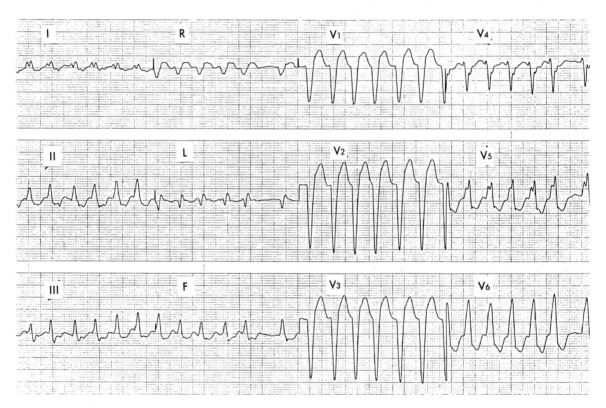

Figure 15C-15.   *Ventricular tachycardia?* or SVT with aberration?

ducted P waves, atrial activity is *not* lacking on this tracing! On the contrary, use of calipers demonstrates the presence of regularly occurring P waves at a rate of 85 beats/minute (arrows in *Figure 15C-14B*). Since none of these P waves conduct, there is *complete AV dissociation*—which virtually *proves* the ventricular etiology of the arrhythmia. Rather than ventricular "tachycardia," however, the relatively

slow ventricular rate (of 110 beats/min) is better described as an *accelerated* idioventricular rhythm (AIVR). This particular patient was asymptomatic and hemodynamically stable at the time this tracing was recorded, so that no treatment (other than *close observation*) was needed.

PROBLEM   *FIGURE 15C-15: Ventricular tachy-cardia?* **or SVT with aberration? (How certain are you of your diagnosis?)**

ANSWER TO FIGURE 15C-15

There is a wide complex tachycardia. The frontal plane axis is normal. QRS morphology is indecisive, and could be consistent with *either* a supraventricular or ventricular etiology. Although there are undulations in the baseline, no definite atrial activity is present. However, in contrast to the last few tracings we have examined, the underlying rhythm in this case is *not* regular. Instead, it is *irregularly irregular*, especially in simultaneously recorded leads aVR, aVL, and aVF. The presence of an irregularly irregular rhythm without definite atrial activity suggests that this is *atrial fibrillation*, in this case with a moderately rapid ventricular response. QRS widening would then be explained by preexisting LBBB. It should again be emphasized that locating a previous ECG to demonstrate the presence of a preexisting bundle branch block would be needed to confirm our diagnosis.

AND a FINAL *(exceedingly tricky)* EXAMPLE OF A WIDE COMPLEX TACHYCARDIA—*FIGURE 15C-16A:* The arrow in this tracing points to a PAC (that peaks the T wave), and *proves* that the run of anomalous beats is supraventricular with aberrant conduction. *Or does it???*

HINT: *Is there evidence of a "marriage" on this tracing?*

ANSWER TO FIGURE 15C-16A

This is a difficult tracing! Nevertheless, definitive evidence of ventricular tachycardia is present.

Morphologically, despite the superficial resemblance of anomalous and sinus conducted beats (both are predominantly negative complexes), their initial deflection is *very* different. Sinus conducted beats manifest a slender, initially positive (r wave) deflection, followed by an almost vertically descending negative (S wave) deflection. In contrast, anomalous beats manifest a totally negative QS configuration with delay and slight slurring of the terminal portion of the S wave (most closely resembling complex **Q** in Fig. 15A-16). This suggests that the anomalous beats represent a run of *right ventricular tachycardia*.

Definitive evidence in support of this impression is forthcoming from analysis of *Figure 15C-16B*, which demonstrates that beat #4 is a *fusion beat*. Note that the PR interval preceding this beat is ever so slightly *shorter* than the PR interval preceding each of the other sinus conducted beats. Furthermore, the morphologic appearance of beat #4 is *intermediate* between that of beats #3 and #5 (it lacks an initial r wave, and is slightly wider than the other sinus conducted beats). The reason the T wave of beat #4 appears peaked (and simulates a PAC) is that this T wave is *also* the result of a "marriage" (i.e., fusion), in this case between the T waves of beats #3 and #5.

There are two final points to make about the run of anomalous beats shown in Fig. 15C-16A. The first regards the *regularity* of this tachyarrhythmia—or more precisely, *the lack thereof!* On close inspection (and with use of calipers), it can be seen that the run exhibits a ***"cool-down"*** *phenomenon* (beginning rapidly at a rate of about 140 beats/min, and then gradually decelerating). By the end of the tracing, the heart rate has slowed to 110 beats/min. What happens beyond this point (i.e., whether the ventricular rate continues to slow down) is not known.

Technically then, the first few beats in the run (i.e., beats #6-8 in Fig. 15C-16B) should be called *ventricular tachycardia*—whereas the latter portion of the run is more properly referred to as AIVR (*accelerated* idioventricular rhythm). Distinction between these two entities is sometimes difficult. Rates over 130-140 beats/minute clearly constitute ventricular tachycardia, whereas rates below 110 beats/minute are clearly termed AIVR. In between lies a "grey zone"—which for the case shown in Fig. 15C-16A might be perceived as a zone of "*transition*." Clinically, AIVR need *not* be treated if the patient is hemodynamically stable, whereas sustained ventricular tachycardia definitely merits treatment.

For academic interest (and to keep you sharp), we include one final finding (that admittedly is of little clinical significance). Return to Fig. 15C-16A. Note that a *notch* can be seen at the peak of the upstroke of the QS complex (i.e., at the junction of the end of the QS complex and the beginning of the ST segment) for *all* but the initial beat in the anomalous run (i.e., for every beat *except* #5 in Fig. 15C-16B). It is likely that this notch represents *retrograde* (i.e., *ventriculo-atrial*) con-

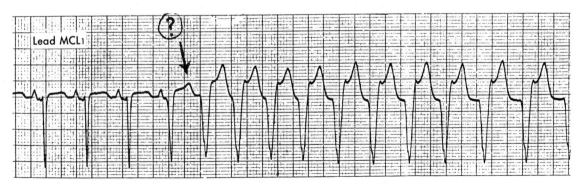

Figure 15C-16A.   The arrow points to a PAC and proves that the run of anomalous beats is of supraventricular etiology. *Or does it???*

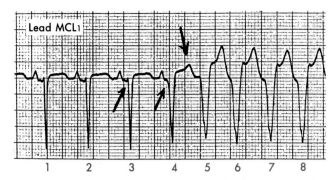

Figure 15C-16B. Focused illustration of the first eight beats in Fig. 15C-16A, proving a ventricular etiology for the run of anomalous beats. Beat #4 is a **_fusion beat_** (and manifests a morphology intermediate between that of beats #3 and #5). The slanted, upward-pointing arrows indicate that the initial deflection of beat #4 is different from that of beat #3, and that the PR interval preceding beat #4 is shorter. The T wave of beat #4 (downward-pointing arrow) is *also* the result of fusion, in this case between the T wave of beats #3 and #5.

duction from ventricular beats (that only becomes established *after* the first beat in the run).

We hope you have enjoyed this chapter. Admittedly, we have included numerous subtle (and some downright tricky) findings to keep things interesting. Much more important than detection and correct diagnosis of all of these findings, however, is *appreciation of the basic principles involved and the clinical approach.* We summarize these basic principles as follows:

i. It *won't* always be possible to differentiate between PVCs and aberrancy.

ii. A beat/rhythm should always be judged as "guilty" (i.e, ventricular in origin) until proven otherwise.

iii. Clinical correlation is key (i.e., hemodynamically unstable patients require immediate cardioversion *regardless* of the etiology of their arrhythmia).

iv. Awareness and application of the basic principles suggested in this chapter (and consolidated in Figs. 15A-14 and 15A-16, and Tables 15B-1 and 15B-2) will usually go a long way toward suggesting the etiology of the arrhythmia with a high degree of certainty.

REFERENCES AND SUGGESTED READINGS

Akhtar M, Shenasa M, Jazayeri M, Caceres J, Tchou PJ: Wide QRS complex tachycardia: reappraisal of a common clinical problem, *Ann Intern Med* 109:905, 1988.

Baerman JM, Morady F, DiCarlo LA, de Buitleir M: Differentiation of ventricular tachycardia from supraventricular tachycardia with aberration: value of the clinical history, *Ann Emerg Med* 16:40, 1987.

Buxton AE, Marchlinski FE, Doherty JU, Flores B, Josephson ME: Hazards of intravenous verapamil for sustained ventricular tachycardia, *Am J Cardiol* 59:1107, 1987.

Curtis AB, Grauer K: Wide complex tachycardia due to coexistent supraventricular and ventricular tachycardia, *J Fam Pract* 30:706, 1990.

Dancy M, Camm AJ, Ward D: Misdiagnosis of chronic recurrent ventricular tachycardia, *Lancet* 2:320, 1985.

Fox W, Stein E: *Cardiac rhythm disturbances: a step-by-step approach,* Philadelphia, 1983, Lea & Febiger.

Grauer K: Differentiating between aberrantly conducted beats and ventricular ectopy, *Cont Ed Fam Phys* 19:85, 1984.

Grauer K: *When 12 leads are better than one.* In *A practical guide to ECG interpretation,* St Louis, 1992, Mosby Year–Book.

Kindwall KE, Brown J, Josephson ME: Electrocardiographic criteria for ventricular tachycardia in wide complex left bundle branch block morphology tachycardias, *Am J Cardiol* 6:1279, 1988.

Langendorf R, Pick A, Winternitz M: Mechanisms of intermittent ventricular bigeminy, I. appearance of ectopic beats dependent upon length of the ventricular cycle, the "rule of bigeminy," *Circulation* 2:422, 1955.

Levitt MA: Supraventricular tachycardia with aberrant conduction versus ventricular tachycardia: differentiation and diagnosis, *Am J Emerg Med* 6:273, 1988.

Marriott HJL: *Practical electrocardiography,* Baltimore, 1982, Williams & Wilkins.

Marriott HJL, Conover MHB: *Advanced concepts in arrhythmias,* St Louis, 1983, Mosby–Year Book.

Morady F, Baerman JM, DiCarlo LA, DeBuitleir M, Krol RB, Wahr DW: A prevalent misconception regarding wide-complex tachycardias, *JAMA* 254:2790, 1985.

Steinman RT, Herrera C, Schuger CD, Lehmann MH: Wide QRS tachycardia in the conscious adult: ventricular tachycardia is the most frequent cause, *JAMA* 261:1013, 1989.

Stewart RB, Bardy GH, Greene HL: Wide complex tachycardia: misdiagnosis and outcome after emergent therapy, *Ann Intrn Med* 104:766, 1986.

Swanick EJ, LaCamera F, Marriott HJL: Morphologic features of right ventricular ectopic beats, *Am J Cardiol* 30:888, 1972.

Vera Z, Cheng TO, Ertem G, Shoalch-var M, Wickramasekaran R, Wadhwa K: His bundle electrocardiography for evaluation of criteria in differentiating ventricular ectopy from aberrancy in atrial fibrillation, *Circulation* 45-46 (Suppl 2):90, 1972 (abstract).

Wellens HJJ, Bar FWHM, Lie KI: The value of the electrocardiogram in the differential diagnosis of a tachycardia with a widened QRS complex, *Am J Med* 64:27, 1978.

CHAPTER 16

MORE ADVANCED CONCEPTS IN ARRHYTHMIA INTERPRETATION

At this point, we'd like to leave our Chapter 15 focus on aberration and explore a number of *more advanced* concepts in arrhythmia interpretation. We emphasize that this material extends well beyond the core of what is needed to successfully complete the ACLS course. It is *not* for the beginning interpreter. However, if you've followed our dis-

cussion of more basic concepts in Chapter 3, and enjoy the clinical challenge of treating patients with cardiac arrhythmias, read on. . . . *

With these words of introduction, it's time to pick up a pair of calipers and enter into the *mindset* of the clinical "arrhythmologist."

SECTION A

TACHYARRHYTHMIAS: REVIEW OF A PRACTICAL CLINICAL APPROACH

Perhaps the greatest challenge faced by the emergency care provider during cardiac resuscitation is the task of interpreting tachyarrhythmias. Institution of the appropriate treatment and the ultimate fate of the patient often hang in the balance. In Chapter 15 we delved into ways of differentiating between aberration and ventricular ectopy, and how to apply such techniques in interpreting wide complex tachyarrhythmias. In this chapter, we expand on this material and place particular emphasis on the diagnosis of supraventricular tachyarrhythmias. Before turning our attention to the electrocardiographic clues for interpretation of specific arrhythmias, however, it might be helpful to review a practical, clinical approach to the problem.

PROBLEM   **Consider the situation posed by a middle-aged man with the tachyarrhythmia shown in *Figure 16A-1*. How would you proceed both *diagnostically* and *therapeutically* if the patient were tolerating this rhythm?**

ANSWER TO FIGURE 16A-1   There is a regular tachyarrhythmia at a rate of about 200 beats/min. Although an upright deflection is seen toward the latter portion of each R-R interval, it is unclear if this positive deflection represents a P wave, the T wave, or both. The critical question that must be addressed is whether the etiology of the tachyarrhythmia is supraventricular or ventricular. Unfortunately, the answer is *not* forthcoming from analysis of the single monitoring lead shown in Fig. 16A-1. One simply *cannot tell* if the QRS complex is wide, since it is virtually impossible to be sure where the QRS complex ends and the ST segment begins. Even if it were known that the QRS complex was wide, the possibility would still exist that the tachyarrhythmia was supraventricular with either preexisting bundle branch block or aberrant conduction.

Initial Priorities

The first thing to do when confronted with any tachyarrhythmia is determine whether the patient is hemodynamically stable. Clinical evidence of **hemodynamic compromise** (i.e., hypotension, chest pain, shortness of breath, depressed mental status) is an indication for immediate cardioversion *regardless* of the etiology of the tachyarrhythmia.

It should be emphasized that hemodynamic stability—

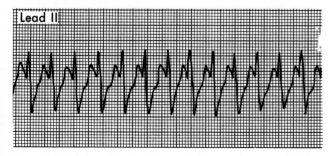

Figure 16A-1.   Middle-aged man with a tachyarrhythmia. He is hemodynamically stable. *How would you proceed both diagnostically and therapeutically?*

---

*Chapters 15 and 16 *complement* each other. Although ideally the material in Chapter 15 will have been read first, it is *not* essential to do so, and you may find it more interesting to work through selected portions of both chapters as clinical questions arise in your practice.

in and of itself—should *never* be taken as evidence against a ventricular etiology. However, once you establish that the patient is hemodynamically stable (as is the case in Fig. 16A-1), at least you have a finite amount of time to:

1. take a deep breath (and gather your thoughts)
2. attempt to narrow down the diagnostic possibilities
3. consider non-pharmacologic diagnostic / therapeutic options (i.e., application of a vagal maneuver, cough version)
4. initiate medical therapy
5. arrange for backup assistance in the event cardioversion is ultimately needed.

Practical Considerations

Practically speaking, if the patient is hemodynamically stable but you are unsure of the etiology of the tachyarrhythmia, there are three basic ways to approach the problem:

Approach #1: Hold off on treatment while you seek more information.

Approach #2: Assume the rhythm to be *supraventricular* and treat accordingly.

Approach #3: Assume the rhythm to be *ventricular tachycardia* and treat accordingly.

Which approach to take will depend on a number of factors, including the patient's clinical condition, the resources you have available, and the relative certainty you feel about the likely etiology of the arrhythmia.

> We have already extolled the virtues of *Approach #3* when the tachyarrhythmia is regular, the QRS complex wide, normal atrial activity is absent, and definitive evidence of a supraventricular etiology is lacking. Clearly, when significant doubt exists about the etiology of an arrhythmia, *the most conservative (and usually the safest) course to follow is to assume that the patient is in ventricular tachycardia and treat accordingly.* Nevertheless, there are times in clinical practice when one or more factors may lead you to believe (or at least strongly suspect) that the rhythm is probably supraventricular. *Approaches #1* and *#2* may become reasonable alternatives at such times.

APPROACH #1: HOLD OFF ON TREATMENT WHILE YOU SEEK MORE INFORMATION

The goal of this approach is to obtain enough information to allow definitive (or at least a more certain) diagnosis. Treatment can then be optimized. Thus for the case presented in Fig. 16A-1, since the rhythm is being tolerated, you might:

a. Obtain a 12-lead ECG to see if P waves are evident in any other leads, or if assessment of QRS morphology in other leads can aid in differentiation.

> As emphasized in Chapter 15, obtaining a 12-lead ECG (especially one with *simultaneously* recorded leads) is often invaluable in suggesting the etiology of the arrhythmia. *In general, when confronted with a tachyarrhythmia of unknown etiology in a hemodynamically stable patient,* **always obtain a 12-lead ECG (if at all possible)!**

b. Search through the patient's chart / medical record for rhythm strips (or a 12-lead ECG) that was recorded *before* the onset of the tachycardia.

> For example in the case presented, if prior rhythm strips obtained while the patient was in sinus rhythm demonstrate a QRS complex of *identical* configuration to that shown in Fig. 16A-1, one could be relatively certain that the arrhythmia is supraventricular.

c. Look at the neck veins and listen to the first heart sound.

> The presence of irregular cannon waves in the neck and / or variation in the intensity of the first heart sound is evidence on physical examination of *AV dissociation*, and almost always means that the rhythm is ventricular tachycardia.*
>
> The converse is not necessarily true. Granted, failure to hear any variation in the intensity of the first heart sound, and either the absence of cannon waves, or recognition of *regular* cannon waves in the neck are physical findings that suggest AV dissociation is *not* present. However, failure to detect these physical signs *in no way* rules out the possibility that ventricular tachycardia is still present. This is because ventricular tachycardia can occur with 1:1 *retrograde* conduction or in association with atrial fibrillation. From a purely practical standpoint, it is often extremely difficult to accurately evaluate a patient for physical signs of AV dissociation under the stressful situation of being confronted with an acutely ill patient who is in a tachyarrhythmia of uncertain etiology. *Even if AV dissociation is present, it is all too easy to miss it by physical examination.* Thus, signs of AV dissociation on physical examination are *only* helpful if they are present. No firm conclusion can be reached if they are absent.

d. Switch monitoring leads.

> Since the rhythm in the case presented (in Fig. 16A-1) was recorded from lead II, rhythm strips should also be obtained from leads MCL_1 and MCL_6.

e. Consider additional (alternate) monitoring lead systems.

> One of the simplest alternate systems to obtain is an **S_5 lead.** With the ECG hooked up to record on standard lead I, the *left* arm (positive) electrode is positioned at the fifth interspace just to the right of the sternum, while the *right* arm (negative) electrode is placed over the manubrium of the sternum. This provides a *bipolar* precordial lead that may sometimes elucidate atrial activity.

---

*Admittedly, a wide complex tachycardia could also result from AV dissociation between an atrial pacemaker and an accelerated junctional rhythm that conducts with aberration. Practically speaking, this is such a rare clinical occurrence that the finding of AV dissociation (either on an ECG or on physical examination) can be used as incriminating evidence of ventricular tachycardia.

f. Consider *statistical likelihood* in light of the clinical setting.

The *overwhelming majority* of adults (middle-aged or older) who present in a regular wide complex tachycardia of uncertain etiology are in ventricular tachycardia—especially if they have a history of underlying cardiac disease (either angina pectoris, prior myocardial infarction, or heart failure)—*regardless* of what their blood pressure is during the arrhythmia.

APPROACH #2: ASSUME A SUPRAVENTRICULAR ETIOLOGY AND TREAT ACCORDINGLY

It might not be unreasonable to assume a supraventricular etiology for the rhythm shown in Fig. 16A-1 if one thought that the QRS complex did not appear to be significantly widened—especially if the patient continued to tolerate the arrhythmia. In conjunction with the rapid heart rate (of about 200 beats/min), these findings could be consistent with a supraventricular etiology (although they definitely do *not* rule out the possibility of ventricular tachycardia). Therefore, *IF it was felt that the rhythm in Fig. 16A-1 was supraventricular*, you might:

a. Apply a **vagal maneuver** (i.e., carotid sinus massage, Valsalva, etc.) under constant ECG monitoring.
b. Try to convert the rhythm medically with an intravenously administered drug effective in treating supraventricular tachyarrhythmias (i.e., verapamil,* adenosine, digoxin, and/or a β-blocker).
c. *Reapply* a vagal maneuver *after* initial administration of the antiarrhythmic agent.
d. Be ready to cardiovert at any time should the patient show signs of hemodynamic compromise.

Practical considerations in the application of vagal maneuvers are discussed a little later in this section. Even if the maneuver fails to convert the tachyarrhythmia, it may still provide useful diagnostic information. The reason for recommending *reapplication* of the maneuver *after* initial administration of the antiarrhythmic agent is the synergism between these two measures. Thus, reapplication of a vagal maneuver later in the therapeutic process (after administration of an antiarrhythmic agent) may succeed in converting the arrhythmia.

Detailed description of benefits and drawbacks of the various antiarrhythmic agents has already been covered (in Chapters 2 and 14). We limit discussion below to a number of selected key features. IV **verapamil** has long been a favored drug for acute treatment of PSVT. It is easy to administer and extremely effective, converting PSVT to sinus rhythm more than 90% of the time. A dose of 5 mg may be given over

a 1-to-2-minute period. Lower doses (2-3 mg) given more slowly (over 3-4 minutes) are advised in the elderly. If there is no response to an initial dose of verapamil in 15-30 minutes, a repeat dose (of 5-10 mg) may be given. The most important point to emphasize about verapamil is that the drug should *never* be given indiscriminately as a *diagnostic maneuver* to a patient with a wide complex tachycardia of unknown etiology. Doing so may have disastrous consequences (i.e., precipitation of ventricular fibrillation) if the tachycardia turns out to be ventricular.

Practically speaking, there should virtually *always* be time to verify QRS duration in other leads (by obtaining a 12-lead ECG) *prior* to administration of verapamil. By definition, if there is not time to do so, the patient is *hemodynamically unstable* and needs to be immediately cardioverted *regardless* of whether the arrhythmia is supraventricular or not.

Adenosine is a newer, attractive alternative therapeutic option to verapamil for acute treatment of PSVT. The drug is well tolerated in most patients, and equally effective as verapamil in converting the arrhythmia. Adenosine is given as a *rapid* (as fast as possible) IV bolus in an initial dose of 6 mg.* If there is no response within 1 to 2 minutes, a second bolus (this time at a dose of 12 mg) should be given. If there is still no response after another 1 to 2 minutes, a third (and final) 12-mg dose of the drug may be given (for a total dose of 6 + 12 + 12 = 30 mg).

The beauty of IV adenosine is that if it is going to work, it will do so within minutes. The half-life of the drug is exceedingly short (*less* than 10 seconds), so that if there has been no response by 1 to 2 minutes after a dose, a second (or third) dose can be given, or another agent may be tried.

Advantages of adenosine over verapamil are that if adverse effects do occur, they are usually short-lived; that the drug is more likely to help diagnostically (by transiently slowing the ventricular response and allowing atrial activity to be seen—even if it doesn't convert the arrhythmia); and that it is less likely to precipitate ventricular fibrillation if given to a patient with a wide complex tachycardia of unknown etiology that turns out to be ventricular tachycardia.

On the other hand, advantages of verapamil are that its therapeutic effect lasts longer than that of adenosine; it is available in an oral dosage form (for long-term antiarrhythmic maintenance and/or prophylaxis); it also slows the ventricular response of atrial fibrillation and atrial flutter (whereas adenosine only works for reentry tachyarrhythmias such as PSVT); and it is less likely than adenosine to cause profound bradycardia (if administered in the manner suggested above).

Less commonly used agents for treatment of PSVT include **digoxin** and **β-blockers.** Digoxin has a slower onset of action than either verapamil or adenosine. Moreover, it would *not* be recommended in this particular case, since the possibility still exists that the rhythm in Fig. 16A-1 is ventricular tachycardia (for which digitalis is contraindicated).

β-blockers may be effective for both supraventricular and ventricular tachyarrhythmias, especially when these arrhythmias are associated with ischemia or increased sympathetic tone. However, IV forms of this class of drug (such as propranolol or esmolol) should *not* be given soon after verapamil because this greatly increases the risk of inducing AV block. (IV verapamil can probably be given safely to patients taking

---

*Although specifics of our discussion on the use of an IV calcium channel blocking agent for treatment of supraventricular tachyarrhythmias in this chapter focuses on verapamil, the recently released **IV form** of **diltiazem** could probably be used in a similar manner—*taking similar precautions*. (See Chapter 14 for full discussion on the use of IV diltiazem.)

---

*Rapid injection of the IV bolus of adenosine should be *immediately* followed by a saline flush to prevent breakdown of any drug that may have gotten caught in the IV tubing.

oral β-blockers provided left ventricular function is normal.) An additional drawback of IV esmolol is its rather complicated dosing regimen.

APPROACH #3: ASSUME A VENTRICULAR ETIOLOGY AND TREAT ACCORDINGLY

Given that the QRS complex in Fig. 16A-1 may be wide (depending on where the QRS ends and the ST segment begins), and given the uncertainty about the presence of atrial activity, the most conservative evaluative approach to this arrhythmia would be to assume a ventricular etiology and treat accordingly:

a. *Ask the patient to cough.*

   Cough version has been used by cardiologists in the catheterization laboratory for years. Although the mechanism of action of the cough is unclear (activation of the autonomic nervous system? enhanced perfusion from the increase in intrathoracic pressure? conversion of the mechanical energy of a cough into electrical energy?), the technique will successfully convert some patients out of ventricular tachycardia, and allow others to maintain consciousness for a short period of time *despite* persistence of their arrhythmia. It merits a trial if the patient is conscious.

b. Consider whether there is time to gather more information.

   Because patients in ventricular tachycardia may sometimes remain conscious and maintain hemodynamic stability for extended periods of time, it may be desirable to consider some of the evaluative measures listed in **Approach #1** (i.e., obtaining a 12-lead ECG, searching for prior tracings on the patient)—*even if you are reasonably sure that the rhythm in question is ventricular tachycardia.* Doing so may allow you to make a more definitive diagnosis, and thus optimize therapy.

c. Begin **lidocaine.** Administer an IV bolus of this drug, and then start an IV infusion.

   Lidocaine is the antiarrhythmic agent of choice for treatment of ventricular tachycardia. The drawback of *empiric* use of the drug (i.e., when you are not *sure* that the rhythm is ventricular tachycardia) is that it is not effective for treatment of supraventricular tachyarrhythmias, and on occasion may paradoxically *increase* the rate of such rhythms.

d. Consider IV **procainamide.**

   This may be the drug of choice for medical treatment of a wide complex tachycardia *when the etiology of the arrhythmia is unclear.* Procainamide is a Type IA antiarrhythmic agent that is equally effective as quinidine for treatment of supraventricular arrhythmias. Because of its effect on conduction properties of the reentry circuit, it may successfully convert some cases of PSVT to sinus rhythm. Thus, procainamide offers the distinct advantage of potential efficacy in treatment of wide complex tachyarrhythmias *regardless* of their etiology. The drug is equally effective as lidocaine in treating ventricular arrhythmias (especially when such arrhythmias are not the result of acute ischemia). Moreover, even if procainamide fails to convert ventricular tachycardia, it is likely to slow the ventricular rate, which may allow the patient to maintain hemodynamic stability despite persistence of the arrhythmia. Finally, pro-

cainamide is also effective in treatment of wide complex tachyarrhythmias that are the result of WPW (with atrial fibrillation or atrial flutter) because it slows *antegrade* conduction down the accessory pathway. It may therefore be the antiarrhythmic agent of choice for *empiric* therapy when a drug is indicated but the etiology of the arrhythmia is uncertain.*

e. Proceed with **synchronized cardioversion.**

   This modality is also effective regardless of the etiology of the tachyarrhythmia. It is indicated if (and as soon as) the patient becomes hemodynamically unstable and/or if there is no response to medical therapy. In the latter case, as long as the patient is tolerating the tachycardia, cardioversion may be performed under *semielective* conditions. That is, the patient may be premedicated with 5 to 10 mg of IV Valium (or other sedating medication), anesthesia personnel can be called to the bedside, and lower energy levels (i.e., 50 joules) may be tried first.† Higher energies (i.e., 100-200 joules) are often selected when cardioversion is used to treat patients with hemodynamically unstable tachyarrhythmias.

After Sinus Rhythm Is Restored

Regardless of the approach selected for management of the tachyarrhythmia shown in Fig. 16A-1, the goal of treatment is the same—*to restore sinus rhythm.* It is important to remember, however, that treatment objectives do not end with achievement of this goal. *Equally important* is the task of *maintaining sinus rhythm* and *preventing a recurrence* of the tachyarrhythmia. Thus, **after sinus rhythm has been restored,** you may want to:

a. Obtain a *post-conversion* 12-lead ECG.

   The post-conversion ECG may be helpful in a number of ways. First, it *documents* that sinus rhythm has been restored. It may also provide a clue to the *precipitating cause* of the arrhythmia (i.e., acute ischemia or infarction, underlying WPW, etc.), and help determine subsequent management (i.e., the need for hospital admission, oral or intravenous antiarrhythmic therapy, etc.). Finally, it may allow *definitive diagnosis of the tachyarrhythmia* to be made *retrospectively* by providing a reference for comparison of the "normal" QRS complex during sinus rhythm with the anomalous QRS complex during the tachycardia.

b. Evaluate the patient for the presence of any potentially ***exacerbating factors*** that could have contributed to producing the arrhythmia. If found, an attempt should be made to correct these if at all possible.

---

*A case can also be made for considering **adenosine** as an alternative agent for empiric treatment of a regular tachyarrhythmia of uncertain etiology. Although the ultrashort half-life of this drug will usually safeguard against deterioration to ventricular fibrillation (if the rhythm turns out to be ventricular tachycardia)—our clear preference for empiric treatment is IV procainamide.

†It should be emphasized that by definition, *there should almost always be time to sedate a conscious patient prior to cardioversion.* Thus, some patients may remain hemodynamically "stable" (i.e., alert, asymptomatic, and apparently perfusing) for a period of time *despite* having a systolic blood pressure of *less* than 90 mm Hg.

Among the potentially exacerbating factors to consider are electrolyte abnormalities (i.e., hypokalemia, hypomagnesemia), ischemia, heart failure, and other severe underlying medical disorders (i.e., hypoxia, sepsis, anemia, etc.). If present, potassium and/or magnesium supplementation; antiischemic therapy (with nitrates, calcium blockers, and/or β-blockers); treatment of heart failure (with digoxin, diuretics, and/or ACE-inhibitors); and/or correction/treatment of other underlying disorders—is (are) essential if recurrence of the tachyarrhythmia is to be prevented.

Another potential exacerbating factor to consider is *proarrhythmia*. At least 5% to 10% of *all* patients treated with antiarrhythmic agents will demonstrate this effect in which the very arrhythmia they are being treated for is paradoxically *exacerbated* by the antiarrhythmic drug. As might be imagined, it is often exceedingly difficult to detect the proarrhythmic effect in an acutely ill patient who presents with a life-threatening arrhythmia. Nevertheless, the possibility of proarrhythmia should at least be considered if patients were on prior antiarrhythmic therapy.

c. Consider appropriate antiarrhythmic therapy.

After evaluating the patient for potential exacerbating factors (and correcting these as much as possible), the key to long-term management (and prevention of recurrence) of arrhythmias such as the one shown in Fig. 16A-1 will rest on having made an accurate diagnosis of the arrhythmia. *Only by knowing what is being treated can treatment be optimized.*

Vagal Maneuvers

Vagal maneuvers have been used in the evaluation and management of patients with cardiac arrhythmias for well over half a century. They remain today an extremely helpful diagnostic/therapeutic tool for tachyarrhythmias in which atrial activity is either absent or only intermittently present.

Vagal maneuvers work by slowing the heart rate and/or prolonging atrioventricular conduction time. These effects can be produced in a number of ways including carotid sinus massage, Valsalva, activation of the diving reflex, induction of gagging, tongue pulling, and "hunkering down," among others. Because of complications and/or patient discomfort, the use of some of these methods has become quite limited (Roberge et al, 1987). For example, application of ocular pressure is no longer recommended since there have been reports of resultant retinal detachment. Induction of gagging and activation of the diving reflex (i.e., facial submersion in ice) are both extremely unpleasant for the patient. Moreover, gagging may produce vomiting with the risk of subsequent aspiration, while activation of the diving reflex may not always be practical (i.e., in a patient who is acutely dyspneic). Tongue pulling is painful. For practical considerations, we therefore restrict our discussion to the following four vagal maneuvers: (1) carotid sinus massage; (2) Valsalva; (3) "hunkering down"; and a less commonly described technique, (4) digital rectal massage.

CHARACTERISTIC CLINICAL RESPONSES TO VARIOUS VAGAL MANEUVERS

The potency of effect from utilization of the various vagal maneuvers will vary depending on operator technique, patient-related factors (which are often intangible), and the particular maneuver selected. Nevertheless, certain cardiac arrhythmias characteristically produce certain clinical responses *(Table 16A-1)*. Thus, vagal stimulation of a patient in **sinus tachycardia** will usually produce gradual heart rate slowing with resumption of the tachycardia upon completion of the maneuver. "Telltale" P waves may become evident during the maneuver, allowing definitive diagnosis and direction of therapy toward alleviating the underlying cause of the sinus tachycardia. In contrast, with an AV nodal reentry tachycardia such as **PSVT,** application of a vagal maneuver will either terminate the tachyarrhythmia, or have no effect at all.

Ventricular tachycardia does not respond to vagal maneuvers.* Clinically therefore, the *lack of response* to a vagal maneuver is of no diagnostic value when applied to a patient in a regular wide complex tachycardia (since both PSVT and ventricular tachycardia may fail to respond). Finally, **atrial fibrillation** and **atrial flutter** generally respond to vagal maneuvers with a decrease in atrioventricular conduction of supraventricular impulses, and a resultant reduction in heart rate. This slowing of the ventricular response may allow atrial activity to become evident and facilitate diagnosis *(Figure 16A-2)*. Resumption of the tachyarrhythmia will occur upon completion of the maneuver.

It should be emphasized that vagal maneuvers may need to be repeated a number of times. In particular, patients with PSVT who fail to respond to initial application of a vagal maneuver may be successfully converted to sinus rhythm on *reapplication* of the vagal maneuver at a later point in the therapeutic process (i.e., *after* administration of an antiarrhythmic agent).

CAROTID SINUS MASSAGE (CSM)

CSM may be the most commonly utilized vagal maneuver by medical personnel. Under constant ECG monitoring, the patient's head is turned to the left and the area of the *right* carotid bifurcation (near the angle of the jaw) is carefully but *firmly* massaged for 3 to 5 seconds. Carotid

---

*There are a number of reports in the literature of vagal maneuvers converting ventricular tachycardia to sinus rhythm (Schweitzer and Teichholz, 1985). This is a *rare* phenomenon. Another phenomenon that may occasionally be produced by application of a vagal maneuver to a patient in ventricular tachycardia is VA dissociation. For practical purposes, however, one would do well *not* to expect vagal maneuvers to have any clinical effect when administered to a patient in ventricular tachycardia.

Table 16A-1

Characteristic Clinical Responses of Various Cardiac Arrhythmias to Vagal Maneuvers	
Tachyarrhythmia	**Response to Carotid Sinus Massage (CSM)**
Sinus Tachycardia	- Gradual slowing with CSM, with resumption of the tachycardia after the maneuver
PSVT	- Abrupt termination of the tachyarrhythmia with conversion to sinus rhythm **or** - No response to CSM
Atrial Flutter or Atrial Fibrillation	- Increased degree of AV block with resultant slowing of the ventricular rate (CSM often permits diagnosis of atrial flutter by allowing clear visualization of flutter waves as the ventricular rate slows)
Ventricular Tachycardia	- No response to CSM

massage should *not* be continued for more than 5 seconds at a time. To be effective, *firm* pressure must be applied—so much so, that you may want to prewarn a conscious patient that the maneuver will be uncomfortable (and may even be a little painful). Massage must be applied in the correct location. All too often, pressure is applied too low (i.e., to the mid-portion of the neck). The carotid sinus (bifurcation) lies *high* in the neck—*just below the angle of the jaw!*

If there is no response to an initial attempt at CSM, additional attempts may be made on the same side of the neck—*always* being sure that *constant ECG monitoring* is ongoing during the procedure—and always being sure to limit the period of pressure application to *no more than* 5 seconds at a time. After several attempts on the right side, the left side may also be tried. *Never massage both carotids at the same time!*

> The reason many clinicians prefer to massage the *right* carotid first is that this side is believed to exert a greater influence on the sinus node, whereas the left carotid is believed to act more on the AV node.
>
> The efficacy of CSM may be increased by placing the patient in a Trendelenburg position of about − 10°, having them take a full inspiration—followed by a full expiration—and then another full inspiration that is held briefly—and then reapplying CSM in the Trendelenburg position if there has been no response. This sequence of maneuvers has been termed **"Augmented Carotid Massage"** (Pomeroy, 1992).

CSM is not a completely benign maneuver, particularly in older individuals (Schweitzer and Teichholz, 1985).

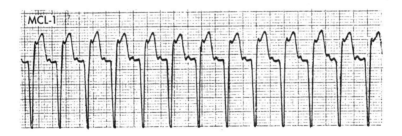

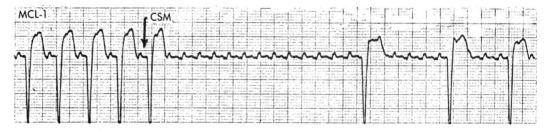

Figure 16A-2. Application of carotid sinus massage (CSM) at the point indicated by the arrow to an elderly man who had been in supraventricular tachycardia. As can be seen, CSM decreased (almost too well in this case) conduction through the AV node, revealing *flutter* waves (at a rate of just under 300 beats/min) that had been obscured by the tachycardia.

Complications that may occur include syncope, stroke (from dislodgement of a carotid plaque), bradyarrhythmias (such as sinus arrest, high-grade AV block, and prolonged periods of asystole), and ventricular tachyarrhythmias (especially in patients with digitalis intoxication). As a result, CSM should probably *not* be attempted in patients with a history of sick sinus syndrome (SSS), cervical bruits, cerebrovascular disease, or when the possibility of digitalis intoxication exists. (Listen to the neck for bruits *before* applying CSM!)

As emphasized earlier, *continuous ECG monitoring must be ongoing while the maneuver is performed*. For documentation purposes (i.e., to *prove* that you didn't massage for *longer* than 5 seconds)—and to assist in interpretation of the response to CSM, the onset and completion of the maneuver should be marked directly on the tracing. The person assigned to watch the monitor is there to alert the operator (and advise *immediate* cessation of massage) if significant slowing occurs (such as was seen in Fig. 16A-2).

VALSALVA

A Valsalva maneuver is performed by having the patient forcibly exhale (bear down) against a closed glottis (as if trying to go to the bathroom) for up to 15 seconds at a time. Although the Valsalva maneuver requires a patient to be alert, cooperative, and able to understand instructions, it is often extremely effective, and may produce even more potent vagal stimulation than CSM (Mehta et al, 1988). Many otherwise healthy individuals with recurrent supraventricular tachyarrhythmias (such as PSVT) will have already taught themselves this maneuver (or the "hunkering down" maneuver) by the time you see them based on their empiric experience that it "makes their palpitations go away."

> An interesting study by Mehta et al (1988) found Valsalva to be the most effective vagal maneuver for terminating AV nodal reentry tachyarrhythmias. The authors postulate the reason for this procedure's superior efficacy compared to CSM is that the increase in systemic blood pressure that occurs during the relaxation phase of Valsalva produces *bilateral* baroreceptor stimulation, compared to the unilateral manual stimulation resulting from CSM. Valsalva was found to be *most effective* when performed in the *supine* position. This is probably because a compensatory increase in sympathetic tone is produced by standing, which partially counteracts the vagotonic (parasympathomimetic) effect of Valsalva.

"HUNKERING DOWN"

Although less formally recognized in the literature, "hunkering down" is an effective, patient-initiated maneuver in which the individual squats, hugs the abdomen with both arms, and bears down (William P. Nelson—

personal communication). Potent vagal stimulation is the result.

DIGITAL RECTAL MASSAGE (DRM)

A less-known (underutilized?) technique for increasing vagal tone is *digital rectal massage* (Roberge et al, 1987). Although not usually thought of by health care providers as a potential therapeutic measure for the treatment of cardiac arrhythmias, DRM is effective (the rectum being richly supplied by sympathetic and parasympathetic nerve fibers), easy to perform, and probably *safer* than CSM when administered to older individuals who might have underlying carotid atherosclerosis (since it obviates the risk inherent with CSM of dislodging a carotid plaque). DRM also offers the advantage of not interfering with resuscitative measures that may be ongoing at other anatomic sites. As with all other vagal maneuvers, *constant ECG monitoring* is advised while the procedure is performed.

ADENOSINE

Although administration of adenosine is *not* a vagal maneuver, we list it here because use of this drug may be helpful in the evaluation of selected patients with supraventricular tachyarrhythmias of uncertain etiology. The almost immediate effect of adenosine in slowing the ventricular response may reveal atrial activity (in a similar manner to the way application of CSM did in Fig. 16A-2), and thus allow definitive diagnosis of the arrhythmia (i.e., *chemical Valsalva*).

Looking for Atrial Activity

Diagnosis of supraventricular tachyarrhythmias often hinges on recognition of atrial activity. Evidence of such atrial activity may be exceedingly subtle and easy to overlook. Before delving into discussion of the various supraventricular tachyarrhythmias, we present two final exercises that focus on recognition of subtle activity.

PROBLEM   **Examine *Figure 16A-3A*: Beats #8-#11 demonstrate normal sinus rhythm at a rate of 80 beats/minute. *Is there evidence of atrial activity during the tachycardia represented by beats #1-#7?***

HINT: How does T wave morphology of the normally conducted beats in Fig. 16A-3A compare to T wave morphology during the tachycardia?

ANSWER TO FIGURE 16A-3A   T wave morphology during the tachycardia is definitely different than after conversion to sinus rhythm (beats #8-11). Arrows in *Figure 16A-3B* demonstrate that the notching and peaking of the ST segment and T wave during the tachycardia is

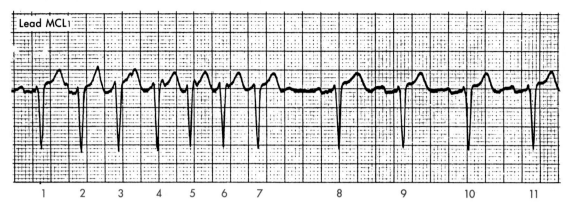

Figure 16A-3A. *Is there evidence of atrial activity during the tachycardia (beats #1-7)?*

due to atrial activity at a rate of approximately 160 beats/minute. (Did you find *all* of the P waves in Fig. 16A-3A—*including the one that notched the terminal portion of the QRS complex of beat #6?*) Although the precise mechanism of this tachycardia is unclear, the rhythm provides an excellent example of the key principle for detecting subtle atrial activity: *Establish normal QRST morphology; then scrutinize the QRS complex, ST segment, and T wave during the tachycardia to see if QRST morphology changes.*

PROBLEM   *Figure 16A-4A is the post-cardioversion rhythm strip of a patient who presented with hypotension from new-onset atrial fibrillation with a rapid ventricular response. Is the patient still in atrial fibrillation? (i.e., Is there evidence of normal [sinus conducted] atrial activity on this post-cardioversion rhythm strip?)*

CLINICAL PEARL: Why is it so very important to

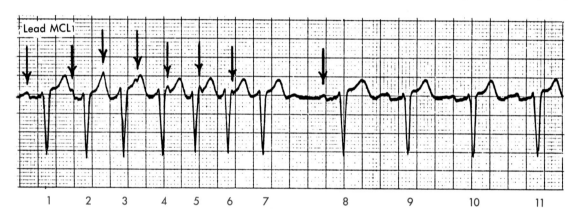

Figure 16A-3B.   Arrows indicate that notching and peaking of the ST segment and T wave during the tachycardia (beats #1-7) in Fig. 16A-3A results from atrial activity at approximately 160 beats/minute.

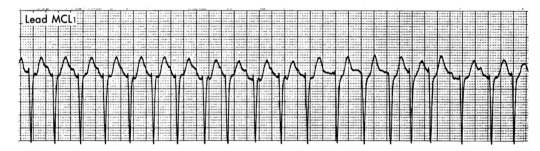

Figure 16A-4A.   Post-cardioversion rhythm strip from a patient who presented with hemodynamically unstable atrial fibrillation. *Is this patient still in atrial fibrillation?*

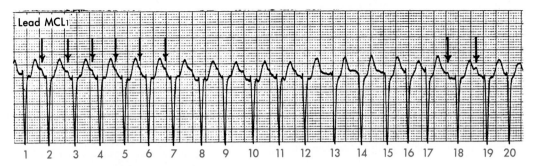

Figure 16A-4B. Although admittedly subtle, arrows indicate that the underlying rhythm in Fig. 16A-4A was sinus tachycardia, which was interrupted by frequent PACs.

determine if normal atrial activity is present on the post-cardioversion rhythm strip?

ANSWER TO FIGURE 16A-4A

Despite the irregular irregularity of a large portion of the rhythm strip shown in Fig. 16A-4A, this patient is *no longer* in atrial fibrillation. Instead, sinus rhythm has returned (as indicated by arrows in *Figure 16A-4B)*, albeit frequently interrupted by PACs. Admittedly, sinus P waves in Fig. 16A-4B are exceedingly subtle. Nevertheless, the consistent positive deflection that deforms the terminal portion of many of the T waves (indicated by the arrows) appears to be real. The importance of this finding is that it confirms the success of cardioversion. *Failure to maintain sinus rhythm would then suggest the need for additional medical therapy (rather than repeat attempts at cardioversion).* On the other hand, failure of cardioversion to at least initially convert the patient to normal sinus rhythm suggests that repeat cardioversion

(perhaps at a higher energy level) may be indicated. It is well to remember that although atrial flutter typically responds to synchronized cardioversion at low energy levels (of 20-50 joules), much higher energy levels (i.e., 200 joules or more) may be needed for cardioversion of atrial fibrillation.

References

Mehta D, Ward DE, Wafa S, Camm AJ: Relative efficacy of various physical manoeuvres in the termination of junctional tachycardia, *Lancet* 1:11881, 1988.

Pomeroy PR: Augmented carotid massage, *Ann Emerg Med* 21:1169, 1992.

Roberge R, Anderson E, MacMath T, Rudoff J, Luten R: Termination of paroxysmal supraventricular tachycardia by digital rectal massage, *Ann Emerg Med* 16:1291, 1987.

Schweitzer P, Teichholz LE: Carotid sinus massage: its diagnostic and therapeutic value in arrhythmias, *Am J Med* 78:645, 1985.

SECTION B

NARROW COMPLEX TACHYARRHYTHMIAS

Classification of tachyarrhythmias is generally easier when the QRS complex is of normal duration. In such cases, evaluation of the rhythm's regularity and identification of atrial activity become the key differentiating factors.

Perhaps the most comforting dividend derived from evaluating narrow complex tachyarrhythmias is knowing that the patient is likely to be hemodynamically stable, and that you will probably have at least some time to carefully analyze the arrhythmia. Nevertheless, three *caveats* are worthy of mention.

1. **Before concluding that a particular tachyarrhythmia is supraventricular, be sure that QRS duration has been evaluated in *more* than one lead.** The QRS complex may appear deceptively narrow if viewed from a single monitoring lead in which the initial or terminal portion of the complex lies on the baseline.

2. *Not all patients with supraventricular tachyarrhythmias will be hemodynamically stable.* This is particularly true for older individuals with underlying cardiac disease. For example, sudden onset of rapid atrial fibrillation may precipitate hemodynamic decompensation in two ways: (1) *loss of the atrial kick* (which accounts for between 5% to 40% of cardiac output); and (2) reduced stroke volume (from the faster heart rate which disproportionately shortens diastolic filling time). Superimposed ischemia and/or acute infarction may further depress an already compromised cardiac output. Thus, careful evaluation of the patient must *always* assume priority (to assure hemodynamic stability) over dissection of the intricacies of the arrhythmia. *Hemodynamic instability is an indication for immediate cardioversion regardless of whether the tachyarrhythmia is supraventricular or not.*

3. **On *rare* occasions, ventricular tachycardia may manifest as a relatively narrow complex tachycardia.** In a fascinating study by Hayes et al (1991), 5% of 106 patients with inducible sustained ventricular tachycardia were found to have documented narrow complex ventricular tachycardia (with a QRS duration of between 0.09 and 0.11 second) on electrophysiologic testing. Origin near the ventricular septum would allow rapid access of the arrhyth-

mogenic focus to the proximal ventricular conduction system, and was felt to explain the relatively short QRS duration in this study. It would also explain why these patients are often refractory to treatment with conventional antiarrhythmic agents that work by prolonging His-ventricular conduction, since doing so may paradoxically *facilitate* initiation into (or maintenance of) a proximally situated reentry circuit.

For the most part, patients in the study with narrow complex ventricular tachycardia had underlying cardiac disease, as well as additional electrocardiographic clues suggestive of a ventricular etiology (i.e., taller left rabbit ear in lead V_1, predominantly negative QRS complex in lead V_6, AV dissociation, or QRS concordance in the precordial leads). Recognition of such clues should therefore prompt consideration of a possible ventricular etiology *regardless* of QRS duration!

Practically speaking, it is likely that the occurrence of narrow complex ventricular tachycardia is *much less common* in general practice than the 5% incidence reported in this study, since study subjects represented a highly select group of patients referred for electrophysiologic testing. Nevertheless, it may be well to keep in mind that **on rare occasions** (*perhaps more so in individuals with a history of recurrent "SVT" that has been "resistant to conventional antiarrhythmic therapy"*), **ventricular tachycardia may masquerade as a relatively narrow complex tachycardia!**

With these three caveats in mind, it's time to evaluate a series of narrow complex tachyarrhythmias:

PROBLEM   *Figure 16B-1* is from an asymptomatic 6-year-old child.

ANSWER TO FIGURE 16B-1   The rhythm is regular. The R-R interval is just *under* 2 large boxes in duration, so that the heart rate is 155 beats/min. Each QRS complex is preceded by a P wave with a fixed PR interval. This is *sinus tachycardia*. The PR interval (0.09 second) is normal considering the age of the child.

Sinus tachycardia needs to be kept in the differential of *all* supraventricular tachycardias. Although usually easy to rec-

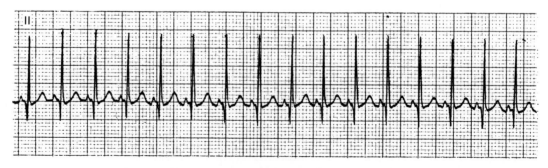

Figure 16B-1.   Narrow complex tachyarrhythmia from an asymptomatic 6 year old child.

ognize (by the presence of an upright P wave in lead II), diagnosis may become difficult with rapid rates, as the P wave may be hidden by the preceding T wave. Clinically, the principal concern in evaluating a patient with sinus tachycardia is to determine its cause (i.e., hyperthyroidism, illness, or exercise), and to correct this if at all possible.

A helpful differential point in the evaluation of supraventricular tachyarrhythmias in adults* is that *sinus tachycardia usually does NOT exceed 150-160 beats/min in a supine patient* (i.e., in an adult who is not exercising).

*All bets are off in children, for whom much faster rates (of up to 200 beats/min or more) may be recorded during sinus tachycardia. (See Chapter 17.)

PROBLEM   **Figure 16B-2A is from a middle-aged adult on digitalis. *What is going on?***

ANSWER TO FIGURE 16B-2A   The rhythm is regular with a ventricular rate of about 115 beats/min. P waves outnumber QRS complexes by two to one, making the atrial rate about 230 beats/min. The QRS complex is narrow, implying a supraventricular mechanism, and each QRS complex is preceded by a P wave with a constant PR interval. Thus P waves *are* related to the QRS complexes, albeit only one of every two P waves is conducted to the ventricles. This is *atrial tachycardia* with *2:1 AV block.*

The finding of atrial tachycardia with AV block in a patient on digitalis should prompt the emergency care provider to highly suspect *digitalis toxicity.* Clinically, the reason it is im-

portant to know if digitalis toxicity is present is because this would entail withholding the drug, whereas treatment of atrial tachycardia not due to digitalis toxicity often consists of *administering* the drug!

Treatment of atrial tachycardia with block also entails correction of accompanying electrolyte disturbances (hypokalemia, hypomagnesemia) that might exacerbate the effect of digitalis toxicity. However, hypokalemia in particular must not be corrected too rapidly because doing so may temporarily worsen the degree of AV block.

PROBLEM   **Examine *Figure 16B-2B*. What clinical condition is suggested by this tracing? *Why?***

ANSWER TO FIGURE 16B-2B   The underlying rhythm is *atrial tachycardia* at a rate of 220 beats/min. *High-grade* (or *high-degree*) *block* is present, since only a small number of atrial impulses are conducted to the ventricles. In addition, there is evidence of *ventricular irritability* (i.e., PVCs). The *combination* of these findings (atrial tachycardia, high-grade AV block, and PVCs) is almost pathognomonic for **digitalis toxicity.**

Differentiating Between Atrial Flutter and Atrial Tachycardia with Block

At times it may be extremely difficult to differentiate between atrial flutter and atrial tachycardia with 2:1 AV block. Again, the clinical importance of making this distinction is that one condition (atrial flutter) is often treated with digitalis, whereas the other (atrial tachycardia with block) is usually treated by *withdrawal* of the drug.

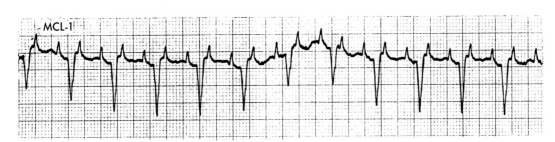

Figure 16B-2A.   Rhythm strip obtained from a middle-aged adult on digitalis.

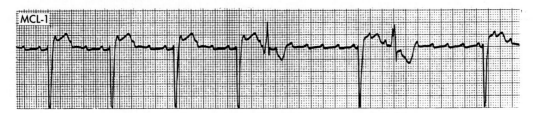

Figure 16B-2B.   *What clinical condition is suggested by this arrhythmia?*

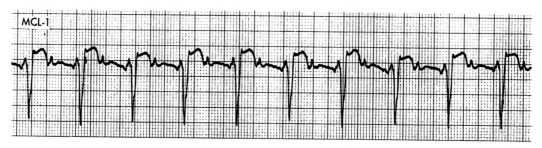

Figure 16B-3A. *Is this arrhythmia likely to be atrial tachycardia with block, atrial flutter, or neither?*

Atrial flutter is characterized electrocardiographically by a sawtooth pattern with an atrial rate of between 250 and 350 beats/min *in the untreated adult.* As emphasized in Section B of Chapter 3, the most common ventricular response to untreated atrial flutter is 2:1 AV conduction (in which the ventricular rate is between 140 and 160 beats/min). Less commonly there may be 4:1 AV conduction (ventricular response ≈ 70-75 beats/min) or variable ventricular conduction. Odd AV conduction ratios (such as 3:1 or 5:1) are rare. The principal exception to the rate parameters cited above is if the patient is being treated with a type I antiarrhythmic agent (quinidine, procainamide, disopyramide) or verapamil, in which case the atrial rate of flutter may *decrease* (and a correspondingly slower ventricular response may be seen). Otherwise, identification of regular atrial activity at a rate of close to 300 beats/min is almost invariably the result of atrial flutter.

The atrial rate with **atrial tachycardia** tends to be slower than for untreated atrial flutter (150-240 beats/min). Electrocardiographically, P waves may or may not be upright in lead II (depending on the site of atrial automaticity). At times (and especially with digitalis toxicity), *both* P wave morphology *and* the atrial rate may vary, whereas these are almost invariably constant for atrial flutter (since flutter is believed to be due to reentry within a *fixed* atrial reentrant circuit). In addition, the *baseline* between P waves tends to be *isoelectric* with atrial tachycardia in contrast to the sawtooth pattern of flutter. Although 2:1 AV conduction is common, any conduction ratio may be present (as was the case for Fig. 16B-2B).

PROBLEM **Examine the arrhythmia shown in *Figure 16B-3A*. Is this likely to be atrial tachycardia with block, atrial flutter, or neither? *Why?***

ANSWER TO FIGURE 16B-3A The rhythm is regular at a rate of about 85 beats/min. There is 2:1 AV

conduction (although this may *not* be readily apparent on initial inspection).

If you had difficulty identifying two P waves for each QRS complex in this tracing, try the following. Set your calipers at *exactly* half of the R-R interval defined by consecutive QRS complexes. Then position the calipers on the point of the P wave that *is* clearly seen (it occurs right after the T wave). The next advance of the calipers will land on the upstroke of the r wave, and this is the other P wave *(Figure 16B-3B)*. Thus, although the QRS complex may appear to be wide in this tracing, it is really of normal duration because the initial positive deflection (that simulates an r wave) is actually a P wave.

Although the atrial rate for the arrhythmia shown in Fig. 16B-3A is *much slower* than one usually sees with flutter, the baseline is *not* isoelectric as one would expect for atrial tachycardia (as it was for Figs. 16B-2A and 16B-2B). As a result, it would *not* be possible to definitively determine the etiology of this arrhythmia from inspection of Fig. 16B-3A alone. In this particular case, it turned out that the patient was in *atrial flutter,* and that the atrial rate had been much faster before long-term treatment with quinidine, digitalis, and verapamil was begun.

Type I antiarrhythmic agents (quinidine, procainamide, disopyramide) should *never* be given to patients in atrial flutter who have not already been digitalized. This is because, in addition to slowing the atrial rate of flutter (decreased atrial automaticity), these agents may also improve AV nodal conduction. Thus a patient who was only able to conduct every other atrial impulse when the rate of flutter was 300/min (2:1 conduction = ventricular response of 150/min) may now be able to conduct 1:1 if the atrial rate is slowed to 200/min (= ventricular response of 200/min). Having digitalis on

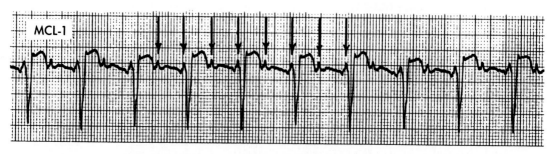

Figure 16B-3B. Arrows indicate that there are two P waves for every QRS complex, with the second P wave simulating an initial positive deflection (r wave) in the QRS complex.

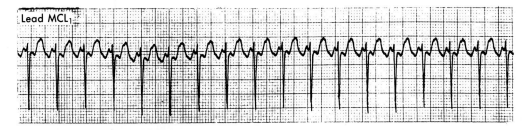

Figure 16B-4A.   Supraventricular tachyarrhythmia. *What is the diagnosis?*

board prevents such increases in the ventricular response from occurring when the type I drug is added.

The clinical dilemma that may sometimes arise is that posed by the situation seen in Fig. 16B-3B—*Is the 2:1 AV conduction the result of atrial flutter (with the atrial rate being slowed by antiarrythmic therapy) or atrial tachycardia with block (as a result of digitalis toxicity)?* Obtaining a serum digoxin level (to rule out the possibility of digitalis toxicity) may help resolve the problem.

PROBLEM   Interpret the supraventricular tachyarrhythmia shown in *Figure 16B-4A.*

ANSWER TO FIGURE 16B-4A   The QRS complex of this tachyarrhythmia is narrow and regular at a rate of about 150 beats/min. *One must therefore be suspicious of atrial flutter with 2:1 AV conduction.* Setting a pair of calipers at precisely *half* the ventricular rate (i.e., half the R-R interval) allows one to walk out atrial activity (the negative deflections) at a rate of 300 beats/min *(Figure 16B-4B)*. A vagal maneuver could be performed if further confirmation was needed.

In our experience, atrial flutter remains one of the most commonly overlooked diagnoses in all of medicine! Unless a high index of suspicion is constantly maintained for the possibility of flutter, the diagnosis will continue to be missed.

> *Always suspect atrial flutter until proven otherwise whenever there is a regular, supraventricular tachycardia at a rate of about 150 beats/min*—especially if normal atrial activity cannot be identified.

As is the case for ventricular fibrillation, atrial flutter may be "set off" by a premature impulse if it arrives at an opportune time during the vulnerable period of repolarization. Consider the interesting tracing shown in *Figure 16B-5.*

After 5 sinus beats, flutter waves suddenly appear (the first one peaks the T wave of the fifth QRS complex).

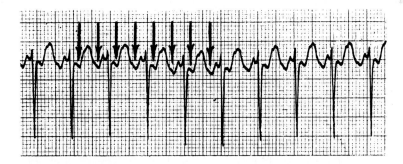

Figure 16B-4B.   Blow-up picture of the regular, supraventricular tachyarrhythmia shown in Fig. 16B-4A. Arrows indicate regular flutter activity at a rate of 300 beats/minute.

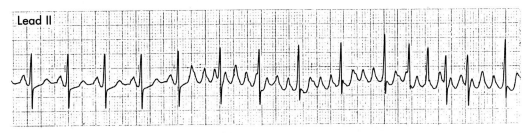

Figure 16B-5.   Precipitation of atrial flutter by the occurrence of a PAC that spikes the T wave of the fifth beat.

Initially 4:1 AV conduction is present, but toward the end of the tracing the ventricular response becomes variable. This particular patient continued to go in and out of atrial flutter numerous times despite intensive medical therapy.

PROBLEM   **Return to the regular supraventricular tachyarrhythmia shown in Fig. 16B-4A. A short while later this patient was observed to be in the rhythm below (Figure 16B-6). What has happened?**

ANSWER TO FIGURE 16B-6   The regular notching that was seen in the baseline of Figure 16B-4A has disappeared, and the rhythm has become ever so slightly irregular. Whether this still represents atrial flutter (now with a somewhat variable ventricular response—in which flutter activity produces a "pseudo-r′ deflection," and also peaks the T wave), or whether the patient has developed atrial fibrillation (with coarse fib waves) is not completely clear.

> Although the rhythm in Figure 16B-6 still looks regular, *it isn't!* If you missed this—go back and *carefully* measure the R-R interval with calipers.

PROBLEM   **Figure 16B-7 was obtained from another patient who was known to be in atrial flutter. What is unusual about this example of atrial flutter?**

ANSWER TO FIGURE 16B-7   The ventricular response is regular at a rate of about 85 beats/min. Three P waves are seen for each QRS complex (i.e., there is 3:1 AV conduction). Thus, the atrial rate of the flutter activity is about 255 beats/min (i.e., 85 × 3 = 255). *It is distinctly unusual for atrial flutter to conduct with an odd conduction ratio.*

> Two additional points may be made about this tracing. First, despite the nearly isoelectic baseline between atrial activity, this rhythm does not represent atrial tachycardia with block. The atrial rate of atrial tachycardia is almost always slower than that shown here (i.e., *less* than 250 beats/min).
>
> Second, despite the abundance of P waves in this tracing, there is definite evidence that some atrial activity *is* being conducted. That is, the PR interval preceding each QRS complex *is* constant. Of academic interest is the fact that the flutter wave closest to the QRS complex is rarely the one that is conducted (since concealed conduction usually delays transmission of atrial impulses to the AV node).

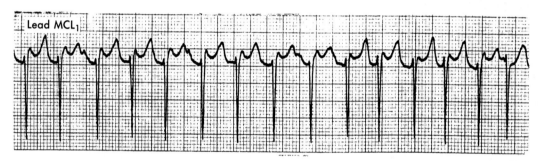

Figure 16B-6.   Follow-up tracing to the rhythm shown in Fig. 16B-4A. *What has happened?*

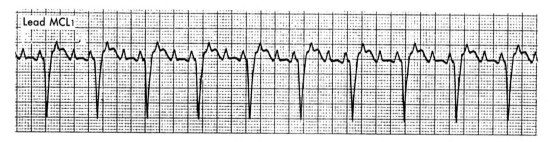

Figure 16B-7.   *What is unusual about this example of atrial flutter?*

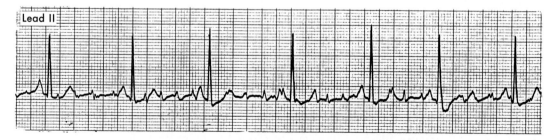

Figure 16B-8A.   Atrial flutter. *Or is this atrial flutter?*

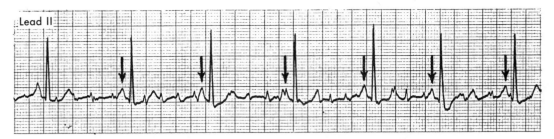

Figure 16B-8B. Arrows indicate the presence of normal, sinus conducted activity (in the form of upright P waves) that is *unaffected* by the smaller irregularly occurring upright deflections.

PROBLEM *Figure 16B-8A illustrates a final example of atrial flutter. Or does it???*

ANSWER TO FIGURE 16B-8A Although at first glance the rhythm again appears to be atrial flutter, this is *not* the case. Use of calipers demonstrates that the upright deflections between QRS complexes are definitely not regular. This makes it exceedingly unlikely that these deflections represent flutter activity, since atrial flutter is almost always a regular rhythm.

The answer is forthcoming in *Figure 16B-8B,* in which arrows indicate the presence of normal sinus-conducted P waves (that are upright with a constant PR interval in this lead II) before each QRS complex. The fact that these sinus P waves are *unaffected* by the smaller, irregularly occurring upright deflections proves that these smaller deflections are the result of *artifact*. The patient in this case had Parkinson's disease, which characteristically produces a tremor at a frequency that approximates the rate of atrial flutter.

Atrial Fibrillation

There often seems to be a reluctance to diagnose atrial fibrillation. This may be because the entity is diagnosed on the basis of *negative* findings (the absence of atrial activity) rather than positive ones. The issue can be simplified by remembering the following: *If the rhythm in question is irregularly irregular and atrial activity is absent, the diagnosis is atrial fibrillation.* Fine (or coarse) undulations may be noted in the baseline (i.e., *"fib"* waves), but no consistent P wave deflections will be seen.

The diagnosis of atrial fibrillation is most easily overlooked when the ventricular response is rapid. The tendency is to assume that the rhythm is regular and diagnose PSVT. As mentioned previously, the clinical importance of differentiating between these two rhythms is that treatment may differ. Although digoxin and verapamil are often effective for treatment of either arrhythmia, many clinicians prefer to use verapamil for PSVT and digoxin for atrial fibrillation. Adenosine is highly effective for PSVT, but it is ineffective treatment of atrial fibrillation (since adenosine is only effective in reentry tachyarrhythmias).

PROBLEM **Apply these concepts to evaluate the supraventricular tachyarrhythmia shown in *Figure 16B-9. Would adenosine be likely to convert this arrhythmia?***

ANSWER TO FIGURE 16B-9 Use of calipers demonstrates an ever so slight (but definite) irregular irregularity to the rhythm. Atrial activity is absent. The diagnosis is therefore *atrial fibrillation,* in this case with a *rapid ventricular response.* Adenosine is unlikely to be effective in converting this arrhythmia to sinus rhythm.

Although adenosine will not be effective in converting a supraventricular tachyarrhythmia such as atrial fibrillation (that is not dependent on a reentry mechanism), it is still sometimes used as a diagnostic maneuver. That is, adenosine will *temporarily* slow the ventricular response which may allow definitive diagnosis by revealing underlying atrial activity. Because of the very short half-life of the drug, the tachyarrhythmia usually resumes within a minute.

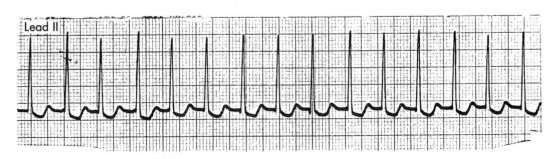

Figure 16B-9. *Would adenosine be likely to convert this supraventricular tachyarrhythmia?*

Three special situations should be kept in mind with respect to atrial fibrillation. We present two of them now, and save the third for later in this chapter.

PROBLEM   Examine the rhythm shown in *Figure 16B-10*. What two clinical conditions might produce this arrhythmia?

ANSWER TO FIGURE 16B-10   The rhythm is irregularly irregular and the ventricular response is slow (between 35 and 55 beats/min). Rapid flutter waves are noted early on, but become less well defined toward the end of the tracing (i.e., atrial *"flutter-fibrillation"*).

> Although some clinicians question whether atrial fibrillation and flutter can coexist, we feel use of this term is justified because it provides the best way to describe the pattern of atrial activity seen in Fig. 16B-10. Clinically, this arrhythmia behaves the same as atrial fibrillation.

The two clinical conditions that are commonly associated with atrial fibrillation and a slow ventricular response are *sick sinus syndrome* and *digitalis toxicity*.

PROBLEM   The second special situation to keep in mind with atrial fibrillation is shown in *Figure 16B-11*. This tracing was obtained after treatment of the patient whose rhythm was shown in Fig. 16B-9.

ANSWER TO FIGURE 16B-11   Although there are fine undulations in the baseline, no consistent atrial activity is seen. The rhythm becomes regular after the third beat. Considering that this patient was previously in atrial fibrillation with a *rapid* ventricular response (Fig. 16B-9)

and was treated (presumably with digoxin), there is now *"regularization"* of the atrial fibrillation. This should strongly suggest digitalis toxicity. The mechanism responsible for regularization of atrial fibrillation is AV block (from excess digitalis) with resultant escape of a regular and slightly accelerated junctional pacemaker (at a rate of 75 beats/min).

Digitalis Toxicity

Even today, digitalis toxicity is one of the most common iatrogenic illnesses that results in admission to the hospital. The disorder may present with anorexia, nausea, vomiting, headache, fatigue, depression, confusion, visual disturbances (especially of color vision), or cardiac arrhythmias. Although anorexia and nausea are usually the first signs, cardiac arrhythmias may sometimes be the *only* manifestation. While almost any cardiac arrhythmia can be seen with digitalis toxicity, those listed in *Table 16B-1* are particularly suggestive of the disorder when they occur in a patient taking the drug.

> Note that we have already seen four arrhythmias in this section that are highly suggestive of digitalis toxicity (Figs. 16B-2A, 16B-2B, 16B-10, and 16B-11). *More will follow before the end of this chapter.*

PROBLEM   The tachyarrhythmia shown in *Figure 16B-12* is also irregularly irregular. *Is this atrial fibrillation?*

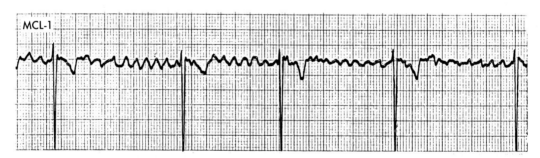

Figure 16B-10.   *What two clinical conditions might produce this arrhythmia?*

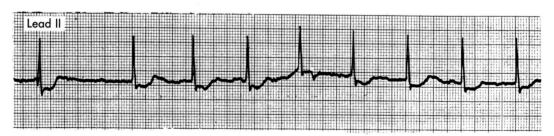

Figure 16B-11.   Rhythm strip obtained after treatment of the arrhythmia shown in Fig. 16B-9.

Table 16B-1

Cardiac Arrhythmias Commonly Associated with Digitalis Toxicity*

• Inappropriate sinus bradycardia
• Sinus pauses or sinus arrest
• Sinoatrial block
• 1° AV block
• 2° AV block, Mobitz type I (Wenckebach)
• Wenckebach-type block with atrial fibrillation or flutter
• Atrial tachycardia with block*
• Atrial fibrillation if there is:
  • a slow ventricular response (<60 beats/min)
  • *regularization* of the ventricular response*
• Accelerated junctional escape rhythms or junctional tachycardia*
• Increased ventricular ectopy, especially if there is:
  • ventricular bigeminy
  • multiform PVCs

*Especially suggestive of digitalis toxicity.

ANSWER TO FIGURE 16B-12   Although the rhythm is irregularly irregular, this is *not* atrial fibrillation because there is evidence of atrial activity. Definite P waves precede each QRS complex. Most of these P waves are positive (with either a pointed or notched configuration), but some are biphasic. P wave morphology constantly varies, and no predominant form is noted. The rhythm is *multifocal atrial tachycardia (MAT)* or *chaotic atrial mechanism.*

Multifocal Atrial Tachycardia (MAT)

MAT is most often seen in patients with chronic obstructive pulmonary disease (COPD). It is important clinically to distinguish this arrhythmia from atrial fibrillation,

since prognosis and treatment of the two conditions differs dramatically. With rapid atrial fibrillation, digitalization constitutes a medical treatment of choice. In otherwise uncomplicated cases (that is, in the absence of acute myocardial infarction, hypoxemia, hyperthyroidism, and hypokalemia), the ventricular response is often used to gauge the amount of IV digoxin that is adminstered. Following an initial loading dose of between 0.5 and 0.75 mg of digoxin, increments of 0.125 to 0.25 mg can be given every few hours until the ventricular response is under control.

In contrast, treatment of MAT *must* be directed at correcting the underlying cause of the arrhythmia (most often hypoxemia). MAT is notoriously resistant to treatment with digoxin. It is easy to imagine what might therefore happen if one fails to recognize this arrhythmia and embarks on a course of vigorous digitalization. Not surprisingly, digitalis toxicity is a leading cause of morbidity and mortality in patients with MAT. The serious nature of MAT is evident from the extremely high mortality rate of 30-50% during the hospital stay in which the disorder is first diagnosed (Kastor, 1990).

The key to diagnosing MAT is to be aware of the settings in which it most frequently occurs (patients with COPD and hypoxia, or occasionally in extremely ill ICU patients). It is definitely more common in older patients (average age 70 years), although the rhythm can also occur in extremely ill children (Kastor, 1990). One may need to look especially hard (in as many monitoring leads as possible) for atrial activity should any of the above individuals present with an irregularly irregular rhythm.

P waves in MAT frequently manifest the pattern of *P-pulmonale* (tall and peaked in the inferior leads), suggesting right atrial enlargement. This is to be expected, considering that most patients with the rhythm have underlying COPD. For example, note how tall and pointed many of the P waves are in the lead II shown below (Fig. 16B-12).

MAT is a rapid rhythm. By definition (i.e., multifocal atrial "tachycardia"), the heart rate *exceeds* 100 beats/min. However, in many cases the overall rate of the rhythm will be less than 120 beats/min, and not demanding of antiarrhythmic therapy per se. If rate control is needed, verapamil is the drug of choice (with or without calcium pretreatment).* Small doses of di-

---

*The beneficial effect of verapamil with MAT is the result of decreasing the *number* of atrial ectopic impulses, and *not* from AV nodal blocking of their conduction (Levine et al, 1985).

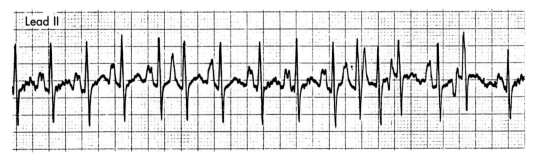

Figure 16B-12.   *Is this irregularly irregular tachyarrhythmia atrial fibrillation?*

goxin can be used (and may exert a synergistic effect with verapamil), but digoxin *must* not be "pushed" until rate control is achieved as it might if atrial fibrillation were present. Ideal treatment of MAT consists of optimizing the patient's underlying medical condition (correcting hypoxemia, treatment of sepsis, shock, pneumonia, etc.) and special attention directed toward normalization of serum electrolyte status (hypokalemia, and especially hypomagnesemia). Administration of IV magnesium may occasionally be helpful even when serum magnesium levels are normal (Kastor, 1990).

A final therapeutic option to consider for MAT is the use of IV β-blockers (i.e., propranolol, esmolol, metoprolol). Although there is justifiable concern in using these agents in patients with significant bronchospasm, their efficacy in suppressing ectopic foci, controlling the ventricular response, and blocking excessive sympathetic tone would seem to make them ideal drugs for treatment of those patients with MAT who do not have pulmonary disease or significant heart failure (Kastor, 1990).

A question that frequently arises is how to differentiate between sinus rhythm with frequent PACs and MAT? Consider the example shown in *Figure 16B-13*.

As was the case for Fig. 16B-12, the rhythm here is irregularly irregular and P waves precede virtually every QRS complex. However, despite the irregularity, the *underlying mechanism* of the arrhythmia appears to be *sinus* (since similar-appearing P waves with a constant PR interval precede beats #1, #2, #5, #6, #7, #9, #10, #14, and #15). This differs from Fig. 16B-12 in which no predominant P wave form was noted.

> Admittedly, distinction between MAT and sinus rhythm with frequent PACs becomes exceedingly difficult at times.

Fortunately, such distinction is mainly of academic interest since clinical behavior of these two arrhythmias is usually similar.

PROBLEM **The woman whose rhythm is shown in *Figure 16B-14* was coughing at the time this tracing was recorded. *Should she be immediately cardioverted?***

ANSWER TO FIGURE 16B-14 Although at first glance this tracing may prompt concern, close inspection reveals baseline aberration with spurious-looking complexes at a rate of *over* 300 beats/min!!! No real tachyarrhythmia has a ventricular rate this fast in adults. The *artifact* totally disappeared as soon as the patient stopped coughing.

PROBLEM **The tachyarrhythmia shown in *Figure 16B-15* is from a middle-aged woman who presented to the emergency department with the sudden onset of palpitations. What is the rhythm? *What is the likely mechanism of the arrhythmia?***

HINT: Is there evidence of atrial activity?

ANSWER TO FIGURE 16B-15 A precisely regular supraventricular tachyarrhythmia at a rate of 180 beats/min is seen. Normal atrial activity is absent. The differential includes:

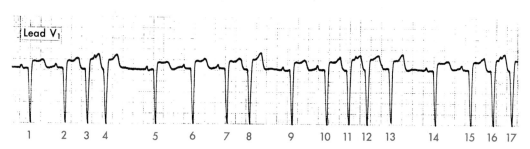

Figure 16B-13. Irregular rhythm. *Is this MAT or sinus rhythm with frequent PACs?*

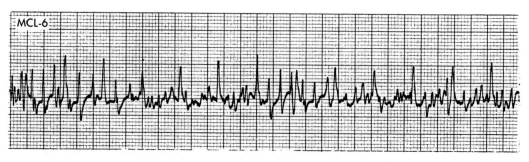

Figure 16B-14. This tracing was obtained from a patient who was coughing. *Should she be immediately cardioverted?*

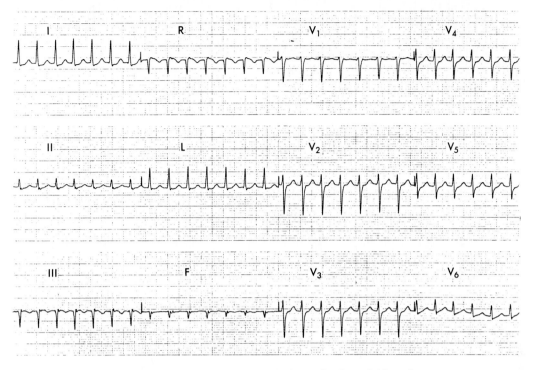

Figure 16B-15. What is the likely mechanism of this tachy-arrhythmia? *Is there evidence of atrial activity?*

i. Sinus tachycardia (unlikely at this heart rate)
ii. Atrial flutter (unlikely because the ventricular response is faster than one expects to see with flutter, and there is no hint of a sawtooth pattern anywhere)
iii. Atrial fibrillation (ruled out by the precise regularity of the rhythm)
iv. PSVT (the most likely diagnosis by the process of elimination).

Paroxysmal Supraventricular Tachycardia (PSVT)

Confirmation of the clinical impression that the rhythm shown in Fig. 16B-15 is PSVT might be forthcoming from application of a vagal maneuver (Valsalva or carotid sinus massage). If the rhythm were sinus tachycardia or atrial flutter, one would expect the ventricular response to slow and atrial activity to emerge. If on the other hand the rhythm was PSVT, CSM would be expected to either convert the tachyarrhythmia to sinus rhythm, or have no effect at all (See Table 16A-1).

CSM had absolutely no effect. The patient was sedated, and on the presumption that the rhythm was PSVT, 5 mg of IV *verapamil* was administered (slowly over a 2-minute period).

In the event that the patient is hemodynamically stable (as will usually be the case for supraventricular tachyarrhythmias), a real benefit may be derived from **sedation.** In addition to relieving the anxiety that so commonly accompanies these tachyarrhythmias, sedation will often reduce *sympathetic* tone.

Enhanced sympathetic tone frequently plays an important role in perpetuating PSVT because it shortens the refractory period of AV nodal tissue and speeds conduction through the area. It also attenuates the effects of the vagus nerve on AV conduction, so that a greater degree of vagal tone may be needed to terminate the arrhythmia (Wasman et al, 1980).

PROBLEM **Over the next 20 minutes the rhythms shown sequentially in *Figures 16B-16A, -16B, -16C, and -16D* were observed. *What has happened?***

ANSWER TO FIGURES 16B-16A, -16B, -16C, and -16D The rate of the tachyarrhythmia progressively decreases until conversion to a sinus mechanism (at a rate of 115 beats/min) finally occurs (Fig. 16B-16D). The heart rate is 180 beats/min in 16B-16A, 145 beats/min in 16B-16B, and 135 beats/min in 16B-16C.

As opposed to vagal maneuvers that tend to convert PSVT in a more abrupt manner (if they work), verapamil typically produces a gradual slowing of the ventricular response until a sinus mechanism is restored (Feigl and Ravid, 1979). This is thought to be due to a verapamil-induced progressive slowing of conduction in the pathway contained within the reentry circuit. Occasionally the rhythm may become slightly irregular (with *alternation* of long and short cycle lengths) prior to termination of the tachycardia. At termination, one or more PVCs are sometimes seen before resumption of sinus rhythm.

Figure 16B-17 is taken from a patient whose PSVT was terminated by CSM. During the 10 beats of PSVT that begin this tracing, a minimal irregularity develops. Then comes a fusion beat with 2 PVCs, followed by a 1-second pause, a sinus beat, 2 more PVCs, and resumption of sinus rhythm.

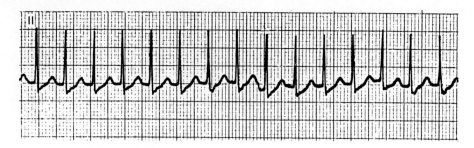

Figure 16B-16A. First in a series of sequential tracings observed after sedation and treatment with IV verapamil. *What happens in Figs. 16B-16B, -16C, and -16D?*

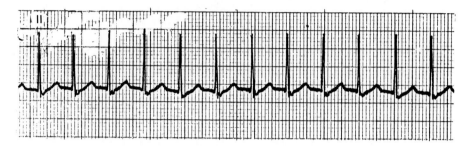

Figure 16B-16B. Second sequential tracing in the series.

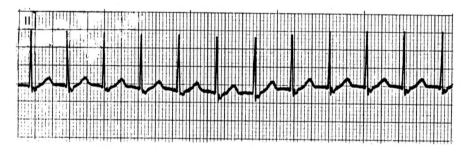

Figure 16B-16C. Third sequential tracing in the series.

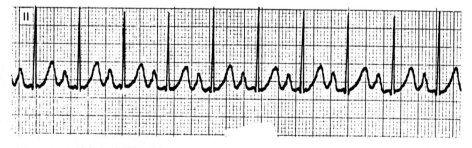

Figure 16B-16D. Fourth sequential tracing in the series.

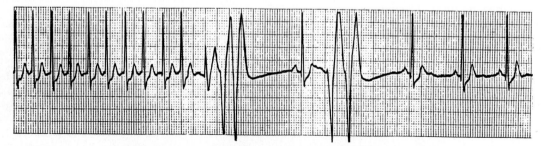

Figure 16B-17. Termination of PSVT by CSM. Ventricular ectopy and a brief pause are seen before resumption of sinus rhythm.

PROBLEM   **Return to the case of the middle-aged woman who presented with the tachyarrhythmia shown in Fig. 16B-15. Now that she has been converted to normal sinus rhythm (Fig. 16B-16D),** *what should you do next?* **Why?**

ANSWER   Obtain a post-conversion 12-lead ECG *(Figure 16B-18)*. Reasons for always obtaining a post-conversion 12-lead ECG include:

  i. To verify (document) the return of normal sinus rhythm
 ii. To look for evidence of an accessory pathway (i.e., WPW)
iii. To rule out ischemia or acute infarction (realizing that T wave inversion on a post-conversion tracing may occasionally be seen simply as an "after-effect" of the rapid rate of the tachycardia)
 iv. To look for *retrospective* clues to the mechanism of the tachyarrhythmia.

In this particular case, note the return of normal upright P waves in lead II of the post-conversion tracing. There is no evidence of WPW (i.e., no delta waves), and no evidence of ischemia or acute infarction. Some of the ST segment depression that had been seen in the lateral leads during the tachycardia (on Fig. 16B-15) was apparently *rate-related*, since it is no longer present on this post-conversion tracing.

MECHANISMS OF SUPRAVENTRICULAR TACHYCARDIAS

There are two principal mechanisms of supraventricular tachycardias: (1) increased automaticity, and (2) reentry. With ***increased automaticity,*** an automatic atrial focus begins to discharge rapidly on its own and usurps the pacemaking function from the SA node. This is the usual mechanism of atrial tachycardia that results from digitalis toxicity. Because the AV node is not involved in perpetuation of the arrhythmia, therapeutic measures designed to decrease AV nodal conduction will not terminate the tachycardia (although they may slow the ventricular response and/or increase the degree of AV block). Instead, treatment of atrial tachycardia must be directed toward correcting the underlying cause of the increased atrial automaticity (i.e., withholding digitalis).

Reentry is the other major mechanism of supraventricular tachycardia. Reentry may occur in a number of sites including the SA node, the atria, the AV node, and between the atria and ventricles via an accessory pathway. Sinoatrial reentry and intra-atrial reentry are both difficult to recognize electrocardiographically (without the benefit of electrophysiologic study), as well as being distinctly uncommon in adults. As a result, we do not address them further in our discussion.

Practically speaking, reentry involving the AV node is *by far* the most common mechanism of supraventricular tachycardia that the emergency care provider will encounter in adults.

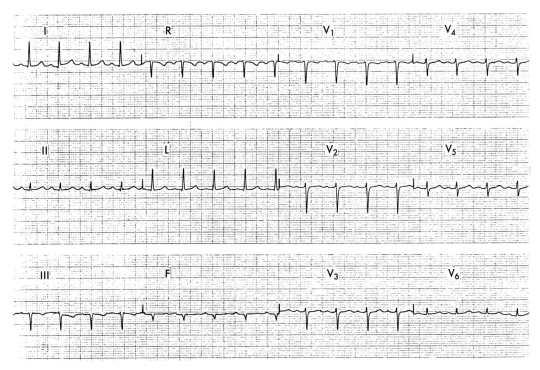

Figure 16B-18.   Post-conversion 12-lead ECG obtained from the patient who presented with the tachyarrhythmia shown in Fig. 16B-15.

The Mechanism of Reentry

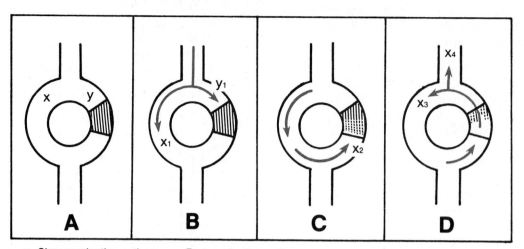

x–Slow conduction pathway   y–Fast conduction pathway

Figure 16B-19A.   Theoretical illustration of a reentry circuit. The three necessary components are: (1) two separate pathways (labeled **x** and **y**); (2) unidirectional block in one of these pathways (represented by the lined area in pathway **y**); and (3) slow conduction along the other pathway.

Three conditions must be present for there to be a reentry circuit:

i. The existence of *two separate pathways* that join to form a closed circuit
ii. Unidirectional block in one of these pathways
iii. Slow conduction along the unblocked pathway

These conditions are illustrated in *Figure 16B-19A.* The two pathways are **x** and **y,** and they meet to form a closed loop (Panel A in Figure). Conduction is slowed down pathway **x.**

A zone of *unidirectional* block exists along pathway **y** (lined area in the Figure).

When an impulse reaches the circuit, it begins to travel down both pathways. Because of the area of block along the faster pathway, conduction of the impulse is unable to complete the circuit (it is stopped at point y_1 in Panel B). However, conduction of the impulse continues along the unblocked pathway (point x_1 in Panel B). In order for the reentry circuit to be established, conduction must be *slow enough* along pathway **x** for the zone of block to have recovered its ability to conduct by the time the impulse labeled x_2 arrives (Panel C). If this

Reentry in PSVT

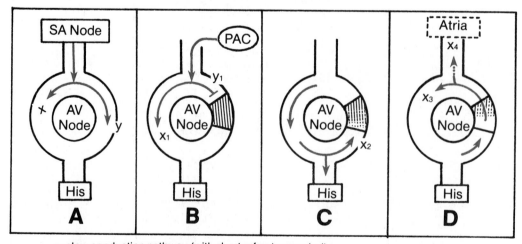

x–slow conduction pathway (with short refractory period)
y–fast conduction pathway (with long refractory period)

Figure 16B-19B.   The theoretical illustration of a reentry circuit that was shown in Fig. 16B-19A is felt to apply to conditions existing at the AV node.

is the case, the impulse can be conducted through this zone, after which it is able to begin traveling around the circuit again (point x_3 in Panel D). Along the way, it may give off a retrograde impulse (x_4 in Panel D).

The three conditions described above that are necessary for reentry are felt to exist at the level of the AV node *(Figure 16B-19B)*. Thus, conduction through the AV node is *not* homogeneous (via a single pathway) as one might imagine. Instead there appears to be a *longitudinal dissociation* of conduction fibers, which results in a functional division into two separate conduction pathways. One of these pathways has a long refractory period and conducts *rapidly* (**y** in Panel A of Fig. 16B-19B). The other has a short refractory period and conducts *slowly* (**x** in Panel A).

Under normal conditions (as one might expect), the impulse is transmitted to the bundle of His by conduction along the faster pathway (Panel A in Fig. 16B-19B).

In Panel B a premature impulse (PAC) occurs. Due to the relatively long refractory period of the fast pathway, the premature impulse is likely to find conduction still blocked down this route when it arrives at the AV node (i.e., it is unable to travel beyond point y_1 in Panel B). However, it is likely that the shorter refractory period of the slow pathway will be over, allowing conduction to proceed via this route toward the bundle of His (x_1 in Panel B).

If conditions are just right, conduction down the slow pathway will outlast the refractory period of the fast pathway. In this case, by the time the impulse reaches point x_2 (Panel C), the fast pathway will have recovered enough to allow *retrograde* conduction. The reentry loop may then be perpetuated if at the time the impulse reaches point x_3, it is able to be conducted again down the slow pathway (Panel D). Along the way an impulse may be conducted (returned) to the atria (Point x_4), producing a *retrograde* P wave on the electrocardiogram (an *echo* beat).

PROBLEM   **Consider the ECG shown in *Figure 16B-20*. Look closely at the QRS complex *during* the** tachycardia. **Is it different at all from the QRS complex during sinus rhythm (beats #1-3)?**

ANSWER TO FIGURE 16B-20   This tracing provides a nice example of how a laddergram may be used to illustrate the mechanism of an arrhythmia. Following three beats of sinus rhythm, a PAC occurs (notching the T wave that precedes beat #4). This first PAC conducts normally to the ventricles. However, a second PAC (that notches the T wave preceding beat #5) apparently sets up the conditions necessary for reentry to occur, and precipitates a run of PSVT at a rate of 180 beats/min.

Close scrutiny of the QRS complex *during* the tachycardia reveals that its appearance is *not* the same as during normal sinus rhythm (beats #1-3). Instead, a distinct notch is present during the tachycardia at the junction of the end of the QRS complex and the beginning of the ST segment (arrow). This notch is the result of retrograde conduction to the atria during the reentry tachycardia (and corresponds to point x_4 in Panel D of Fig. 16B-19B).

Several points may be made about this tracing. Note first how the reentry cycle is initiated by a PAC (corresponding to Panel B in Fig. 16B-19B). Note also that the PR interval of this PAC is *prolonged* compared to the PR interval of the normal sinus beats! This reflects the path of this impulse, which is being conducted down the *slow* pathway (corresponding to point x_1 in Panel B of Fig. 16B-19B). It is then conducted to the ventricles at the same time as it returns up the fast pathway (Panel C). Because conduction goes down the *slow* pathway and back up the fast pathway, this type of PSVT is known as the **slow-fast form.** It is by far the most common type in adults. (As we will see momentarily, there is also a *fast-slow* form of PSVT in which conduction first goes down the fast pathway and comes back up the slow pathway.)

ATRIAL ACTIVITY IN PSVT

The presence of atrial activity, its polarity, and its location relative to the QRS complex provide important clues to the mechanism of PSVT *(Figure 16B-21)*. With normal sinus

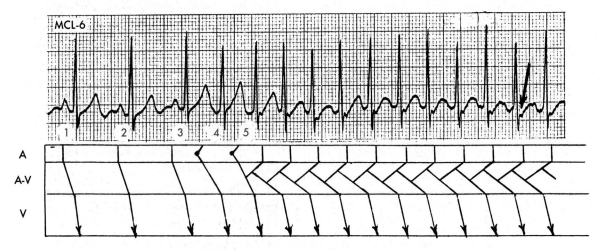

Figure 16B-20.   *Is there evidence of atrial activity during the supraventricular tachyarrhythmia that begins after beat #5?*

Atrial Activity in PSVT

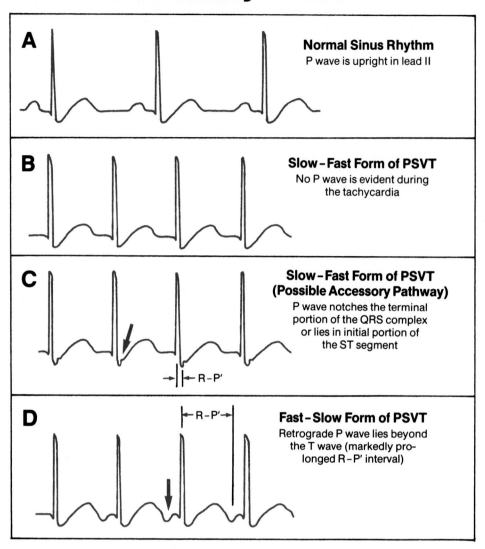

Figure 16B-21.   Atrial activity in PSVT.

rhythm, P waves will be upright in lead II (Panel A in this Figure). They will also be upright and normal in appearance with the uncommon reentry tachycardias in which the reentry circuit is contained within the SA node or the atria, since the impulse arises from the same location as it does for sinus rhythm.

In contrast, for PSVT involving the AV node, P waves will be inverted in lead II, reflecting the fact that they are being conducted in a retrograde manner. Most of the time with the *slow-fast* form of PSVT, the P wave is conducted so rapidly in the retrograde direction (since it is being conducted via the fast pathway) that it coincides with the QRS complex and is not visible on the surface ECG (Panel B). If retrograde conduction takes slightly longer, however, a retrograde P wave may be seen to notch the terminal portion of the QRS complex or the initial portion of the ST segment (Panel C). Patients with accessory pathways (WPW) may demonstrate this pattern when they develop PSVT that conducts down the normal pathway (via the AV node) and retrograde up the accessory pathway. Because the reentry circuit of patients with an accessory pathway is longer than that for patients whose reentry

circuit is contained entirely *within* the AV node, retrograde atrial conduction may be delayed long enough that the retrograde P wave notches the middle or terminal portion of the ST segment. Finally, with the *fast-slow* form of PSVT (i.e., conduction down the fast pathway and back up the slow pathway), retrograde atrial conduction will be delayed by the greatest degree. In this case, the RP′ interval* is significantly prolonged (and the inverted P wave occurs only *after* the T wave) due to the very long time required for retrograde conduction to occur over the slow pathway (Panel D).

PROBLEM   **Examine *Figure 16B-22A*. What type of PSVT is present?**

ANSWER TO FIGURE 16B-22A   This is the *fast-slow* form of PSVT. As indicated in the laddergram shown

---

*The ***RP′ interval*** refers to the interval from the R wave of the QRS complex until the electrocardiographic marker (P′) of retrograde atrial activity.

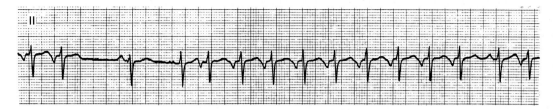

Figure 16B-22A.   *What type of PSVT is present?*

in Figure 16B-22B, beat #3 is sinus conducted. Beat #4 is conducted by a P wave with a different morphology (i.e., an ectopic P wave). Following this, the tachycardia begins. As can be seen, the RP′ interval is greatly prolonged, reflecting the *delay* in retrograde transmission of the impulse over the slow pathway.

> It is of interest that the tachycardia in Fig. 16B-22B is not only initiated by a PAC, but it is also terminated by a PAC (that produces a slight peak in the T wave of the third to last beat). Because of the reentry nature of the arrhythmia, premature impulses are likely to alter conduction properties of at least a portion of the reentry circuit and abruptly (i.e., *paroxysmally*) either initiate or terminate the cycle.

Clinically, the reason it may be important to differentiate between the fast-slow form of PSVT (seen in Fig. 16B-22A) and the much more common slow-fast form (seen in Fig. 16B-20) is the different response to therapy. In general, the less common fast-slow form of PSVT is much more difficult to treat. Although similar antiarrhythmic medications are used in long-term management, recurrences are often so frequent with the fast-slow form that this arrhythmia is sometimes called an "incessant" tachycardia.

> The "incessant" tachycardia (fast-slow form) of PSVT is seen much more often in children than in adults.

PROBLEM   **Return one last time to the case of the middle-aged woman whose presenting ECG was shown in Fig. 16B-15 (on page 565).** *Do you now see a clue on this tracing that suggests the mechanism of the arrhythmia?*

ANSWER   Review of the tachyarrhythmia shown in Fig. 16B-15 reveals that there *is* evidence of retrograde atrial activity during the tachycardia. Although admittedly subtle, a notch is present in the terminal portion of the QRS complex in leads II, III, and aVF on this tracing that is *not* present on the post-conversion tracing shown in Fig. 16B-18. This identification of retrograde atrial activity virtually confirms the reentry nature of the tachyarrhythmia, and supports the use of management measures predicated on interrupting AV nodal reentry (i.e., vagal maneuvers, adenosine, verapamil, digoxin, and/or β-blockers).

> Lest there be any doubt about the presence of retrograde atrial activity during the tachyarrhythmia shown in Fig. 16B-15, we provide blow-up pictures of several key leads from the 12-lead ECGs during the tachycardia and after conversion to normal sinus rhythm. Thus, *Figure 16B-23A* is a blow-up picture of leads II, III, aVL, and aVF from the post-conversion tracing shown previously in Fig. 16B-18. The arrow in lead II documents return of normal sinus activity. Similarly, *Figure 16B-23B* is a blow-up picture of these same four leads from the 12-lead tracing during the tachycardia (i.e., from Fig. 16B-15). Arrows in Fig. 16B-23B clearly demonstrate notching in the terminal portion of the QRS complex *during* the tachycardia that is *not* present in Fig. 16B-23A after conversion to sinus rhythm. This notching represents retrograde atrial activity.

Our reason for focusing on such subtle evidence of atrial activity during the run of PSVT is threefold:

i. It makes analyzing these tachyarrhythmias a much more interesting task.

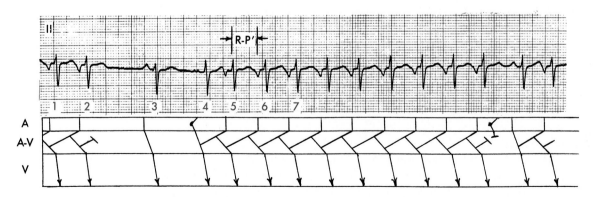

Figure 16B-22B.   Laddergram demonstrating a reentry tachycardia that is precipitated by an ectopic P wave (beat #4), and which manifests a prolonged R-P′ interval (suggestive of the fast-slow mechanism form of PSVT).

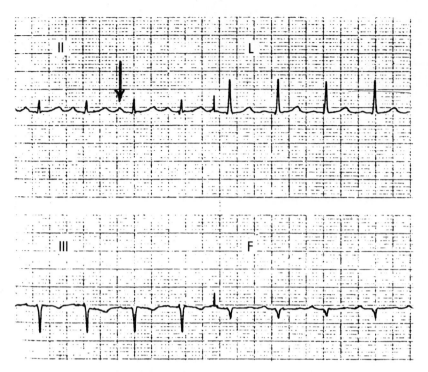

Figure 16B-23A. Blow-up picture of leads II, III, aVL, and aVF of the post-conversion tracing (shown in Fig. 16B-18). The arrow in lead II documents return of normal sinus activity.

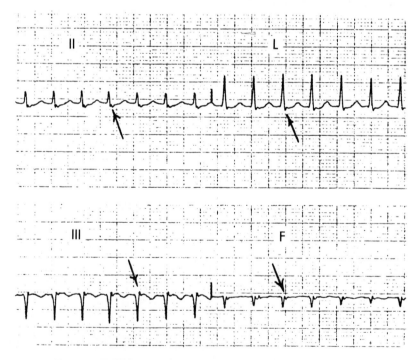

Figure 16B-23B. Blow-up picture of the same leads shown in Fig. 16B-23A, retrospectively demonstrating that notching (arrows) of the terminal portion of the QRS complex *during* the tachycardia (in Fig. 16B-15) is the result of retrograde atrial activity.

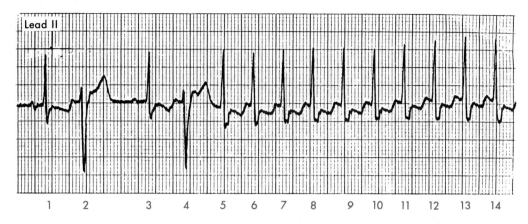

Figure 16B-24A. *Is there a clue to the mechanism of the run of PSVT (beats #5-14)?*

ii. Detection of retrograde atrial activity during the tachycardia provides an extremely helpful clue to the mechanism of the arrhythmia (and therefore to its likely response to therapy).

iii. As we will see in Section C of this chapter, the presence and location of retrograde atrial activity during the run of PSVT also provides a helpful clue to the likelihood of the existence of an accessory pathway.

PROBLEM **Try one final example of PSVT. Is there a clue to the mechanism of the run of PSVT (beats #5-14) in *Figure 16B-24A? Might the second PVC (beat #4) in this tracing be playing a role in initiation of the reentry tachycardia?***

HINT: Is there evidence of atrial activity associated with this second PVC?

HINT TO THE HINT: Is the T wave of the second PVC (the T wave of beat #4) different than the T wave of the first PVC (the T wave of beat #2)?

ANSWER TO FIGURE 16B-24A   The rhythm begins with a sinus-conducted beat (#1), followed by a PVC (beat #2), another sinus-conducted beat (#3), and a second PVC (#4)—after which the run of PSVT begins. Note that the S wave of the QRS complex *during* the tachycardia (beats #5-14) is *wider* than the S wave of the two sinus-conducted beats (#1 and #3). This S wave widening probably reflects *retrograde atrial activity* (back up the fast pathway), and suggests that beats #5-14 represent the slow-fast form of PSVT.

The laddergram shown in *Figure 16B-24B* provides insight to the onset of the tachycardia. Note the negative deflection that deforms the T wave of the second PVC, after which the run of PSVT begins. This negative deflection is probably the result of *retrograde* atrial conduction, which then initiates the reentry tachycardia.

Although far from being a simple tracing, Fig. 16B-24B illustrates that reentry tachycardia may be initiated by PVCs as well as by PACs.

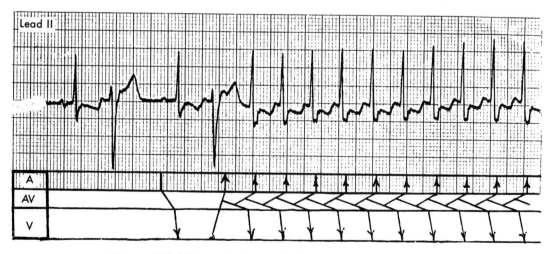

Figure 16B-24B. Laddergram of the arrhythmia shown in Fig. 16B-24A, suggesting that retrograde atrial conduction from the second PVC initiates the run of reentry tachycardia.

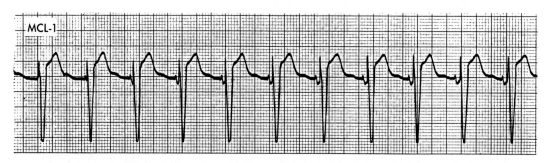

Figure 16B-25.   *What is the likely mechanism of this narrow complex arrhythmia?*

PROBLEM   **We conclude this section with the narrow complex arrhythmia shown in *Figure 16B-25*. What is the likely mechanism of this rhythm? *What clinical conditions are most commonly associated with this arrhythmia?***

ANSWER TO FIGURE 16B-25   The rhythm becomes regular after the first complex at a rate of 95 beats/min. The QRS is 0.10 second in duration, or at the upper limit of normal. Atrial activity is evident; however, the PR interval constantly varies! At least in the initial part of the tracing the PR interval is far too short to allow normal conduction. Therefore, *AV dissociation is present.* The underlying rhythm is *junctional tachycardia.* This rhythm most often occurs in the setting of digitalis toxicity, but it may also be seen in association with acute inferior infarction, or after open heart surgery.

The mechanism of junctional tachycardia is *increased automaticity.* Because retrograde block in the AV node is frequently seen with this arrhythmia, the SA node is able to continue firing at its own inherent rate. AV dissociation is the usual result. *The presence of AV dissociation per se effectively rules out any type of reentry tachycardia!*

Strictly speaking, it would be more correct to refer to the arrhythmia shown in Fig. 16B-25 as an *accelerated* junctional rhythm rather than junctional tachycardia since the heart rate is less than 100 beats/min. Clinical implications of an accelerated junctional rhythm and junctional tachycardia are the same.

References

Feigl D, Ravid M: Electrocardiographic observations on the termination of supraventricular tachycardia by verapamil, *J Electrocardiol* 12:129, 1979.

Hayes JJ, Stewart RB, Greene L, Bardy GH: Narrow QRS ventricular tachycardia, *Ann Intern Med* 114:460, 1991.

Kastor JA: Multifocal atrial tachycardia, *N Engl J Med* 322:1713, 1990.

Levine JH, Michael JR, Guarnieri T: Treatment of multifocal atrial tachycardia with verapamil, *N Engl J Med* 312:21, 1985.

WIDE COMPLEX TACHYARRHYTHMIAS: ADDITIONAL CONCEPTS

Since we covered recognition of wide complex tachyarrhythmias in depth in the previous chapter, we limit our discussion here to a few new concepts.

PROBLEM   *Figure 16C-1A shows a regular, wide complex tachycardia. What is the likely etiology of this arrhythmia? Would you expect it to be helpful to obtain the patient's old chart?*

ANSWER TO FIGURE 16C-1A   A regular tachyarrhythmia is seen at a rate of 140 beats/min. As noted, the QRS complex is widened. P waves appear to be present and *related* (by a fixed PR interval) to the QRS complex. However, atrial activity is *not* normal, since these P waves are *negative* in this lead II monitoring lead. Therefore the rhythm *cannot* be sinus tachycardia.

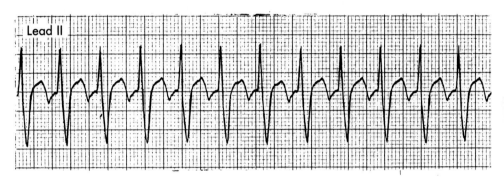

Figure 16C-1A.   *What is the likely etiology of this wide complex tachycardia?* The patient is hemodynamically stable.

Despite the suggestion of regular and related atrial activity, the presence of QRS widening should still raise the possibility of ventricular tachycardia. Obtaining this patient's old chart proved to be invaluable in this regard. In it were numerous 12-lead ECGs which documented an *identical* (widened) QRS morphology in lead II during sinus rhythm—*virtually proving that the rhythm shown in Fig. 16C-1A was supraventricular.* This narrowed down the diagnostic possibilities to three entities:

  i. PSVT (of the fast-slow type)
 ii. Junctional (or low atrial) tachycardia (with inverted P waves in this lead II)

iii. Atrial flutter (which should be most strongly considered in view of the heart rate that is close to 150 beats/min)

It would be difficult to distinguish between these three possibilities based on this tracing alone. Administration of a vagal maneuver increased the degree of AV block, and revealed the rhythm to be atrial flutter. The patient reverted to sinus rhythm following treatment *(Figure 16C-1B)*.

Note that the P wave is now upright (as it should be in lead II) in this post-conversion tracing. Note also that the QRS complex during sinus rhythm (in Fig. 16C-1B) is

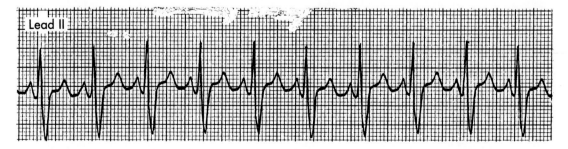

Figure 16C-1B.   Follow-up tracing to the wide complex tachyarrhythmia shown in Fig. 16C-1A. Sinus rhythm has been restored.

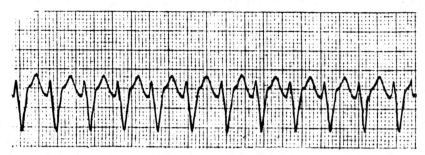

Figure 16C-2.   Rhythm strip obtained from an elderly lady with new-onset "fluttering" in her chest. *Should she be treated for PSVT?*

truly *identical* in appearance to the QRS complex during the tachycardia (in Fig. 16C-1A).

> It should be emphasized that recognizing the presence of a supraventricular tachyarrhythmia (such as atrial flutter) by itself does *not* rule out the possibility of coexistent ventricular tachycardia (Curtis and Grauer, 1990). Atrial tachycardia, atrial flutter, and atrial fibrillation may *all* occur concomitantly with ventricular tachycardia. Thus, the KEY for establishing the supraventricular nature of the arrhythmia shown in Fig. 16C-1A was obtaining the patient's old chart which contained numerous old ECGs with an identical (widened) QRS morphology.

PROBLEM   **The rhythm strip shown in *Figure 16C-2* is from an elderly lady with new-onset "flut-**

tering" in her chest. **She was not in distress, did not complain of chest pain, and had a blood pressure of 90/60 mm Hg at the time this tracing was recorded. Treatment for PSVT was begun.** *Do you agree*?

ANSWER TO FIGURE 16C-2   Despite minimal symptoms and the relatively normal appearance of the QRS complex, the *inescapable* fact is that *the QRS complex is wide* (at least 0.13 second in duration)! Moreover, atrial activity is absent. One must therefore consider the following 5 entities:

   i. Ventricular Tachycardia
  ii. VENTRICULAR TACHYCARDIA

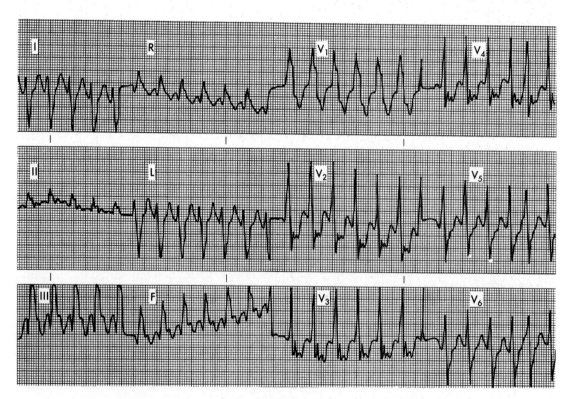

Figure 16C-3.   12-lead ECG obtained from the elderly lady whose lead I rhythm strip recording was shown in Fig. 16C-2.

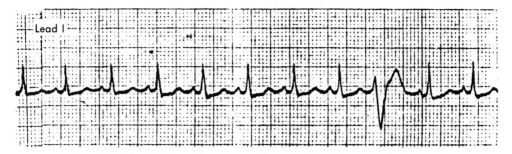

Figure 16C-4.   Subsequent lead I rhythm strip recording from the elderly lady who had initially presented with the tachyarrhythmia shown in Fig. 16C-2.

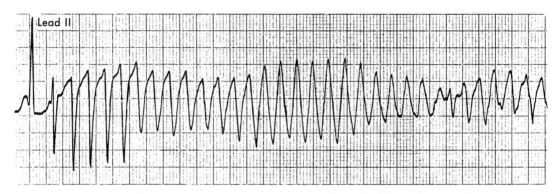

Figure 16C-5.   Initial rhythm strip recording from an unresponsive patient who had overdosed on an unknown medication. *How should this arrhythmia be treated?*

iii. **VENTRICULAR TACHYCARDIA**
iv. SVT with preexisting bundle branch block
v. SVT with aberrant conduction

PROBLEM   **Since the patient was tolerating the arrhythmia, a 12-lead ECG was obtained (*Figure 16C-3). Does this 12-lead tracing help in the differential?***

ANSWER TO FIGURE 16C-3   A fairly regular, wide complex tachycardia is seen without evidence of normal atrial activity. There are two strong clues that this is *ventricular tachycardia*: the taller *left* rabbit ear in lead V_1 (similar to complex **G** in Fig. 15A-14), and the bizarre (markedly rightward) frontal plane axis.

> Note that there is notching in the ST segment in leads II, V_2, V_3, and V_4. Although this could conceivably represent 1:1 *retrograde* (VA) conduction, it is hard to be sure of this finding, and it therefore is of little help in the differential.

PROBLEM   **Before any treatment was given, the patient spontaneously converted to the rhythm shown in *Figure 16C-4*. Does this support your previous suspicion?**

ANSWER TO FIGURE 16C-4   The rhythm is sinus tachycardia at a rate of 115 beats/min. The anomalous beat toward the end of the tracing is clearly a PVC in the context of this rhythm strip. Since this beat is *identical* in

morphology to the wide complex tachycardia seen earlier (in Fig. 16C-2), it *proves* that the patient had been in ventricular tachycardia all along.

> The cases in Figs. 16C-1A and 16C-2 highlight the potential utility of prior recordings for making a definitive (albeit sometimes retrospective) diagnosis of the etiology of a wide complex tachycardia. In addition, the second case provides yet another example of a patient remaining in ventricular tachycardia despite stable hemodynamic status.

PROBLEM   **No history was obtainable from the next patient, whose initial rhythm strip recording is shown in *Figure 16C-5*. The patient had taken an overdose of an unknown medication. The bottle of pills was empty. *How should this arrhythmia be treated?***

ANSWER TO FIGURE 16C-5   The initial beat in this tracing is narrow and upright. It is presumably a supraventricular impulse, although admittedly, additional rhythm strips would be needed to verify this presumption.

Following this beat, the action begins. The QRS complex widens, and a very rapid tachyarrhythmia with a "slinky"-like configuration and *alternating polarity* (first negative—then positive—then negative again toward the end of the tracing) is seen. The pattern is characteristic of **torsade de pointes**.

Torsade de Pointes

Originally described by the French physician Dessertenne in 1966, torsade de pointes all too often goes unrecognized and is treated incorrectly as "ordinary" ventricular tachycardia or ventricular fibrillation. This can have profound consequences for the patient who may be shocked countless times in an attempt to convert this arrhythmia. Drugs such as quinidine and procainamide that usually are effective in suppressing ventricular ectopy paradoxically exacerbate the arrhythmia.

Torsade de pointes frequently is associated with a long QT interval on the baseline ECG. The arrhythmia is thought to be triggered by the occurrence of a PVC at a relatively late point during the repolarization process. Paroxysms of ventricular tachycardia with alternating polarity ensue. These paroxysms often terminate spontaneously, but frequently recur until the underlying predisposing cause of QT prolongation has been corrected.

The most important causes of torsade de pointes are those conditions that produce QT interval prolongation *(Table 16C-1)*. Overdose from phenothiazines or tricyclic antidepressants is a common precipitating event. Electrolyte disturbance (especially hypokalemia or hypomagnesemia) exacerbates the problem. Of the antiarrhythmic agents, quinidine is by far the most common precipitant. Toxic levels of this drug need *not* be present for QT prolongation to occur (which places the onus on the clinician to periodically check for QT prolongation in patients on maintenance antiarrhythmic therapy).

Since the best treatment of torsade de pointes lies in prevention, it is important to be able to recognize QT prolongation. Although complex tables (encompassing patient age, sex, and heart rate) have been developed which precisely define normal limits for QT interval duration, awareness of a simple "rule of thumb" can greatly facilitate determining if this interval is prolonged:

Table 16C-1

Causes of QT Prolongation and Torsade de Pointes

Drugs:
- type IA antiarrhythmic agents (quinidine, procainamide, and disopyramide)
- amiodarone (less common)
- phenothiazines (especially with overdose)
- tricyclic antidepressants (especially with overdose)

Electrolyte disturbances:
- hypokalemia
- hypomagnesemia

Intrinsic heart disease:
- ischemic heart disease
- myocarditis

Central nervous system catastrophe:
- subarachnoid hemorrhage
- cerebrovascular accident

Liquid protein diet *(not used much anymore)*

Congenital QT prolongation syndrome *(rare)*

In general, the QT interval should normally measure *less* than one half the R-R interval.*

*This rule of thumb is less reliable if the heart rate is over 100 beats/min.

Application of this general rule is illustrated in *Figure 16C-6A*. Thus, the QT interval is clearly normal (i.e., *less than half the R-R interval*) in the lefthand panel of this figure, and obviously prolonged in the righthand panel. Reference to this patient's 12-lead ECG *(Figure 16C-6B)* indicates

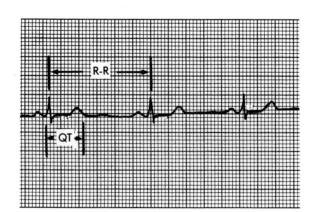
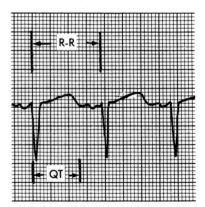

Figure 16C-6A. The QT interval normally measures *less* than one-half the R-R interval. Thus, the QT interval is normal in the lefthand panel of this figure, but clearly prolonged in the righthand panel.

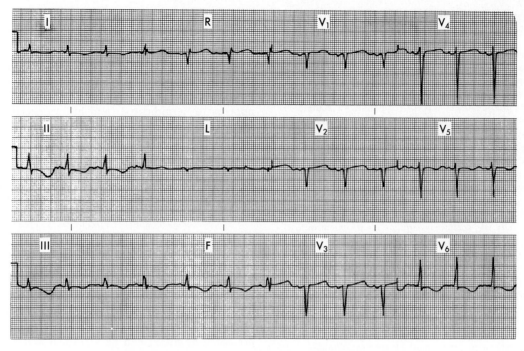

Figure 16C-6B.   12-lead ECG from the patient whose V₃ lead was shown in the righthand panel of Fig. 16C-6A. The QT interval is markedly prolonged.

how striking QT interval prolongation was in this particular case.*

TORSADE DE POINTES: TREATMENT CONSIDERATIONS

The goal of treatment of torsade de pointes is twofold: (1) to eliminate predisposing factors if at all possible, and (2) to suppress (or at least control) the arrhythmia until the QT interval returns to normal. Type I antiarrhythmic agents (quinidine, disopyramide, and procainamide) prolong the QT interval, and are absolutely *contraindicated* in the treatment of this disorder. *Isoproterenol* prevents bradycardia (which may precipitate torsade) and shortens the QT interval; it has been recommended in the past as a drug of choice. However, use of this drug in the presence of rapid heart rates such as that seen in Fig. 16C-5 (or in patients who may have underlying cardiac disease) is controversial at best, and may be potentially lethal if the rhythm turns out to be ventricular tachycardia instead of torsade. Lidocaine, bretylium, and phenytoin have little effect on the QT interval, and have met with mixed success (Parrish et al, 1982; Kim and Chung, 1983).

---

*Obtaining a 12-lead ECG is far superior to assessing QT interval duration from inspection of a single monitoring lead. This is because the full electrocardiogram provides 11 additional viewpoints. Measurement of QT interval duration is recommended in the lead that suggests the *greatest* degree of QT interval prolongation. A lead such as aVL in Fig. 16C-6B should not be used since the boundaries of the QT interval are not well seen.

Cardioversion may be required for episodes of torsade de pointes that become sustained. Despite success in most cases, it should be remembered that cardioversion will usually be no more than a temporizing measure because of the arrhythmia's disturbing tendency to recur.

The drug emerging as the treatment of choice for torsade de pointes is **magnesium** (Tzivoni et al, 1984, 1988; Perticone et al, 1986). Although the precise mechanism for its action in the treatment of this disorder is unclear, a number of investigators have reported excellent results with empiric use of this agent *regardless* of whether serum magnesium levels were low at the time of administration.

The optimal protocol for magnesium administration in the setting of torsade remains controversial. Perticone et al (1986) recommend initial infusion at a relatively slow rate (≈50 mg/min) to minimize the likelihood of developing adverse effects (flushing, hypotension, or decreased myocardial contractility). In a small series of patients, initial infusion at this rate was 100% successful in abolishing torsade within 30 minutes of administration. In their study, this initial infusion of magnesium was continued for 2 hours at 50 mg/minute, and then followed by prophylactic administration of 5-6 grams of magnesium sulfate over the next 3 to 4 days.

Tzivoni et al (1988) report equal success in a small series of patients with torsade following bolus administration of magnesium sulfate (2 gm given IV over 1-2 minutes and repeated 5-15 minutes later if there was no response). Torsade was abolished within minutes in all cases. Patients were then continued on prophylactic magnesium infusion (at a low infusion rate of 3-20 mg/min) over the next 1 to 2 days until QT interval prolongation resolved (to a QT interval of <0.50 second). Adverse effects were minimal other than a short-lasting flushing sensation.

Additional points of interest brought out from this study by Tzivoni were:

i. Serum magnesium levels prior to development of torsade were *normal* in all patients studied.

ii. *Hypokalemia* (serum potassium <3.5 mEq/L) was *common*. Potassium replacement was given when appropriate, but this treatment was *not* responsible for acute resolution of the arrhythmia (because IV magnesium therapy had already corrected torsade *before* potassium was given).

iii. Despite marked QT interval prolongation prior to treatment, shortening this interval was *not* the mechanism responsible for magnesium's success (because IV bolus therapy did not significantly alter QT interval duration).

iv. Despite 100% efficacy in treatment of torsade, magnesium sulfate was completely *ineffective* for treatment of patients with polymorphous ventricular tachycardia in which there was no QT prolongation. Conventional antiarrhythmic therapy (with lidocaine or procainamide) was successful in these cases.

v. The optimal dose of magnesium sulfate is not yet known. However, for potentially *life-threatening arrhythmias* (such as torsade), higher doses may be needed (i.e., 1-2 gm IV over 1-2 minutes, and repeated 5-15 minutes later if the arrhythmia persists)—and a lower dose administered over a longer period of time might not be as effective (Banai and Schuger, 1989).

Based on these results, we suggest strong consideration of *empiric therapy* with *magnesium sulfate* for patients with torsade de pointes, especially when the torsade is associated with QT interval prolongation. Although important to measure and follow both serum potassium and magnesium levels, empiric therapy with magnesium sulfate appears to be indicated (and has an excellent chance of being successful) *regardless of whether serum magnesium levels are normal or low.*

Serum magnesium levels do *not* accurately reflect total body magnesium content. This is because the overwhelming majority of body magnesium is contained within the intracellular compartment (Gums, 1987). Serum magnesium levels reflect *extracellular* magnesium. As a result, it is essential to appreciate that *serum magnesium levels may be normal despite significant body depletion of this cation!*

If administration of magnesium fails to control sustained episodes of torsade, *sequential overdrive pacing* becomes the intervention of choice. Pacing at a rate of 80 to 120 beats/min usually allows control of the arrhythmia until the precipitating factor can be identified and corrected (and the QT interval has a chance to come back toward normal).

Table 16C-2

Suggested Approach to Treatment of Torsade de Pointes*

1. Place the patient on continuous ECG monitoring (with special attention directed at monitoring the QT interval)
   - Obtain a 12-lead ECG as soon as the patient is hemodynamically stable as a baseline (for assessing the QT interval in *all* 12 leads), and to rule out other cardiac abnormalities (such as bundle branch block, ischemia, or acute infarction) that might also affect QT interval duration.

2. Discontinue/avoid all drugs that may further lengthen the QT interval and perpetuate/predispose to torsade:
   - type IA antiarrhythmic agents (quinidine, procainamide, disopyramide)
   - phenothiazines
   - tricyclic antidepressants

3. Correct electrolyte abnormalities (especially hypokalemia and hypomagnesemia)

4. Consider empiric therapy with magnesium sulfate (*even if serum magnesium levels are normal!*)
   - **Magnesium sulfate** (10% solution) may be administered by **bolus** (1-2 gm given IV over 1-2 minutes, and repeated 5-15 minutes later if no response) or by **infusion** (at 50 mg/min over 2 hours). In either case, consideration should be given to *prophylactic* magnesium therapy by continuous infusion (adding 2-4 gm of magnesium sulfate to the patient's daily IV maintenance fluids) *or* intermittent bolus therapy (giving 2-4 gm IM daily) over the ensuing 1 to 2 days.

5. *Cardioversion* as needed when the ventricular tachyarrhythmia is sustained.

6. *Sequential overdrive pacing* if the patient fails to respond to magnesium sulfate, especially if episodes of torsade are sustained and appear to be precipitated by bradycardia.

7. Consider other measures:
   - Lidocaine
   - Phenytoin
   - Isoproterenol

*The best treatment of torsade is prevention (i.e., awareness of potentially predisposing factors shown in Table 16C-1 and careful monitoring of patients at highest risk of developing this disorder).

Table 16C-2 incorporates the concepts we have discussed into a suggested approach for treatment of torsade de pointes. (*Additional discussion on the use of magnesium as an antiarrhythmic agent is found in Chapter 2, and in Section B of Chapter 12; full discussion of the management of TCA Overdose is found in Section G of Chapter 13.*)

ADDENDUM TO ANSWER TO FIGURE 16C-5

Even though the etiology of the overdose in this particular case was unknown, serum electrolytes (including serum magnesium) should be obtained, and empiric therapy with magnesium sulfate (according to recommendations in Table 16C-2) strongly considered while more information is gathered.

We conclude this section with another interesting (and important) variation of a wide complex tachyarrhythmia.

PROBLEM **The rhythm shown in *Figure 16C-7A* is from a middle-aged woman with new-onset palpitations. She was otherwise not in distress, did not complain of chest pain, and had a blood pressure of 90/60 mm Hg at the time this tracing was recorded. The rhythm was diagnosed as atrial fibrillation with a rapid ventricular response, and treatment with IV digoxin was begun. *Would you have done the same?***

ANSWER TO FIGURE 16C-7A   The rhythm is rapid and irregularly irregular. No atrial activity is seen. Although the QRS complex is definitely widened, the gross irregularity of the rhythm makes ventricular tachycardia unlikely. This leaves *atrial fibrillation* as the probable diagnosis.

PROBLEM   **What is distinctly unusual about this as an example of atrial fibrillation?**

ANSWER   The rate. Under normal conditions with atrial fibrillation, the refractory period of the AV node does not allow more than 150 to 200 impulses/minute to be conducted to the ventricles. The ventricular response is clearly faster than this in certain parts of this tracing. In such places, the R-R interval is just over one large box in duration, which corresponds to a heart rate of about 250 beats/min. This is too fast for atrial impulses to be transmitted over the normal (AV nodal) conduction pathway. The most reasonable explanation is that atrial im-

pulses must be *bypassing* the AV node and conducted to the ventricles via an *accessory pathway* with a much shorter refractory period.

PROBLEM   **The patient's old hospital chart was found to contain a 12-lead ECG obtained at a time when she was in normal sinus rhythm *(Figure 16C-7B)*. Does this make her underlying diagnosis more evident?**

ANSWER TO FIGURE 16C-7B   The rhythm in this 12-lead ECG is fairly regular at a rate of between 50-60 beats/min. The QRS complex is wide. Nevertheless, each QRS is preceded by a P wave with a constant (albeit shortened) PR interval. Since the P wave is upright in lead II, the mechanism must be sinus (in this case, sinus bradycardia and arrhythmia).

Note that the initial portion of the upstroke of the QRS complex in many of the leads (especially I, aVL, and V_2-V_6) is *slurred*. This slurring represents a *delta wave*. The finding of delta waves (together with *QRS widening* and *PR interval shortening*), is characteristic of the ***Wolff-Parkinson-White (WPW) Syndrome***.

Wolff-Parkinson-White (WPW) Syndrome

WPW is a syndrome in which one or more accessory conduction pathways exist that allow an alternate route for transmission of the electrical impulse from the atria to the ventricles. It has an approximate incidence of 2 per 1,000 individuals in the general population. This is infrequent enough to account for the lack of clinical experience many emergency care providers have in direct management of such patients, but not so uncommon that the entity can be ignored. Most emergency care providers will encounter *at least several patients* with the syndrome each year, a small number of whom may present with potentially life-threatening tachyarrhythmias such as the one shown in Fig. 16C-7A.

Conduction of the sinus impulse in patients with WPW may be via the normal (AV nodal) pathway, down the accessory tract, or it may alternate between the two. These patients are prone to develop atrial tachyarrhythmias in which a reentry circuit is set up between the normal AV nodal pathway and the accessory tract. With PSVT, this most often results in antegrade (i.e., forward) conduction *down* the AV nodal pathway (producing a *narrow* QRS complex during the tachycardia) and retrograde conduction back up the accessory pathway

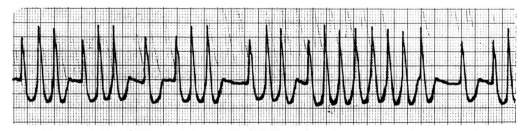

Figure 16C-7A.   Rhythm strip obtained from a middle-aged woman with new-onset palpitations. *Should she be treated with IV digoxin?*

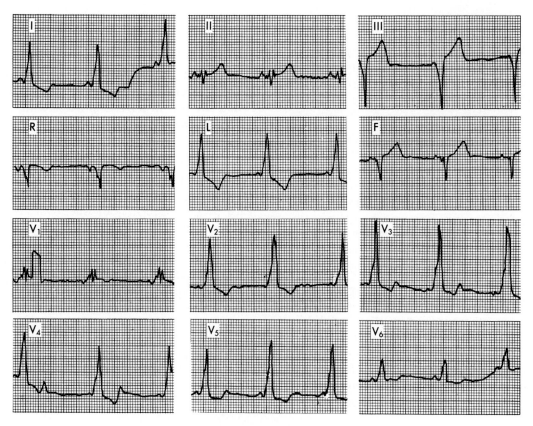

Figure 16C-7B.   12-lead ECG obtained from the chart of the middle-aged woman who presented with the tachyarrhythmia shown in Fig. 16C-7A. *What is her underlying diagnosis?*

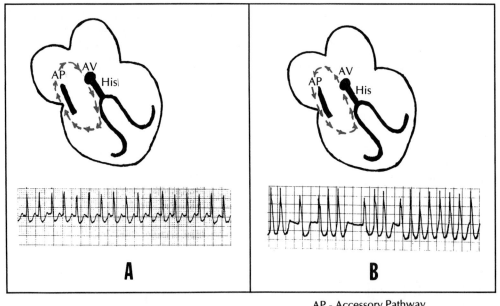

AP - Accessory Pathway
AV - AV Nodal Pathway
His - Bundle of His

Figure 16C-8.   Pathways of conduction of supraventricular tachyarrhythmias in patients with WPW. With PSVT (Panel **A**), antegrade conduction of the impulse is almost always transmitted down the normal AV nodal pathway, and retrograde via the accessory pathway. In contrast, with atrial fibrillation (Panel **B**) or atrial flutter, transmission of the impulse is almost always conducted *down the accessory pathway*, and retrograde via the AV nodal pathway.

(Panel A in Fig. 16C-8). PSVT is by far the most common tachyarrhythmia observed in patients with WPW. It is usually well tolerated by the patient.

In contrast, with atrial fibrillation in WPW, antegrade transmission of the impulse is almost always conducted down the *accessory* tract, with retrograde conduction back to the atria over the AV nodal pathway. *Antegrade conduction over the accessory pathway results in QRS widening during the tachycardia.* Because of the short refractory period of the accessory pathway, there may be 1:1 conduction of atrial impulses during atrial fibrillation, resulting in a ventricular response that exceeds 250 beats/min (Panel B in Fig. 16C-8). Such rapid rates may not be well tolerated (i.e., the ventricles may not be able to adequately contract at this rate), and as a result the rhythm can deteriorate into ventricular fibrillation.

Although less commonly seen than atrial fibrillation, atrial flutter may also occur in patients with WPW. As with atrial fibrillation, antegrade transmission of atrial impulses is almost always down the accessory pathway when patients with WPW develop atrial flutter. As a result, there may be 1:1 AV conduction (so that the ventricular response may be as fast as 250-350 beats/min).

Although digoxin and verapamil are both extremely effective medications for slowing the ventricular response of rapid atrial fibrillation, they are *contraindicated* when atrial fibrillation occurs in association with WPW.* This is because *digoxin and verapamil may further accelerate conduction down the accessory pathway and exacerbate the arrhythmia.*

The goal of treating rapid atrial fibrillation with WPW is to prevent facilitation of antegrade conduction down the accessory pathway. This can be done by increasing the *antegrade refractory period* of the accessory pathway. Drugs that exert a beneficial effect on this refractory period include procainamide (which is the drug of choice for emergency treatment), other IA agents (quinidine, disopyramide), amiodarone, IC agents (such as flecainide, encainide, and propafenone), and to a lesser extent lidocaine. Consequently, the medical treatment of choice for the tachyarrhythmia shown in Fig. 16C-7A would be to administer an IV loading dose of **procainamide.**

Administration of IV β-blockers (i.e., propranolol, esmolol) may be a helpful adjunct to procainamide (Wellens et al, 1987; Michelson, 1989). Many factors influence conduction properties of the accessory pathway, including the degree of underlying autonomic tone. In particular, antegrade conduction down the accessory pathway may be *accelerated* by an increase in sympathetic tone (Wellens et al, 1987). Sudden onset of a rapid tachyarrhythmia (such as atrial fibrillation or flutter in a patient with WPW) may produce an increase in sympathetic discharge either as a manifestation of anxiety (from the palpitations), or as a compensatory response in an attempt to maintain a normal systolic blood pressure. β-blockade may blunt this sympathetic response, and thus prevent catecholamine-induced shortening of the antegrade refractory period.

It should be emphasized that immediate cardioversion is indicated if hemodynamic decompensation occurs at any time during the treatment process. A trial of medical therapy (i.e., administration of IV procainamide with or without a β-blocker) is a reasonable alternative in patients who are not hemodynamically compromised, although it should be realized that pharmacologic therapy may occasionally produce hypotension and/or postconversion depression of electrical or mechanical function (Michelson, 1989).

Although *overt evidence* of WPW (as manifested by delta waves, PR interval shortening, and QRS widening) is relatively uncommon in the general population (2 per 1,000 incidence), there appears to be a greater incidence of individuals with *concealed* accessory pathways. The term **"concealed"** implies that under normal conditions, *conduction over the accessory pathway only occurs in retrograde fashion.* Since there is no antegrade (forward) conduction down the accessory pathway, these individuals manifest none of the ECG findings of WPW cited above. As a result, there is no way to identify the existence of an accessory pathway in these otherwise healthy individuals as long as they remain in normal sinus rhythm. Nevertheless, because they harbor an alternate route for conduction (the concealed accessory pathway), they maintain the potential to develop reentry tachyarrhythmias.

As we have emphasized in Fig. 16B-21, identification of atrial activity and its relationship to the QRS complex may provide valuable clues to the mechanism of PSVT. Thus, notching of the terminal portion of the QRS complex and/or initial portion of the ST segment (as was seen during the PSVT shown in Figs. 16B-15 and 16B-20) suggests a reentry mechanism of the "slow-fast" type.

PROBLEM   **Examine the 12-lead ECG shown in *Figure 16C-9*, obtained from a 30-year-old woman with "palpitations." She is otherwise healthy. *Is there a clue to the mechanism of her arrhythmia?***

HINT: Does retrograde atrial activity in Fig. 16C-9 (indicated by the arrows) occur later (i.e., with a longer RP′ interval) than the retrograde atrial activity seen in Figs. 16B-15 and 16B-20? *If so, why might this be?*

ANSWER TO FIGURE 16C-9   The rhythm of this supraventricular tachyarrhythmia is regular at a rate of just over 150 beats/min. Arrows indicate retrograde atrial activity that notches the mid-portion of the ST segment in the inferior leads. Most of the time, retrograde atrial activity with PSVT of the slow-fast type will occur sooner, and either be hidden within the QRS complex (Panel B in Fig. 16B-21), or notch the terminal portion of the QRS or the initial portion of the ST segment (Panel C in Fig. 16B-21). The possibility of a *concealed accessory pathway* should be considered when retrograde atrial activity during PSVT occurs as late in the ST segment as it does in Fig. 16C-9.

It is not generally appreciated that as many as 30% of adults with PSVT have a *concealed* accessory pathway. As already noted, conduction during PSVT in such individuals is almost always *orthodromic* (i.e., down the normal AV nodal pathway

---

*Because atrial flutter also almost always conducts down the accessory pathway, digoxin and verapamil are also contraindicated for treatment of this arrhythmia when it occurs in association with WPW. Instead, recommended medical therapy for atrial flutter in patients with WPW is similar to that recommended for atrial fibrillation with WPW (i.e., with antiarrhythmic agents that slow antegrade conduction down the accessory pathway).

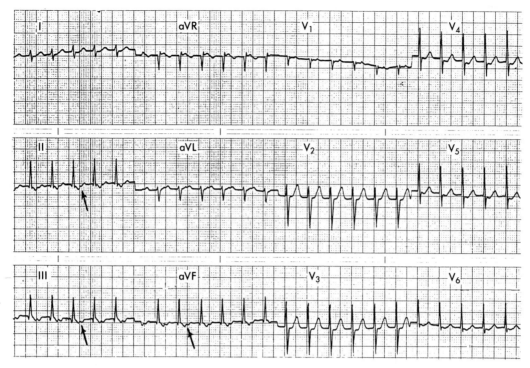

Figure 16C-9. 12-lead ECG obtained from a 30 year old woman with palpitations. *Why might the retrograde atrial activity (indicated by the arrows in the inferior leads) occur so late after the QRS complex?*

and back up the accessory pathway), and the QRS complex remains narrow. *As long as the accessory pathway remains concealed, management of these tachyarrhythmias is identical to that of the more typical slow-fast form of PSVT in which the reentry circuit is contained entirely within the AV node* (i.e., application of vagal maneuvers, adenosine, verapamil, digoxin, etc.). The problem is that occasionally a patient who was thought to have purely orthodromic PSVT may spontaneously develop atrial fibrillation during treatment (Michelson, 1989). Considering that drugs such as digoxin and verapamil can potentially accelerate conduction down the accessory pathway, disastrous consequences could result.

Practically speaking, it will *NOT* be necessary in most cases to address the supraventricular tachycardias with nearly as much sophistication as we have in Sections B and C of this chapter. Clinically in the acute care setting, treatment of a narrow complex PSVT tends to be similar *regardless* of whether the mechanism is the typical slow-fast form of PSVT, the fast-slow form, reentry utilizing an SA-nodal or intra-atrial circuit, or orthodromic PSVT in patients with an accessory pathway *with the rare exception of those patients who have an accessory pathway and are predisposed to developing atrial fibrillation.*

Putting WPW into Clinical Perspective

We terminate this section by attempting to place the syndrome of WPW in a proper clinical perspective. As stated by Fisch (1990), "WPW fascinates the cardiologist, electrocardiographer, electrophysiologist, and cardiovascular surgeon alike and to a degree that, at first glance, appears to be out of proportion to its overall importance." It should be remembered that this syndrome is relatively uncommon, and that the overwhelming majority of *asymptomatic individuals* with either overt ECG evidence of WPW or with concealed accessory pathways have an excellent long-term prognosis (Leitch et al, 1990; Krahn et al, 1992). The clinical dilemma is that on rare occasions, sudden cardiac death may be the initial manifestation of WPW (Klein et al, 1989). In such cases, the mechanism for sudden cardiac death is almost invariably the result of sudden development of very rapid atrial fibrillation (as in Fig. 16C-7A), with deterioration to ventricular fibrillation (Klein et al, 1989). On other infrequent occasions, patients with WPW may present to an emergency facility with atrial fibrillation and a very rapid ventricular response. *The principal purpose of our discussion of WPW in this chapter is simply to highlight how to recognize and treat this potentially life-threatening presentation of this fascinating syndrome.*

Long-term management of patients with WPW has been the source of much controversy. The key issues to address are whether patients with this syndrome who are at greatest risk of sudden death can be readily identified, and if so, can treatment improve their prognosis. As already emphasized, the overall risk of sudden death in patients with WPW is exceedingly low (an estimated 1 death per 1,000 years of patient follow-up—Klein et al, 1989). This risk is even lower for the overwhelming majority of patients with WPW who are asymptomatic, do not have a positive family history of sudden death, and do not have underlying cardiac disease (and are thus better able to tolerate the exceedingly rapid tachyarrhythmias). Another possible reason for the excellent overall long-term prognosis of patients with WPW is that with time, a significant percentage of such patients lose their capacity for antegrade conduction over the accessory pathway. This may result in a correspondingly lower risk of developing a rapid ventricular response should atrial fibrillation develop (Klein et al, 1989; Fisch, 1990).

Interestingly, a surprising number of patients who initially present with electrocardiographic evidence of WPW demonstrate *intermittent* preexcitation when followed over a period of years. Moreover, many such individuals manifest a tendency for the disorder to disappear with time (Krahn et al, 1992). In contrast, and despite the presumed congenital origin of accessory pathways, electrocardiographic evidence of WPW may be delayed and only make its first appearance in a patient's later years. Whether intermittence of preexcitation is the result of slowed conduction through the AV node (leading to preferential conduction over the accessory pathway), impaired capacity for antegrade conduction over the accessory pathway, fluctuation in the degree of underlying sympathetic tone, and/or other unidentified "triggering" factors is unclear (Krahn et al, 1992).

Fortunately, electrophysiologic studies may provide an abundance of clinically useful information regarding the conduction properties of the accessory pathway in patients with WPW. Such information includes determination of whether retrograde conduction is possible, which tachyarrhythmias are inducible, whether there is more than one accessory pathway, and the shortest effective refractory period of the accessory pathway (i.e., the shortest R-R interval between preexcited beats during rapid atrial fibrillation). Results from such studies may afford invaluable insight into a patient's likely clinical course and prognosis. For example, patients with a shortest preexcited interval of ≤220 msec appear to be at highest risk of sudden death, those with a shortest preexcited interval of between 220 to 250 msec are at somewhat lower risk, and those with a shortest preexcited interval of >300 msec are at almost negligible risk (Klein et al, 1989). However, because the *overall risk of sudden death* is so low to begin with in asymptomatic patients with WPW, mass screening and invasive investigation with electrophysiologic testing of such patients does *not* appear to be justified (Klein et al, 1989; Michelson, 1989; Fisch, 1990). Despite its ability to predict which patients are at greatest risk of developing serious arrhythmias, it is unable to predict with any reliability whether these arrhythmias will occur (Beckman et al, 1990).

In contrast, full electrophysiologic investigation is indicated for otherwise healthy, active individuals with WPW who develop *symptomatic* tachyarrhythmias. This is because it appears that a majority of individuals with even a *single* episode of rapid atrial fibrillation will eventually have a recurrence of this potentially life-threatening arrhythmia (Beckman et al, 1990). Options for treatment of such individuals are exciting and include medical treatment (which may control tachyarrhythmias in many patients) and surgical or ablative treatment. Referral to a specialized center for identification and localization of the problematic accessory pathway(s) with subsequent surgical interruption and/or ablation is curative in a high percentage of cases, and may obviate the need for any antiarrhythmic therapy at all.*

References

Banai S, Schuger C: Magnesium sulfate is the treatment for torsades de pointes if the right dose is given, *Am J Cardiol* 65:266, 1989.

Beckman KJ, Gallastegui JL, Bauman JL, Hariman RJ: The predictive value of electrophysiologic studies in untreated patients with Wolff-Parkinson-White syndrome, *J Am Coll Cardiol* 15:640, 1990.

Calkins H, Sousa J, El-Atassi R, Rosenheck S, Buitleir M, Kou WH, Kadish AH, Langberg JJ, Morady F: Diagnosis and cure of the Wolff-Parkinson-White syndrome or paroxysmal supraventricular tachycardias during a single electrophysiologic test, *N Engl J Med* 324:1612, 1991.

Curtis AB, Grauer K: Wide complex tachycardia due to coexistent supraventricular and ventricular tachycardia, *J Fam Prac* 30:706, 1990.

Fisch C: Clinical electrophysiological studies and the Wolff-Parkinson-White pattern, *Circulation* 82:1872, 1990.

Gums JG: Clinical significance of magnesium: a review, *Drug Intell Clin Pharm* 21:240, 1987.

Jackman WM, Wang X, Friday KJ, Roman CA, Moulton KP, Beckman KJ, McClelland JH, Twidale N, Hazlitt HA, Prior MI, Margolis PD, Calame JD, Overholt ED, Lazzara R: Catheter ablation of accessory atrioventricular pathways (Wolff-Parkinson-White syndrome) by radiofrequency current, *N Engl J Med* 324:1605, 1991.

Kim HS, Chung EK: Torsade de pointes: polymorphous ventricular tachycardia, *Heart Lung* 12:269, 1983.

Klein GJ, Prystowsky EN, Yee R, Sharma AD, Laupacis A: Asymptomatic Wolff-Parkinson-White: should we intervene? *Circulation* 80:1902, 1989.

Krahn AD, Manfreda J, Tate RB, Mathewson FAL, Cuddy TE: The natural history of electrocardiographic preexcitation in men: the Manitoba follow-up study, *Ann Intern Med* 116:456, 1992.

Leitch JW, Klein GJ, Yee R, Murdock C: Prognostic value of electrophysiology testing in asymptomatic patients with Wolff-Parkinson-White pattern, *Circulation* 82:1718, 1990.

Michelson EL: Clinical perspectives in management of Wolff-Parkinson-White syndrome, part I: recognition, diagnosis, and arrhythmias, *Mod Conc Cardiovasc Dis* 58:43, 1989.

Michelson EL: Clinical perspectives in management of Wolff-Parkinson-White syndrome, part II: diagnostic evaluation and treatment strategies, *Mod Conc Cardiovasc Dis* 58:49, 1989.

Parish C, Wooster WE, Braen GR, Robertson HD: Les torsade de pointes, *Ann Emerg Med* 11:143, 1982.

Perticone F, Adinolfi L, Bonaduce: Efficacy of magnesium sulfate in the treatment of torsade de pointes, *Am Heart J* 112:847, 1986.

Tzivoni D, Keren A, Cohen AM, Loebel H, Zahavi I, Chenzbraun A, Stern S: Magnesium therapy for torsades de pointes, *Am J Cardiol* 53:528, 1984.

Tzivoni D, Banai S, Schuger C, Benhorin J, Keren A, Gottleib S, Stern S: Treatment of torsade de pointes with magnesium sulfate, *Circulation* 77:392, 1988.

Wellens HJJ, Brugada P, Penn OC: The management of preexcitation syndromes, *JAMA* 257:2325, 1987.

---

*Recently, Jackman et al (1991) have demonstrated that catheter delivery of radiofrequency current guided by direct recordings of accessory pathway activation may be effective in up to 99% of cases with no mortality and a significantly lower morbidity than surgical ablation of the previously used technique of catheter ablation with high-energy shocks. As suggested by the results of Calkins et al (1991), the day may not be far off when diagnosis *and* cure of symptomatic WPW patients with supraventricular tachyarrhythmias is accomplished by a single electrophysiologic study (i.e., without the need for serial EP studies, long-term drug therapy, and separate surgical ablation).

SECTION D

AV BLOCKS—AND A STEP BEYOND

In Section D of Chapter 3 we introduced basic concepts in the diagnosis of the AV blocks. We would now like to pick up from that point and explore some of the difficulties encountered when an arrhythmia suspected of having some degree of AV block fails to "obey all of the rules."

The ability to accurately diagnose the AV blocks (like all other arrhythmias) depends on the use of a systematic approach.

The **4-Step Systematic Approach** we suggest looks for:
  i. Regularity of the rhythm (of *both* atrial and ventricular rhythms)
  ii. Evidence of atrial activity (P waves)
  iii. QRS widening
  iv. A relationship between P waves and the QRS complex (*"Who's married to whom?"*)

As emphasized in Chapter 3, it doesn't matter in which order these four points are addressed, as long as *each* of the points are considered in evaluation of *each* arrhythmia encountered. Identification of atrial activity (i.e., *"Cherchez le P"*) and its relationship to the QRS complex are particularly important in the diagnosis of AV blocks.

> In addition to these four points, assessment of **hemodynamic status** is an integral part of the interpretation. Thus, determination that a heart block is "only first degree" would

be of little consolation if the patient was unresponsive, hypotensive, and had a heart rate of 20 beats/minute.

As a "warmup" to this chapter, examine the following two tracings. *Pay particular attention to the atrial activity.*

HINT: Neither of these tracings demonstrate significant AV block.

PROBLEM   Examine *Figure 16D-1.* **"Cherchez le P"** (i.e., *Look for P waves*). Qu'est-ce qui se passe avec les P? (i.e., *What happens to these P waves?*)

ANSWER TO FIGURE 16D-1   P waves are readily identifiable in this tracing—*but their morphology continually changes!* The first two complexes (beats #1 and #2) are preceded by a peaked P wave and are conducted with 1° AV block (PR interval = 0.22 second). P wave morphology then changes and takes on a biphasic configuration for beats #3-7, all of which are conducted with a normal PR interval. A negative P wave precedes beat #8, followed by resumption of the peaked P wave configuration and acceleration of the rate. This figure illustrates a *wandering atrial pacemaker, sinus bradycardia,* and *sinus arrhythmia*—all components of the *sick sinus syndrome.*

> Did you note that the amplitude of the peaked P wave preceding beat #2 was slightly *less* than that of the P wave preceding beat #1? If this is a real finding (i.e., if it is *not* due to patient movement or baseline artifact), it may either represent an additional focus of atrial activity, or an *atrial* fusion beat (i.e., the "offspring" of a "marriage" between the P waves preceding beats #1 and #3).

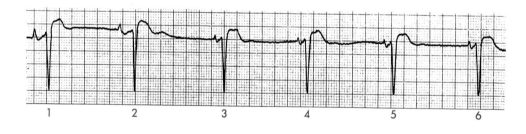

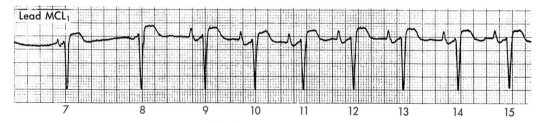

Figure 16D-1.   Continuous rhythm strip from an MCL₁ monitoring lead. *Describe the atrial activity.*

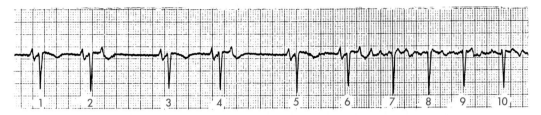

Figure 16D-2.   *What happens to the P waves in this arrhythmia?*

PROBLEM   **Examine *Figure 16D-2*. Once again, *what happens to the P waves?***

ANSWER TO FIGURE 16D-2   Initially there is a "regular irregularity" to the rhythm. Sinus rhythm is identified by recognition of an upright P wave with a fixed PR interval in front of beats #1 through #6. The underlying sinus rate is 70 beats/min (as determined by the R-R interval between beats #1-2, #3-4, and #5-6). The third, sixth, and ninth P waves are *early* and peak the T waves of beats #2, #4, and #6. Since every third P wave is a PAC, the underlying rhythm is *atrial trigeminy*. The first two premature P waves (the ones that follow in the T wave of beats #2 and #4) are *blocked*. The third (that peaks the T wave of beat #6) precipitates a few beats of *atrial flutter* that rapidly deteriorates into *atrial fibrillation* with a controlled ventricular response (beats #7-10).

> It is well to remember *before* we launch into our more sophisticated discussion of the AV blocks that **the commonest cause of a pause is a blocked PAC** (and *NOT AV block*)! This is seen in Fig. 16D-2 where the relatively short pauses (that punctuate the R-R intervals between beats #2-3 and #4-5) are initiated by a spiked T wave (the T wave of beats #2 and #4) that is the result of a blocked PAC.
>
> Clinically, since the initial (underlying) arrhythmia in this example is atrial trigeminy (or more simply, frequent PACs), and since atrial fibrillation is precipitated by a PAC (that occurred on the vulnerable period), antiarrhythmic therapy directed at suppressing this enhanced atrial automaticity (i.e., use of type IA agents such as quinidine or procainamide) might be appropriate.

Now that you're attuned to carefully looking for P waves (and alerted to potential pitfalls in diagnosis such as changing P wave morphology and blocked PACs), on to the subtleties of the AV blocks themselves . . . . .

Simplifying Classification of the AV Blocks

As indicated in Section D of Chapter 3, classification of the AV blocks may be simplified by the following approach:

> i. Look initially to see if **1° AV block** is present. (This is usually easy to recognize.)
> ii. Look next to see if **3° AV block** is present. (This is *also* usually easy to recognize.)
> iii. If neither 1° nor 3° AV block is present, but beats are being dropped due to *AV block*, the block *must* be a **2° AV block**.

PROBLEM   **First-degree AV block will *not* always be easy to recognize. Consider the 12-lead ECG shown in *Figure 16D-3A*. What is the rhythm?**

ANSWER TO FIGURE 16D-3A   The rhythm is regular at 95 beats/min, and the QRS complex is of normal duration. It is hard to determine if atrial activity is present. In lead II (which is usually the best lead for identifying atrial activity), all that is seen is an upright deflection at the midpoint of the R-R interval. For all the world, this deflection looks like a T wave. If lead II was the only monitoring lead available, one would have to interpret the rhythm as an *accelerated* AV nodal rhythm (regularly occurring narrow QRS complex without atrial activity).

A different impression might be obtained from inspection of lead V_1 (which usually is the next best lead to choose when searching for P waves). Here, the upright deflection that occurs in the middle of the R-R interval looks much more like a P wave than a T wave. Were this the case, then the rhythm would be sinus with 1° AV block. The point to emphasize is the *impossibility* of distinguishing between these two entities on the basis of the ECG shown in Fig. 16D-3A alone!

PROBLEM   **A short while later, the rhythm strip shown in *Figure 16D-3B* was recorded from this same patient. *Does this rhythm strip clarify what the rhythm was in Fig. 16D-3A?***

ANSWER TO FIGURE 16D-3B   The heart rate has decreased, and P waves can now be clearly seen notching each T wave (arrows). *The patient had been in 1° AV block all along!*

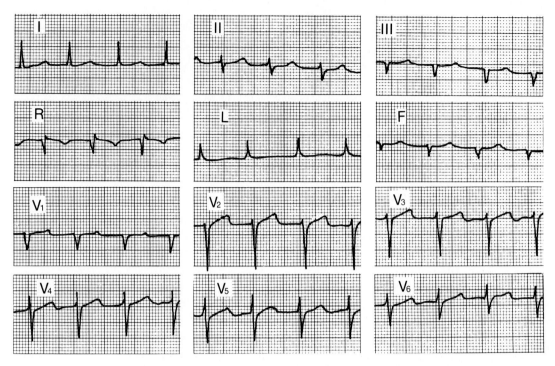

Figure 16D-3A. 12-lead ECG. *What is the rhythm?*

First-degree AV block is almost always an extremely easy rhythm to identify. In reality, it is nothing more than a sinus rhythm in which the PR interval is prolonged. All atrial impulses are conducted to the ventricles with 1° AV block—*it's just that they take a little longer to get there!*

The above example illustrates the exception to the rule that 1° AV block is easy to recognize, and shows how P waves may occasionally be hidden by T waves when the PR interval becomes markedly prolonged.

PROBLEM **How long can the PR interval be prolonged and *still* conduct?**

ANSWER Very long. Normal SA node–initiated impulses have been observed to conduct with PR interval prolongation of *more than* 1 second (Marriott—personal communication).

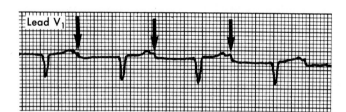

Figure 16D-3B. Rhythm strip obtained a short while later from the patient whose 12-lead tracing was shown in Fig. 16D-3A. Arrows indicate that P waves had been hiding from within the T wave.

PROBLEM **Moving up in the severity of AV block, examine the tracing shown in *Figure 16D-4A*. Does this represent 3° (complete) AV block?**

ANSWER TO FIGURE 16D-4A In Section D of Chapter 3 we listed the criteria for diagnosing complete (3°) AV block:

i. Atrial regularity (usually)
ii. Ventricular regularity (usually)
iii. Complete AV dissociation *despite* adequate opportunity for normal conduction to occur (usually implying a heart rate of *less than* 45 beats/min).

Although 3° AV block may exist in association with sinus arrhythmia and/or an irregular junctional or ventricular escape pacemaker, in most cases *both* the atrial and ventricular rhythms will be regular (or at least *almost* regular) with this conduction disorder. This provides a helpful clue to the diagnosis of AV block: *If the ventricular rhythm is not regular, it is likely that the rhythm is something OTHER than 3° AV block* (such as a complex form of 2° AV block).

The third criterion stated above is critical. It is impossible to diagnose 3° AV block with certainty unless there is evidence on the tracing that P waves are unable to conduct *despite more than adequate opportunity to do so.* Practically speaking, it is hard to guarantee "adequate opportunity to conduct" when the rate of the escape pacemaker is *more than* 45 beats/minute.

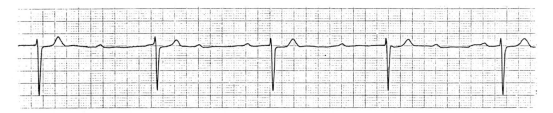

Figure 16D-4A.   *Is this 3° (complete) AV block?*

Each of the three conditions listed above as requirements for the diagnosis of complete AV block are present in Fig. 16D-4A. That is:

i. The ventricular rate is regular (at a rate of about 30 beats/min).

ii. The atrial rate is also regular (at a rate of about 75 beats/min) as indicated by the arrows in *Figure 16D-4B*.

iii. None of the P waves conduct (i.e., there is *complete AV dissociation*), despite more than adequate opportunity to do so.

Although P waves cannot be identified in every spot where an arrow is placed in Fig. 16D-4B, one can assume that they are present since the regularity of those P waves that are evident continues throughout. One would *not* expect P waves highlighted by arrows #2, #4, #7, and #9 to conduct since the PR interval for this atrial activity is either too short or occurs during the refractory period (i.e., during the T wave). Similarly, the P wave highlighted by arrow #11 (and possibly also the P wave highlighted by arrow #6) might not necessarily

be able to conduct if a significant degree of 1° AV block was present. However, one would certainly expect *at least one* of the remaining P waves (highlighted by arrows #1, #3, #5, #8, or #10) to occur at a time when conduction is possible if the degree of AV block were not complete. Since the ventricular rate remains regular throughout (and P waves continue to "march through the QRS complex"), there is no conduction, and the degree of AV block must be complete.

The level of the AV block in this example is probably *below* the AV node because the QRS complex appears to be wide (more than half a large box in duration, or at least 0.11 second) and the ventricular response so slow.

PROBLEM   **Examine *Figure 16D-5*. Is this also complete AV block?**

ANSWER TO FIGURE 16D-5   No. The first three beats appear to be sinus conducted with a marked 1° AV block (PR = 0.62 second). The QRS complex is wide, suggesting underlying bundle branch block. *Asystole* (not complete AV block) follows.

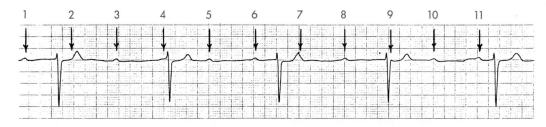

Figure 16D-4B.   Arrows indicate that the degree of AV block in Fig. 16D-4A is complete. The atrial rate is regular and completely dissociated from the QRS complex despite having more than adequate opportunity to conduct in several places on the tracing.

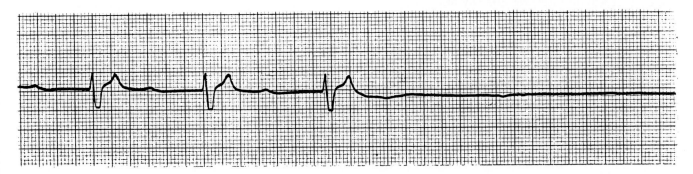

Figure 16D-5.   *Is this complete AV block?*

AV Dissociation

Perhaps the area that causes the greatest confusion regarding the AV blocks concerns the diagnosis of AV dissociation. We might start with the definition:

AV dissociation is a *secondary* rhythm disturbance (*never* a primary disturbance) that occurs when the atria and ventricles fail to respond to the same impulse and beat independently (Lipman et al, 1984).

One should therefore *never* say that a rhythm *"is"* AV dissociation, but rather that AV dissociation is present because of _____ (= the primary disorder).

The three principal reasons why AV dissociation may occur are:

---

i. **Default** (from slowing of the sinus pacemaker)
ii. **Usurpation** (from a junctional or ventricular pacemaker that accelerates enough to take over (i.e., "usurp") the primary pacemaker function
iii. **AV block** (which produces a slowing of the ventricular response by preventing conduction of one or more sinus impulses).

It should be apparent from the above list that AV block is only one of the conditions that cause AV dissociation. Since there are two other conditions that can cause AV dissociation (usurpation and default), *AV block (complete or otherwise), cannot be synonymous with AV dissociation.*

PROBLEM   **AV dissociation is present in *Figure 16D-6*. What is its cause? Is *3°* (complete) AV block present?**

TECHNICAL (SEMANTIC) CONCERN: What is the correct way to interpret this rhythm?

ADDITIONAL CLINICAL CONCERNS: Does the patient whose rhythm is shown in Fig. 16D-6 need a pacemaker? *What underlying clinical condition(s) should be suspected?*

ANSWER TO FIGURE 16D-6   The QRS complex is narrow and the ventricular rate fairly regular at 115-120 beats/min. P waves precede the first few complexes but become lost in the QRS after beat #7. Although the PR interval appears to be short (0.10 second) for beats #1-4, these P waves could possibly still be conducting. However, conduction is definitely *not* possible for the P waves preceding beats #5-7 (as the PR interval is just *too short* for these beats). *AV dissociation* is therefore present—at least *temporarily* (i.e., P waves are at least temporarily unrelated to QRS complexes). The cause of AV dissociation in this case is *usurpation* by an *accelerated junctional pacemaker* that takes over the pacemaking function.

The semantically correct interpretation of the rhythm shown in Fig. 16D-6 is **junctional *tachycardia*** (because this is the *primary* rhythm disturbance). As a result of the accelerated junctional rate, there is **AV dissociation** (which is a *secondary* phenomenon). Since the rate of the accelerated junctional pacemaker *exceeds* 100 beats/min, the primary rhythm disturbance is best termed junctional *tachycardia*.

Clinically, the common causes of accelerated junctional rhythms or junctional tachycardia are digitalis toxicity, inferior myocardial infarction, and the postoperative state following open heart surgery.

It is important to emphasize that there is no evidence at all of any form of AV block on this tracing! That is, *P waves are never shown to fail to conduct at a time when they should conduct.*

Admittedly, one could not rule out the possibility that some degree of AV block may be present in Fig. 16D-6. All one can say is that the rate of the junctional escape rhythm in this tracing is too fast to allow determination if any degree of AV block is present. Clinically, the issue is somewhat academic since a pacemaker would not be required as long as the patient remained hemodynamically stable and could be closely observed until the underlying cause of the accelerated junctional rhythm resolved.

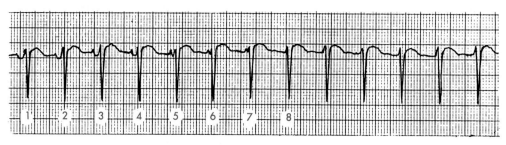

Figure 16D-6.   What is the cause of AV dissociation in this rhythm? *Is there evidence of AV block?*

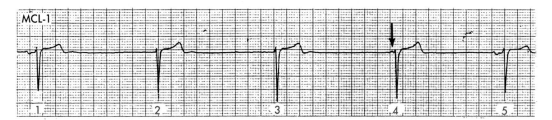

Figure 16D-7. Is there evidence of AV dissociation on this tracing? *Is there complete AV block?*

PROBLEM **Interpret the rhythm shown in *Figure 16D-7?* Is there evidence of AV dissociation? *Is 3° (complete) AV block present?***

HINT: What is the *primary* rhythm disturbance?

ANSWER TO FIGURE 16D-7 Hopefully you did not interpret this rhythm simply as "AV dissociation." AV dissociation *is* present—however (as always), it is a *secondary* disorder. The underlying rhythm in Fig. 16D-7 appears to be an *AV nodal escape rhythm* at the slow rate of 33 beats/min (as seen from beats #2 and #3). Note that sinus conduction had started this tracing (beat #1), but that atrial activity then disappeared until just before beat #4. This P wave (arrow) is definitely too close to the next QRS complex to conduct—therefore, AV dissociation is present. The sinus pacemaker speeds up at this point (the R-R interval between beats #4-5 is less than the R-R interval during the junctional rhythm), and sinus conduction is able to resume with beat #5. The fact that P wave morphology and the PR interval preceding beats #1 and #5 are identical strongly supports our contention that these are normally conducted sinus beats.

The correct interpretation of this rhythm is therefore that a slow *AV nodal escape rhythm* is present, arising by *default* of the sinus pacemaker (from marked sinus bradycardia and/or a sinus pause)—and which produces *transient* AV dissociation. Complete AV block is not present. It *can't* be, since there is evidence of normal conduction on the tracing (i.e., beats #1 and #5 are sinus-conducted). Another clue to the absence of 3° AV block is apparent simply from inspection of the tracing—*the ventricular response is not regular.* Thus, correction of the primary rhythm disturbance (in this case, sinus bradycardia) may be all that is needed to eliminate failed conduction of supraventricular impulses.

Note that we have referred to the escape rhythm here as being *AV nodal* because the QRS complex is narrow and similar in appearance to the sinus-conducted beats. However, one really cannot determine the site of the escape pacemaker with any certainty. Potential pacemaking cells exist throughout the myocardium. As long as the impulse arises *from somewhere in the conduction system* (the AV node, the bundle of His, or the bundle branches), the QRS complex may appear similar in morphology to the sinus-conducted beats. In this case, the fact that the rate of the escape pacemaker is slower than the usual rate of an AV nodal rhythm (40-60 beats/min) suggests that its focus may arise *below* the AV node.

Note also that although QRS morphology of the escape beats (#2, #3, and #4) is similar to that of the sinus-conducted beats (#1 and #5), it is *not* identical (it differs in that the S wave is slightly deeper). Such subtle differences in QRS morphology often exist between sinus-conducted beats and escape beats originating from the AV node or slightly lower in the conduction system. As we will see later in this chapter, *recognition of such subtle differences in QRS morphology may sometimes provide an important clue as to whether a particular P wave is conducting!*

PROBLEM **Interpret the rhythm shown in *Figure 16D-8A.* Is there evidence of atrial activity?**

HINT: Look *carefully* at the first beat.

ANSWER TO FIGURE 16D-8A At first glance, this appears to be either a junctional or accelerated ventricular escape rhythm (depending on whether the QRS complex was felt to be wide or not). The KEY to interpretation of the rhythm lies with assessment of the first beat. The very narrow, pointed upright deflection that precedes this beat looks very much like a P wave. If this

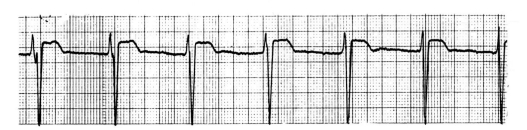

Figure 16D-8A. *Is there evidence of atrial activity in this tracing?*

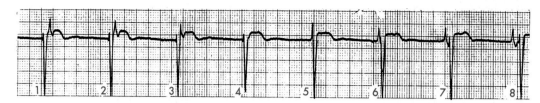

Figure 16D-8B.   Follow-up tracing from the patient whose rhythm was shown in Fig. 16D-8A. *Does this clarify the situation?*

were so, the PR interval preceding this first QRS complex would be exceedingly short and unlikely to conduct. After the first beat, atrial activity seemingly disappears. However, in view of the fact that the first QRS complex in this tracing has only a small (3 mm) r wave, the much larger (6 mm-plus) upright deflection seen at the onset of the other complexes in this tracing may represent more than just the QRS. That is, if the P wave that precedes the first QRS complex occurred *just a little bit later*, the resultant complex might then look like all of the other beats in this tracing.

PROBLEM   *Figure 16D-8B* **was obtained from the same patient shortly thereafter.** *Does it clarify the situation?*

ANSWER TO FIGURE 16D-8B   Atrial activity (in the form of a tall, pointed P wave) is much more evident on this follow-up tracing. It can now be seen that an underlying *AV nodal rhythm* exists with an almost perfectly regular rate of 52-53 beats/min. P waves are totally unrelated to the QRS complex—they follow the QRS in the beginning of the tracing (beats #1, #2, and #3), then get lost within the QRS (beat #4), *superimpose* on the initial part of the QRS (beats #5 and #6), and finally precede the QRS with a short PR interval (beats #7 and #8). This confirms our previous suspicion that P waves were present all along in Fig. 16D-8A (and superimposed on the QRS). When atrial and junctional pacemakers are unrelated but operate at nearly identical rates (as they do here), the condition is known as **isorhythmic AV dissociation**.

> Occasionally, atrial and junctional pacemakers continue to beat at nearly the same rate for extended periods of time, resulting in a rhythm in which P waves move "in and out" of the QRS complex. This phenomenon has been colorfully

termed *accrochage* by the French from their verb *s'accrocher* (to cling to). Despite slight variation in the rate of one or both competing pacemakers, each remains almost in phase with the other, *as if some unseen force was acting to keep the two together*. The situation is somewhat akin to a horse race in which the two front-runners remain neck and neck down the home stretch, each trying to eke out ahead of the other.

PROBLEM   **Having recognized the presence of isorhythmic dissociation in Figs. 16D-8A and 16D-8B, how would you render your interpretation of these rhythms?**

HINT: What is the *primary* rhythm disturbance in each case?

ANSWER   The primary rhythm disturbance in Figs. 16D-8A and 16D-8B is *sinus bradycardia*. As a result of sinus slowing (i.e., of "default" of the sinus pacemaker), AV dissociation occurs as the pacemaking function is naturally taken over by the slightly faster AV nodal escape rhythm (that is discharging appropriately at a rate of between 40 to 60 beats/min).

> Despite the fact that *none* of the P waves in either tracing are conducted (with the possible exception of beat #8 in Fig. 16D-8B), there is absolutely no evidence of any degree of AV block! On the contrary, the fact that the AV nodal rhythm takes over the pacemaking function may be a good thing, since it provides a regular ventricular response at a reasonable heart rate. Without establishment of this escape rhythm, it is possible that the ultimate rate of the defaulting sinus pacemaker would have been much slower.

PROBLEM   **Examine the rhythm shown in *Figure 16D-9*. Is there AV dissociation? Is there evidence of AV block?**

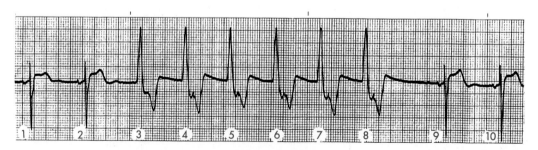

Figure 16D-9.   *Is there AV dissociation?* Is there evidence of AV block?

ANSWER TO FIGURE 16D-9   Following two sinus beats, the QRS complex widens and changes dramatically in appearance. Beats #3-8 obviously arise from a ventricular focus (wide, bizarre-looking QRS complex, no reason for aberrancy). These beats represent a run of *accelerated idioventricular rhythm (AIVR)* that takes over the pacemaking function because its intrinsic rate (80 beats/min) is faster than the rate of the sinus pacemaker.

Although AIVR is often an escape rhythm (that arises in response to slowing of the sinus pacemaker), this is not the case here. Instead, the first beat in the run (#3) occurs somewhat early (i.e., slightly *before* the next expected sinus beat). That is, the R-R interval between beats #2-3 measures *less* than the R-R interval between sinus conducted beats in the tracing (#1-2 and #9-10)—so that the beat that initiates the run of AIVR (#3) actually "usurps" the rhythm from the sinus pacemaker.

> Note notching in the ST segment after the first beat in the run of AIVR (i.e., for beats #4-8). This represents *retrograde* conduction to the atria from the idioventricular focus. As a result of this retrograde conduction the SA node is suppressed and prevented from discharging during the run. Thus, preservation of retrograde (VA or ventriculoatrial) conduction in this case *prevents* AV dissociation from taking place! A short pause follows the last beat in the run (#8), during which time the SA node is able to recover before resuming the pacemaking function (with beat #9).
>
> Contrast this situation with one in which retrograde conduction to the atria is blocked (such as occurs with the example of complete AV block that we reviewed in Fig. 16D-4A). Under the circumstances of complete (antegrade *and* retrograde) AV block, the SA note will continue to discharge at its own inherent rate, and complete AV dissociation will result (Fig. 16D-4B).

There is no indication of any degree of AV block in Fig. 16D-9, as all sinus initiated impulses (beats #1, #2, #9, and #10) are conducted to the ventricles with a normal PR interval.

The Many Faces of Wenckebach

In Section D of Chapter 3 we listed the following as characteristic features (i.e., "footprints") of 2° AV block Mobitz type I (Wenckebach):

> i. Regularity of the atrial rate
> ii. Group beating
> iii. Progressive lengthening of the PR interval until a beat is dropped
> iv. Duration of the pause (that contains the dropped beat) of *less* than twice the shortest R-R interval

In addition to the above, one might add:

> v. Progressive *shortening* of the R-R interval *within* groups of beats.

These features are illustrated in *Figure 16D-10*. Note that as the PR interval lengthens from beats #2-4, the R-R interval *shortens* (i.e., the R-R interval between beats #2-3 is greater than that between #3-4).

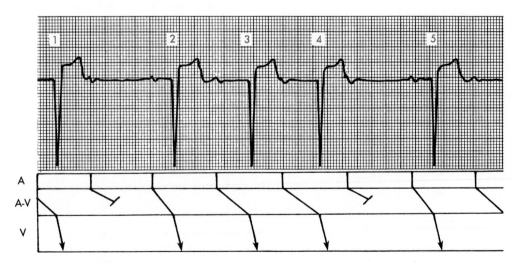

Figure 16D-10.   Second-degree AV block, Mobitz type I (Wenckebach). Each of the five characteristic "footprints" of Wenckebach cited above are present.

Note also in Fig. 16D-10 that the pause containing the dropped beat (the R-R interval between beats #4-5) is *less* than twice the shortest R-R interval (the R-R between beats #3-4). The reason for this is that the greatest *increment* (increase) in the PR interval usually occurs between the first and second beats of a Wenckebach group. In contrast, with Mobitz II 2° AV block, the PR interval for consecutively conducted QRS complexes remains constant, so that the pause which contains the dropped beat will be *equal* to twice the R-R interval. Finally, with phenomena such as sinus exit block or sinus pauses (which may both be manifestations of the sick sinus syndrome), and with blocked PACs (that reset and often suppress the SA node), the pause that contains the dropped beat is likely to be *greater* than twice the shortest R-R interval.

Up until now we have restricted our use of the term, "Wenckebach" to refer to 2° AV block occurring *at the level of the AV node*. We have also used "Wenckebach" as a synonym for 2° AV block of the Mobitz I type. Actually, many other examples of "Wenckebach-like" conduction exist, including:

i. Sinoatrial (SA) block with Wenckebach exit block
ii. Wenckebach AV conduction (which may occur at as many as *three* different levels within the AV node!) in the presence of atrial fibrillation or flutter
iii. Wenckebach AV conduction in the presence of atrial tachycardia
iv. Junctional rhythms with *retrograde* Wenckebach
v. Wenckebach periodicity arising from *within* a bundle branch (producing progressively increasing degrees of bundle branch block on successive beats)
vi. Ventricular tachycardia with retrograde Wenckebach exit block
vii. Many others . . . . .

Potentially, Wenckebach periodicity can occur in *any* segment of the conduction system that is capable of developing block (Conner, 1987). In depth discussion of these Wenckebach phenomena obviously extends beyond the scope of this book. Nevertheless, a relevant (and all too commonly ignored) clinical point worthy of emphasis is that recognition of the typical "footprints" of Wenckebach periodicity should prompt suspicion of the presence of this conduction disturbance *even when P waves are absent!*

As indicated in Table 16B-1, Wenckebach conduction disturbances are one of the most typical manifestations of digitalis toxicity. Recognition of Wenckebach periodicity in a patient who is being treated with digitalis should therefore raise a RED FLAG for the possibility of digitalis toxicity.

As helpful as recognition of the "typical footprints" is, it is well to remember that *not all arrhythmias obey all of the rules*, and not all of the footprints will be present in every case. In fact, a majority of arrhythmias that manifest Wenckebach periodicity will lack one or more of the "classic criteria" (Conner, 1987). For example, if an underlying sinus arrhythmia is present in a patient with Mobitz I 2° AV block, the atrial rhythm will not be regular (by definition), the R-R interval may not progressively decrease within each Wenckebach group, and the pause may not be less than twice the shortest R-R interval. Moreover, other arrhythmias can sometimes mimic certain aspects of Wenckebach periodicity such as a group beating (i.e., atrial bigeminy or trigeminy, blocked PACs, etc.). Nevertheless, keeping a watchful eye out for "the footprints" will yield surprising dividends in arrhythmia diagnosis.

PROBLEM   Next, consider *Figures 16D-11* and *16D-12A,* taken from an elderly woman with a known history of *atrial fibrillation* and congestive heart failure. *Is she still in atrial fibrillation?*

ANSWER TO FIGS. 16D-11 AND 16D-12A
Fine undulations in the baseline and the absence of definite P waves in this lead II monitoring lead suggest that the underlying rhythm is still atrial fibrillation. One is struck, however, by the *regular* irregularity of the ventricular response (*group beating!*). Long and short cycles alternate in Fig. 16D-11, while in Fig. 16D-12A typical features of Wenckebach periodicity are seen (group beating, progressively *decreasing* R-R intervals, pause duration of *less* than twice the shortest R-R interval). *Thus despite persistence of atrial fibrillation, there appears to be Wenckebach conduction!*

As alluded to earlier, the clinical significance of recognizing Wenckebach conduction in the setting of atrial fibrillation for a patient on digitalis is the same as that for recognizing "regularization" of the ventricular response—*it strongly suggests digitalis toxicity* (Table 16B-1).

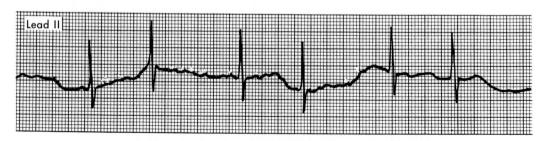

Figure 16D-11.   Rhythm strip from an elderly patient with congestive heart failure. *Is she in atrial fibrillation?*

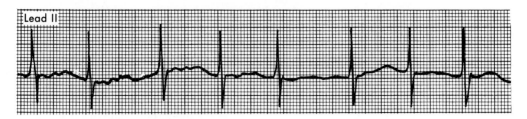

Figure 16D-12A.   Companion rhythm strip to Fig. 16D-11.
Is this atrial fibrillation?

The mechanism responsible for group beating in Fig. 16D-12A is illustrated in the laddergram shown in *Figure 16D-12B.* As noted, underlying atrial fibrillation is still present (fine undulations in the baseline, absence of P waves in lead II). As a result of digitalis toxicity, complete AV block is present (i.e., *none* of the atrial impulses are able to penetrate through the AV node to the ventricles). In response to the complete AV block, an AV nodal pacemaker takes over. And, as a result of digitalis toxicity, this escape pacemaker is not only accelerated, but also man-

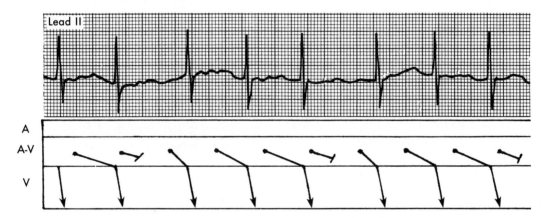

Figure 16D-12B.   Laddergram of the rhythm shown in Fig. 16D-12A. Underlying atrial fibrillation is present. Wenckebach periodicity (group beating, progressively *decreasing* R-R intervals, pause duration *less* than twice the shortest R-R interval) is the result of complete AV block and an accelerated AV nodal rhythm with Wenckebach exit block out of the AV node.

ifests Wenckebach exit block *out of the AV node*—producing the group beating seen in Fig. 16D-12B.

> We emphasize that being able to draw the laddergram shown in Fig. 16D-12B is *not* necessary for recognition of Wenckebach conduction. All that is needed is a discerning look at the overall pattern of the rhythm in Figs. 16D-11 and 16D-12A. Consistency to this degree in the regularity of each group would be exceedingly unlikely for a random rhythm such as atrial fibrillation. Postulating the existence of AV block

with some type of organized junctional response (i.e., Wenckebach exit block conduction) is by far the most reasonable explanation.

PROBLEM   **The rhythm shown in *Figure 16D-13A* was obtained from an elderly woman with a history of syncope. Among her multiple medications was her "heart pill." *What do you suspect is going on?***

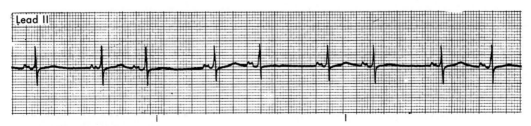

Figure 16D-13A.   Rhythm obtained from an elderly woman with a history of syncope. She is on digitalis. *What do you suspect is going on?*

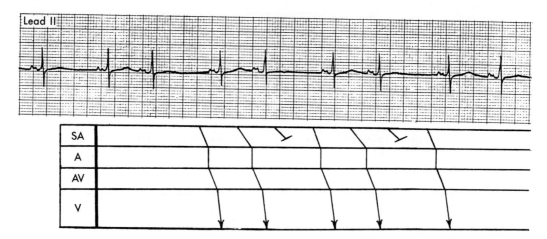

Figure 16D-13B.   Laddergram of the tracing shown in Fig. 16D-13A demonstrating SA block with Wenckebach conduction *out of* the SA node (i.e., Wenckebach exit block). SA nodal impulses are progressively delayed until one is blocked. Wenckebach periodicity is preserved (i.e., there is group beating and the pause containing the dropped beat is less than twice the shortest R-R interval).

HINT: Is there a pattern to the arrhythmia?

EXTRA HINT: The rhythm is *not* atrial bigeminy (i.e., every other beat is *not* a PAC!). It also is not *AV* nodal Wenckebach (i.e., it is *not* 2° AV block of the Mobitz I type).

ANSWER TO FIGURE 16D-13A   The most remarkable finding on this tracing is the presence of **group beating**—in this case with alternating long-short cycles. This should immediately suggest the possibility of some type of Wenckebach conduction.

Proceeding with the Four-Question Approach, the QRS complex is narrow, and normal-appearing P waves (with a normal PR interval) precede each QRS complex. Thus, the underlying rhythm is sinus. Although a possible explanation for the early beats is that they are simply PACs, this would seem less likely in view of the identical P wave morphology compared to the normal sinus P waves.

The laddergram shown in *Figure 16D-13B* offers an alternative explanation—*Wenckebach exit block out of the **SA node*** (i.e., SA block). With this conduction disturbance, the SA node continues to discharge at a regular rate. However, conduction of each impulse is progressively delayed, until finally an impulse is unable to get out of the SA node (i.e., "exit block"). The cycle then repeats itself.

Note that in addition to the usual A, AV, and V tiers in this laddergram, we have included a fourth tier labeled SA (sinoatrial tier). Events that occur within this tier are *not* seen on the surface ECG. Nevertheless, incorporation of the SA tier into Fig. 16D-13B is essential for illustrating the progressive delay of SA nodal impulses until one is finally blocked.

SA block with Wenckebach conduction (exit block) differs from AV nodal Wenckebach in that the atrial rate is *not* regular (since SA nodal impulses are *delayed* until one

is blocked), and the PR interval does *not* prolong (since each SA nodal impulse that does get out of the SA node is then conducted normally).* However, other elements of Wenckebach periodicity are preserved (i.e., group beating, pause containing the dropped beat of less than twice the shortest R-R interval).

As might be imagined, SA block may be a manifestation of the sick "sinus" syndrome. As is the case for other types of Wenckebach conduction, when seen in a patient taking digitalis, toxicity should be considered.

We emphasize that SA block is *not* a common conduction disturbance, and that its mechanism is somewhat complex. Nevertheless, it does occur, and it may have important clinical implications. Recognition of group beating is the KEY to suspecting the diagnosis.

We continue to illustrate some of the "many faces" of Wenckebach over the next few examples, in which typical features are not always evident.

PROBLEM   **Consider the rhythm shown in *Figure 16D-14*. Do you suspect some type of Wenckebach conduction? (i.e., Is there a *pattern* to the irregularity?)**

HINT TO THE MECHANISM: Are all QRS complexes identical in morphology? *Are all QRS complexes conducted?*

---

*It is somewhat hard to determine if the PR interval in Fig. 16D-13A is truly constant or increases slightly (due to some ever so subtle alteration in QRS complexes). *For simplicity,* we have assumed the former and drawn the laddergram accordingly—although admit the possibility that *in addition* to underlying SA block, a degree of AV Wenckebach may also be present.

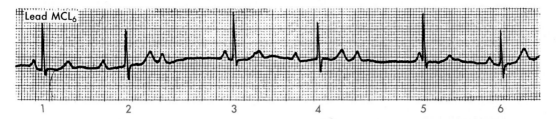

Figure 16D-14.   *Do you suspect some type of Wenckebach conduction?*

ANSWER TO FIGURE 16D-14   Once again, the most striking finding on this tracing is the presence of *group beating*—which should again lead you to suspect that a type of Wenckebach conduction disturbance *may* be present. P wave morphology is constant but the P-P interval varies, suggesting that *sinus arrhythmia* is the underlying rhythm. Beats *are* being dropped (i.e., one would definitely expect the P waves following beats #2 and #4 to conduct). Since complete AV block is unlikely (because the ventricular response is so variable), this tracing probably represents a type of 2° AV block. The narrow QRS and the presence of group beating suggest Mobitz I as the prime suspect.

The KEY lies with analysis of beats #1, #3, and #5. On close inspection it can be seen that QRS morphology of each of these beats differs slightly from that of beats #2, #4, and #6 (the latter three beats having a shorter R wave and slightly deeper S wave). The PR interval preceding beat #5 is *definitely too short to conduct*. This implies that this beat (and probably *also* the other two beats like it [beats #1 and #3]) are *junctional escape beats*. Supporting this contention is the fact that the R-R interval of the two escape beats that are seen on this tracing (the R-R interval between beats #2-3 and #4-5) is the same, and corresponds to a junctional escape rate of 38 beats/min.

> It is important to appreciate that the emergence of escape beats in this tracing is *appropriate*—and that without them the ventricular response would be even slower. However, their presence makes definitive diagnosis of the conduction disturbance a difficult task from this tracing alone.

Subsequent rhythm strips on this patient confirmed our suspicion that the arrhythmia was indeed 2° AV block, Mobitz type I (Wenckebach).

> This tracing is an excellent example of how in addition to group beating, recognition of subtle differences in QRS mor-

phology between junctional and sinus conducted beats may also provide a major clue to diagnosis.

PROBLEM   **What is the cause of the pause (between beats #7-8) in *Figure 16D-15? Could Wenckebach be present?***

ANSWER TO FIGURE 16D-15   By far, the commonest "cause of a pause" is a blocked PAC. However, this is *not* the cause of the pause that occurs between beats #7-8 in this tracing!

Following seven supraventricular beats that manifest a fairly constant R-R interval comes a pause. P waves with a prolonged PR interval (*1° AV block*) are evident in front of beats #1-5. Continuation with calipers set at the P-P interval beyond this point reveals a notch in the T wave of beat #5, no overt evidence of atrial activity in the T wave of beat #6, peaking of the T wave of beat #7, and an undisguised P wave (that occurs precisely on time) in front of beat #8. Thus the atrial rate remains perfectly regular, and the P wave hidden within the T wave of beat #7 is not conducted.

> The reason that the cause of the pause in this case is *not* a blocked PAC is that the P wave that is hidden within the T wave of beat #7 is *not* premature! (Instead, the atrial rhythm remains regular throughout the tracing.)

The relationship between P waves and the QRS complex is not all obvious on initial scanning of this tracing, since it is hard to determine if the PR interval is progressively increasing from beats #1-7. However, close inspection of the PR interval just *before* the pause, and comparison of this with the PR interval at the end of the pause (i.e., the PR interval that precedes beat #8) reveals a definite difference. Similarly, comparison of the PR interval preceding

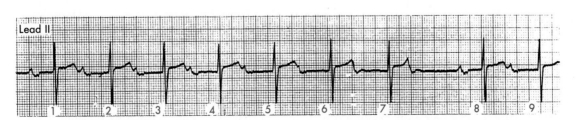

Figure 16D-15.   *Could the cause of the pause in this tracing be due to Wenckebach?*

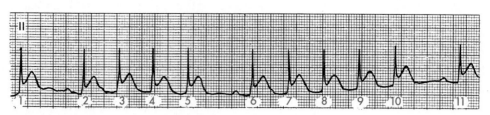

Figure 16D-16A. Rhythm strip from a patient with an acute inferior infarction. *Can you explain the irregularity of the ventricular response?*

the first beat in the sequence (beat #1) with the PR interval of the last beat in the sequence before the pause (#7) suggests that the PR interval *must be lengthening* until the beat is dropped. Therefore, the rhythm is 2° AV block, Mobitz type I (Wenckebach).

> Recognition of long Wenckebach cycles such as the one shown here is often quite difficult because PR interval prolongation from beat to beat may not be at all obvious. The KEY to diagnosis rests on three principles:
>
> i. First, rule out the commonest cause of a pause (i.e., a blocked PAC)
> ii. Look for the other "footprints" of Wenckebach (i.e., regular atrial rhythm, pause duration of less than twice the shortest R-R interval)
> iii. Compare the PR interval just *before* the pause with the PR interval at the *end* of the pause to see if it has lengthened.

PROBLEM   *Figure 16D-16A was taken from a patient with an acute inferior infarction. Can you explain the irregularity of the ventricular response?*

HINT #1:   Do you see groups of beats?
HINT #2:   Are any beats definitely conducted?
HINT #3:   Are any other "footprints" present?
HINT #4:   Does the clinical setting (acute inferior myocardial infarction) provide an additional clue?
HINT #5:   *See Table 3D-2.*

ANSWER TO FIGURE 16D-16A   This is a difficult tracing. Nevertheless, there are a number of clues to the etiology of this arrhythmia:

i. Group beating is present (albeit the groups contain different numbers of beats). Identical intervals between these groups (i.e., identical R-R intervals between beats #1-2, #5-6, and #10-11) suggest that this grouping is *not* simply by chance. *Recognition of group beating and the clinical setting (acute inferior infarction) are the KEY clues suggesting the etiology of this arrhythmia.*
ii. Beats #2, #6, and #11 *definitely* appear to be conducted (since the PR interval preceding each of these beats is the same). These beats are conducted with *1° AV block* (PR interval = 0.27 second).

iii. In addition to group beating, two of the other typical "footprints" of Wenckebach are present: (1) the atrial rate is regular (*see below*), and (2) the pause containing the dropped beat is *less* than twice the shortest R-R interval. Additional electrocardiographic findings consistent with 2° AV block, Mobitz type I (Wenckebach) are the presence of 1° AV block, and the fact that the QRS complex is narrow.
iv. As implied above, 2° AV block, Mobitz type I is a frequent complication of acute inferior infarction (since the inferior wall of the left ventricle and the AV node are *both* almost always supplied by the right coronary artery).

Taken together, the *combination* of these findings should make you strongly suspect 2° AV block of the Wenckebach type—*even if you are unsure of how to prove this suspicion.*

> Our explanation of this arrhythmia is somewhat complex, and is best understood by illustration with a laddergram (*Figure 16D-16B*). Despite the fact that ST segment elevation from the acute inferior infarction obscures atrial activity, the likely location of P waves can still be deduced. Working on the assumption that the arrhythmia *may* be Mobitz I, this would mean that the atrial rate should be regular and that dropped P waves should be contained within the T waves of beats #5 and #10 in Figure 16D-16A. Looking at the entire first Wenckebach cycle (encompassing beats #2-6), *five* P waves should be contained inside—three P waves that precede beats #3, #4, and #5 (and are hidden in the T wave), the nonconducted P wave (that is hidden in the T wave of beat #5), and the one clearly seen P wave (that precedes beat #6). Dividing this entire cycle length (the interval from the R wave of beat #2 until the R wave of beat #6) by five should therefore yield the P-P interval of the underlying sinus rate (if the atrial rate is regular). Starting with the P wave that is clearly seen (the P wave preceding beat #2), *presumed* atrial activity can now be plotted out and the laddergram completed. *That these suppositions are probably accurate is supported by subtle notching of the T wave of beats #2 and #6 at PRECISELY the place where one would expect the next P wave to occur (arrows in Fig. 16D-16B), and* the fact that the atrial rate marches out perfectly for the entire rhythm strip.

Construction of this laddergram admittedly extends well beyond the scope of this text. Nevertheless, the important point to remember is that although the *footprints* of Wenckebach may be subtle, they can usually be identified if looked for. Doing so, and considering the clinical context (in this case, acute inferior infarction), may suggest the diagnosis

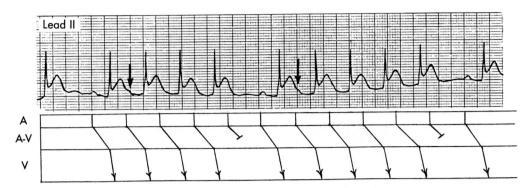

Figure 16D-16B. Laddergram of the arrhythmia shown in Fig. 16D-16A. Arrows indicate P waves that are partially hidden within the terminal aspect of preceding T waves. Second degree AV block of the Wenckebach type is suggested by the presence of typical "footprints" (regular atrial rate, progressively increasing PR interval, pause duration of less than twice the shortest R-R interval), 1° AV block, and narrow QRS complex that all occur in the clinical setting of acute inferior infarction.

even when atrial activity is partially hidden and the mechanism of the arrhythmia is complex.

When (and Why) to Suspect Mobitz II

Up until this point we have concentrated our attention on the diagnostic features of Mobitz I 2° AV block. We conclude this section by focusing on the other major form of 2° AV block: Mobitz II.

We start with the definition:

> **Mobitz II 2° AV block** is said to occur when atrial impulses are blocked in the setting of *CONSECUTIVELY* conducted beats that manifest a *constant PR interval*.

PROBLEM   **Almost every other beat in *Figure 16D-17* is dropped. *Is this Mobitz II?***

HINT: Does the PR interval remain constant *throughout* the entire rhythm strip? (i.e., Does the PR interval remain

constant when *CONSECUTIVELY conducted beats are seen???*)

ANSWER TO FIGURE 16D-17   Although it is hard to be certain of where the QRS ends and the ST segment begins, the QRS complex in this tracing appears to be slightly prolonged. The atrial rate remains regular throughout at 75 beats/min. For the first four beats, every other P wave is blocked. For those beats that are conducted (#1, #2, #3, and #4), the PR interval remains constant. If the rhythm strip ended here (i.e., *after* beat #4), it would be *impossible* to distinguish between the Mobitz I and Mobitz II forms of 2° AV block. Moreover, because of QRS widening (and to a lesser extent the normal PR interval), one would have to be concerned about the possibility of Mobitz II.

As emphasized in Section D of Chapter 3, definitive differentiation between Mobitz I and Mobitz II may not be possible in the setting of 2° AV block when there is *pure* 2:1 AV conduction. This is *not* the case here, however, since the telltale sign of Wenckebach (PR interval lengthening) surfaces at the end of the tracing (the PR interval preceding beat #5 lengthens with respect to the PR interval preceding beat #4). Because it is exceedingly unlikely for a patient to switch abruptly from Mobitz I to Mobitz II, the conduction disturbance shown in Fig. 16D-17 almost certainly represents Wenckebach (*not* Mobitz II!) with 2:1 and 3:2 AV conduction.

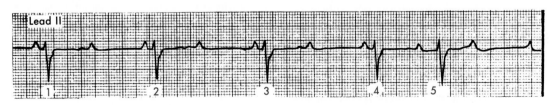

Figure 16D-17.   *Is this Mobitz II 2° AV block?*

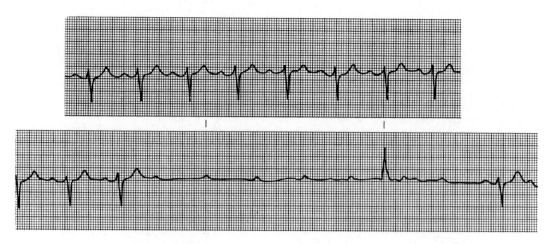

Figure 16D-18. Rhythm strip from a patient with acute anterior infarction. Sudden development of Mobitz II 2° AV block with a long period of ventricular standstill.

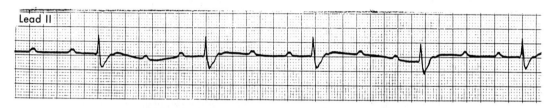

Figure 16D-19. *What kind of AV block is present?*

The KEY to arriving at the *correct diagnosis* in this case resides with the definition given above for *Mobitz* II: *CONSECUTIVELY conducted beats* manifesting a *constant PR interval MUST* be seen before one can conclude that any nonconducted atrial impulses are the result of Mobitz II 2° AV block. When there is *pure* 2:1 AV conduction, *consecutively* conducted beats will never be seen (by definition). As a result, one cannot determine if the PR interval is prolonging before a beat is dropped—so that one cannot rule out the possibility of Mobitz I 2° AV block with 2:1 AV conduction.

Clinically, Mobitz II is *far less common* than Mobitz I. *Figure 16D-18,* taken from a patient with an acute anterior infarction, illustrates why prompt recognition of this uncommon conduction disturbance is essential when it does occur.

ANSWER TO FIGURE 16D-18   Initially the patient is in sinus rhythm. Then, with nary a warning, comes a 4-second period of *ventricular standstill* that is finally terminated by a ventricular escape beat. This behavior is typical of Mobitz II 2° AV block, which may sometimes very suddenly and dramatically progress to either complete AV block or ventricular standstill. The clinical setting in which this conduction disorder is most likely to occur is acute anterior infarction. Recognition of Mobitz II 2° AV block is a definite indication for pacemaker therapy (insertion of a transvenous pacemaker, or at least active standby with an external pacemaker).

PROBLEM   **We conclude this section with the arrhythmia shown in *Figure 16D-19*. What kind of AV block is present?**

ANSWER TO FIGURE 16D-19   The ventricular response is regular at a rate of just under 40 beats/min. The atrial rate is also regular at 115 beats/min (with a partially hidden P wave notching the terminal portion of each QRS complex). Complete (3°) AV block is not present because despite conduction of only one out of every three P waves, a relationship *does* exist between those P waves that are conducted and the QRS (i.e., the PR interval remains constant!). Although one cannot rule out the possibility of Mobitz I (since *consecutively* conducted beats are never seen before a beat is dropped), QRS widening and the high-grade nature of the conduction disturbance make it likely that the anatomic level of the block is low. Our interpretation would be:

- *2° AV block with 3:1 AV conduction (i.e., high-grade AV block)—probable Mobitz II.*

Section E offers a **Final Challenge** in diagnosis of the AV blocks. *Are you up to the challenge?*

REFERENCES

Conner RP: The Wenckebach phenomenon, *Heart Lung* 16:506, 1987.

SECTION E

AV BLOCKS: A FINAL CHALLENGE

In an attempt to consolidate the information presented in Section D of this chapter, we offer a **Final Challenge in AV Block.** Many of these tracings contain subtle findings, and some are downright tricky. To keep you "honest" we intentionally include a number of exceedingly deceptive *mimics* of AV block among the examples of the various forms of AV block. *Are you up to the challenge?*

PROBLEM   **A pause occurs after beat #9 in *Figure 16E-1*. Is this pause the result of 2° AV block?**

ANSWER TO FIGURE 16E-1   The first four beats in this tracing are sinus conducted. Beat #5 is a PAC (with the premature P wave subtly notching the terminal portion of the preceding T wave). Following this comes a ventricular couplet (beats #6 and #7), two more sinus beats, and then the pause. . . . .

The most common cause of a pause is a blocked PAC!

In our experience, the most common reason *(by far!)* for misdiagnosis of either 2° or 3° AV block is failure to recognize the presence of one or more blocked PACs. Sur-

prisingly often such PACs will be obvious (if looked for), although occasionally they may only be recognizable as a subtle notching in the preceding T wave. This is the case here. Comparison of the "normal" T wave (i.e., the T wave of beats #1, #2, #3, and #8) with the T wave of beat #9 (at the onset of the pause) reveals this notching.

> Note that the PR interval of the beat that terminates the pause (beat #10) is short. This is a *junctional escape beat* that discharged before the P wave that precedes it was able to conduct to the ventricles. The fact that the QRS complex of beat #10 is narrow and similar (but *NOT* identical) in morphology to the other sinus-conducted beats on this tracing (its S wave is not quite as deep) is additional evidence in support of this being a junctional beat.

PROBLEM   **Almost every other P wave in *Figure 16E-2* is not conducted. *Does this represent 2:1 AV block of the Mobitz I or Mobitz II type?***

ANSWER TO FIGURE 16E-2   Neither. There is no evidence of any AV block on this tracing.

The most common cause of a pause is a blocked PAC!

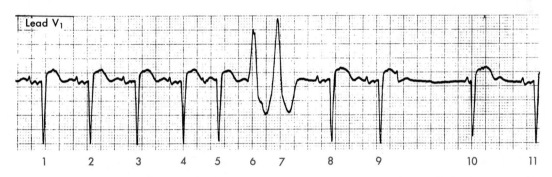

Figure 16E-1.   *Is the pause between beats #9-10 the result of 2° AV block?*

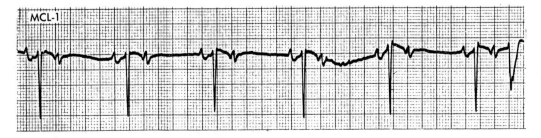

Figure 16E-2.   *Does this rhythm represent Mobitz I or Mobitz II 2° AV block?*

In general, the atrial rate will be regular with either Mobitz I or Mobitz II 2° AV block (unless there is an underlying sinus arrhythmia). The atrial rate in Fig. 16E-2 is far too irregular for this to be a form of AV block. Instead, every other P wave occurs *early*. This suggests that the underlying rhythm is *atrial bigeminy* (i.e., every other P wave is a PAC), in which all of the PACs are blocked except for the last one (that conducts with a LBBB pattern of aberration). *Atrial bigeminy with blocked PACs is one of the most common mimics of 2:1 AV block.*

> Two additional subtle points provide further support for the diagnosis of atrial bigeminy:
>
> i. Morphology of the early-occurring P waves appears to be ever so slightly different than that of those P waves that are conducted normally (which all seem to have a wider terminal negative component). If the rhythm was a form of AV block, all of the P waves should look the same.
>
> ii. The morphologic appearance of the last QRS complex on the tracing is consistent with an aberrantly conducted supraventricular impulse (similar initial r wave deflection, rapid initial descent of the S wave). The presence of one PAC should raise the possibility of other PACs on the tracing.

PROBLEM   Does the arrhythmia shown in *Figure 16E-3* represent a form of AV block?

ANSWER TO FIGURE 16E-3   The ventricular rhythm is definitely irregular in this tracing. Nevertheless, the QRS complex is narrow, and each QRS *is* preceded by a P wave (albeit with a long and *changing* PR interval). Normal-appearing (i.e., upright) P waves are seen in this lead II monitoring lead at a slightly variable rate (of between 55-62 beats/minute).

Three P waves are not conducted (the P waves that follow beats #3, #4, and #5). However, the cause of the pauses in this example does *not* appear to be due to blocked PACs since the non-conducted P waves are not premature and their morphology is *identical* to that of the sinus conducted P waves on this tracing. Mentally subtracting these P waves from the T wave at the onset of each pause leaves us with a flat ST segment and T wave that appears to be identical to the "normal" T wave (i.e., the T wave that follows beats #1 and #2).

The KEY resides in focusing on the PR interval that precedes beats #1-3: *the PR gradually prolongs until a beat is*

dropped! Two of the other "footprints" are present: (1) the R-R interval progressively decreases (albeit ever so slightly) from beats #1-2 to beats #2-3; and (2) the pause containing the dropped beat (i.e., the R-R interval between beats #3-4) is *less* than twice the shortest R-R interval. Thus, the rhythm in Fig. 16E-3 is 2° AV block, Mobitz type I (Wenckebach) with 4:3 and 2:1 AV conduction.

> Two other findings that are consistent with Mobitz I 2° AV block are that the QRS complex is narrow and that there is also 1° AV block for the first beat in each Wenckebach sequence (i.e., for beats #1, #4 and #5). Although hard to determine from this short tracing, there is also the suggestion of "group beating" (with the R-R interval between beats #3-4 and #4-5 being almost the same).
>
> As noted above, the P-P interval varies slightly. This is most likely the result of a ***ventriculophasic sinus arrhythmia.*** Slight variation in the atrial rate is commonly seen with either AV block or AV dissociation in the setting of a slow ventricular response. Although the precise mechanism for this phenomenon is not entirely clear, it may reflect rate-related alterations in coronary perfusion. Thus in this particular example, shorter P-P intervals surround QRS complexes, whereas the P-P intervals that are contained within the pauses (i.e., the P-P intervals *between* beats #3-4 and 4-5) are *longer*—presumably because coronary perfusion is decreased during this time.

A final "footprint" of Wenckebach that we have not previously discussed is present on this tracing: ***PR/RP reciprocity.*** As a natural result of Wenckebach conduction, *the shorter the* **RP interval,** *the longer the next* **PR interval** will be (and vice versa). RP interval shortening causes the P wave to occur at a relatively *earlier* point in the refractory period. As might be expected, this tends to produce a greater degree of prolongation of the next PR interval.

> For example, in Fig. 16E-3, the RP interval following beat #1 (i.e., the interval from the R wave of beat #1 until the next P wave) is slightly *longer* than the RP interval that follows beat #2. *This explains why the PR interval that precedes beat #3 is slightly longer than the PR interval that precedes beat #2!* That is, the *shorter* **RP interval** (that follows beat #2) is associated with a correspondingly *longer* **PR interval** preceding the next beat (preceding beat #3).

Despite the fact that *RP/PR reciprocity* is fundamental to the diagnosis of AV nodal Wenckebach, many clinicians are unfamiliar with this concept. Practically speaking, it is *not* essential to invoke this concept for diagnosis of the overwhelming majority of cases of Mobitz I 2° AV block. This is because the other more commonly cited "foot-

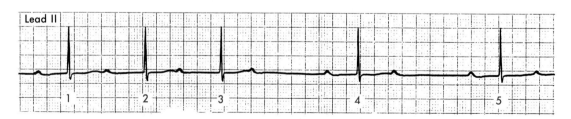

Figure 16E-3.   *Does this arrhythmia represent a form of AV block?*

prints" almost always provide more than ample information to make the diagnosis. However, on occasion (as in Fig. 16E-3), recognition of RP/PR reciprocity may provide an extremely helpful clue that 2° AV block of the Wenckebach type is either present, or that the patient *has the potential* to develop Wenckebach conduction.

PROBLEM   Does the arrhythmia shown in *Figure 16E-4* represent a form of AV block?

ANSWER TO FIGURE 16E-4   On initial inspection this arrhythmia may appear to resemble the arrhythmia just discussed (in Fig. 16E-3). This is *not* the case! Although the ventricular rhythm is once again irregular and the QRS complex is narrow, any resemblance between Figs. 16E-3 and 16E-4 ends here. Small, upright deflections that *simulate* P waves are noted to occur between each R-R interval, *but these deflections appear more related to the QRS complex that precedes them* rather than to the subsequent QRS complex (i.e., the R-"P" interval is *fixed!*). The ventricular response is too irregular for this to be a junctional rhythm with a retrograde P wave. Thus, the rhythm is *atrial fibrillation* with a controlled ventricular response. The small upright deflections following each QRS complex are T waves *(and not P waves!)*.

PROBLEM   Does the arrhythmia shown in *Figure 16E-5* represent a form of AV block?

ANSWER TO FIGURE 16E-5A   On initial inspection, there is the suggestion of group beating. The QRS complex is narrow and the ventricular rhythm irregular. Some P waves are clearly evident—others appear to notch the terminal portion of the T wave. Underlying *sinus arrhythmia* is present, since the atrial rate is slightly

irregular. P waves *do* precede each QRS complex, however, and within each group of beats the PR interval lengthens until a beat is dropped. This is *2° AV block, Mobitz type I*. The reason the diagnosis may not be initially apparent is the result of the sinus arrhythmia, fairly slow atrial rate, and underlying 1° AV block.

Three additional "footprints" of Wenckebach are present on this tracing and help solidify the diagnosis:

 i. Progressively decreasing R-R intervals
 ii. Pause duration of *less* than twice the shortest R-R interval
 iii. *RP/PR reciprocity* (see our Answer to Fig. 16E-3).

In Figure 16E-5B, recorded from the same patient, arrows highlight the P waves. The relationship of these P waves to the QRS (progressively lengthening PR interval within each group until a beat is dropped) is now more readily recognized.

PROBLEM   Does the arrhythmia shown in *Figure 16E-6* represent a form of AV block?

ANSWER TO FIGURE 16E-6   Initially there is sinus bradycardia at a rate of about 48 beats/min. There follows a short pause which is terminated by a *junctional escape rhythm* (beginning with beat #4) at the slightly slower rate of 45 beats/min. Retrograde conduction to the atria occurs with the junctional rhythm. There is no evidence of any AV block.

The reason for the short pause (after beat #3) in the sinus rhythm is not apparent. It may be as "innocent" as transient slowing of the SA nodal pacemaker, or as worrisome as sinus arrest. Takeover of the pacemaking function by the junctional escape rhythm is not only appropriate in this case, but also *protective* (since it ensures that the ventricular response will not drop below 45 beats/min).

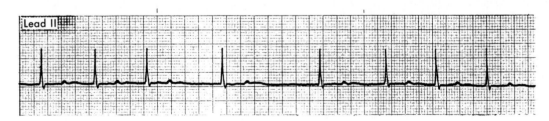

Figure 16E-4.   *Does this arrhythmia represent a form of AV block?*

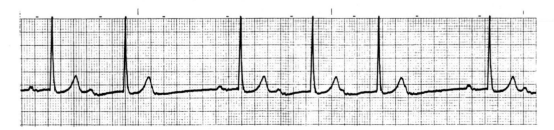

Figure 16E-5A.   *Does this arrhythmia represent a form of AV block?*

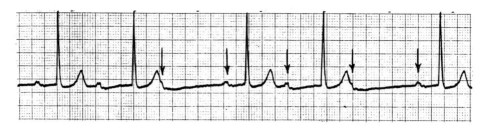

Figure 16E-5B. Follow-up rhythm strip to Fig. 16E-5A. Arrows highlight atrial activity. Progressive lengthening of the PR interval until a beat is dropped is now more apparent.

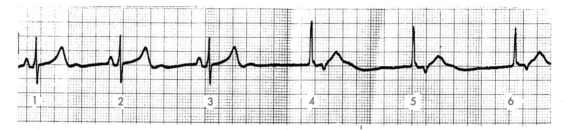

Figure 16E-6. *Does this arrhythmia represent a form of AV block?*

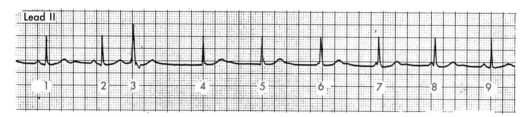

Figure 16E-7A. Does this arrhythmia represent a form of AV block? *Do any of the P waves fail to conduct at a time when they would be expected to conduct?*

Note that QRS morphology of the junctional beats (#4, #5, and #6) differs slightly from QRS morphology of the sinus-conducted beats.

PROBLEM Does the arrhythmia shown in *Figure 16E-7A* represent a form of AV block?

HINT #1: Do any of the P waves fail to conduct at a time when they would be expected to conduct?

HINT #2: Is there evidence of atrial activity after beat #3? *If so, in what direction?* (What effect might this atrial activity have on the SA node?)

ANSWER TO FIGURE 16E-7A The first two beats in this tracing are sinus conducted. There follows a PVC (beat #3) and a change in the underlying rhythm. That is, no P wave is seen to precede beats #4 and #5, and only a portion of the P wave precedes beats #6-8. Thus, beats #4-8 represent a *junctional escape rhythm* (narrow, normal-appearing QRS complex, absent P wave or PR interval too short to conduct). Normal sinus rhythm resumes with the last beat on the tracing (beat #9).

Reference to the laddergram shown in *Figure 16E-7B*

clarifies the mechanism for the arrhythmia. It is likely that the shallow negative deflection that follows the PVC represents *retrograde* atrial activity. Retrograde atrial conduction would be expected to depolarize the atria and reset the SA node, thereby delaying discharge of the next sinus impulse. Thus, there is a normal, physiologic explanation for the short pause that follows the PVC. Because the duration of this pause (6 large boxes or 1.20 second) is *greater* than the R-R interval of the junctional escape focus, the junctional escape rhythm temporarily takes over until the SA node recovers sufficiently to resume its pacemaking function (with beat #9).

Because the PR interval preceding beats #6-8 in Fig. 16E-7A is too short to conduct, these P waves are *unrelated* to the QRS complex. Thus by definition, there is *AV dissociation*—in this case due to the temporary "default" of the SA nodal pacemaker. However, there is absolutely no evidence of any degree of AV block since the reason for development of AV dissociation is physiologic (i.e., *suppression* of SA nodal activity as a result of retrograde conduction from the PVC), and *none* of the non-conducted P waves occur at a time when they should be expected to conduct.

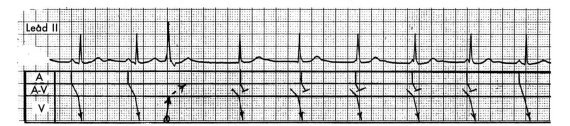

Figure 16E-7B.   Laddergram of the arrhythmia shown in Fig. 16E-7A. Retrograde atrial conduction from the PVC delays discharge of the SA nodal pacemaker and allows the junctional escape focus to take over. Normal sinus rhythm resumes with the last beat on the tracing.

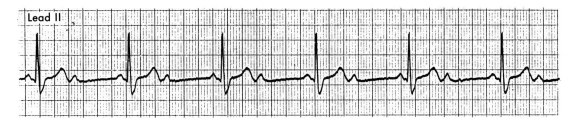

Figure 16E-8.   *Does this arrhythmia represent a form of AV block?*

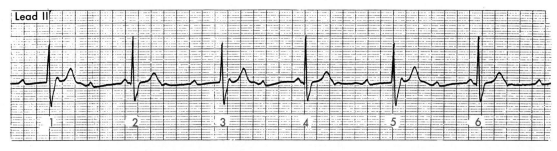

Figure 16E-9A.   Follow-up rhythm strip to Fig. 16E-8. *Has this patient now developed 3° (complete) AV block?*

PROBLEM   Does the arrhythmia shown in *Figure 16E-8* represent a form of AV block?

ANSWER TO FIGURE 16E-8   As opposed to the example of "pseudo 2:1 AV block" that we presented in Fig. 16E-2, the atrial rate here is truly regular (at a rate of 90 beats/min). The ventricular response is also regular (at a rate of about 45 beats/min), the QRS complex is wide, and each QRS is preceded by a P wave with a fixed (and normal) PR interval. Since every other P wave is non-conducted, there is *2° AV block with 2:1 AV conduction*.

You may be bothered by the slight variation in P wave morphology between conducted and non-conducted P waves. Unfortunately, *no rhythm strip is perfect.* It is likely that the slightly greater amplitude and peaking of non-conducted P waves (the P waves immediately following T waves) is due to *superposition* upon much smaller U waves that almost imper-

ceptibly lie below.* Complicating matters further, morphology of those P waves that are conducted also changes slightly from beat to beat as the result of baseline artifact. However, *because atrial activity is so regular in Fig. 16E-8, the 2:1 AV block is likely to be real (and not the result of atrial bigeminy with blocked PACs).*

As emphasized earlier, it is often impossible to distinguish between the Mobitz I and Mobitz II forms of 2° AV block in the presence of 2:1 AV conduction. In this particular example, QRS widening and the normal PR interval preceding conducted beats are two factors in favor of Mobitz II *(see Table 3D-2).*

PROBLEM   **A short while later, this same patient was observed to be in the rhythm shown in *Figure 16E-9A*. Has the patient now developed 3° (complete) AV block?**

---

*Small U waves *are* seen to follow some of the T waves in the next tracing recorded from this same patient (Fig. 16E-9A) in places where they are no longer obscured by atrial activity.

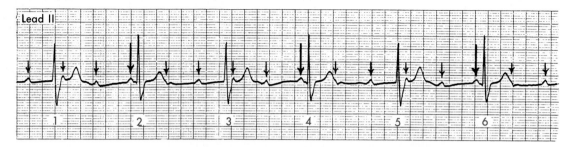

Figure 16E-9B. Explanatory tracing illustrating the mechanism of the arrhythmia shown in Fig. 16E-9A. Arrows indicate atrial activity. Large arrows indicate P waves that are conducting.

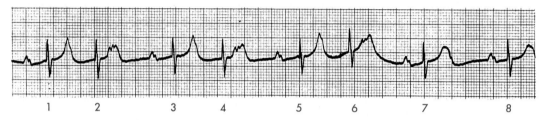

Figure 16E-10A. *Does this arrhythmia represent a form of AV block?*

ANSWER TO FIGURE 16E-9A Although at first glance it may appear that 3° AV block has developed, this is *not* the case! Our first clue that the rhythm shown in Fig. 16E-9A is *not* 3° AV block is that the ventricular rhythm *is no longer regular!* The answer is forthcoming in *Figure 16E-9B*.

Careful measurement with calipers reveals that R-R intervals between beats #1-2, #3-4 and #5-6 are all *shorter* than the R-R interval of the escape rhythm (the R-R interval between beats #2-3 and #4-5). Atrial activity remains regular in Fig. 16E-9B (arrows), albeit at a slightly *faster rate* (105 beats/min) than was present in Fig. 16E-8. *Beats #2, #4, and #6 are conducted!* P waves preceding each of these beats (large arrows) demonstrate a fixed and identical PR interval to the PR interval that preceded *each* of the conducted beats in Fig. 16E-8. Further support that these beats are truly conducted arises from the fact that the QRS complex of each of these beats differs ever-so-slightly from the QRS complex of non-conducted beats #1, #3, and #5 (which have a slightly shorter R wave and deeper S wave), and that each of the conducted beats occurs early compared to the R-R interval of the non-conducted escape rhythm.

> This tracing provides another excellent example of how seemingly minor differences in QRS morphology may sometimes provide a major clue to whether certain beats are being conducted.

Although the subtleties of this arrhythmia are admittedly complex, the KEY point is that the rhythm shown in Fig. 16E-9A is *not* complete AV block—and that careful assessment of the regularity of the ventricular response is an easy-to-determine parameter that leads the way to this conclusion.

PROBLEM **Does the arrhythmia shown in *Figure 16E-10A* represent a form of AV block?**

ANSWER TO FIGURE 16E-10A Yes, although this may not be readily apparent on initial inspection of this tracing. The QRS complex is narrow and the ventricular rate irregular. Once again, the KEY to interpretation of the rhythm lies with recognition of group beating. This should suggest the possibility of Wenckebach. Definite P waves are present in front of beats #1, #3, #5, #7, and #8. Note that the PR interval preceding each of these beats is fixed and prolonged (i.e., there is *1° AV block*). The question is whether other P waves are present on the tracing. The varying appearance of T waves (which are alternately peaked and notched early in the tracing, and ultimately become rounded) suggests that additional P waves may well be hiding within these T waves (and altering their appearance). That this is in fact the case can be verified by setting calipers to an interval that equals the distance between the P wave that precedes beat #3 and the point at the apex of the T wave of this beat. Doing so enables one to "walk out" the atrial rate for the rest of the tracing *(Figure 16E-10B)*.

It is apparent from Fig. 16E-10B that atrial activity is indeed regular. Focusing on QRS complexes within each group, it can now be seen that each QRS *is* preceded by

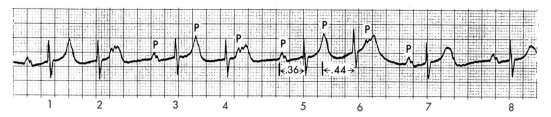

Figure 16E-10B. Explanatory tracing illustrating the mechanism of the arrhythmia shown in Fig. 16E-10A. P wave regularity is now evident.

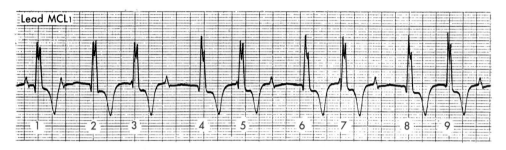

Figure 16E-11A. *Is the group beating in this tracing due to Mobitz I?*

a P wave, and that the PR interval progressively increases (for example, from 0.36 to 0.44 second for beats #5 and #6) until a beat is dropped (the P wave that notches the T wave of beat #6 is not conducted). Thus the rhythm is *2° AV block, Mobitz type I (Wenckebach)* with 3:2 and 2:1 AV conduction.

> In addition to group beating and regularity of the atrial rate, the pause containing the dropped beat in Fig. 16E-10P is *less* than twice the shortest R-R interval.

PROBLEM **Group beating is again present in *Figure 16E-11A. Is this also due to Mobitz I 2° AV block?***

ANSWER TO FIGURE 16E-11A The answer is *not at all* apparent from initial inspection of this tracing.

Nevertheless, the remarkable consistency of the group pattern in Fig. 16E-11A has to heighten one's index of suspicion for the possibility of Wenckebach conduction.

QRS complexes are wide. The initial deflection of the QRS varies slightly from beat to beat (with beats #3, #5, and #7 *all* manifesting a small initial positive deflection). *This small initial positive deflection may represent atrial activity!* Practically speaking, use of calipers and construction of a laddergram are essential for understanding the mechanism of this complex arrhythmia.

> The KEY for constructing the laddergram is to determine the atrial rate. The best way to do this is to find a place on the tracing in Fig. 16E-11A where *consecutive* P waves can clearly be seen. The only place this occurs involves the two P waves that sandwich beat #1. Assuming this distance to be the P-P interval, regular atrial activity can now be mapped out for the rest of the tracing *(Figure 16E-11B)*.

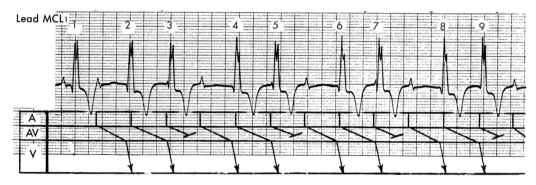

Figure 16E-11B. Laddergram of the tracing shown in Fig. 16E-11A. Atrial activity is regular, and the PR interval within groups prolongs until a beat is dropped.

Using the laddergram as a reference, it can be seen that P waves are hidden within the QRS complex of beats #2, #4, #6, #8, and #9. P waves produce a small positive deflection that is *superimposed* on the initial portion of the QRS complex of beats #3, #5, and #7. Again, using the laddergram as a reference, it can be seen that each QRS complex *is* preceded by a P wave, and that the PR interval within each group of beats prolongs until a beat is dropped. Thus the rhythm is *2° AV block, Mobitz type I (Wenckebach)* with 3:2 AV conduction. The reason for QRS widening is preexistent RBBB.

> This tracing is difficult to interpret for a number of reasons including QRS widening, the rapid atrial rate (of about 120 beats/min), and *marked* PR interval prolongation of the first conducted beat in each sequence—*all* of which act to conceal much of the atrial activity. Without use of calipers and the benefit of the laddergram shown in Fig. 16E-11B, it would be virtually impossible to prove the presence of Mobitz I 2° AV block, and equally difficult to accept that the P waves preceding beats #2, #4, #6, and #8 are *all* conducting, and that the PR interval is prolonged as much as it is (to *at least* 0.45 second)! Nevertheless, even *without* the laddergram and a pair of calipers, some type of Wenckebach conduction should be suspected simply from the regular irregularity (group beating) seen on the tracing.

PROBLEM   **The rhythm shown in *Figure 16E-12A* was obtained from an elderly woman with a long history of congestive heart failure and atrial fibrillation. She is on multiple medications. *What do you suspect is going on clinically?***

ANSWER TO FIGURE 16E-12A   The QRS complex is narrow. Although there are fine undulations in the baseline, no definite P waves are seen on this tracing. The R-R interval varies slightly from beat to beat, although the degree of irregularity is *not nearly* what one would expect for a patient in atrial fibrillation. Thus, there is **"regularization"** of atrial fibrillation. In a patient taking digitalis (as is likely here considering the clinical scenario), this strongly suggests toxicity.

> Among the many electrocardiographic manifestations of digitalis toxicity are AV block and accelerated junctional rhythms. This may result in "regularization" of atrial fibrillation if the irregularly occurring supraventricular impulses (from the atrial fibrillation) are prevented from passing through the AV node (due to *AV block*), and an escape rhythm arises (*accelerated* junctional rhythm) to take over the pacemaking function. The rate seen here (approximately 90 beats/min) is significantly faster than the usual AV nodal escape rate of 40-60 beats/minute, and definitely qualifies as an accelerated junctional response.

PROBLEM   **A short while later, a much more irregular rhythm was obtained from this same patient (Figure 16E-12B). Has she gone "back" into atrial fibrillation?**

ANSWER TO FIGURE 16E-12B   As noted, the rhythm has clearly become more irregular. Nevertheless, there is a distinct pattern to the irregularity. "Regularization" is seen for the initial four beats of the tracing (with an R-R interval similar to that noted in Fig. 16E-12A). This is followed by group beating (alternating long-short cycles for beats #5-6 and #7-8), and ends with a cycle of three beats (#9-11) that demonstrate typical Wenckebach periodicity (progressively *decreasing* R-R interval within a cycle).

Note that for *each* of the three "groups" of beats on the tracing (i.e., for beats #5-6, #7-8, and #9-11), the pauses

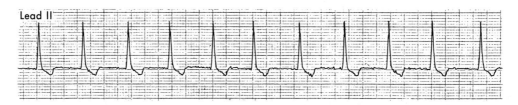

Figure 16E-12A.   Rhythm strip from a patient with a long history of congestive heart failure and atrial fibrillation. *What do you suspect is going on clinically?*

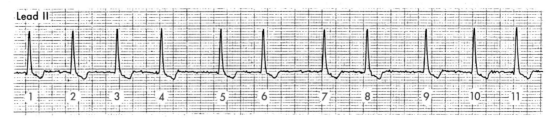

Figure 16E-12B.   Follow-up rhythm strip to Fig. 16E-12A on the elderly woman with a history of congestive heart failure. *Has she gone "back" into atrial fibrillation?*

(i.e., the longer R-R intervals that occur *between* beats #4-5, #6-7, and #8-9) are not only approximately the same in duration, but also measure *less* than twice the shortest R-R intervals. In addition, note that the "shortest" R-R interval of each group (the R-R interval between beats #5-6, #7-8, and #10-11) is virtually *the same* as the R-R interval of the accelerated junctional response during regularization (the R-R interval between beats #1-2, #2-3, and #3-4). The overall pattern of these relationships is much too unusual to simply be the result of chance, and strongly suggests Wenckebach conduction. In this case, the Wenckebach conduction occurs as junctional impulses are transmitted *out of* the AV node (i.e., Wenckebach "exit block"). Together with Fig. 16E-12A, this pattern overwhelmingly suggests digitalis toxicity *(see Table 16B-1)*.

PROBLEM   **The rhythm shown in *Figure 16E-13* is another example of group beating. Is this also the result of Wenckebach?**

ANSWER TO FIGURE 16E-13   Despite the presence of group beating, there is no evidence of AV block on this tracing. Once again, *the most common cause of a pause . . . . .* and, premature P waves *can* clearly be seen to notch the T waves of beats #2 and #6. Thus, the rhythm is sinus with blocked PACs.

> AV nodal Wenckebach is not present because the atrial rate is not regular (the P waves that notch the T waves of beats #2 and #6 definitely occur *early*), and the PR interval does not prolong.
>
> Of interest, note that the PR interval preceding beat #7 is shorter than the PR interval of the sinus conducted beats on the tracing. This implies that beat #7 is a *junctional escape beat* that occurs *before* the P wave preceding it is able to conduct to the ventricles. Considering that the R-R interval preceding this escape beat (the R-R interval between beats #6-7) is about 6.5 large boxes, the rate of this junctional escape focus is appropriate (i.e., well within the range of 40-60 beats/min).

> Clinically, *blocked PACs are seen far more commonly than AV block*. Because non-conducted PACs frequently produce grouping of beats, this rhythm disturbance may superficially mimic AV nodal Wenckebach.

PROBLEM   **Is the group beating shown in *Figure 16E-14A* the result of Mobitz I 2° AV block?**

ANSWER TO FIGURE 16E-14A   Once again despite group beating, Wenckebach is not present. The QRS complex is narrow and the underlying rhythm is sinus. Two short pauses are seen (between beats #2-3 and #5-6), and *the most common cause of a pause . . .* Note that the T waves of beats #2, #5, and #8 all have an extra notch or peak that the "normal" T waves do not have. This is due to a blocked PAC. As was the case for Fig. 16E-13, other reasons can be cited for why this rhythm disturbance is not Wenckebach, including irregularity of the atrial rate and the absence of PR interval prolongation within each group.

PROBLEM   **A short while later, the rhythm shown in *Figure 16E-14B* was recorded on the same patient. *What has happened?***

ANSWER TO FIGURE 16E-14B   Once again the QRS complex appears normal, and the underlying rhythm is sinus. Beat #4 is early. Although this beat is wider, its initial deflection (slope *and* direction) is *identical* to that of the normally conducted beats. Note that the T wave preceding this beat is peaked compared to the T wave of normally conducted complexes. Beat #4 is a PAC conducted with aberration. In contrast, peaking of the T wave

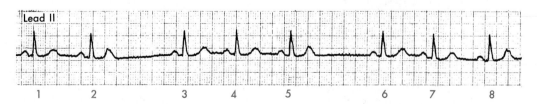

Figure 16E-13.   *Is the group beating seen in this tracing the result of Wenckebach?*

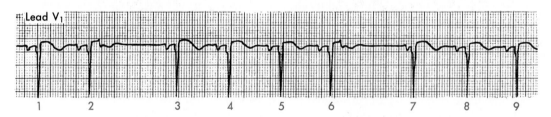

Figure 16E-14A.   *Is the group beating seen here the result of Wenckebach?*

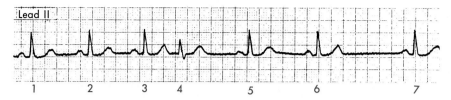

Figure 16E-14B.   Follow-up rhythm strip to Fig. 16E-14A.
What has happened?

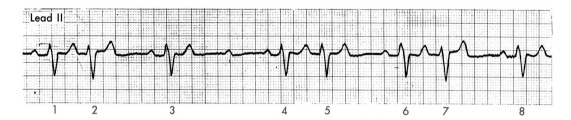

Figure 16E-15.   *Is this example of group beating the result of Wenckebach?*

of beat #6 (and the pause that follows) is the result of the same phenomenon seen in Fig. 16E-14A—*Non-conduction of a PAC.*

> The reason the first premature P wave in this tracing conducts but the second does not may be explained by *cycle-sequence comparison* (as was discussed in Section A of Chapter 15). Although the coupling intervals of each of these PACs is identical, the R-R interval *preceding* beat #6 is longer than the R-R interval preceding beat #3. As a result, the absolute refractory period following beat #6 will be slightly longer (Ashman phenomenon).

PROBLEM   **The rhythm shown in *Figure 16E-15* is a final example of group beating. *Is this pattern the result of Wenckebach?***

ANSWER TO FIGURE 16E-15   This is a difficult tracing, since no definite P waves are seen in front of beats #2, #5, and #7. The KEY is provided by the long R-R interval in which *two P waves occur in a row* before beat #4. Using this distance as the P-P interval, the atrial rate can be mapped out across the entire tracing (with the "missing" P waves plotting out at points that all correspond to the apex of the T waves). Thus, the atrial rhythm *is* regular. Several beats are dropped, which means that a type of 2° AV block must be present. Since the QRS complex is widened and each QRS is preceded by a P wave with a *fixed* PR interval, this probably represents Mobitz II.

> Additional reasons why this conduction disturbance is not Wenckebach are that pauses containing the dropped beat(s) are *not* less than twice the shortest R-R interval, and that *consecutively* conducted complexes are seen (beats #1 and 2; #4 and 5; and #6 and 7) in which the PR interval does not prolong.

PROBLEM   **Interpret the rhythm shown in *Figure 16E-16*. Is there evidence of AV block? (If so, of what type?) *What clinical condition is suggested by this arrhythmia?***

ANSWER TO FIGURE 16E-16   The QRS complex is narrow and the ventricular rate regular at 100 beats/min. The atrial rate is also regular, with two P waves occurring for each QRS. The relation of P waves to the QRS is constant, suggesting that every other atrial impulse is being conducted. Rather than Mobitz I or Mobitz II 2° AV block, however, the underlying problem appears to be *atrial tachycardia* (at a rate of 200 beats/min), in this case associated with *2:1 AV block.*

> Atrial tachycardia with block (formerly known as PAT with block) is one of the most typical manifestations of digitalis toxicity *(see Table 16B-1)*, although on occasion this arrhythmia may be seen in a patient who is not taking the drug.

The other diagnostic possibility to consider for the arrhythmia shown in Fig. 16E-16 is atrial flutter with 2:1 AV conduction. Against flutter is the atrial rate (which is well *below* the expected rate of 300 beats/min) and the lack of a clear sawtooth pattern. However, the possibility of atrial flutter could not be ruled out if the patient was on antiarrhythmic medication (that might slow the atrial rate) on the basis of this rhythm strip alone.

We conclude this section with a few clinical vignettes.

PROBLEM   **A middle-aged man presents to the Emergency Department with a several-hour history of severe chest pain. Blood pressure is 100/70 mm Hg, the chest pain has stopped, and he appears fairly comfortable at the time you arrive. His admission**

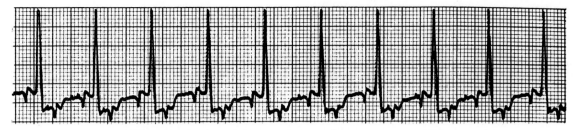

Figure 16E-16. Is there evidence of AV block? *What clinical condition is suggested by this arrhythmia?*

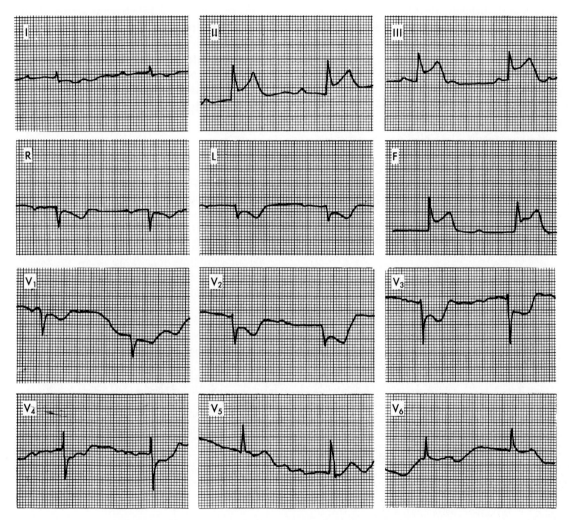

Figure 16E-17. 12-lead ECG obtained from a middle-aged man with severe chest pain. *How would you interpret this tracing?*

ECG is shown in *Figure 16E-17. How would you interpret this tracing?*

ANSWER TO FIGURE 16E-17   The QRS complex is narrow, and the rhythm fairly regular at a rate of between 45-50 beats/min. The PR intervals appear to vary in the different leads, indicating *AV dissociation*. ST segment elevation in leads II, III, and aVF; reciprocal ST segment depression in the anterolateral leads; and the clinical history all suggest *acute inferior infarction*.

PROBLEM   **Does the rhythm strip shown in *Figure 16E-18A* clarify the reason for the AV dissociation?**

ANSWER TO FIGURE 16E-18A   It can now be seen that the atrial rate is regular (at 80 beats/min), and

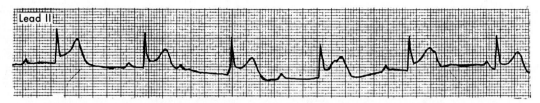

Figure 16E-18A. Rhythm strip obtained from the middle-aged man whose 12-lead ECG was shown in Fig. 16E-17. *Does this rhythm strip clarify the reason for AV dissociation?*

that P waves "march through" the QRS complexes *(Figure 16E-18B)*. Several of these P waves occur at points during the R-R interval where one would expect them to conduct if conduction was possible. Although our criteria for diagnosing 3° AV block are not completely met (the ventricular rate is a bit *over* 45 beats/min, and this rhythm strip is not really long enough to convincingly demonstrate the occurrence of P waves in *all* phases of the R-R interval), Fig. 16E-18B suggests that *3° AV block with a junctional escape pacemaker* may be present.

> Clinically, AV conduction disturbances in the setting of acute inferior infarction are often transient and may not require treatment as long as the patient is asymptomatic and remains hemodynamically stable. At least for the moment, this appears to be the situation in this case. Were the patient to develop chest pain, hypotension, ventricular ectopy, or other signs of hemodynamic compromise, treatment would be indicated. Atropine is the drug of choice. If atropine is ineffective, pacemaker therapy (insertion of a transvenous pacemaker or application of an external pacemaker) would be required.

PROBLEM The rhythm strips shown in *Figures 16E-19A* and *16E-19B* were recorded sequentially from a patient admitted several hours earlier for suspected acute myocardial infarction. *How would you interpret the rhythm?* What treatment would be indicated if the patient were asymptomatic and hemodynamically stable?

ANSWER TO FIGS. 16E-19A AND 16E-19B
No P waves are seen in either rhythm strip. The QRS complex is narrow for the first four beats in Fig. 16E-19A, during which time the rhythm is junctional with a slightly accelerated ventricular response (at about 65 beats/min). Beat #5 in this tracing occurs early and initiates a regular rhythm with a wider QRS complex of a completely different configuration. This is an *accelerated idioventricular rhythm (AIVR)*. It speeds up slightly but continues throughout Fig. 16E-19B.

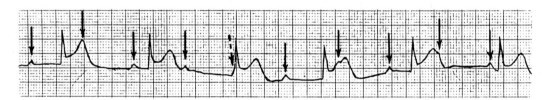

Figure 16E-18B. Arrows indicate that the atrial rate in Fig. 16E-18A is regular, and that P waves "march through" the QRS complexes.

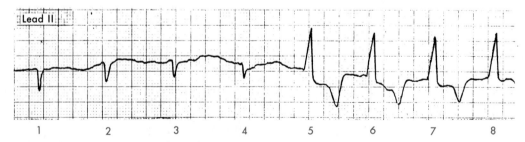

Figure 16E-19A. Rhythm strip recorded from a patient suspected of acute myocardial infarction. *How would you interpret the rhythm?*

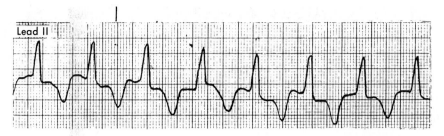

Figure 16E-19B.   Sequential rhythm strip to Fig. 16E-19A.

Four therapeutic options exist for managing AIVR:
  i. Lidocaine
  ii. Defibrillation (or synchronized cardioversion)
  iii. Atropine
  iv. *Benign neglect*

AIVR is commonly observed in the setting of acute myocardial infarction. It is usually a transient rhythm disorder that rarely results in adverse hemodynamic effects. Practically speaking, the risk of deterioration to ventricular fibrillation is minimal. Therefore in the asymptomatic, hemodynamically stable patient, the fourth option (*benign neglect*) is usually the treatment of choice.

AIVR most often occurs as an escape rhythm that arises in response to a failing SA or AV nodal pacemaker. As a result, treatment with lidocaine, defibrillation or synchronized cardioversion are not recommended as long as the patient remains hemodynamically stable because any of these actions may suppress (or *eliminate*) the *only* perfusing rhythm the patient has.

Occasionally, AIVR may also be seen as a "usurping" rhythm when the accelerated ventricular rate *overrides* the supraventricular pacemaker. This is the case in Fig. 16E-19A, in which a junctional rhythm at a rate of 65 beats/min is superseded by AIVR at 70 beats/min. If hypotension did occur with this rhythm, *atropine* would become the treatment of choice in the hope of stimulating the supraventricular pacemaker to overtake the ventricular rhythm.

> Most patients maintain adequate perfusion with AIVR. However, because the "atrial kick" is lost with this ventricular rhythm, some patients may develop hypotension.

PROBLEM   **A short while later the patient became hypotensive and atropine was given (*Figure 16E-20*). Was the atropine effective?**

ADDITIONAL QUESTION   **What is beat #6?**

ANSWER TO FIGURE 16E-20   AIVR at a rate of about 75 beats/min is again seen for the first five beats of the tracing. This is followed by resumption of the supraventricular rhythm at a rate of about 130 beats/min. Because P waves are still absent, this rhythm is probably junctional tachycardia. Although resumption of a supraventricular pacemaker and acceleration of the heart rate are both indicators of a favorable response to atropine, the response is not ideal since sinus rhythm (and the associated atrial kick) did not return.

> The QRS complex of beat #6 (and possibly also beat #7) manifest a morphology intermediate between that of the ventricular beats (#1-5) and the supraventricular beats (#8-12). They are *fusion beats*.

PROBLEM   **The final patient in this section is a 40-year old man admitted for acute inferior infarction. He is asymptomatic and hemodynamically stable. How would you interpret his initial rhythm strip (*Figure 16E-21A*)?**

ANSWER TO FIGURE 16E-21A   The QRS complex is narrow and the ventricular rate irregular. Group beating is present, raising the possibility of Wenckebach. The atrial rate is regular at 80 beats/min (*Figure 16E-21B*). Each QRS complex is preceded by a P wave, and the PR

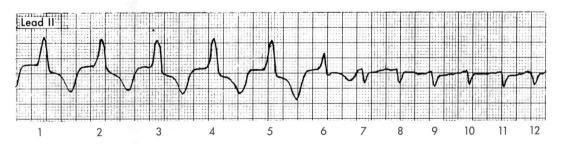

Figure 16E-20.   Follow-up tracing to Fig. 16E-19B after administration of atropine. *Was the atropine effective?*

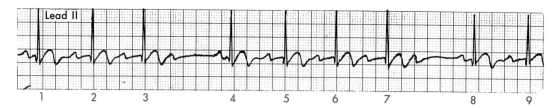

Figure 16E-21A.   Initial rhythm strip from a 40 year old man admitted for acute inferior infarction. *How would you interpret this arrhythmia?*

interval progressively increases within each group until a beat is dropped. This is *2° AV block, Mobitz type I (Wenckebach).*

It is of interest that *all* of the electrocardiographic and clinical **"footprints" of Wenckebach** are present on this tracing.

  i. Group beating
  ii. Progressively increasing PR interval within each group until a beat is dropped
  iii. Progressively *decreasing* R-R interval within each group
  iv. Regular atrial rate
  v. Pause duration of *less* than twice the shortest R-R interval
  vi. RP/PR reciprocity
  vii. Narrow QRS complex
  viii. Evidence of acute infarction (developing q wave, ST segment coving, and T wave inversion) in this inferior lead

PROBLEM   **The patient is treated with atropine. A short while later he is observed to be in the rhythm shown in *Figure 16E-22A.* Is he now in 3° (complete) AV block?**

ANSWER TO FIGURE 16E-22A   Regularly occurring atrial activity (now at a rate of 85 beats/min) continues. P waves "march through" the QRS complex without the slightest relation to it. Yet the R-R interval is *not* regular as one would expect if the AV block were

complete. This suggests that some type of 2° AV block is present.

Figure 16E-22B demonstrates the regularity of the atrial rate in this rhythm. The PR interval preceding beats #2 and #5 is definitely *too short* to conduct (arrows in Fig. 16E-22B). This suggests that beats #2 and #5 are *junctional escape beats* that occur as a result of the brief pause in the rhythm. Since the R-R interval preceding these beats is the same as the R-R interval between beats #3-4 and #6-7, it is likely that this constant R-R interval reflects the rate of the *junctional escape rhythm* (which is 47 beats/min). By the same token, beats #4 and #7 may also be junctional escape beats, although it is impossible to know for sure from this short rhythm strip. What can be said with certainty, however, is that the R-R interval shortens before beats #3 and #6. This strongly suggests that these beats are sinus conducted (albeit with 1° AV block). Thus, *intermittent AV dissociation* (rather than complete AV block) is present on this tracing.

Note that *none* of the P waves that fail to conduct in Fig. 16E-22B occur at a time when they would be expected to conduct. Therefore, the degree of underlying AV block is unknown, and not necessarily severe.

Although the mechanism for this arrhythmia is rather complex, the point to emphasize is that the rhythm in Fig. 16E-22A is *not* 3° AV block and does *not* necessarily require

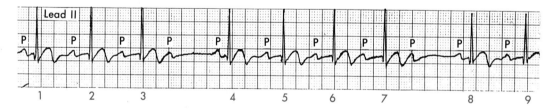

Figure 16E-21B.   Explanatory tracing indicating that the atrial rate is regular at 80 beats/min. The PR interval progressively increases within each group until a beat is dropped.

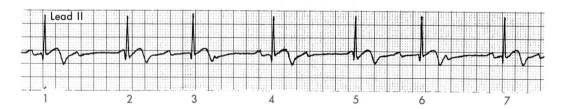

Figure 16E-22A.   Follow-up tracing to Fig. 16E-21A after administration of atropine. *Is the patient now in 3° (complete) AV block?*

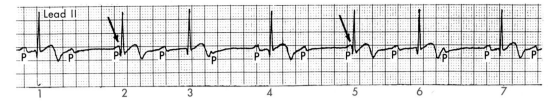

Figure 16E-22B. Explanatory tracing indicating that the atrial rate in Fig. 16E-22A is still regular. Arrows highlight the exceedingly short PR interval that precedes beats #2 and #5 (and which is clearly too short to conduct).

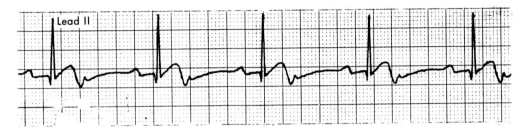

Figure 16E-23A. Follow-up tracing to Fig. 16E-22A after more atropine is given. *Has the degree of AV block "worsened" since Fig. 16E-21A?*

a pacemaker (provided that the ventricular response of the junctional escape focus remains adequate to maintain stable hemodynamic status).

PROBLEM   **More atropine is given. The result is the rhythm shown in *Figure 16E-23A. Has the degree of AV block "worsened" since Fig. 16E-21A*?**

ANSWER TO FIGURE 16E-23A   2:1 AV conduction is now present, with every other P wave producing a notch in the terminal portion of the QRS complex.

> If you are having difficulty identifying the second P wave, set your calipers to precisely one-half the R-R interval (= 0.58 second). Regularly occurring P waves can now be mapped out on the tracing *(Figure 16E-23B)*.

Despite the fact that fewer beats are being conducted on Fig. 16E-23A compared to Fig. 16E-21A, the degree of AV block has *not* necessarily worsened!!!! The only thing that we know has changed since Fig. 16E-21A is the *atrial rate.* At an atrial rate of 80 beats/min (as was present in Fig. 16E-21A), the patient's AV node was able to conduct most atrial impulses. As the atrial rate increased to 85 beats/min (Fig. 16E-22A), fewer impulses were conducted. Finally with an atrial rate of 105 beats/min (Fig.

16E-23A), only one out of every two impulses can be conducted. *It is entirely possible that this patient would still be capable of a much more favorable conduction ratio if the atrial rate had remained at 80 beats/min.*

Use of atropine may be a two-edged sword. The drug works by both increasing the rate of the SA nodel pacemaker *and* improving conduction through the AV node. This particular case is an example in which the former effect of atropine (increasing the atrial rate) predominates, paradoxically exacerbating the patient's condition (since the effective ventricular response decreased as the atrial rate increased!).

Returning to the initial scenario in this case, it should be noted that the patient was asymptomatic and hemodynamically stable in a Wenckebach rhythm with an adequate ventricular response (Fig. 16E-21A). *No atropine at all was indicated at this point.* Second-degree AV block of the Mobitz I type is a common accompaniment of acute inferior infarction that often resolves without the need for any treatment.

Finally, one should remember that in addition to classifying the AV blocks by degree, it is essential to specify the atrial and ventricular response. The patient in this case manifested Mobitz I 2° AV block throughout. However, clinical implications of 2:1 AV conduction and the slower ventricular response seen in Fig. 16E-23A may differ significantly from clinical implications when the AV conduction ratio is more favorable.

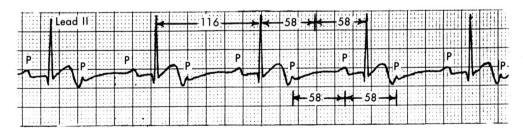

Figure 16E-23B. Explanatory tracing to Fig. 16E-23A illustrating continuation of regular atrial activity (with a P-P interval of 0.58 second).

SECTION F

A BRIEF VIEW AT INTERPRETING PACEMAKER RHYTHMS

Interpretation of pacemaker rhythms is a topic unto itself. As a result of the ever increasing sophistication of newer devices (including programmable dual-chambered pacemakers and permanent pacemakers capable of altering parameters in response to patient activity), interpretation of complex pacemaker rhythms has become an exceedingly challenging task.

Our goals for this section are modest. We do not review all of the types of cardiac pacemakers, as such discussion would extend well beyond the scope of this book. Instead, we focus on the principal concern of most emergency care providers: *To determine if a pacemaker is functioning.*

Pacing nomenclature uses a series of letters to describe pacing features of a particular device. For example, function of the standard demand pacemaker is designated by the letters **V-V-I**, where the first letter indicates the chamber *paced* (in this case, the **V**entricles), the second letter indicates the chamber *sensed* (also the **V**entricles), and the third letter indicates that the pacemaker is *Inhibited* if a spontaneous beat occurs.

This is in contrast to **D-D-D** pacemakers that have **D**ual pacing capability (of *both* the atria *and* ventricles), **D**ual sensing capability (of *both* the atria *and* ventricles), and the **D**ual capability of being *either* inhibited *or* triggered by a spontaneous beat. DDD pacemakers offer the distinct advantage of being more physiologic. They preserve *sequential* depolarization (of atria—then ventricles), and thus maintain the "atrial kick" (which contributes 5-40% of cardiac output, an amount that may be essential for certain older individuals with only marginal left ventricular function). As might be imagined, operation and circuitry of DDD pacemakers is more complex, and interpretation of tracings (which may contain a multitude of atrial and ventricular spikes dependent on sensing intervals that are *not* always known) is correspondingly more difficult.

Interpretation of pacemaker rhythms in the demand (VVI) mode is far simpler. Fortunately, this is the mode most commonly encountered by the emergency care provider—and the one we concentrate on in this section.

Assessment of Pacemaker Function

Assessment of pacemaker function in the demand mode can be simplified by the approach suggested in *Table 16F-1.*

Utilization of this basic approach may be facilitated by application of two basic concepts:

i. *Imagining YOURSELF as the pacemaker.* How would YOU act if you were a pacemaker whose "sole function in life" was to observe (i.e., *sense*) the patient's underlying rhythm, assuming you were programmed to "take over" (i.e., *pace*) whenever (if ever) the patient's spontaneous rhythm slowed down.

ii. *Keeping in mind that MOST of the time, the pacemaker will be right.* Pacing devices are truly amazing. In general, their accuracy is uncanny. As a result, we prefer to give the pacemaker "the benefit of the doubt" (and *look extra hard* for a reason to explain why the pacemaker acted as it did), *before* concluding that the device malfunctioned.

Pacemakers are *NOT* always right, and at times they do malfunction. Considering the potentially disastrous consequences of pacemaker malfunction, prompt recognition is essential. Nevertheless, keeping in mind that "more of the time the pacemaker will be right" may be extremely helpful in interpreting the significance of questionable findings on pacemaker tracings.

Table 16F-1

Suggested Approach for Assessment of Pacemaker Function in the Demand Mode*

1. Seek out *all* pacemaker spikes on the tracing:
  • Are all pacer spikes **capturing?**
 	
2. Determine the rate at which the pacemaker is set.
  • Do all *successively occurring* pacemaker spikes occur at *precisely* this rate?
 	
3. Look for *spontaneous beats.*
  • Try to determine the spontaneous (underlying) rhythm.
 	
4. Determine if spontaneous beats are **sensed:**
  • Is the pacemaker **inhibited** by a faster rhythm?
  • Does the pacemaker "take over" when spontaneous beats slow down?
 	
5. Save evaluation of unexplained phenomena as the last step in the process.
  • Remember the most likely causes of such phenomena (i.e., PVCs, pacer *fusion* complexes).

*Use of calipers is *essential* for accurate assessment of pacemaker function.

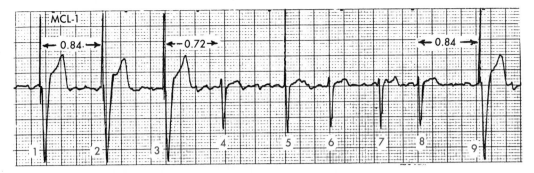

Figure 16F-1.   Rhythm strip from a patient with a demand (VVI) pacemaker. *Is the pacer functioning appropriately?*

PROBLEM   **Examine *Figure 16F-1*, obtained from a patient with a demand (VVI) pacemaker. *Is the pacemaker functioning appropriately?***

ANSWER TO FIGURE 16F-1   Applying the approach suggested by Table 16F-1 for assessment of pacemaker function, we can state the following:

1. Five pacemaker spikes are seen on this tracing (the tall vertical lines at the onset of complexes #1, #2, #3, #5, and #9). It is clear that each of these pacer spikes (*except #5*) *captures* the ventricles (evidenced by the observation that *each* of the spikes is immediately followed by a widened QRS complex and its associated T wave).

   Events surrounding the pacer spike associated with complex #5 are much harder to explain. As a result, we defer interpretation of this complex until the end of our analysis.

2. The rate at which a demand (VVI) pacemaker is set can be determined by measuring the interval between *successive* pacer spikes.

   For most patients, the pacing rate will usually be set at between 70-75 beats/min (corresponding to a pacing interval of about 0.80-0.85 second, or just over four large boxes in duration). However, slower or faster pacing rates are sometimes chosen in an attempt to optimize hemodynamics (depending on the clinical setting, the reason for insertion of the pacemaker, and the nature of the underlying conduction disturbance).

   The ***pacing interval*** in Fig. 16F-1 is 0.84 second (just over four large boxes), and corresponds to a pacing rate of 72 beats/min.

   Successive pacing spikes are seen for the first three beats in the tracing. Note that the pacing interval (i.e., the interval between the pacer spikes that separate complexes #1 and #2; and #2 and #3) remains *precisely* the same. This is as it should be for all successive pacer spikes on a rhythm strip obtained from a patient with a demand pacemaker. Variation in the pacing interval may be an indication of battery failure.

3. Four spontaneous beats are seen on this tracing. That is, beats #4, #6, #7, and #8 are all similar-appearing, narrow QRS complexes that are not associated with a pacer spike. There is no regularity in the oc-

currence of these spontaneous beats, and no definite P waves are seen, suggesting that the underlying rhythm is atrial fibrillation.

4. Spontaneous beats appear to be sensed. This is best evidenced by complex #9 in which the pacer spike occurs 0.84 seconds after the r wave of the preceding spontaneous beat. *If you were a pacemaker whose sole function in life was to wait up to 0.84 second before firing (to see if a spontaneous beat occurred), wouldn't you have acted accordingly?*

   It is important to appreciate that the ***sensing interval*** will not always be perfectly predictable. This is because it will not always be possible to determine the exact point in the QRS complex that is being sensed. As a result, it may sometimes appear that the pacemaker is sensing the patient's spontaneous rhythm either a little too early or a little too late. Awareness of this potential variation in the sensing interval, and keeping in mind that the pacemaker "will usually be right" should greatly assist in interpreting the significance (if any) of small variations in the sensing interval.

   Additional evidence in favor of adequate pacemaker sensing is the fact that no pacemaker spikes are seen to interrupt the spontaneous rhythm between beats #5-8. During this time, spontaneous beats occur at a rate that exceeds 72 beats/min (the rate at which the pacemaker is set). *If you were a pacemaker told not to discharge as long as spontaneous beats kept occurring at an interval that did not exceed 0.84 second, wouldn't you also remain silent with the occurrence of beats #5-8?*

5. Evaluation of complex #5 has been intentionally saved for last. If we excluded analysis of this complex from our interpretation, we could confidently state the following about the tracing shown in Figure 16F-1:

Demand (VVI) pacemaker at a rate of 72 beats/min that appears to be functioning (i.e., *sensing and capturing*) appropriately.

The difficulty interpreting complex #5 is that the QRS and T wave associated with this pacer spike resemble the QRS and T wave of spontaneous beats much more than the pacemaker-initiated complexes. This suggests that despite the fact that the pacemaker fired (and produced a spike), it did *not* succeed in capturing the ventricles. Since *everything else* on the tracing suggests that the pacemaker is functioning appropriately, it is likely that some reason exists to explain why the pacemaker acted as it did. Possibilities include:

   i. That a spontaneous beat occurred at a moment that was too late to prevent the pacer spike, but in time to prevent pacemaker-initiated depolarization of the ventricles. That this might be the case is all the more likely considering the underlying rhythm, since prediction of when the next spontaneous beat should occur is impossible in the presence of atrial fibrillation.

   ii. That complex #5 is a *pacemaker fusion beat* (produced by the near simultaneous occurrence of a spontaneous beat and a pacemaker-initiated complex). In support of this supposition is the ever-so-subtle (but real) observation that the S wave of complex #5 is slightly *deeper* than the S wave of each of the other spontaneous beats on the tracing (as might be expected if a slight degree of fusion with a pacemaker-initiated complex occurred).

Since both of these possibilities are plausible explanations for the appearance of complex #5—and in view of the appropriate sensing and capture evident on the remainder of the tracing—one could surmise that the pacemaker is *probably* functioning properly. Proof would require additional tracings.

   It should be apparent from this example that *both* paced and spontaneous beats must be present on a particular rhythm strip for *complete* assessment of pacemaker function (i.e., assessment of *both* sensing and pacing capability). If only paced complexes are seen, one will only be able to judge the adequacy of ventricular capture. On the other hand, if only spontaneous beats are seen, nothing can be said about the adequacy of ventricular capture (i.e., about the pacemaker's ability to pace). In this latter case, however, the *rate* of the spontaneous rhythm may provide some insight (at least indirectly) about the adequacy of sensing.

PROBLEM   **Imagine you are caring for a patient *known* to have a demand (VVI) pacemaker set at 75 beats/min. Could anything be said about the pace-**maker's *sensing function* if the patient presented in a normal (regular) sinus rhythm at a rate of 80 beats/min? *What if the rate of the sinus rhythm was 70 beats/min?* (Assume that no pacer spikes are seen on either rhythm strip.)**

ANSWER   If a demand (VVI) pacemaker set to discharge at a rate of 75 beats/min was sensing appropriately, the pacemaker should be *inhibited* by a faster spontaneous rhythm and stimulated (to take over) by a slower rhythm. One would therefore *not* expect to see any pacemaker spikes at all if the patient presented in a regular spontaneous rhythm at 80 beats/min (since this is *faster* than the pacing rate). Although the finding of a faster spontaneous rhythm would at least provide some *indirect* evidence of appropriate sensing function, it unfortunately does *not* rule out the alternative possibility that the pacemaker *is not functioning at all*. For example, if the pacemaker was completely *turned off* and the patient happened to be in a normal sinus rhythm at 80 beats/min, an identical rhythm strip might also be seen. Thus, in order to *directly* demonstrate adequate sensing function, pacer spikes *and* spontaneous beats must *both* be seen on the tracing.

   On the other hand, one could definitely say that something must be wrong if a patient known to have a demand (VVI) pacemaker set at 75 beats/min presents in a spontaneous rhythm at a rate of 70 beats/min. In this case the pacemaker *should have sensed the decrease in rate, taken over the pacemaking function,* and *maintained* the heart rate at *precisely* 75 beats/min.

PROBLEM   **The rhythm strip shown in *Figure 16F-2* was obtained from a patient in cardiac arrest. An emergency transvenous pacemaker has just been inserted.**

   1. *Is the pacemaker functioning appropriately?*
   2. What is beat X?
   3. What should be done clinically?

ANSWER TO FIGURE 16F-2   Regular pacemaker spikes at a rate of 95 beats/min are seen. Despite this, there is no evidence of ventricular *capture*, and the patient remains in asystole. Beat **X** represents an agonal complex that the pacemaker failed to sense.

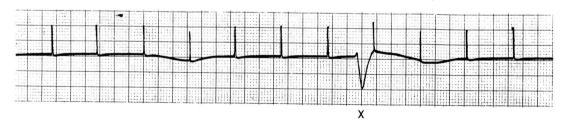

X

Figure 16F-2.   Rhythm strip obtained from a patient in cardiac arrest. *Is the pacemaker functioning appropriately?* What is beat **X**? *What should be done clinically?*

Pacemaker spikes that capture the ventricles should produce a QRS complex and a T wave. Because of the ventricular origin of paced beats, the QRS complex they produce should be wide. In contrast to the paced beats in Fig. 16F-1 (#1, #2, #3, and #9), however, the baseline in Fig. 16F-2 remains flat throughout the tracing (with the exception of the one agonal complex marked **X**).

Clinically, the first thing to do is to maximize the amplitude of the pacing stimulus (and/or reposition the pacing electrode) in an attempt to capture the ventricles. If this not rapidly effective, the patient must be treated for asystole with immediate resumption of CPR (since there is no perfusion with the rhythm shown in Fig. 16F-2), epinephrine (in increasing doses), atropine (as appropriate), and/or other measures as suggested in the Algorithm for treatment of asystole (Figure 1D-1). Practically speaking, persistence of asystole with failure to capture portends an ominous prognosis.

PROBLEM   **The rhythm shown in *Figure 16F-3* was also obtained from a patient in cardiac arrest. An external pacemaker has just been applied. *Is it functioning appropriately?***

ANSWER TO FIGURE 16F-3   The initial three complexes on the tracing demonstrate a paced rhythm (with appropriate capture) at a rate of 70 beats/min. Thereafter, pacemaker spikes cease. A long pause (of *more than 3 seconds!*) ensues, followed by two agonal beats (#4 and #5) and another pause at the end of the tracing. For this patient in cardiac arrest, cessation of pacemaker spikes (pacemaker malfunction) in association with an underlying agonal rhythm portends an ominous prognosis.

PROBLEM   **Do the demand (VVI) pacemakers shown in *Figures 16F-4* and *16F-5* appear to be functioning appropriately?**

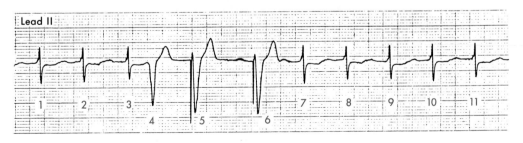

Figure 16F-3.   Rhythm strip obtained from another patient in cardiac arrest. *Is the external pacemaker functioning appropriately?*

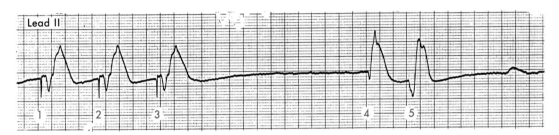

Figure 16F-4.   *Does this demand (VVI) pacemaker appear to be functioning appropriately?*

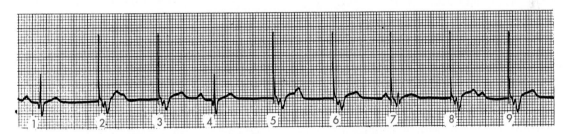

Figure 16F-5.   *Does this demand (VVI) pacemaker appear to be functioning appropriately?*

BONUS (Challenge) QUESTION *Can you determine the underlying rhythm in each case?*

ANSWER TO FIGURE 16F-4

Pacemaker spikes precede complexes #2, #3, and #5-9. Adequate ventricular *capture* is present, since a QRS follows each pacemaker spike. The rate of the pacemaker is 72 beats/min (corresponding to an R-R interval between *successive* pacemaker spikes of 0.84 second).

Beats #1 and #4 represent spontaneous QRS complexes. Each is preceded by a P wave with a constant (albeit slightly prolonged) PR interval, suggesting that these P waves are conducted. The pacemaker appropriately *senses* these QRS complexes, as evidenced by the fact that it does not fire until 0.84 second after each spontaneous beat.

> It is difficult to determine the underlying rhythm (and the reason for pacemaker insertion) solely from the information provided by Fig. 16F-4. P waves occur throughout this rhythm strip, although the atrial rate is *not* regular. As noted above, P waves preceding beats #1 and #4 are conducted with 1° AV block. Additional P waves appear to notch the T waves of pacemaker-initiated complexes #2 and #5, precede the pacemaker spike of complex #7, and follow the T wave of complex #8. Since one would at least expect this last P wave to conduct (and it doesn't), some type of 2° AV block is likely to be present.

In summary, although some questions remain about the rhythm shown in Fig. 16F-4 (i.e., the mechanism of the underlying arrhythmia and the reason for pacemaker insertion), the pacemaker appears to be functioning (sensing *and* capturing) appropriately.

ANSWER TO FIGURE 16F-5

Only two pacemaker spikes are seen in this tracing (preceding complexes #5 and #6). The interval separating these spikes (i.e., the **pacing** or **sensing interval**) is 0.84 second, suggesting that the pacemaker has again been set to discharge at a rate of 72 beats/min. Both of these spikes *capture* the ventricles.

The underlying rhythm is fairly regular at a rate of about 100 beats/min. The QRS complex of the underlying rhythm is narrow, consistent with a supraventricular mechanism.

> P waves are *not* readily apparent, *with two exceptions!* Careful inspection of the R-R interval between beats #6-7 reveals a small amplitude, upright deflection immediately following the peaked T wave of the pacemaker-initiated complex. That this small upright deflection preceding beat #7 is really a P wave (conducting in this case with 1° AV block) is supported by the finding of a similar appearing small, upright deflection *just before* the pacer spike of complex #6, and the fact that the P-P interval between these two P waves (0.60 second, or three large boxes) is virtually the *same* as the R-R interval separating each of the spontaneous beats on this tracing! Thus, the underlying rhythm is sinus tachycardia with 1° AV block (in which the small amplitude P waves preceding beats #1-3 and #8-11 are hidden within the flattened T wave of each preceding beat!). Since the rate of the underlying spontaneous rhythm (about 100 beats/min) is clearly *faster* than the pacing rate

(72 beats/min), no pacemaker spikes appear during the spontaneous rhythm. This provides *indirect* evidence of appropriate sensing function.

This leaves beat #4 as the last finding to explain on this tracing. Beat #4 is wide, early, and is not preceded by a premature P wave—suggesting that it is a PVC. This PVC is *not* sensed by the pacemaker, however, since the pacer spike of complex #5 occurs well *before* the expected sensing interval (i.e., the interval between beat #4 and the pacer spike of complex #5 is clearly *less* than 0.84 second).

> If the pacemaker had sensed this PVC (beat #4), it should have waited an additional 0.84 second before discharging the next pacemaker spike. Instead, the pacemaker sensed beat #3, as evidenced by the fact that the interval between beats #3-5 *exactly* equals the pacing/sensing interval (of 0.84 second)!

Clinically, it is hard to be certain from this single tracing that the pacemaker is malfunctioning. This is because except for beat #4, adequate pacing (i.e., capture) and sensing appear to be present. There may (?) be some physiologic reason that beat #4 is not sensed (i.e., occurrence in the refractory period of beat #3). Clearly, additional evidence (in the form of more tracings) is needed before a definite conclusion can be reached. Nevertheless, the possibility of pacemaker malfunction needs to be considered.

> A final, incidental finding on this tracing is the different amplitude of the two pacer spikes. Variation in pacer spike amplitude is common and most often reflects positional changes rather than pacemaker malfunction.

PROBLEM

The final tracing in this section was obtained from a middle-aged man complaining of "palpitations." A permanent pacemaker had been inserted years earlier. *Is the pacemaker functioning appropriately? Can you think of any reasons that might explain why the pacemaker acted as it did for beats #3-5? (i.e., Is it possible that this pacemaker is functioning appropriately after all?)*

HINT: The patient remembers being told that a "special pacemaker" was being implanted that would allow him to remain active (Fig. 16F-6).

ANSWER TO FIGURE 16F-6

Pacemaker spikes precede *each* of the nine complexes on this tracing (i.e., there is *100% capture*). There are no spontaneous beats. Of concern, however, is the marked variation in the R-R interval of the first five paced beats in this tracing. Clearly, if this was a demand (VVI) pacemaker, the varying pacing interval would indicate severe malfunction.

An alternative explanation (*suggested by the HINT*) is possible. Certain types of newer pacing devices are able to alter the rate of ventricular pacing in reponse to patient movement. Heart rate acceleration of these pacemakers allows such individuals to remain more active by appro-

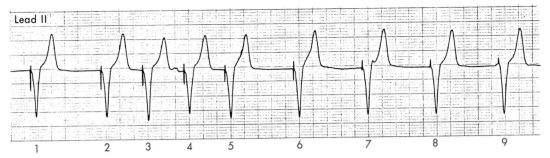

Figure 16F-6. Rhythm strip obtained from a middle-aged man with palpitations. Is the pacemaker functioning appropriately? *Could the pacemaker be functioning appropriately?*

priately increasing cardiac output in response to activity. Thus, if instead of a demand (VVI) pacemaker, an activity-related pacemaking device had been implanted in this patient, the rhythm shown in Fig. 16F-6 could reflect appropriate pacemaking function (100% capture) with heart rate acceleration in response to activity.

In the absence of any spontaneous beats, it is virtually impossible to determine the true underlying rhythm in Fig. 16F-6. There are, however, several indications of atrial activity. The most apparent of these is the P wave that precedes complex #4. Careful inspection of the T wave of complex #7, and the pacemaker spike of complex #9 reveals evidence of additional atrial activity. Setting one's calipers to the *lowest common denominator* of these three signs of atrial activity (i.e., setting the calipers to 0.94 second) and *walking out* this interval suggests that an underlying regular atrial rhythm at about 65 beats/min may be present. None of these P waves would occur at a time when they would be expected to conduct, however, so that no conclusion can be drawn as to the underlying rhythm disturbance (and reason for pacemaker implantation).

The KEY point emphasized by this tracing is the difficulty that may be encountered in the interpretation of pacemaker rhythms when the type and specifications of the pacemaker are unknown!

As stated in our introduction to this section (and summarized by the approach suggested in Table 16F-1), interpretation of pacemaker rhythms in the demand (VVI) mode is usually straightforward (and relatively easy to master). Fortunately, this is by far the most common mode of pacing encountered by the emergency care provider in the setting of cardiac arrest.

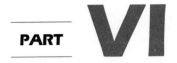

PART **VI**

Pediatric Resuscitation

Chapter opener

CHAPTER 17

PEDIATRIC RESUSCITATION

Dan Cavallaro, REMT-P
Ken Grauer, MD
Jorge Gourid, MD
Al Saltiel, MD

SECTION A

PEDIATRIC AIRWAY MANAGEMENT

Cardiopulmonary arrest is a relatively infrequent event in children. Practically speaking, except for those working in specialized pediatric settings, exposure to cardiopulmonary emergencies in children is likely to be limited. As a result, many emergency care providers are not completely comfortable managing this disorder.

The purpose of this chapter is to present a basic approach for recognition and treatment of cardiac and/or respiratory difficulty in children. In doing this, we will emphasize the differences between adult and pediatric patients as they relate to management of acute cardiac and/or airway related emergencies. We focus on Pediatric Airway Management in **Section A,** and consolidate this information into an Algorithm in **Section B.** Assessment of Pediatric Circulatory Status and Drugs in Emergency Cardiac Care are covered in **Section C.** We conclude the chapter with an overview of Pediatric Arrhythmias in **Section D.**

Priorities of Pediatric Resuscitation

Most cardiopulmonary arrests that occur in children are secondary to hypoxemia from respiratory distress. In response to severe hypoxemia, the heart slows, and marked bradycardia is frequently seen. *Asystole is the most common terminal event in pediatric cardiac arrest.* This is in marked contrast to cardiopulmonary arrest in adults, in whom ventricular tachycardia/fibrillation rather than bradycardia is much more likely to be the precipitating mechanism.

Unfortunately, meaningful survival from pediatric resuscitation is poor. The pediatric heart generally responds better to resuscitative measures than the adult heart. However, by the time pediatric cardiac arrest occurs, most children will have already been hypoxic for an extended period of time and suffered severe (and often irreversible) neurologic damage. Thus, the emphasis in resuscitation of children must be directed toward *early recognition* of the

signs and symptoms of respiratory distress with specific efforts aimed at improving ventilation and oxygenation.

It is not generally appreciated that after infancy, the major causes of morbidity and mortality in children are *accidents* and *injuries* (Luten, 1989). In many cases, these occurrences are preventable. Considering the poor outlook for survival once pediatric arrest does occur, the emphasis for health care providers *must* begin well before the considerations discussed in this chapter. Educating parents and encouraging them to adopt relatively simple preventive measures may be lifesaving. Examples include routine use of seat-belts (to minimize the extent of injury in motor vehicle accidents), use of bike helmets, and "child-proofing" the home (to reduce the chance of accidental poisoning, burns, self-inflicted gun-shot wounds, and electrocution). If there is a swimming pool, adequate barriers to prevent entry of a stray child are essential. *Young children cannot be left unattended.* Finally—encouraging parents to become trained in BLS (including application of the Heimlich maneuver) may prove lifesaving in the event of respiratory arrest (from accidental poisoning or drowning) or foreign body obstruction.

It is important to realize that respiratory depression severe enough to cause cardiopulmonary arrest in children is usually secondary to some other cause. Examples include infection (pneumonia, sepsis), metabolic or electrolyte abnormalities (hypoglycemia, hypocalcemia), sudden infant death syndrome (SIDS), toxic drug ingestion, electrical shock, cardiac arrhythmias, congestive heart failure, poisoning, drowning, allergic reactions, trauma, shock, and cardiac tamponade. Successful resuscitation often ultimately depends on identification and treatment of the underlying cause.

Recognition of Respiratory Distress in Children

Before discussing management of the airway, it may be helpful to review the signs and symptoms of respiratory distress in children. Recognition of clues available from careful physical examination often allows determination of the underlying pathophysiology causing the respiratory distress, as well as assessment of the severity of the condition *(Table 17A-1).*

Simple inspection provides a wealth of information regarding the effort (work) of breathing and the adequacy of air exchange. Despite natural inclinations to the contrary, *forcing oneself to spend a focused moment VISUALLY ASSESSING the child BEFORE performing other parts of the physical examination and BEFORE initiating therapeutic intervention is an important KEY to successful resuscitation.*

LEVEL OF CONSCIOUSNESS

Four of the five assessment parameters listed in Table 17A-1 are evident on inspection. Of these, appearance and level of consciousness are probably the easiest to assess. The child who is alert and still playful or cheerful is unlikely to be in severe distress. In contrast, decreased responsiveness (as indicated by agitation or lethargy) is a worrisome sign, and suggests development of hypoxia, hypercarbia, or both. Unless ventilatory status can be rapidly improved, intubation will often be needed.

SKIN COLOR/CYANOSIS

Assessment of color may provide an indication of the adequacy of air exchange. Ideally, mucous membranes and skin color will be pink, although it is important to emphasize *that the finding of good color alone cannot be taken as definitive evidence of adequate oxygenation.* Development of **cyanosis** depends on the presence of an increased *amount* of reduced (unsaturated) hemoglobin in the blood (or more precisely, in the superficial capillaries). Children who are severely anemic are much less likely to demonstrate cyanosis regardless of the severity of their pulmonary condition. This is because anemic patients have less circulating hemoglobin, and therefore are correspondingly less likely to develop the critical *amount* of reduced hemoglobin needed to produce the dusky, blue tint of cyanosis in the skin.

Cyanosis may be *central* (due to a low oxygen saturation content in arterial blood) or *peripheral* (due to an unusually high oxygen extraction ratio from peripheral areas such as the nails or lips). Often, both types are present (i.e., *mixed cyanosis*). Children with congenital heart disease who have large right-to-left shunts typically develop central cyanosis in which the dusky discoloration involves not only the extremities, but also the mucous membranes within the mouth and the skin of the trunk. In contrast, cyanosis that develops as a result of *stagnation* of blood (as typically occurs in low flow states such as shock) is peripheral.

Table 17A-1

Signs and Symptoms of Respiratory Distress in the Pediatric Patient				
	MILD Respiratory Distress	**MODERATE Respiratory Distress**	**SEVERE Respiratory Distress**	**RESPIRATORY FAILURE**
Appearance/Level of Consciousness	• Alert	• Alert or may be confused	• Lethargic	• Unresponsive
Skin Color and Color of Mucous Membranes	• Pink	• Pink or cyanotic	• Cyanotic	• Cyanotic
Respiratory Rate	• Mildly increased	• Mild to moderately increased	• Markedly increased	• Decreased or apneic
Work of Breathing	• Subcostal retractions	• Subcostal retractions • Intercostal and sternal retractions • Nasal flaring	• Subcostal retractions • Intercostal and sternal retractions • Nasal flaring • Suprasternal retractions	• Decreased respiratory effort or none
Heart Rate	• Mildly increased	• Mild to moderately increased	• Markedly increased	• Decreased

Clinically, cyanosis is usually best observed in peripheral areas (such as the feet and hands), and in places where the skin is relatively thin and unpigmented where superficial capillaries carrying reduced hemoglobin are close to the surface (i.e., the cheeks, ears, lips, nail beds, and mucous membranes of the mouth). It is not well seen in the conjunctive or sclera. Practically speaking, it is not always easy to detect cyanosis, particularly in blacks, if lighting is less than optimal, and/or in the excitement and flurry of activity commonly present in an emergency situation. However, *if cyanosis is detected it is highly likely that the child is in trouble!*

PATTERN OF RESPIRATION

The pattern of respiration may be insightful. A pattern of rapid, shallow breathing typically suggests parenchymal pulmonary disease such as pneumonia or pulmonary edema. In contrast, a pattern of more deliberate, slower and deeper respiration is more likely to reflect airway obstruction. Extrathoracic obstruction (as may be caused by croup, tracheal stenosis, foreign body obstruction, etc.) typically produces a prolonged *inspiratory* phase (since the upper airway narrows on inspiration). In contrast, the intrathoracic obstruction of an asthmatic prolongs *expiration.*

Work of breathing may be assessed by the extent of accessory muscle recruitment (Table 17A-1). Increased diaphragmatic effort is an early indicator of respiratory distress, and is reflected by subcostal retractions. Intercostal muscles are usually called into play next; intercostal retractions and nasal flaring suggest moderate respiratory distress. Finally, accessory muscles of the abdomen and neck are recruited, the latter producing suprasternal retractions. This suggests severe respiratory distress and possible impending respiratory failure.

Auscultation of the chest helps determine the adequacy of air movement through the respiratory passages. Initially when large airways become narrow, gas movement becomes noisy and stridor may be heard. With further narrowing, air flow becomes turbulent, and wheezing may be heard. Ultimately with critical narrowing of large airways, airflow becomes minimal and no sounds are heard. This explains why silence is such an ominous auscultatory finding in a patient with asthma.

> Remember that the chest wall of children is thin, and sounds are easily transmitted. As a result, it may be possible to hear "normal" breath sounds over areas of the chest wall that overlie lung which is either collapsed, or infiltrated with pneumonia.

Transmural airway pressures vary during the different phases of respiration. During inspiration, extrathoracic airways narrow. As a result, a partially obstructed airway may become narrow and produce stridor. *Inspiratory stridor suggests upper airway obstruction.* In contrast, intrathoracic airway diameters become smaller with expiration. This explains why asthmatic obstruction typically produces expiratory wheezing.

> The importance of SERIAL EXAMINATION in assessing the degree of cardiopulmonary distress cannot be overemphasized.

Cardiopulmonary processes are *dynamic.* Worsening (especially if progressive) of the assessment parameters listed in Table 17A-1 may indicate a need for intensive intervention that was not apparent from initial evaluation. Serial notation of heart rate and respiratory rate (carefully *counted* over a period of at least 30 seconds) is an extremely useful way to objectively document disease progression.

> Norms for heart rate and respiratory rate vary greatly with the age and activity of the child. During the first year of life, a respiratory rate of 30 to 40/minute and a heart rate of 150 beats/minute (or more) are *not* outside the range of normal (especially if the child is crying). After the first year of life, norms for respiratory rate at rest drop into the 20 to 30/minute range (Rowe, 1987). Heart rates exceeding 100 beats/minute are still commonly encountered (Garson, 1983). Much more important than the specific number of respirations or heart beats per minute at any one instant in time is the **trend** (i.e., **serial examination**) of these parameters assessed in conjunction with the patient's appearance, level of consciousness, color, and effort (work) of breathing (Table 17A-1).

UPPER AIRWAY OBSTRUCTION FROM INFECTIOUS DISEASE

The term **"croup"** is applied to a number of infectious processes of the upper airway that produce a brassy *(croupy)* cough, inspiratory stridor, hoarseness, and signs of respiratory distress. Two entities in this syndrome that the emergency care provider must be comfortable differentiating between are acute epiglottitis and laryngotracheobronchitis (LTB). The former condition (epiglottitis) may have potentially serious consequences, while the latter (LTB) condition is much more likely to be self-limiting.

LTB is a viral form of croup that is most commonly seen between 3 months and 3 years of age. These patients present with a several-day history of low-grade fever and URI symptoms (rhinorrhea, sore throat) that progresses into a brassy or barking cough with gradually increasing respiratory difficulty. They rarely appear toxic, and conservative therapy (cool mist) is often all that is needed. Adjunctive therapy in children who are hospitalized may include racemic epinephrine by aerosol and a single dose of corticosteroids.

In contrast, **acute epiglottitis** is a bacterial infection (most commonly due to *Haemophilus influenzae,* type b). It occurs in a somewhat older age group (2-7 years of age), and is much more abrupt in onset. Within hours these children develop high fever, sore throat, dysphagia, and marked respiratory distress. These children are much more ill-appearing than are children with LTB. Typically the child with epiglottitis sits bolt upright with head and neck protruding forward to assist in breathing *(Figure 17A-1)*. Drooling is common because of the inability to swallow secretions. The spontaneous cough of LTB is not seen. Instead the voice is muffled as if someone had put a pillow over the child's head. As the degree of airway obstruction worsens, air exchange becomes progressively more difficult.

Clinically, LTB is a far more common condition. However, due to the emergent nature of its counterpart, it is essential for the emergency care provider to be able to recognize acute epiglottitis when it does occur. Lateral neck X-ray films may sometimes be helpful in this regard, although there may not always be time for X-rays to be taken. If the clinician is at all suspicious of this entity, *absolutely* no manipulation of the airway is advised *(not even to visualize the pharynx!)*. Instead the child must be kept as calm as possible *(no venipunctures!)*, and immediate consultation with an anesthesiologist for endotracheal intubation is in order. Many clinicians also prefer to call a surgeon in the event that emergency tracheotomy is necessary. *The child must be closely monitored at all times!*

An interesting clinical study by Mauro et al (1988) described a sequential protocol for visualization of the epiglottis in the ED. Although direct inspection by physical examination may be quicker, less expensive, and more definitive than obtaining lateral X-ray films of the neck, the procedure is definitely not without danger. In an accompanying editorial, Fulginiti (1988) cautions "as countless others have repeated for decades . . . . that children for whom the diagnosis of supraglot-

titis is considered should not have the epiglottis inspected for fear of a vasovagal response that would result in immediate and irreversible cardiorespiratory collapse, respiratory obstruction, and death." Fulginiti adds that, "In practice . . . most pediatricians . . . . would not attempt inspection of the oropharynx in a child for whom they suspect the presence of inflamed supraglottic structures."

Practically speaking, our feeling is that rather than attempting to make a definitive diagnosis, the role of the emergency care provider is to *identify* those children *at risk* of having acute epiglottitis, and to ensure prompt evaluation by the most appropriate health care provider(s) skilled in evaluation and definitive management of this disorder.

Once control of the airway has been achieved, treatment with antibiotics is begun.

Epiglottitis has largely become a *preventable* disease. Vaccination against Haemophilus is now available and effective during the first year of life (Medical Letter, 1991).

FOREIGN BODY OBSTRUCTION

Evaluating a spontaneously breathing patient with suspected foreign body obstruction must be done with extreme care. This is because of the ever present danger of converting a partial airway obstruction to one that is complete.

In general, children with partial airway obstruction are managed in the same manner as adults: the patient should be allowed to cough in the hope that the foreign body will be expelled. *As long as ventilation remains effective, invasive maneuvers are not indicated.* Instead, the emergency care provider should strive to keep the child as calm as possible (letting the parent comfort or hold the child if feasible) while protecting the patient from further injury and maintaining a readiness to intervene at any moment should complete obstruction occur. If partial airway obstruction persists, definitive diagnostic and therapeutic procedures may need to be implemented.

Airway Management and Ventilation

The most important priority in cardiopulmonary resuscitation of children is to effectively manage the airway. Accomplishing this goal alone is often sufficient to resuscitate the child without the need to resort to pharmacologic intervention.

OXYGENATION OF THE SPONTANEOUSLY BREATHING PATIENT

All patients with respiratory distress should receive supplemental oxygen. However, pediatric patients do not always tolerate conventional supplemental oxygen devices that are used in adults. As a result, special attention must be directed at selecting an appropriate method for oxygen delivery based on the child's age, clinical status, and oxy-

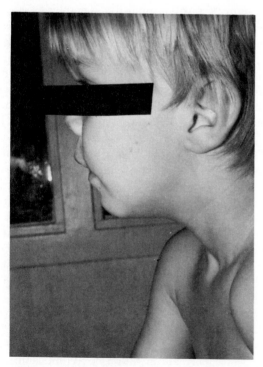

Figure 17A-1. Characteristic posturing of a child with epiglottitis.

gen requirements. In general, delivery of supplemental oxygen to children is provided by one of five methods:

  i. Nasal cannula
 ii. Simple oxygen masks (i.e., a face mask *without* the use of an oxygen reservoir)
iii. Non-rebreather oxygen mask (i.e., a face mask *with* use of an oxygen reservoir)
 iv. Oxygen hoods
  v. Oxygen tents

Nasal cannulas and **simple oxygen masks** are examples of readily available low-flow devices that are generally well tolerated in children and in some infants. The major limitation of a nasal cannula is that its effectiveness is less than optimal in the child who is breathing primarily through the mouth. This restricts its use in children with nasal congestion from an upper respiratory infection or with congenital abnormalities. High flow oxygen delivery is not recommended with nasal cannulas because it may be excessively irritating and dry out the nasal mucosa.

> Unfortunately, infants (i.e., children less than 1 year of age) will usually not tolerate a nasal cannula or oxygen (face) mask as well as older children. Two techniques that may be tried to facilitate oxygen delivery in infants and younger children who are not critically ill are:
>
> i. Having a parent be the one to place and maintain the oxygen mask on the face while holding and comforting the child.
> ii. Using the **"blow-by"** technique in which oxygen flow from oxygen supply tubing is directed toward the child's nose and mouth. Having a parent hold and comfort the patient may again prove invaluable in enticing the child to accept the oxygen.

For children unable to tolerate a nasal cannula or mask, use of an *oxygen hood (Figure 17A-2)* or *tent* may be needed.

The **oxygen hood** is a Plexiglas device designed to fit comfortably over the child's head. It requires a much smaller amount of oxygen than does the **tent** which encloses the child's entire body.

> It is important to recognize that the final concentration of oxygen delivered to the patient is a function of both the minute ventilation and how effectively the oxygen is being delivered. For example, a patient with a minute ventilation of 10 L/min who receives oxygen at a rate of 4 L/min will ultimately receive a mixture of oxygen and room air. In this particular case, the mixture will be approximately 40% oxygen and 60% room air.
>
> A patient with a nasal cannula who is breathing through the mouth will also receive an unpredictable concentration of oxygen. In order to deliver a more reliable concentration of oxygen, high flow devices such as a **face shield** (i.e., a large mask that is less confining for the patient and allows for more controlled oxygen delivery) or a partial rebreathing (or non-rebreathing) mask should be used *(Figure 17A-3)*. These methods allow the comfortable delivery of high gas flows, and may prevent significant mixing with room air or rebreathing of exhaled gases. The resultant delivered concentration of oxygen to the patient's lungs is high.

In older children, a nasal cannula is usually preferable to a simple face mask because it is less confining (and

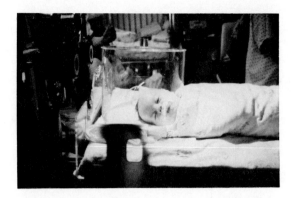

Figure 17A-2.   Oxygen hood.

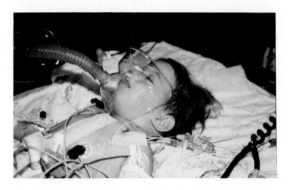

Figure 17A-3.   Use of a face shield is less confining than an oxygen mask, and allows for controlled delivery of high flow oxygen.

therefore better tolerated) and provides equally good oxygen concentrations. In more acutely ill *older* children who require higher concentrations of supplemental oxygen, the **non-rebreathing oxygen face mask** becomes the ventilatory adjunct of choice. An additional advantage of both the nasal cannula and non-rebreathing oxygen mask is that they are usually well tolerated even when worn for an extended period of time.

Initial Management of the Nonbreathing Pediatric Patient

More intensive airway management is required for the patient who is not spontaneously breathing. The first priority is to open the airway. A favored method for accomplishing this is the *jaw thrust*, performed by placing both hands on the patient's head while using the index fingers to displace the mandible anteriorly. This action lifts the tongue off the hypopharynx *(see Figure 7-3 in the Airway chapter)*.

A second method for opening the airway is to carefully slide a small rolled washcloth (or your hand) under the patient's shoulders. This allows the head to slightly tilt back on its axis until the jaw forms a 90° angle to the long axis of the body *(Figure 17A-4)*. This posture is known as

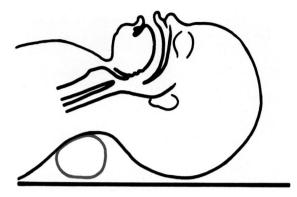

Figure 17A-4.   Sniffing position.

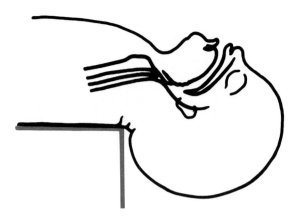

Figure 17A-5.   Anatomical airway obstruction created by hyperextension of the head.

the "sniffing position," since the relationship of the head on the neck is similar to that assumed when smelling an object. Anatomically this action lifts the epiglottis away from the laryngeal opening, and patency of the airway is restored.

> Contrary to popular belief, hyperextending the head of a pediatric patient will *not* ensure patency of the airway. All too often it produces the opposite effect, creating soft tissue airway obstruction by allowing the tongue and epiglottis to fall back over and cover the tracheal opening *(Figure 17A-5).*

A number of anatomical considerations explain why upper airway obstruction occurs so much more commonly in children than in adults:

   i. The tongue and occiput (back part of the head) are relatively larger in children.
   ii. The epiglottis and larynx both lie more anterior and cephalad.
   iii. The airway itself is proportionately smaller.

The relatively large occiput causes the head of the unconscious supine child to flex forward. Soft tissue airway obstruction (occulsion of the small pediatric airway by the relatively large tongue and anteriorly lying epiglottis) is the usual result *(Figure 17A-6).*

Ventilation of Pediatric Patients

There are two basic methods for ventilating pediatric patients: the self-inflating resuscitation bag and the flow-inflation bag.

> Oxygen-powered mechanical breathing devices *(Elder/Robert Shaw valves)* such as the manually triggered units used by emergency prehospital care personnel have *no role* in ventilation of pediatric patients.

The **self-inflating resuscitation bag (bag-valve-mask** or **BVM)** is a unit consisting of a bag, an adapter that can be attached to a mask or endotracheal tube, and a reservoir *(see Figure 7-20 in Chapter 7).* In order to provide elevated concentrations of oxygen, the reservoir must be attached to a high-flow supplemental source of oxygen.

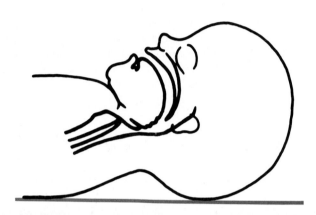

Figure 17A-6.   Anatomical airway obstruction created by flexion of the head.

> Many different bag sizes exist. The one chosen should depend on the size of the child and the tidal volume you want to deliver.

Pop-off valves (which open when a certain airway pressure is attained) may cause problems in the pediatric setting. This is because higher airway pressures are sometimes needed to ventilate patients through the small endotracheal tubes that are used in children. (Should your equipment contain a pop-off valve, it can be bypassed in this setting.)

The **flow-inflation anesthesia bag (Mapelson-D bag)** requires much more skill to operate than does a BVM. It consists of an anesthesia bag, a piece of plastic tubing (approximately 1 foot long), an exhaust valve, and a multipurpose adaptor. The adaptor is usually attached to the oxygen source, a manometer, and an endotracheal tube *(see Figure 7-22 in Chapter 7).* An advantage of this device over the standard BVM is that you can apply CPAP (continuous positive airway pressure) or PEEP (positive endexpiratory pressure). In addition, ventilation with high oxygen concentrations (of almost 100%) is assured. In contrast, the concentration of oxygen delivered with the BVM is somewhat uncertain because the amount of entrained room air is highly variable.

It should be emphasized that the Mapelson-D bag should be operated only by individuals highly trained in its use. In the hands of an inexperienced provider, the risk of complications (i.e., barotrauma with resultant tension pneumothorax) is great. In order to prevent such injury, experienced clinicians often place a manometer into the circuit so that airway pressure can be observed during ventilation.

Adjuncts for Maintaining a Patent Airway

Of the three mechanical adjuncts for ventilation discussed in the chapter on airway management (Chapter 7), only two are used in children. Our comments here are limited to how these modalities apply to children.

Nasopharyngeal and oropharyngeal airways may be of value for initial management of the pediatric airway. Many clinicians prefer to maintain the airway of the spontaneously breathing patient with a **nasopharyngeal trumpet.** This is particularly valuable for the child with a depressed level of consciousness who still retains a sensitive gag reflex. Caution is advised when using this device in young children, however, since the small diameter and relatively long length of the trumpet may paradoxically increase the risk of airway obstruction and stimulate the gag reflex.

For unconscious patients, the **oropharyngeal airway** may be extremely helpful as the initial means of maintaining a patent airway. *Individuals obtunded to the point of being able to tolerate an oropharyngeal airway need definitive management (and protection of the airway) with endotracheal intubation.*

As for adults, there are two methods for inserting the oral pharyngeal airway in children. In the first method, the airway is inserted in an upside down position into the patient's mouth. It is then rotated at the same time as it is slipped into position *(see Figs. 7-11A, B, and C).* In the second method, a tongue blade is used to depress the tongue while the device is inserted into the oral pharynx *(Figures 17A-7A, 17A-7B, 17A-7C, and 17A-7D).*

The *esophageal obturator airway (EOA)* is contraindicated in children under 16 years of age. The risk of esophageal and tracheal damage is simply unwarranted when this device is used in the pediatric age group.

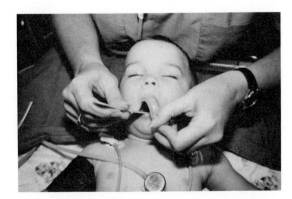

Figure 17A-7A.   The patient's mouth is opened by depressing the chin. The tongue blade is now carefully inserted into the mouth.

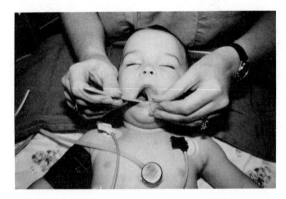

Figure 17A-7C.   While continuing to depress the tongue, the oral airway is carefully slipped over the tongue and into the oral pharynx.

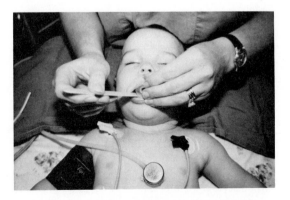

Figure 17A-7B.   Once in the mouth, the tongue blade is used to depress the tongue. This is done by gently pressing against the floor of the mouth. Preparation is made to insert the oral airway.

Figure 17A-7D.   Final position after insertion of the oral airway demonstrating how the flanged portion of the airway rests flush with the patient's lips. While holding the airway in place, the tongue blade may now be removed.

Endotracheal Intubation

The definitive method for managing the *unprotected* airway in the obtunded or unconscious patient is endotracheal intubation. This holds true *regardless* of whether the patient is still spontaneously breathing or not.

Advantages of endotracheal intubation are that:
  i. The airway is protected from aspiration
  ii. Positive pressure ventilation may be given without the risk of gastric insufflation
  iii. An effective alternate route is provided for administering drugs in the event that IV access is lost.

Although the technique for endotracheal intubation of an infant or child is similar to that for an adult, several important differences do exist.

Suctioning the patient prior to intubation is an advisable preparatory measure for both adults and children. Unfortunately, standard suctioning tubing may be somewhat cumbersome when used in pediatric patients.

In adults, *either* a straight *or* curved laryngoscope blade is used, depending on the personal preference of the operator. In contrast, a *straight* blade is generally preferred for intubating very small children or infants. The straight blade is wider and facilitates lifting the tongue out of the line of vision, thus allowing better visualization of the vocal cords. This consideration becomes less important for older children, for whom either blade may be used.

SIZING OF THE ENDOTRACHEAL (ET) TUBE

The size of the ET tube required varies with the age of the child. In most cases, the appropriate size can be estimated by selecting an ET tube of approximately the same diameter as the patient's little fingernail *(Figure 17A-8)*. An even easier way to estimate the size of the ET tube is to gauge tube diameter by the size of the child's external nares. A tube that fits well in the nares is almost always of the appropriate size for the laryngeal opening.

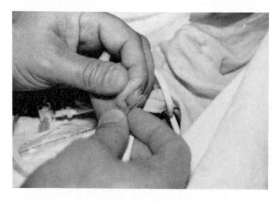

Figure 17A-8.   Estimation of ET tube size by inspection of the diameter of the child's little finger nail.

Premature and full-term newborn infants require ET tubes ranging from 2.5- to 3.5-mm in diameter; a 3-year-old child usually requires a 4.5- to 5.5-mm diameter tube; while a 6-year-old child generally requires a 5.5- to 6.5-mm diameter tube.

TECHNIQUE FOR ENDOTRACHEAL INTUBATION OF CHILDREN

As is the case for adults, the initial step in the intubation process is preoxygenation *(Figure 17A-9)*. This is accomplished by carefully hyperventilating the child with 100% oxygen *prior* to intubation. Insertion of an oral pharyngeal airway will usually facilitate ventilation.

After the child has been adequately oxygenated, the mouth is opened widely with the right hand while the laryngoscope (held in the left hand) is carefully inserted into the right side of the patient's mouth *(Figure 17A-10)*. The tongue is displaced to the left side of the patient's mouth as the laryngoscope is inserted *(Figure 17A-11)*. Insertion of the blade is continued until the epiglottis is visualized *(Figure 17A-12)*. *It is essential not to hyperextend the child's head while attempting to visualize the epiglottis*. Placing the operator's right hand on the child's chin may help stabilize the head *(Figure 17A-13)*.

When using the straight blade, the epiglottis is gently lifted *anteriorly (Figure 17A-14)*. The ET tube is then passed from the right corner of the mouth and threaded through the tracheal

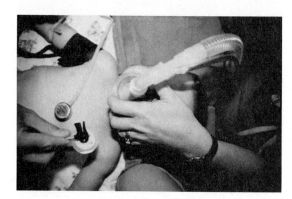

Figure 17A-9.   The initial step in the intubation process is pre-oxygenation.

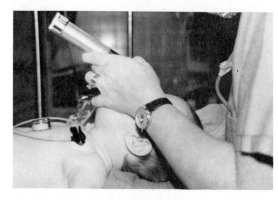

Figure 17A-10.   While maintaining the head in the sniffing position, the laryngoscope is carefully inserted into the right side of the mouth.

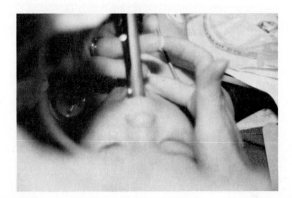

Figure 17A-11. The tongue is displaced to the left side of the patient's mouth as the laryngoscope is inserted.

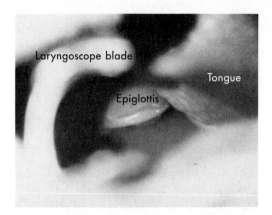

Figure 17A-12. Insertion of the laryngoscope blade is continued until the epiglottis is visualized.

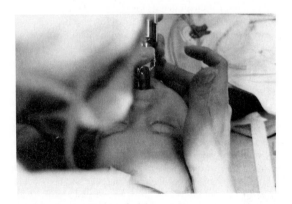

Figure 17A-13. Illustration demonstrating how the patient's head may be stabilized with the operator's right hand while the laryngoscope blade is lifted to visualize the cords.

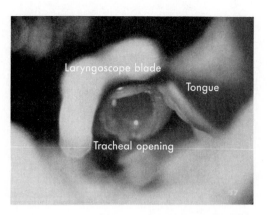

Figure 17A-14. Use of the straight blade to lift the epiglottis and expose the aperture of the trachea. (The epiglottis is hidden from view by the straight blade in this picture.)

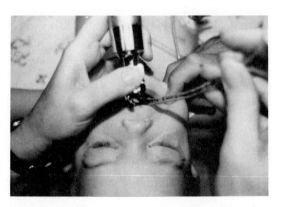

Figure 17A-15. The endotracheal tube is passed from the right corner of the mouth and threaded through the tracheal opening.

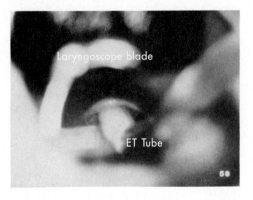

Figure 17A-16. The endotracheal tube is inserted into the trachea under direct vision.

opening *(Figure 17A-15)*. The operator should be certain to clearly visualize the ET tube passing *through* the vocal cords *(Figure 17A-16)*.

Once the ET tube is in place, the laryngoscope may be carefully removed. The ET tube should be held in place by the operator's right hand while the laryngoscope is removed so as not to accidentally extubate the child. It is important to

secure the ET tube in place with tape to prevent accidental extubation and/or inadvertent movement of the tube *(Figure 17A-17)*. The patient can then be ventilated manually (with a BVM device—*Figure 17A-18*) or mechanically (by connecting the ET tube to a ventilator—*Figure 17A-19*).

The procedure for intubation is the same if a *curved* blade is used, except that the tip of the blade is now placed in the

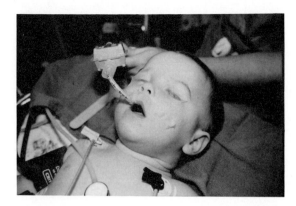

Figure 17A-17. The endotracheal tube is secured in place with tape to prevent accidental extubation and/or inadvertent movement of the tube.

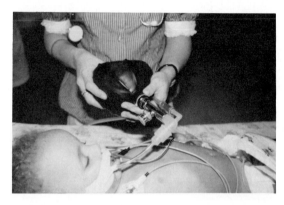

Figure 17A-18. Manual ventilation of the patient after intubation.

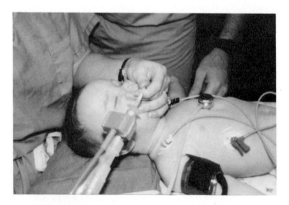

Figure 17A-19. Mechanical ventilation of the patient after intubation performed by connecting the endotracheal tube directly to the ventilator circuit.

vallecula instead of underneath the epiglottis. As in adults, the blade must then be lifted *forward and upward* in order to visualize the cords.

ET tube placement should always be confirmed immediately after intubation by auscultation (for the presence of good, bilateral breath sounds). Definitive confirmation is obtained by ABG analysis and/or chest X-ray.

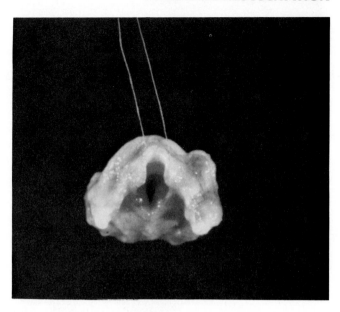

Figure 17A-20. Anatomical specimen demonstrating the omega-shape of the pediatric epiglottis.

SPECIAL CONSIDERATIONS FOR INTUBATION OF CHILDREN

Several important differences exist between the airway of children and adults. The pediatric epiglottis is a much more flimsy structure than its adult counterpart. It is also omega-shaped, whereas the curvature of the adult epiglottis is much less pronounced *(Figure 17A-20)*. As a result, the pediatric epiglottis must be manipulated with extreme care.

Another difference between the pediatric and adult airway is that the laryngeal opening is much smaller in children. This makes it more difficult to pass the ET tube through the cords. Unlike in adults, the smallest part of the pediatric airway is the *cricoid* cartilage! Thus in children, *successfully passing the tube through the cords does not necessarily constitute successful intubation.* In view of this, it is always a good idea to have additional endotracheal tubes (0.5 mm smaller and 0.5 mm larger than anticipated) on hand during the intubation phase.

As already noted, the small size of the pediatric chest results in close approximation of auscultatory fields. Breath sounds may therefore be easily transmitted from the esophagus to the lung fields. More than simply auscultating over the lung fields, one must verify that air sounds are not being heard over the stomach. With proper tube placement, the chest should rise symmetrically during ventilation. If the child had become bradycardic prior to intubation, heart rate should rapidly return toward normal if the ET tube has been properly placed.

Recognition and Treatment of Tension Pneumothorax

Positive pressure ventilation must be administered with great care in children. Failure to do so may result in rupture of the pleura (i.e., pneumothorax), especially in asthmatics who are particularly susceptible to this complication. If unrecognized and positive pressure ventilation is continued, *tension* pneumothorax may develop.

Tension pneumothorax typically manifests clinically by sudden deterioration of hemodynamic and respiratory function. If undetected, it is a potentially fatal iatrogenic complication that may lead to cardiovascular collapse and cardiac arrest. With each additional breath given, the volume of air in the pleural cavity (and resultant intrathoracic pressure) continue to rise. Venous return is impeded, and cardiac output drops dramatically.

A high index of suspicion is often needed to make the diagnosis of tension pneumothorax. Hyperresonance and decreased breath sounds over the affected hemithorax, in association with the clinical setting described above (i.e., sudden deterioration of hemodynamic and respiratory function in an intubated child) should lead one to suspect the diagnosis. Unfortunately, clinical signs are less reliable in smaller children and infants. If respiratory distress is marked, there may not be time to obtain a confirmatory chest X-ray. In such cases, the *only* way to make the diagnosis (and save the patient's life) may be to proceed with needle thoracostomy.

> Needle thoracostomy of children is accomplished by insertion of a small (19 to 21 gauge) butterfly needle attached to a syringe *(Figure 17A-21)* into the 4th IC (intercostal) space at the midaxillary line *(Figure 17A-22)*. If tension pneumothorax is present, the clinician will be rewarded by the release of air under pressure *(Figure 17A-23)*. As much air as possible should be aspirated. Because tension pneumothorax is more common on the right, needle insertion is often tried first on this side of the chest. If no improvement is noted, the left side should be needled as well. Needle insertion should be directed to pass just *over* the rib so as to avoid the neurovascular bundle that runs underneath. If time allows, the area should be cleansed with antiseptic solution prior to needle insertion.

Of cardiopulmonary arrests that occur in asthmatic children, tension pneumothorax is a surprisingly common cause. Awareness of this fact justifies presumptive needle

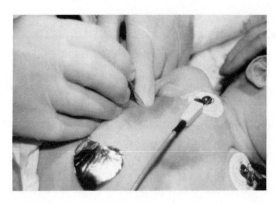

Figure 17A-22.   The butterfly needle is inserted into the 4th intercostal space at the midaxillary line.

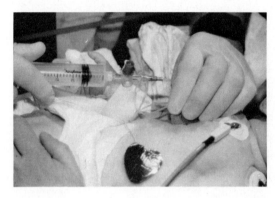

Figure 17A-23.   Illustration demonstrating how air can be evacuated from the pleural space once the needle has been inserted.

thoracostomy when conventional measures fail to resuscitate the child and there is insufficient time to confirm the diagnosis by chest X-ray.

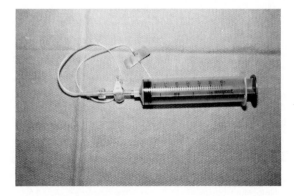

Figure 17A-21.   Illustration of equipment (butterfly needle, stopcock, and attached syringe) used for decompression of tension pneumothorax in children.

> A final word of caution is in order. At times the endotracheal tube may slip from its correct position in the trachea into a mainstem bronchus or into the esophagus. Inadequate ventilation with rapid clinical deterioration may result. *Slippage of the ET tube with inappropriate repositioning (into a mainstem bronchus or the esophagus) may be extremely difficult to differentiate clinically from sudden development of tension pneumothorax.* Both conditions may produce diminished (or absent) breath sounds on one or both sides of the chest. If time permits, a chest X-ray will clarify the situation. However, the emergency care provider may be confronted with life-threatening clinical deterioration of the patient that doesn't allow time to obtain a chest X-ray. In this case the ET tube should be visualized with a laryngoscope. Evidence supporting proper ET tube placement is provided by verifying that the tube passes through the vocal cords and noting the placement marks on the tube itself (which help determine the correct depth of insertion). If this procedure suggests proper ET tube position, it is likely that tension pneumothorax is the cause of respiratory difficulty. Presumptive needle thoracostomy is then indicated.

SECTION B

ALGORITHM FOR MANAGEMENT OF THE PEDIATRIC AIRWAY

We consolidate our approach to management of the pediatric airway in the algorithm shown in *Figure 17B-1*. The first step is to determine whether the child is spontaneously breathing **(1)**. If so, attention is directed at evaluating the parameters of respiratory distress listed in Table 17A-1. If the child is conscious, alert, spontaneously breathing in a normal fashion, and ventilation appears to be adequate **(1—2—3)**, supplemental oxygen may be all that is needed for the moment. Further evaluation of the severity and cause of respiratory difficulty (chest X-ray,

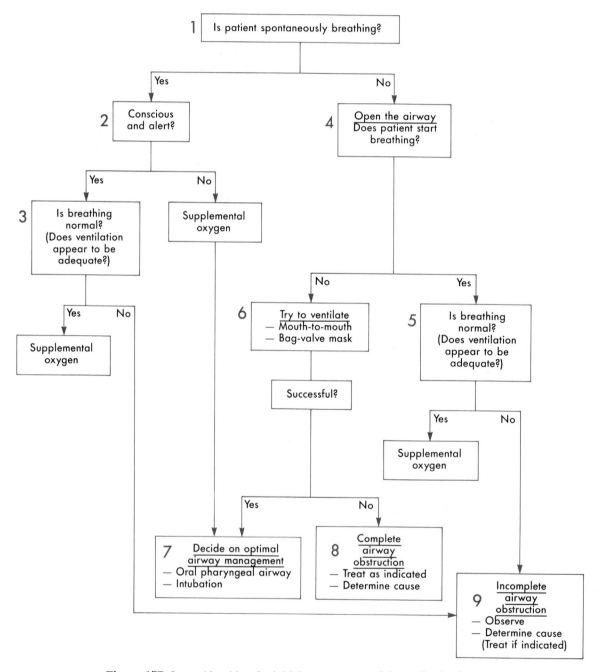

Figure 17B-1.   Algorithm for initial management of the pediatric airway.

ABG analysis, etc.) may proceed in a less urgent manner.

If the patient is not breathing, the first priority is to *open the airway*. Ventilation is then reassessed **(4)**. If normal ventilation resumes, again all that may be needed for the moment is supplemental oxygen **(5)**. However, if the patient does not begin to breathe after the airway is opened, *artificial ventilation* (by mouth-to-mouth or BVM) must be attempted **(6)**.

A good rule of thumb is to "ventilate for gentle chest rise," and to check skin color and mucous membranes for improvement.

If artificial ventilation results in adequate ventilation, efforts should be directed toward definitive management of the airway with endotracheal intubation **(4—6—7)**. In contrast, if the rescuer is unable to successfully ventilate the patient, *complete airway obstruction* must be suspected **(4—6—8)**. *Reposition the patient's head in an attempt to open the airway*. If this is unsuccessful, maneuvers for treating foreign body obstruction should be tried. In the infant under 1 year of age, this includes back blows and chest thrusts. For older children, abdominal thrusts and/or chest thrusts should be used.

If the patient begins to breathe after the airway is opened but continues to demonstrate respiratory difficulty, *partial airway obstruction* should be suspected **(4—5—9)**. Similarly, if the patient is conscious and spontaneously breathing but in an abnormal fashion, there may also be partial obstruction **(1—2—3—9)**. Partial airway obstruction may be caused by either soft tissue obstruction (such as the tongue) or a foreign body. In the latter case, coughing should be encouraged in the hope that the foreign body will be expelled. *As long as the patient is adequately ventilating, no immediate intervention is required*. However, continued close observation is mandatory, however, since partial airway obstruction may at any time become complete.

Finally, if the patient is spontaneously breathing but not alert, more definitive measures are needed to protect the airway **(1—2—7)**. This would entail at least a nasopharyngeal airway for the *semiconscious* patient who retains a sensitive gag reflex and endotracheal intubation for the *unconscious* individual.

SECTION C

ASSESSING PEDIATRIC CIRCULATORY STATUS/ DRUGS IN EMERGENCY CARDIAC CARE

Once control of the **A**irway has been achieved, and adequate ventilation (**B**reathing) assured, attention is directed toward evaluating **C**irculatory status. The most important parameters to assess in this regard are listed in *Table 17C-1.*

Recognition of Cardiovascular Distress in Children

A variety of disease entities may compromise cardiac output. This results in activation of *physiologic compensatory* mechanisms aimed at maintaining blood pressure and preserving blood flow to essential organs. Hemodynamic effects of these compensatory mechanisms on the patient are often readily identified on physical examination, facilitating accurate clinical assessment of cardiovascular function.

One of the earliest changes accompanying a decrease in cardiac output is catecholamine release. This results in an increase in heart rate and arteriolar vasoconstriction. The greater the reduction in cardiac output, the more intense this cardiovascular compensation is likely to be. As shown in Table 17C-1, cardiopulmonary distress is indicated by progressively increasing tachycardia and signs of peripheral vasoconstriction (weak peripheral pulses, cool distal extremities and sluggish capillary refill). With more severe

degrees of cardiopulmonary compromise, central pulses diminish, blood pressure drops and the skin becomes mottled. Ultimately, compensatory mechanisms are no longer able to sustain systemic blood pressure, and frank shock develops.

SPECIFIC ASSESSMENT PARAMETERS
Pulse Assessment

In addition to noting the presence and quality of the pulse, it is essential to accurately determine heart rate. Rates considered normal for adults may represent marked *bradycardia* in children.

As already discussed in Section A, normal values for heart rates in infants and children are surprisingly higher than what one might expect. Thus, the mean heart rate of a 4-month-old child is between 120-140 beats/minute. Heart rates of up to 120 beats/min are still considered normal for children 1 to 2 years of age. Mean heart rate does not drop below 100 beats/min until approximately 8 years of age. *A heart rate of 80 beats/min in the setting of cardiopulmonary arrest must be interpreted as relative bradycardia for most children.*

It is particularly important to pay attention to heart rate during attempts at endotracheal intubation. Should one encounter difficulty intubating a patient in respiratory distress, the attempt should be immediately terminated if heart rate drops below 80 beats/min in infants and 60 beats/min in

Table 17C-1

Signs and Symptoms of Cardiovascular Distress in the Pediatric Patient			
	MILD Cardiopulmonary Distress	**MODERATE Cardiopulmonary Distress**	**SEVERE Cardiopulmonary Distress**
Heart Rate	• Slight increase	• Moderate increase	• Marked increase
Pulses	• Weak peripheral pulses	• Weak proximal pulses	• Absent central pulses
Blood Pressure	• Normal	• Normal or mildly decreased	• Definite hypotension
Peripheral Perfusion	• Normal warmth or slight cooling of extremities • Normal (pink) color of skin and mucous membranes	• Definite cooling of extremities • Extremities may be mottled • Sluggish capillary refill	• Cold extremities • Mottled extremities • Peripheral cyanosis • Poor capillary refill
Respiratory Rate	• Slight increase *(see Table 17A-1)*	• Moderate increase	• Marked increase

children. In such cases, conventional means of ventilation (BVM) should be resumed *at least* until heart rate and blood pressure are restored to more appropriate levels.

The best method for determining the pulse in infants and small children is to palpate for the brachial pulse (Cavallaro and Melker, 1983). This can be done by externally rotating the hand and placing the fingers just below the brachial muscle in the midhumerus area *(Figure 17C-1).*

> Because of the short, chubby neck of infants, location of the carotid pulse is extremely difficult to identify in this age group. Infants simply "don't have necks." In children more than 1 year of age, either the carotid or brachial pulse may be used.
>
> In the past, the femoral pulse has been used as an alternative site for palpating a pulse. The drawback of this practice is that the pulse palpated in the femoral area during external chest compressions may sometimes be the femoral *vein* rather than the artery!

Blood Pressure

Normal blood pressures in children are somewhat lower than those for adults. For example, a systolic blood pressure of 80 mm Hg is *normal* for a 5-year-old child. A simplified method for determining hypotension based on the age of the child has been suggested by the American Heart Association. They define hypotension if systolic blood pressure is less than 70 mm Hg plus 2 times age in years. Thus, the lowest acceptable blood pressure in a 3-year-old child would be 76 mm Hg (70 + [2 × 3]).

It is difficult to accurately determine blood pressure in infants and young children. This may be due to improper cuff size and/or difficulty hearing Korotkoff sounds. Care must be taken to use a cuff that covers approximately two-thirds to three-quarters of the arm as measured from elbow to axilla. Choosing a cuff too narrow may result in artificially elevated blood pressure readings, while selecting a cuff too wide may have the opposite effect. In the event that Korotkoff sounds are inaudible, use of a *palpable* systolic blood pressure suffices. If available, a Doppler may be invaluable.

Peripheral Circulatory Changes

Peripheral circulatory changes are assessed by noting skin temperature (warm, cool, cold), skin color, and *capillary refill time*. The latter is determined by applying just enough pressure to the nailbeds or skin on the toes or fingertips to cause blanching—and then releasing the pressure. The time required for the capillaries to refill should be measured. Capillary refill is described as brisk if it occurs within 1 second, and sluggish if it requires more than 3 seconds.

External Chest Compressions

If no pulse is present, external chest compressions must be started. The rate recommended for compressions is *at least* 100 times per minute for infants, and 80-100 times per minute for children 1 year of age or older. For chest compressions to be effective, the sternum must be de-

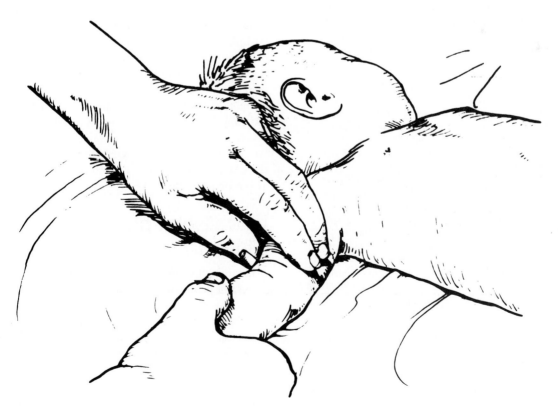

Figure 17C-1.   Palpating the brachial pulse.

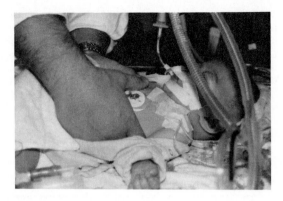

Figure 17C-2.   Circumferentially applied chest compression in an infant.

pressed at least 0.5 to 1 inch for infants, 1 to 1.5 inches for children between 1 and 8 years old, and 1.5 to 2 inches for children older than 8.

As discussed in Chapter 10 on New Developments in CPR, we now know that compression of the heart between the sternum and vertebral column is probably not the principal mechanism for blood flow with CPR in most adults. Instead, the pressure gradient that develops between the intrathoracic and extrathoracic compartments appears to be much more important. The opposite may be true for infants. Because of the compliance and small size of the infant chest wall, actual compression of the heart *may* occur and could be a major mechanism for blood flow in this age group.* As a result, external chest compressions must be of adequate depth in order to be effective. Direct cardiac compression may also be important in older children, although it is still unclear at what age this ceases to be the major mechanism for blood flow.

> An interesting change in basic life support guidelines deals with the recommended hand position for performing external chest compression in infants. In the past it was thought that the infant heart was situated higher in the chest than the heart of older children and adults. Because of this, it was recommended that external chest compressions be delivered over the middle third of the sternum (parallel to the nipple line). This recommendation has been refuted (Orlowski, 1986). We now know that the heart of infants lies over the *lower* third of the sternum, just as it does for older children and adults. Consequently, finger position for external chest compression in infants should be 1 fingerbreadth *below* the nipple line.
>
> Two methods have been recommended for performance of chest compression in small children and infants. One method uses two fingers (the index and middle fingers) to compress the chest. In the second method, both hands of the rescuer are placed circumferentially around the thorax, and the thumbs (which are placed on the sternum) are used to compress the chest *(Figure 17C-2)*. Recent evidence suggests that the latter technique (circumferential application of chest

---

*Preliminary findings of a study utilizing echocardiography during performance of CPR in infants and neonates suggests that direct cardiac compression may *not* be the primary mechanism for blood flow during CPR in this age group (Personal communication—Giroud and Cavallaro).

compression) may generate better hemodynamics during CPR (David, 1988).

Useful Drugs in Pediatric Resuscitation

As we have emphasized, most pediatric resuscitations can be successfully managed by improving oxygenation and ventilation without the need for pharmacologic intervention. However, drug therapy may occasionally be needed to accelerate the heart rate, improve perfusion, and correct hypotension.

Nonpediatric emergency care providers are often uncomfortable calculating the dosages of drugs used in children, particularly when called on to do so during the stress of a pediatric emergency. For this reason it may be advisable to post a chart of commonly used drugs and dosages for pediatric resuscitation in a readily visible location. We indicate one way of displaying this information in *Table 17C-2*, which we show at the end of this chapter.

> Detailed discussion of indications, mechanism of action, and precautions for drugs used in cardiac arrest and emergency cardiac care was covered in Chapters 2 and 14. We do not repeat that information here.

Practically speaking, there are only two truly essential drugs in pediatric resuscitation: *epinephrine* and *oxygen*. Atropine may temporarily reverse bradycardia, but this does not correct (and may only serve to mask) the usual underlying cause of the slow heart rate—hypoxemia from respiratory insufficiency. Dopamine may be a useful agent in the post-resuscitation management of selected pediatric patients, but it is not commonly used during the actual arrest itself. Sodium bicarbonate, lidocaine, and isoproterenol are included in our table for completeness, but these drugs are only rarely used in pediatric resuscitation at the present time.

Establishment of IV Access in Children

Establishing intravenous access is an important component of pediatric resuscitation in the event that drug or fluid administration is necessary. Unfortunately, securing adequate IV access in children is often problematic for the nonpediatric-oriented health care provider. This task may be made even more difficult in the setting of cardiopulmonary arrest by hypotension and/or endogenous release of catecholamines with resultant vasospasm.

In this next section, we review our approach to establishing a suitable route for IV access in children. It should be emphasized at the outset that the focus in pediatric resuscitation must *never* be on establishment of IV access alone. Instead, early control of the airway so as to be able to adequately oxygenate the child is the key. Accomplishment of this goal is much more likely to bring a child back than is administration of drugs.

Routes for Drug Administration

PERIPHERAL VENOUS ACCESS

Peripheral venous access is most often chosen as the initial route for drug and fluid administration. The three sites most commonly selected are:

   i. Antecubital veins
  ii. Long saphenous vein
 iii. External jugular vein

> The favored site for peripheral venous access in adults and normovolemic children has been the dorsum of the hand. Practically speaking, cannulation of these veins on the chubby hand of a hemodynamically compromised child frequently is all but impossible.

Antecubital veins are easily accessible in children and are cannulated in the same fashion as for adults. They serve as an effective route for administering fluid and drugs during pediatric resuscitation.

Another frequently used site of venous access is the *long saphenous vein*. The advantage of this site is that the vein is easy to locate, lies superficially, and is simple to cannulate. The long saphenous vein can be found just anterior to the medial malleolus. From there it runs straight up along the medial aspect of the leg. Unfortunately, due to decreased venous return from subdiaphragmatic veins, the value of this route during cardiac arrest has now become questionable.

The *external jugular* vein is commonly overlooked by the non-pediatric-oriented emergency care provider as a suitable site for venous access in children. This is unfortunate because the site is surprisingly easy to cannulate in children over 1 year of age (especially if they are crying!). Simply place the child in slight Trendelenburg position and rotate the head to the opposite side. This should distend the vein and make it readily visible. Even though the external jugular is classified as a peripheral vein, fluid and drugs administered by this route reach the central circulation almost as quickly as they do when given through a central line. One should therefore strongly consider this site early in the resuscitation phase.

ENDOTRACHEAL DRUG ADMINISTRATION

If difficulty is encountered in obtaining venous access, the endotracheal route provides a very effective alternative for drug administration. Medications that may be given by this route are easily remembered by the mnemonic **A—L—E** (**A**tropine, **L**idocaine, and **E**pinephrine).

CENTRAL LINES

Although central venous access is generally accepted as the ideal method for administering drugs and fluids during cardiopulmonary resuscitation, many clinicians are not comfortable with central venous cannulation of a pediatric arrest victim. A major reason for this is the high complication rate seen when placement of central lines is attempted by those not highly skilled with this technique.

> The *subclavian vein* is probably the most commonly chosen site for obtaining central venous access in adults. However, cannulation of this vein is fraught with danger (frequent occurrence of pneumothorax) for the inexperienced pediatric care provider. The *internal jugular* vein is not a wise choice for the inexperienced either because the short, stubby neck of infants and young children make this vein almost inaccessible. As for adults, the *femoral vein* is no longer recommended as a site for fluid or drug administration due to decreased subdiaphragmatic venous return during cardiac resuscitation.

Intraosseous Access

The intraosseous route for fluid and drug administration was first described in the 1940s. With the advent of Teflon and polyvinyl-chloride catheters, this route was almost forgotten until recently. In view of the difficulty in obtaining intravenous access in hemodynamically compromised infants and small children, interest in the intraosseous technique has recently been revived.

Compelling reasons to *strongly consider* the intraosseous route when immediate vascular access is required include:
   i. Minimal complications
  ii. Rapid administration of intravenous fluids, blood products, and drugs (catecholamines, sodium bicarbonate)
 iii. Ease of insertion. (With practice, intraosseous access may be established in seconds!)

> Practically speaking, it often takes surprisingly long to achieve intravenous access in children during emergency situations. In a study by Kanter et al (1986), more than 1.5 minutes were needed to establish a line in 76% of patients, and greater than 5 minutes were needed in 34% of patients.

As a result of their study, these authors (and others) suggest that if a peripheral line cannot be started within 1 to 2 minutes, strong consideration be given to use of the intraosseous method—especially if the child does not respond rapidly after establishing adequate ventilation (Kanter et al, 1986; Seigler et al, 1989; Fiser, 1990).

> The beauty of the intraosseous technique is that the marrow cavity functions like a "rigid vein" that does not collapse, even in the presence of profound hypovolemia and shock (Fiser, 1990). Absorption is rapid from the marrow sinusoids of long bones because they drain directly into medullary venous channels that enter the systemic circulation.

TECHNIQUE FOR OBTAINING INTRAOSSEOUS ACCESS

The preferred site for attempting intraosseous cannulation in children is the tibia. Prior to cannulation, the area should be prepped and draped in the usual fashion. The area can be infiltrated with a local anesthetic. The procedure is performed with a bone marrow aspiration needle *with* stylet. The purpose of the stylet is to prevent the lumen of the needle from becoming clogged with bony fragments during insertion. Although some clinicians suggest using a spinal needle, we have found the procedure much easier to perform with a bone marrow aspiration needle.

The needle is inserted 1 to 2 fingerbreadths below the tibial tubercle on the anteromedial (flat) surface of the tibia *(Figures 17C-3A and 17C-3B)*. While supporting the lower leg with one hand, be sure to insert the needle while directing it either perpendicular or in a slightly caudal orientation until the periosteum is reached *(Figure 17C-4)*. This orientation for the angle of insertion is important to avoid damaging the growth plate.

At this point, it may be necessary to apply a boring or screwing motion to introduce the needle into the bone *(Figure 17C-5)*. A slight "give" in resistance signals entry into the

marrow. Correct placement is confirmed by aspiration of blood and bony debris into a syringe *(Figure 17C-6)*. This is followed by a saline flush to clear the needle of debris.

Standard IV tubing can now be connected to the needle and the site is ready for drugs and fluid administration *(Figure 17C-7)*.

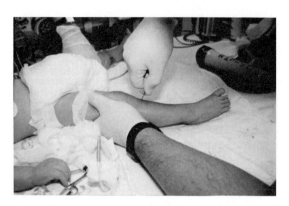

Figure 17C-4.   The lower leg is supported with one hand as the needle is inserted with the other hand. In this illustration, the needle is being advanced perpendicular to the orientation of the tibia.

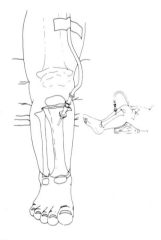

Figure 17C-3A.   Schematic illustration of the proper positioning for insertion of the intraosseous needle.
(Reproduced with permission from the collection of Rick Wiebly, MD).

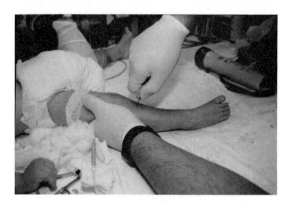

Figure 17C-5.   Once the periosteum is reached, it may be necessary to apply a boring or screwing motion to introduce the needle in the bone. A slight "give" in resistance signals entry into the marrow.

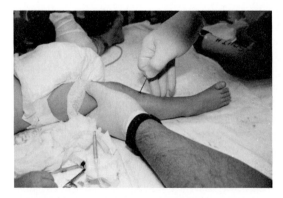

Figure 17C-3B.   Technique for obtaining intraosseous access. The needle is inserted 1-2 fingerbreadths below the tibial tubercle on the anteromedial (flat) surface of the tibia.

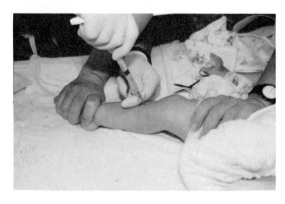

Figure 17C-6.   Correct placement is confirmed by aspiration of blood and bony debris into a syringe.

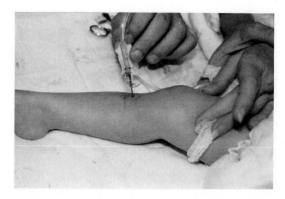

Figure 17C-7. After the intraosseous needle has been flushed with saline, standard IV tubing is connected to the needle. The site is now ready for drugs and fluid administration.

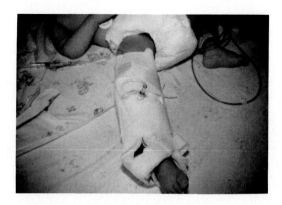

Figure 17C-9. A stack of 4 × 4's is used to protect the needle, and an arm board stabilizes the leg.

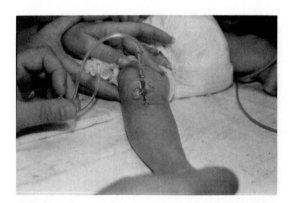

Figure 17C-8. Because of the long length of the bone marrow needle left exposed and its precarious location, special care is needed in securing the needle and preventing it from being bumped or dislodged.

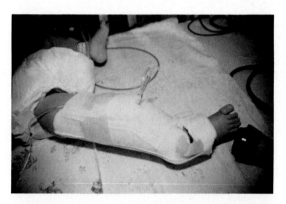

Figure 17C-10. Side view of the technique (shown in Fig. 17C-9) for stabilizing the intraosseous needle.

A word of caution is in order. Because of the long length of the bone marrow needle left exposed and its precarious location *(Figure 17C-8)*, special care is needed in securing the needle and preventing it from being bumped or dislodged. This may be accomplished by placing a stack of 4 × 4's around the needle to stabilize it. An arm board may then be secured under the child's lower extremity to hold the 4 × 4's in place and prevent flexing of the child's leg *(Figures 17C-9 and 17C-10)*.

In general, complications from intraosseous infusion are infrequent. They may include subcutaneous or subperiosteal infiltration of fluid or leakage from the puncture site. Localized cellulitis, abscess formation, and osteomyelitis all occur with an incidence of less than 1%. Complications are further minimized by removing the intraosseous needle as soon as conventional IV access can be established—preferably within 1 to 2 hours (Fiser, 1990).

Defibrillation and Cardioversion

As we have already emphasized, bradycardia or asystole secondary to respiratory arrest is the terminal event in the overwhelming majority of pediatric arrests. Ventricular fibrillation is seldom seen. Consequently, pediatric defibrillation is rarely needed. If defibrillation is necessary, the energy recommended for the initial countershock attempt is 2 joules/kg. If unsuccessful, this energy level should be doubled (to 4 joules/kg) for repeat defibrillation. Thus, for a 1-year-old child weighing 10 kg (22 lb), an energy of 20 joules should be used initially, and additional attempts would be with 40 joules.

On rare occasions, synchronized cardioversion may be needed to convert supraventricular or ventricular tachyarrhythmias to normal sinus rhythm. The recommended energy dose for cardioversion of children is 0.2 to 1.0 joules/kg.

Cardioversion is not an innocuous procedure. Moreover, many children tolerate tachyarrhythmias (of 200 beats/min or more) surprisingly well. As a result, it may be preferable for the adult-oriented emergency care provider to resist the urge to cardiovert a child unless the patient is manifesting signs of profound shock. Help (in the form of an experienced pediatric care provider) will usually be accessible long before this point is reached.

When defibrillating or cardioverting an infant or small child, it is important to use pediatric defibrillator paddles

(Figure 17C-11). The reason smaller paddles are needed is that they decrease transthoracic resistance and reduce the chance of electrical arching between the paddles. Unfortunately, pediatric paddles are not universally available in non-pediatric-oriented facilities. As a result, adult-oriented care providers may not be familiar with the technique of pediatric defibrillation/cardioversion.

Pediatric defibrillator paddles must first be attached to standard adult paddles before they can be used. This is easily done by sliding each pediatric paddle over an adult paddle *(Figure 17C-12)* until it locks into place *(Figure 17C-13)*. The defibrillator may then be charged and discharged in the same manner as for adults.

There are two equally acceptable methods of paddle placement for pediatric defibrillation/cardioversion: the standard (sternum-apex) position *(Figure 17C-14)* or the anterior-posterior position *(Figure 17C-15)*.

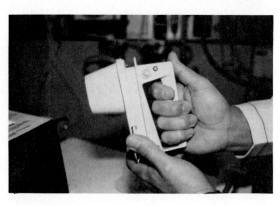

Figure 17C-13.   Final position of the pediatric paddle locked into place on the adult paddle.

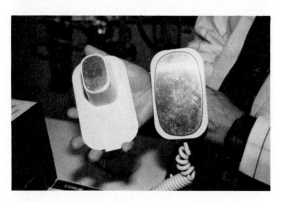

Figure 17C-11.   Comparison of pediatric and adult defibrillator paddles. The surface area of a pediatric paddle (left in the figure) is significantly smaller than that of an adult paddle.

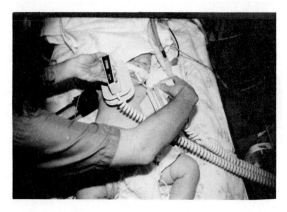

Figure 17C-14.   Standard (sternum-apex) paddle placement position for pediatric defibrillation/cardioversion.

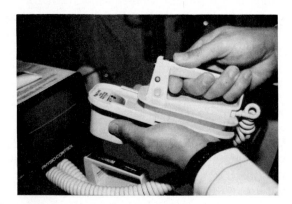

Figure 17C-12.   Sliding the pediatric paddle over the adult paddle.

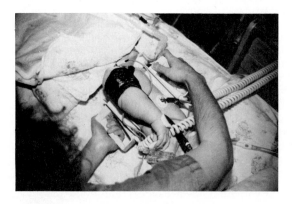

Figure 17C-15.   Anterior-posterior paddle placement position for pediatric defibrillation/cardioversion.

Table 17C-2

Pediatric Drug Dosages

EPINEPHRINE

At the time of this writing, the optimal dose of epinephrine in children remains uncertain. In a relatively small study of witnessed cardiac arrests in children (median age 2.5 to 3 years), Goetting and Paradis (1991) found **High-Dose Epinephrine (HDE** = 0.1 to 0.2 mg/kg) to be superior to **Standard-Dose Epinephrine (SDE)** for treatment of refractory bradycardia or asystole. They suggest that if two standard doses of epinephrine fail to satisfactorily increase perfusion pressure within 5 minutes, that additional standard doses of epinephrine are unlikely to do so either. To minimize the chance of developing neurologic injury, they recommend consideration of HDE at this point.

In an accompanying editorial, Brown and Kelen (1991) caution against generalizing the results from this limited study. Additional prospective, controlled clinical trials will be needed to determine the true efficacy of HDE for refractory pediatric arrest, especially with respect to preserving neurologic function. Until such trials are performed, SDE should probably continue to be used initially (for at least two doses)—perhaps with consideration of HDE in patients who fail to respond.

Dosing of epinephrine by the **intraosseous** *route* is still somewhat empiric. Although standard dosing (i.e., 0.01 mg/kg) may be tried initially, it appears that higher doses (of 0.1 mg/kg or more) may be needed to achieve optimal coronary perfusion in the arrested heart (Spivey et al, 1992). Similarly, it appears that higher than usual doses may be needed for optimal pharmacologic effect when epinephrine is administered by the **endotracheal (ET)** *route* (Crespo et al, 1991). As a result, one may choose to administer HDE doses of drug endotracheally if lower doses are ineffective.

To minimize the volume of diluent, it may be preferable to use a 1:1,000 solution of epinephrine when HDE doses are selected.

SDE Dose = 0.01 mg/kg   **HDE Dose** = 0.1 to 0.2 mg/kg
(Comes in 10-ml syringes [0.1 mg/1 ml] of 1:10,000 soln)

Weight of Patient	SDE Dose for IV Bolus (= 0.01 mg/kg)	HDE Dose for IV Bolus (= 0.1 to 0.2 mg/kg)
10 kg	0.1 mg (1 ml)	1-2 mg
20 kg	0.2 mg (2 ml)	2-4 mg
30 kg	0.3 mg (3 ml)	4-6 mg
Adult	0.5-1 mg (5-10 ml)	5-10 mg

IV Infusion Dose (for **SDE**) = 0.1-1.0 μg/kg/min
   Mix 0.6 × body weight (kg) in mg in 100 ml of D5W.
   Then 1 drop/min = 0.1 μg/kg/min; Titrate to effect.

Weight of Patient	How to Mix	Initial Rate*	Maximum Rate**
10 kg	6 mg in 100 D5W	1 drop/min (= 0.1 μg/kg/min)	10 drops/min
20 kg	12 mg in 100 D5W	1 drop/min (= 0.1 μg/kg/min)	10 drops/min
30 kg	18 mg in 100 D5W	1 drop/min (= 0.1 μg/kg/min)	10 drops/min
Adult	1 mg in 250 D5W	15-30 drops/min (1-2 μg/min)	10 drops/min

*NOTE: When infusing the small quantities of drug required for pediatric IV infusions, it is essential to use an infusion pump to ensure accuracy.
Higher doses may be used for **HDE IV Infusion....

Table 17C-2

Pediatric Drug Dosages—cont'd

ATROPINE:

Dose = 0.02 mg/kg (Comes in 10-ml Bristoject [0.1 mg/1 ml])
   (Minimum dose = 0.1 mg; maximum single dose = 1 mg)
      May repeat 0.02 mg/kg q 5 min up to 1 mg (for child) and 2 mg (for adolescent)

Weight of Patient	Single Dose (IV or ET)
10 kg	0.2 mg
20 kg	0.4 mg
30 kg	0.6 mg
Adult	0.5-1.0 mg

SODIUM BICARBONATE:

Respiratory failure is the most common cause of cardiac arrest in children. The most important treatment priority is to improve ventilation, not to administer sodium bicarbonate. Epinephrine is the drug of choice for the arrested heart. Sodium bicarbonate should be considered only if the arrest is prolonged, or if the patient was known to have an underlying metabolic acidosis.

Dose = 1 mEq/kg (50 ml of 8.4% soln = 50 mEq)

Weight of Patient	Dose (IV or Intraosseous)
10 kg	10 mEq (1/5 ampule)
20 kg	20 mEq (2/5 ampule)
30 kg	30 mEq (3/5 ampule)
Adult	50-100 mEq (1-2 ampules)

Table 17C-2

Pediatric Drug Dosages—cont'd

LIDOCAINE:

Dose = 1 mg/kg IV bolus

Weight of Patient	Dose for IV Bolus
10 kg	10 mg
20 kg	20 mg
30 kg	30 mg
Adult	50-100 mg

IV Infusion Dose = 20-50 μg/kg/min
　　Mix 120 mg in 100 ml of D5W = 1200 μg/ml
　　　Then 1 drop/kg/min = 20 μg/kg/min (Initial rate)
　　　2.5 drops/kg/min = 50 μg/kg/min (Maximum rate)

Weight of Patient	How to Mix	Initial Rate*	Maximum Rate
10 kg	120 mg in 100 D5W	10 drops/min	25 drops/min
20 kg	120 mg in 100 D5W	20 drops/min	50 drops/min
30 kg	120 mg in 100 D5W	30 drops/min	75 drops/min
Adult	1,000 mg in 250 D5W	30 drops/min = 2 mg/min	4 mg/min

*****NOTE:** When infusing the small quantities of drug required for pediatric IV infusions, it is essential to use an infusion pump to ensure accuracy.

DOPAMINE:

IV Infusion Dose = 2-20 μg/kg/min
　　Mix 6 mg × body weight (kg) in 100 ml of D5W.
　　　Then 1 drop/min = 1.0 μg/kg/min
　　　　5 drops/min = 5 μg/kg/min (= usual initial rate)
　　　　20 drops/min = 20 μg/kg/min = maximum rate)

Weight of Patient	How to Mix	Initial Rate*	Maximum Rate
10 kg	60 mg in 100 D5W	5 drops/min (50 μg/min)	20 drops/min
20 kg	120 mg in 100 D5W	5 drops/min (100 μg/min)	20 drops/min
30 kg	180 mg in 100 D5W	5 drops/min (150 μg/min)	20 drops/min
Adult	200 mg in 250 D5W	30 drops/min (400 μg/min)	Titrate up

*****NOTE:** When infusing the small quantities of drug required for pediatric IV infusions, it is essential to use an infusion pump to ensure accuracy.

Table 17C-2

Pediatric Drug Dosages—cont'd

ISOPROTERENOL:

IV Infusion Dose = 0.1-1.0 μg/kg/min
  Mix 0.6 mg × body weight (kg) in 100 ml of D5W.
    Then 1 drop/min = 0.1 μg/kg/min; Titrate to effect.

Weight of Patient	How to Mix	Initial Rate*	Maximum Rate
10 kg	6 mg in 100 D5W	1 drop/min (= 0.1 μg/kg/min)	10 drops/min
20 kg	12 mg in 100 D5W	1 drop/min (= 0.1 μg/kg/min)	10 drops/min
30 kg	18 mg in 100 D5W	1 drop/min (= 0.1 μg/kg/min)	10 drops/min
Adult	1 mg in 250 D5W	30 drops/min (2 μg/min)	20 μg/min

*__NOTE:__ When infusing the small quantities of drug required for pediatric IV infusions, it is essential to use an infusion pump to ensure accuracy.

DEFIBRILLATION:

Dose = 2 J (joules)/kg for initial countershock.
  If this is unsuccessful, double the dose (to 4 J/kg) and repeat × 2.

Weight of Patient	Initial Shock (2nd-3rd Shock)
10 kg	20 J (then 40 J- 40 J)
20 kg	40 J (then 80 J- 80 J)
30 kg	60 J (then 120 J- 120 J)
Adult	200 J (then 300 J- 360 J)

OXYGEN:

Inadequate oxygenation is the most common cause of cardiac arrest in children!

SECTION D

PEDIATRIC ARRHYTHMIAS:
HOW CHILDREN ARE DIFFERENT

Children are not just little adults. Nowhere is this more evident than in the area of pediatric arrhythmia interpretation. Although terminology used to define pediatric and adult arrhythmias is similar, both the spectrum of arrhythmias encountered and the priorities for treatment differ significantly.

Basic concepts in arrhythmia interpretation were presented in Chapter 3. The purpose of this section is neither to duplicate that material, nor to attempt to make the reader an expert in pediatric electrocardiography. Instead, our goal is to discuss the more important and clinically relevant differences between pediatric and adult arrhythmias as they pertain to pediatric resuscitation.

Pediatric Norms

Pediatric norms for heart rate and interval (PR and QRS) duration differ markedly from those of adults. This becomes readily apparent on inspection of the rhythm strip shown in *Figure 17D-1* taken from a healthy infant.

Practically speaking, extensive knowledge of pediatric arrhythmias is *not* essential for successful management of cardiopulmonary resuscitation in children. This is because pediatric cardiopulmonary arrest will almost always be preceded by ventilatory insufficiency—leading to hypoxia, bradycardia, and asystole as the terminal event. Ventricular tachycardia, ventricular fibrillation, and the gamut of more complex arrhythmias encountered in emergency cardiac care of adults are distinctly uncommon in the resuscitation of previously healthy children.*

Principles for management of pediatric arrhythmias are also quite different than for adults. The majority of pediatric arrhythmias are supraventricular (Dick and Campbell, 1984). Most are surprisingly well tolerated, and many are the result of another underlying disorder (i.e., hypoxemia, acid-base disturbance, electrolyte disorder, shock, infection, etc.). *Optimal treatment of pediatric arrhythmias ideally consists of identification and correction of the underlying cause.* Pharmacologic therapy tends to be needed much less often than for adults.

*Although still decidedly less common than in adults, ventricular arrhythmias are more likely to be seen in children with underlying heart disease (i.e., cardiomyopathy, congenital heart disease) and/or following cardiac surgery.

PROBLEM   **In what ways is this tracing different from that of a normal adult?**

ANSWER TO FIGURE 17D-1   The rhythm is sinus at a rate of about 140 beats/min, the PR interval is 0.11 second, and the QRS is 0.05 second in duration. *All of these parameters are normal for an infant!*

> In contrast, in adults the heart rate for normal sinus rhythm varies between 60 and 99 beats/min, the PR interval is between 0.12 and 0.20 second, and the QRS complex is usually not so narrow.

Table 17D-1 demonstrates the pediatric norms for heart rate and interval duration. From this table it can be seen that heart rates of up to 180 beats/min are still normal for children during the first year of life. During this time, *mean* heart rate is between 120-140 beats/min. Heart rates below 90 beats/min constitute sinus *bradycardia* (although it is *not* uncommon for the heart rate of term and especially preterm infants to drop below 80 beats/min during sleep).

> It should be emphasized that the values shown in Table 17D-1 represent pediatric norms for heart rate in children who are *awake!* Heart rates often drop substantially during sleep—to as low as 60 beats/min for a 2-year-old, and as low as 40 beats/min for a 12-year-old (Garson, 1984).

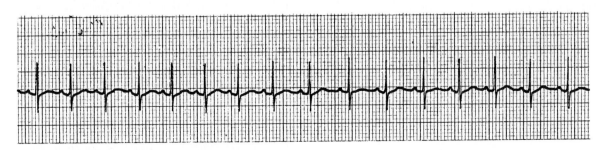

Figure 17D-1.   Rhythm strip obtained from a healthy infant.

Table 17D-1

Pediatric Norms			
Age	**Heart Rate** (beats/min)	**PR Interval** (sec)	**QRS Duration** (sec)
Newborn to 1 yr	90-180	0.07-0.16	0.03-0.08
1-3 yr	70-150	0.08-0.16	0.04-0.08
4-10 yr	60-130	0.09-0.17	0.04-0.09
>10 yr	60-110	0.09-0.20	0.04-0.09
Adapted from Garson A: *The electrocardiogram in infants and children: a systematic approach*, Philadelphia, 1983, Lea & Febiger.			

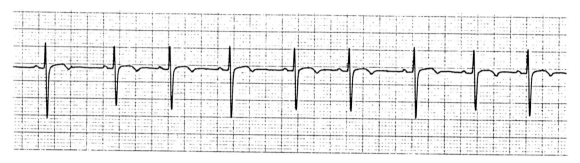

Figure 17D-2.   *Is this tracing abnormal for a 7-year-old child?*

Normal duration of the PR interval in infants and children is significantly less than for adults. Thus a PR interval of 0.08 second is perfectly normal for a 3-year-old, whereas it might suggest an accessory pathway (WPW) in an adult. By the same token, the upper limits of normal for the PR and QRS intervals in children are also less than for adults. Appreciation of this fact is important clinically, since values considered normal for adults are often prolonged for pediatric patients.

Reference to Table 17D-1 makes it evident that a PR interval of 0.18 second is abnormally long for a child under 10 years of age. Such prolongation would constitute 1° AV block in this age group. Similarly, a QRS duration of 0.10 second is also abnormal in a child this age and suggests some type of intraventricular conduction disturbance.

PROBLEM   **Interpret the arrhythmia shown in *Figure 17D-2*. Is this tracing abnormal for a 7-year-old child?**

ANSWER TO FIGURE 17D-2   Although the rhythm is irregular, each QRS complex is preceded by a P wave with a constant PR interval. This is *sinus arrhythmia*. Note the change in QRS amplitude from beat to beat that reflects the child's respiration.

SINUS ARRHYTHMIA

As discussed in Section A of Chapter 3, *sinus arrhythmia is an extremely common **normal** finding among older children and young*

adults. Its principal significance is that it not be confused with a disease state. Sinus arrhythmia is thought to be due to variations in autonomic tone and is often related to respiration. Heart rate tends to increase in a gradual manner with inspiration and decrease with exhalation. A repetitive pattern (group beating) is frequently seen (Figure 17D-2). The arrhythmia does not occur as often in younger children and infants, since respiratory variation in autonomic tone is likely to be much less pronounced in the younger age group.

One should be aware that slight irregularity is commonly present with normal sinus rhythm. A difference of *at least* 0.08 second should exist between the shortest and longest R-R intervals before one diagnoses sinus *arrhythmia*.

Escape Rhythms and AV Dissociation

The sinoatrial (SA) node is the principal pacemaker of the heart. Under usual circumstances, it suppresses all other cardiac tissue with its inherent automaticity. In an awake child with normal sinus rhythm, the SA node fires at a rate of between 60 and 180 beats/min depending on the age and activity of the child (Table 17D-1). If for any reason the principal pacemaker slows markedly or fails to fire at all, another *(subsidiary)* pacemaker will have to take over. The resulting rhythm is known as an *escape* rhythm.

Table 17D-2 shows the usual escape rates of subsidiary pacemakers in the atria, AV node, and ventricles for children and adults.

Table 17D-2

Usual Rates of Subsidiary Pacemakers		
Site of Escape Focus	Up to 3 Yrs (beats/min)	Over 3 Yrs & Adults (beats/min)
Atria	80-100	50-60
AV node	50-80	40-60
Ventricles	40-50	30-40

Adapted from Garson A: *The electrocardiogram in infants and children: a systematic approach*, Philadelphia, 1983, Lea & Febiger.

According to the table, were the sinus rate to slow down in a child less than 3 years of age, a subsidiary pacemaker in the atria should take over at a rate of between 80 to 100 beats/min. If this did not occur, one would then expect an escape rhythm to arise from the site that was "next in line" in the pacemaking hierarchy—the AV node. For a child under 3, the usual rate of a subsidiary pacemaker from this site is between 50 to 80 beats/min. The lowest escape focus—a site in the ventricles—is left as a final safeguard in the event no escape rhythm is forthcoming from either the atria or AV node. The rate of an idioventricular escape rhythm in a child under 3 is usually between 40 to 50 beats/min. As can be seen from the table, *the rate of subsidiary pacemakers for children after about 3 years of age is similar to that for adults.*

It is important to emphasize that escape rhythms are extremely common in otherwise healthy children and usually do not represent a disease state. This is particularly true for escape rhythms that occur during sleep, when variations in vagal tone frequently result in sinus slowing. In one study, 45% of healthy teenagers demonstrated sinus slowing and at least three consecutive beats of an AV nodal escape rhythm during Holter monitoring (Scott et al, 1980). In contrast, persistent AV nodal rhythm is distinctly uncommon in otherwise normal children during the waking hours.

Bundle Branch Blocks

As indicated in Table 17D-1, an intraventricular conduction disturbance may be present in a child despite the fact that the QRS complex is not "wide" by adult standards. *Right bundle branch block (RBBB)* is by far the most common type encountered. This conduction disturbance is usually seen in congenital heart disease, after surgical procedures (especially those involving the right ventricle), or associated with inflammatory diseases such as myocarditis or endocarditis.

Left bundle branch block (LBBB) is rare in children. Observation of a tachyarrhythmia with QRS morphology of an LBBB-type pattern should prompt the emergency care provider to consider ventricular tachycardia or WPW (with anterograde conduction down the accessory path-

way). In either case, immediate attention (and intervention) is mandatory.

AV Block

The atrioventricular (AV) node is under strong influence from the autonomic nervous system. Thus conduction through the AV node may be speeded up or slowed down by alterations in sympathetic or parasympathetic tone.

As discussed in Chapter 3, the PR interval encompasses the period from initial activation in the SA node until the time of ventricular activation. This includes travel of the depolarization impulse through the atria, AV node, and ventricular conduction system (bundle of His, bundle branches). Because the speed of conduction is by far slowest through the AV node (0.3 m/sec, compared to 1.5 m/sec through the atria and 2-4 m/sec through the His-Purkinje system), a major portion of the PR interval reflects travel through this structure. Disorders affecting the AV node are therefore the most common causes of PR interval prolongation.

FIRST-DEGREE AV BLOCK

The criteria for *1° AV block* are age related. For example, a PR interval of 0.17 second is prolonged for children under four and represents 1° AV block in this age group (Table 17D-1). Clinically, this conduction disturbance is encountered in patients with digitalis intoxication, atrial septal defect (due to alteration of normal atrial anatomy), Ebstein's anomaly, inflammatory cardiac disease (viral myocarditis, acute rheumatic fever, or Kawasaki's disease), cardiomyopathy, after surgery for congenital heart disease, or as a normal variant. There usually is no functional importance attached to this finding.

Because of autonomic influence on the AV node, children with high degrees of resting vagal tone (as is so frequently found in the athletically inclined male adolescent) not uncommonly demonstrate 1° AV block. The PR interval may even lengthen and shorten *spontaneously* in such individuals as a normal response to variations in autonomic tone during respiration.

SECOND-DEGREE AV BLOCK

The two types of 2° AV block are Mobitz type I and Mobitz type II. As in adults, *Mobitz type I (Wenckebach)* is by far the most common form.

Clinically, Mobitz I tends to occur with the same conditions that are associated with 1° AV block. Although it may be caused by disease states, normal individuals with increased resting vagal tone frequently manifest this disorder. *The significance of Mobitz I 2° AV block is most strongly related to the clinical setting in which it occurs.* It should therefore be interpreted as a benign normal variant when seen in otherwise healthy, athletically inclined adolescents. In contrast, development of Mobitz I in a patient with underlying cardiomyopathy must be viewed with much more concern.

Mobitz II 2° AV block is distinctly uncommon in children. Rarely, it may be seen postoperatively. Because of the high risk of abrupt cessation of intraventricular conduction, pacemaker therapy must be actively considered. Unfortunately, external pacing in children is problematic at the present time because of the lack of suitably sized external pacing electrodes and excessive skeletal muscle stimulation during pacing with the larger pads that are currently used.

THIRD-DEGREE (COMPLETE) AV BLOCK

Complete (3°) AV block in children may be either congenital or acquired. Either form is uncommon in this age group. However, when 3° AV block does occur in children, clinical manifestations and treatment will depend on the type.

The incidence of **congenital 3° AV block** is 1 per 20,000 live births (Roberts, 1983). It occurs in about 5% of all children born with congenital heart disease, and is surprisingly common in children born to mothers who have systemic lupus erythematosus. The disorder is thought to be due to abnormal development of the conduction system or intrauterine infection. Because the level of congenital 3° AV block is almost always at the AV node, the QRS complex is narrow and a junctional escape pacemaker (at a rate of between 50-80 beats/min) takes over the pacemaking function. An interesting phenomenon seen in children with congenital 3° AV block is that the ventricular response may increase appropriately with activity. Syncope is rare, especially in those individuals in whom the heart rate does not drop below 50 beats/min. In the absence of other significant cardiac abnormalities, stroke volume and cardiac output may increase as the child grows, allowing many individuals to remain relatively asymptomatic (Roberts, 1983).

> The prognosis of congenital 3° AV block appears to be related to the age of the child when the conduction defect is first discovered. Development of congestive heart failure with a significantly increased mortality is much more common in children for whom complete heart block is diagnosed at birth. In contrast, the outlook is much better if the diagnosis is made after the first year of life. Although still a matter of controversy, asymptomatic children (with no signs of heart failure) who demonstrate a narrow QRS complex escape rhythm and a resting heart rate of over 50 beats/min with an appropriate increase in rate in response to exercise may not need to be paced (Karpawich et al, 1981; Garson, 1983).
>
> On the other hand, pacing is usually needed for younger infants (especially neonates) because they generally require a faster heart rate to maintain their cardiac output. Unfortunately, as we have previously indicated, the problems associated with external pacing in children limit its applicability in this situation.

Acquired 3° AV block tends to occur at a lower level in the conduction system than does the congenital form of this disorder. As a result, the QRS complex is most often wide and the ventricular response slow (under 40 beats/min). Unlike congenital 3° AV block, the ventricular response in the acquired form does not increase with activity. Syncope is therefore common, and pacemaker insertion is usually essential.

> Although acquired 3° AV block may be due to infection, it much more commonly results from cardiac surgery. In a significant percentage of surgical patients, the conduction disturbance is transient and only temporary pacing is required. If the conduction defect persists beyond 10 days, however, it is likely that permanent pacing will be required.

Premature Atrial Contractions

Premature atrial contractions (PACs) are commonly found in otherwise normal children. This is especially true for *newborn* infants who almost uniformly demonstrate at least some PACs if monitored continuously. These premature beats are felt to reflect either increased atrial automaticity or AV nodal reentry from the relative immaturity of the AV node. Although usually of little clinical significance, PACs may predispose to development of supraventricular tachyarrhythmias (PSVT or atrial flutter) in certain infants.

Ten to 20% of older children demonstrate PACs. Although occasionally due to metabolic abnormalities (hypoglycemia, hypokalemia, hypocalcemia), hypoxemia, drugs (digitalis), or cardiac surgery, such PACs usually occur in otherwise healthy children and are most often benign. Unless symptoms are present, neither additional work-up nor treatment is indicated.

PROBLEM   **Interpret the rhythm shown in *Figure 17D-3*, taken from a young child. Are there multiple PACs?**

ANSWER TO FIGURE 17D-3   The rhythm illustrates the difficulty one may sometimes have in differentiating between sinus arrhythmia and sinus rhythm with frequent PACs. The rhythm in this figure is not regular. Although P wave morphology varies slightly from beat to beat, all of the P waves (with the notable exception of the P wave preceding beat #6) have a similar shape (upright and with a *small*, rounded deflection) and a constant PR interval. The underlying rhythm here is *sinus arrhythmia*. P waves *may* vary slightly in morphology with sinus rhythm or sinus arrhythmia as they do here. Beat #6 is a *PAC*.

> Practically speaking, it will rarely matter in an asymptomatic child whether an irregularity in a rhythm is due to sinus arrhythmia or sinus rhythm with PACs. Treatment will usually not be needed in either case.

Supraventricular Tachycardia

As discussed in Chapter 3, the term *supraventricular tachycardia* is a general one that encompasses all tachyarrhythmias in which the impulse originates at or above the AV

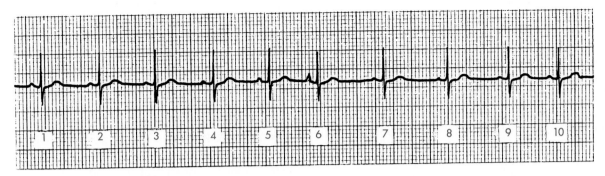

Figure 17D-3.   Rhythm strip obtained from a young child. *Are there multiple PACs?*

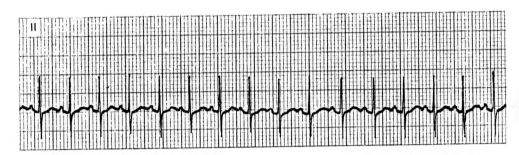

Figure 17D-4.   Rhythm strip obtained from a 4-year-old child. *What is the cause of the rapid rate?*

node. As is the case for adults, the types of supraventricular tachycardias in children are many and include:

  i. Sinus tachycardia
 ii. Junctional tachycardia
iii. Atrial fibrillation or flutter with a rapid ventricular response
 iv. Ectopic atrial tachycardia (EAT)
  v. Paroxysmal supraventricular tachycardia (PSVT)

PROBLEM   **The rhythm in *Figure 17D-4,* taken from a 4-year-old, is quite rapid. In which of the above categories does it fit?**

ANSWER TO FIGURE 17D-4   The rhythm is regular at a rate of about 170 beats/min. The QRS complex is narrow and consistently preceded by an upright P wave with a normal PR interval. This is *sinus tachycardia.* The example again illustrates the point that the upper limit for sinus tachycardia in infants and children may be substantially higher than it is for adults.

SINUS TACHYCARDIA

We have previously defined the lower limits for sinus tachycardia in Table 17D-1, in which we gave the usual expected range for heart rate at various ages. Sinus tachy-

cardia should not exceed 200 beats/min in children over 1 year of age; however, rates of up to 260 beats/min have been observed on rare instances (i.e., with severely ill children with sepsis) in infants (Garson, 1983).

As in adults, the key to sinus tachycardia is to determine (and correct) the underlying cause. When due to illness, serial changes in heart rate may reflect the status of the patient's clinical condition. That is, further acceleration of the rate is often associated with worsening of the condition, while slowing of the rate toward normal suggests improvement.

JUNCTIONAL (AV NODAL) TACHYCARDIA

The term junctional "tachycardia" is somewhat of an anomaly, since heart rate with this rhythm does *not* exceed the normal maximum sinus rate for age. It would therefore be better to describe these arrhythmias as *accelerated junctional (AV nodal) rhythms.*

Table 17D-2 defines the usual rates of subsidiary pacemakers for children under and over 3 years of age. Thus for an AV nodal rhythm in a 2-year-old to be "accelerated," the rate would have to be greater than 80 beats/min. Since these arrhythmias (by definition) do not exceed the normal maximum rate for sinus rhythm at the child's particular age, this means that the heart rate range for this 2-year-old with accelerated AV nodal rhythm is between 70-150 beats/min (Table 17D-1). Similarly, the heart rate range for an accelerated AV nodal rhythm in a 5-year-old would be between 60-130 beats/min.

Morphologically, the rhythm is regular in accelerated AV nodal rhythms, and the QRS complex is narrow and similar to the QRS of sinus-conducted beats (unless aberrant conduction is present). Atrial activity is abnormal and reflects the junctional origin of the arrhythmia. Thus, P waves may be inverted (either preceding the QRS with a short PR interval or retrograde), absent (if retrograde P waves occur at the same time as the QRS), or entirely dissociated from the QRS (AV dissociation by *usurpation*— see Section B in Chapter 16).

> Clinically, *accelerated* AV nodal rhythms are not usually seen in normal children. They most commonly occur in the immediate postoperative period after surgery for congenital heart disease, but may also be seen with rheumatic fever, myocarditis, or digitalis toxicity. Treatment is of the underlying condition.

ATRIAL FIBRILLATION

Atrial fibrillation is rare in infants and young children. The rate of the fibrillating atria may be exceedingly rapid (between 400-700 beats/min), with an accompanying ventricular response of between 120-200 beats/min.

> When atrial fibrillation does occur in the pediatric age group, it is frequently associated with either structurally abnormal heart disease or WPW. This has important clinical implications, since treatment of WPW with either digoxin or verapamil may result in further acceleration of conduction down the accessory pathway with disastrous consequences (Vetter, 1985; McGovern et al, 1986). In contrast, in the absence of WPW, digoxin is the drug of choice for treatment of chronic atrial fibrillation.

ATRIAL FLUTTER

Although it occurs more frequently than atrial fibrillation, *atrial flutter* is still quite uncommon in the pediatric age group. This tachyarrhythmia differs in several ways from its usual appearance in adults.

PROBLEM   **Typical morphologic characteristics of atrial flutter in the pediatric age group are illustrated by the rhythm shown in *Figure 17D-5*. How does this differ from atrial flutter in adults?**

ANSWER TO FIGURE 17D-5   Although the typical sawtooth pattern of atrial flutter is easily recognized in Fig. 17D-5, the atrial rate clearly exceeds 300 beats/min (as the R-R interval of each flutter wave is definitely *less* than one large box). Moreover, the ventricular response (albeit controlled) is irregular.

Atrial flutter in children is distinguished by:
   i. A faster atrial rate
  ii. The frequent occurrence of variable ventricular conduction
 iii. Periods of 1:1 conduction

> While the atrial rate of flutter in children is often around 300 beats/min (as it is in adults), it may be much faster. Rates of up to 450 beats/min have been recorded (Garson, 1984). *It is because of this variability in the atrial rate that atrial flutter in children should be diagnosed by its morphology (sawtooth pattern) and not by its rate.*
>
> Although 2:1 atrioventricular conduction may be seen in children, more commonly the ventricular response is variable (irregular). The point to appreciate is that the ventricular response to atrial flutter may at times be extremely rapid, and periods of 1:1 conduction may occur.

Atrial flutter in children tends to occur in three clinical settings (Garson, 1983):
   i. In hydropic newborns who have had intrauterine tachyarrhythmias
  ii. In otherwise normal infants less than 6 months of age (especially when frequent PACs were observed during the neonatal period)
 iii. In children over 1 year of age who have underlying heart disease (cardiomyopathy, congenital heart disease)

The arrhythmia is *not* benign (due to the very rapid ventricular rates that may occur), and it should be treated. Acute therapy entails medications (such as digoxin or verapamil), overdrive pacing, or synchronized cardioversion.

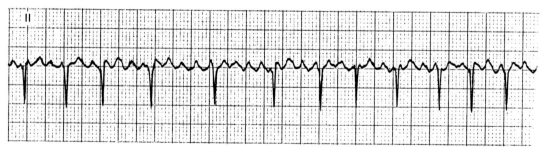

Figure 17D-5.   Example of atrial flutter in a child. *How does this differ from the usual appearance of atrial flutter in adults?*

In discussing the remaining supraventricular tachycardias, two principal mechanisms should be considered: *increased automaticity* and *reentry*. Determining which of these mechanisms is operative is instrumental in understanding the behavior of a particular arrhythmia and in predicting its response to therapy.

ECTOPIC ATRIAL TACHYCARDIA (EAT)

The mechanism of *ectopic atrial tachycardia (EAT)* is increased automaticity. An ectopic atrial focus begins to fire on its own and overtakes control of the pacemaking function (from the SA node) as it gradually speeds up its rate of discharge. Electrocardiographically, abnormal P waves (different in morphology from the sinus-conducted P waves) precede each QRS complex. A "warm-up" phase to the tachycardia may be seen, reflecting the fact that the automatic focus gradually accelerated its rates of discharge *(Figure 17D-6)*. Vagal maneuvers may or may not temporarily slow the tachycardia, but they do not terminate it since the AV node is not involved in perpetuation of the rhythm.

PAROXYSMAL SUPRAVENTRICULAR TACHYCARDIA (PSVT)

In contrast, the mechanism of *PSVT* is reentry. When this mechanism is operative, the impulse is caught in a perpetual cycle in which it continuously circulates within a reentry circuit (Figure 17D-6).

> The site of reentry for PSVT is most commonly the AV node. Occasionally, however, reentry may occur elsewhere (in the SA node, the atria, or through an accessory pathway).

As implied in its name, PSVT most often begins abruptly (—it is "paroxysmal"). It frequently is initiated by a PAC that sets up the cycle of continuous circulation within the reentry circuit. P waves are usually not seen during the tachycardia, although occasionally they may deform the terminal portion of the QRS complex.

Because the AV node is intimately involved with perpetuation of the tachycardia, vagal maneuvers (by slowing conduction through the AV node) may be successful in terminating the arrhythmia. Similarly, a fortuitously timed premature impulse (PAC, PJC, or PVC) may momentarily alter conduction properties of the AV node and also terminate the arrhythmia. This is in contrast to the case with EAT in which the automaticity of the ectopic focus is unaffected by premature beats.

PSVT terminates as abruptly as it begins. Once the reentry circuit is interrupted, the cycle is broken and the SA node may resume its normal function. This differs from the situation with EAT, which resolves by gradual deceleration ("cool-down") of the ectopic pacemaker.

> Catching the onset and termination of the tachycardia often provides a golden opportunity for electrocardiographic differentiation between PSVT and EAT. The former condition is typically initiated by a PAC with a different morphology (that occurs at a critical moment in the cardiac cycle, allowing the conditions of reentry to become established). PSVT terminates as abruptly as it begins (which may be evidenced on the ECG by a PAC or PVC after which the tachycardia stops).

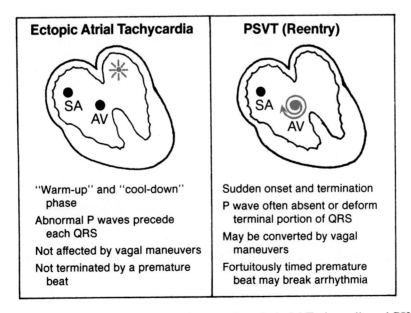

Figure 17D-6.   Clinical comparison between Ectopic Atrial Tachycardia and PSVT.

In contrast, EAT is not initiated by a PAC. Instead there is usually a gradual "warm-up" (acceleration) of the tachycardia in which P wave morphology at the onset is identical to P wave morphology throughout the tachycardia. Termination of the tachycardia is not abrupt either, but rather is most often marked a gradual "cool-down" until resumption of normal sinus rhythm (noted by a change in P wave morphology back to that of the normal sinus-conducted beats).

PROBLEM Examine *Figure 17D-7*, taken from a previously well child who *suddenly* developed palpitations. What is the likely mechanism of this arrhythmia?

ANSWER TO FIGURE 17D-7 The rhythm is regular at a rate of 195 beats/min. The QRS complex is narrow, and no P waves are evident. The differential includes:

    i. Sinus tachycardia
    ii. Atrial flutter
    iii. EAT
    iv. PSVT

Although the rate seen here is more rapid than one usually expects for sinus tachycardia, one cannot absolutely rule out this possibility, since rates of up to 220 beats/min have been recorded in children. However, this diagnosis is unlikely because there is no evidence of atrial activity and the child was perfectly well until the sudden onset of this arrhythmia. *Children with rapid sinus tachycardia are almost always ill from some other cause!*

In adults, the diagnosis of atrial flutter must be included in the differential of regular supraventricular tachycardias when the ventricular response is about 150 beats/min. Because the atrial rate of flutter is often *greater* than 300 beats/min in children (up to 450 beats/min), this rule of thumb does not apply. However, an *irregular* ventricular response is most commonly seen with atrial flutter in children. In this tracing the rhythm is regular without even the slightest hint of atrial activity. It is therefore unlikely that the rhythm represents atrial flutter.

This leaves us with differentiating between ectopic atrial tachycardia (EAT) and PSVT. As we have noted, the

onset of the rhythm with EAT is often gradual, and ectopic (abnormal) P waves are usually clearly visible on the ECG. In contrast, PSVT tends to have a much more abrupt onset, and P waves are either not evident or they deform the terminal portion of the QRS complex. *PSVT is therefore the most likely diagnosis of the arrhythmia.*

PSVT is a much more common cause of an *acute* tachycardia than EAT. This is fortunate because PSVT is usually much easier to treat. All one has to do is interrupt the reentry circuit (even momentarily), and the arrhythmia is terminated. Measures that may be effective include vagal maneuvers, digoxin, verapamil, propranolol, and adenosine.*

EAT, on the other hand, is a "chronic" arrhythmia that is often resistant to therapy. Although medications may slow the arrhythmia, they usually will not terminate it. Moreover, episodes of ectopic atrial tachycardia tend to be prolonged and frequently recur. As a result, EAT has been called an "incessant" tachycardia (defined as the presence of the arrhythmia *more than 10% of the time* during any 24-hour period). Whereas the long-term outlook for patients with this arrhythmia had been bleak in the past, promising results are now being obtained by definitive therapy with cryoablation and/or surgical excision of the ectopic focus. Considering the disappointing response of EAT to medical therapy, and that chronicity of this arrhythmia with persistent tachycardia may lead to development of congestive cardiomyopathy and heart failure, enthusiasm for definitive means of treatment is likely to continue (Gillette et al, 1985; Gillette, 1989).

Although PSVT is usually well tolerated by otherwise healthy adults, it is important to appreciate that this arrhythmia is often *not* so benign when it occurs in infants or small children. If allowed to persist, infants in particular face a great risk of developing congestive heart failure. The younger the infant, the higher the ventricular rate (espe-

---

*Although *verapamil* has been a drug of choice for treatment of PSVT in adults, the drug should be used with extreme caution in younger children, especially if they are acutely ill (Shahar et al, 1981; Porter et al, 1983). Excessive heart rate slowing, decreased contractility, and profound hypotension (from vasodilatation and negative inotropy) can occur with potentially disastrous consequences in such patients (Gillette, 1989).

Recently, enthusiasm has grown for the use of *adenosine* as treatment of PSVT in pediatric patients. The drug is extremely effective and appears much less likely to produce adverse hemodynamic effects in infants or young children than verapamil. Even if adverse effects do occur, the exceedingly short half-life of adenosine tends to limit their duration (Reyes et al, 1992).

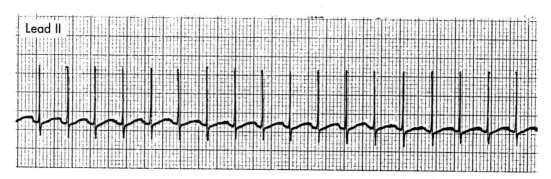

Figure 17D-7. Rhythm strip from a child with new-onset palpitations. *What is the likely mechanism of the arrhythmia?*

cially if over 180 beats/min), and the longer the duration of the tachycardia (especially if for more than 24 hours), the more likely and the sooner congestive heart failure will develop (Mehta et al, 1983; Gillette, 1989). If the infant doesn't readily respond to conservative measures (vagal maneuvers such as application of an ice pack to the face for about 15 seconds) or pharmacologic therapy (adenosine, digoxin)—and/or hemodynamic compromise develops, emergency cardioversion may be needed.

> In the newborn, PSVT (with rates of up to 300 beats/min!) is sometimes recognized only after a child becomes listless and stops feeding. The diagnosis is easy to overlook since normal heart rates in children this age are rapid (and increase even more if crying occurs during an examination). *Suspect PSVT if the tachycardia persists when the infant is asleep or at rest.* Develop the habit of routinely *counting* the heart rate on physical examination of infants and young children.

TACHYCARDIAS ASSOCIATED WITH ACCESSORY PATHWAYS

The full-blown syndrome of WPW (delta wave, short PR interval, and prolonged duration of the QRS) is relatively rare in children, with a reported incidence of only 0.15% (Garson, 1984). About two thirds of these individuals have no evidence of underlying cardiac abnormality, while congenital heart disease (especially Ebstein's anomaly or tricuspid atresia) is present in the remainder.

Electrocardiographically, WPW is diagnosed in children in the same manner as for adults, with the exception that the PR interval and the QRS complex may be shorter in duration and the delta wave may be less obvious.

> Despite the fact that outright ECG evidence of an accessory pathway is so uncommon, *concealed* accessory pathways exist in a significant percentage of children. The reason delta waves are not seen on the ECG of such individuals is that conduction is preferentially channeled down the normal pathway (through

the AV node, the His, and the bundle branches—*Panel A of Figure 17D-8*). However, the accessory pathway (AP) participates with the AV node in forming a reentry circuit.

With PSVT, the QRS complex during the tachycardia usually remains narrow (and the accessory pathway remains *concealed*) since conduction is in an *antegrade* direction (i.e., down the normal pathway, and back up the AP—*Panel B of Figure 17D-8*).

The clinical significance of concealed accessory pathways lies with their potential to conduct in the opposite direction (antegrade down the AP, and back up the normal pathway—*Panel C of Figure 17D-8*). In this case the QRS complex would be *wide* during the tachycardia. While antegrade conduction is rare with PSVT, it is not at all uncommon in the presence of atrial fibrillation or atrial flutter. Unknowingly administering digoxin or verapamil in such cases may further accelerate antegrade conduction down the accessory pathway and precipitate ventricular fibrillation!

Great strides have been made in the surgical treatment of patients with WPW. Intraoperative electrophysiologic studies as are currently performed in specialized centers are able to localize and interrupt the accessory pathway (whether manifest or concealed) in up to 95% of cases in children who are 3 months of age or older (Gillette, 1989). The decided advantage of surgical intervention over medical treatment is that the patient can be *cured* instead of being subjected to the lifelong need of taking antiarrhythmic medication with its associated cost, risk of adverse effects, and less than optimal success rate.

Ventricular Arrhythmias

As is the case for adults, the significance of PVCs in children is most strongly related to the clinical setting in which it occurs. Although occasional PVCs are commonly seen in children, frequent and complex ventricular ectopy is distinctly unusual in the absence of underlying heart disease. *Asymptomatic occurrence of isolated PVCs in otherwise healthy children is almost always benign!*

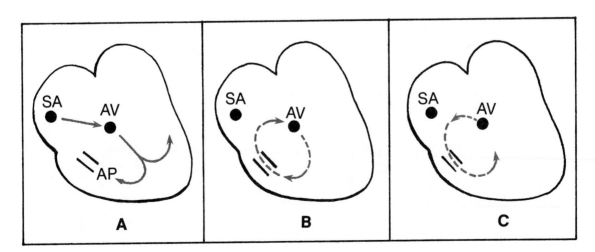

Figure 17D-8. Conduction possibilities in the presence of an accessory pathway *(AP)*. *See text.*

Because of the generally benign nature of PVCs in the pediatric age group, treatment is rarely (if ever) indicated in the absence of symptoms—even when ventricular ectopy is frequent!

ECG DIAGNOSIS OF PVCS IN CHILDREN

ECG diagnosis of ventricular arrhythmias in children differs from diagnosis of such arrhythmias in adults in a number of interesting ways.

PROBLEM   **Examine the rhythm shown in** *Figure 17D-9,* **taken from an acutely ill 2-year-old child. Is the sixth complex wide enough to be a PVC?**

ANSWER TO FIGURE 17D-9   The underlying rhythm is sinus tachycardia at a rate of 200 beats/min. The sixth complex differs markedly from all of the other beats in this rhythm strip, and it is not preceded by a P wave. Yet at most, it is "only" 0.09 second in duration! *Can it be a PVC?*

Before answering this question, it may be helpful to once again return to Table 17D-1 presented at the beginning of this chapter. Note that the normal QRS duration for a 2-year-old is between 0.04 and 0.08 second. Thus, the sixth complex in Fig. 17D-9 *is* wide, considering the child's age. This beat is a PVC.

> From this example one can easily imagine how ventricular tachycardia in a child might be mistaken by an adult-oriented emergency care provider as a supraventricular tachycardia. *Wide* is a relative term. It is important to remember that 0.09-0.10 second represents definite QRS widening in children. (Garson has reported a case of ventricular tachycardia in a 2-day-old in which the QRS complex of the tachyarrhythmia was *only* 0.05 second!!!)

DIFFERENTIATION BETWEEN PVCS AND ABERRANCY

One of the most difficult problems in arrhythmia recognition in adults is differentiating between PVCs and supraventricular premature beats that conduct aberrantly.

Features useful in this differentiation were detailed in Section A of Chapter 15. They include:

   i. Morphological clues (especially a RBBB pattern in a right-sided monitoring lead)
  ii. Similar initial deflection to the normal beats
 iii. Recognition of a *premature* P wave
 iv. Width of the QRS complex
  v. Presence of a full compensatory pause
 vi. Rate of the tachycardia
vii. Presence of AV dissociation

Virtually all bets are off in children!!!!

As noted above, QRS duration is of little assistance since premature complexes as narrow as 0.09 second (or less) may be "wide" in certain age groups. QRS morphology is simply too variable in children for one to place any stock in morphological clues such as a RBBB pattern or a similar initial deflection. Compensatory pauses are meaningless, because a majority of children demonstrate retrograde conduction (which resets the sinus cycle) and the ubiquity of sinus arrhythmia makes it impossible to know which cycle to count. Finally, the rate of a tachycardia is of little assistance, since ventricular tachycardia as fast as 428 beats/min has been recorded in children!

In reality, aberrant conduction is relatively uncommon in children (Garson, 1983). This helps simplify the problem. If a premature complex is wide (considering the age of the child) and no *premature* P wave can be clearly identified, one must work on the assumption that the beat is a PVC.

As an extension to these tenets, consider the case of the *regular wide complex tachycardia.* In adults, the differential for this type of tachyarrhythmia includes:

   i. Supraventricular tachycardia with aberrant conduction
  ii. Supraventricular tachycardia with preexisting bundle branch block
 iii. Ventricular tachycardia

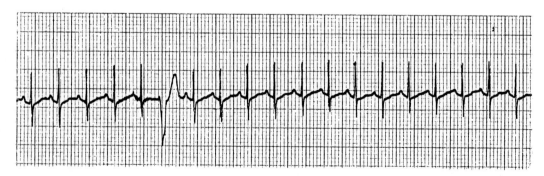

Figure 17D-9.   Rhythm strip obtained from a 2-year-old. *Is the sixth complex wide enough to be a PVC?*

For all practical purposes, this differential can be narrowed even further in children. Intraventricular conduction defects are uncommon in pediatrics (except in the postoperative period or in children with congenital heart disease). Since aberrant conduction is also uncommon, this means that *regular, wide complex tachyarrhythmias in children will most often be due to ventricular tachycardia* (especially if a narrow QRS was present during normal sinus rhythm)!

> At times it may be invaluable to have access to previous rhythm strips on a particular patient to see if the QRS complex had previously been wide during sinus rhythm, or to study the morphology of beats that could clearly be identified as PVCs. In the absence of such evidence, one should suspect that wide tachycardias are ventricular in origin.
>
> Ventricular tachycardia does *not* always produce symptoms in children. As was the case for PVCs, *the significance of ventricular tachycardia also depends on the clinical setting in which it occurs.* Thus, although children with idiopathic ventricular tachycardia should be referred for appropriate evaluation, treatment of otherwise healthy children will not be necessarily needed in the absence of symptoms.
>
> In contrast, ventricular tachycardia is more likely to be seen in children with an underlying cardiac disorder (i.e., congenital heart disease, following cardiac surgery, cardiomyopathy, prolonged QT syndrome, cardiac tumor, digitalis toxicity, etc.). Such individuals are more likely to be symptomatic (with compromised hemodynamics), and treatment is often indicated (Hakim, 1988).

Overall Perspective of Arrhythmias Encountered in Pediatric Resuscitation

Even though we have greatly simplified our discussion of arrhythmia recognition in children, *we have delved into much greater detail than is necessary for managing the overwhelming majority of cardiac arrests in children.* Some general concepts bear repeating:

i. The pediatric heart responds to hypoxemia by slowing its rate. As a result, *bradycardia and asystole are far and away the most common arrhythmias associated with cardiopulmonary arrest in children.*

Except in children with underlying organic heart disease (i.e., cardiomyopathy, congenital heart disease), *asystole* is almost always a *secondary* manifestation of hypoxemia that develops in response to the inciting event (i.e., drowning, trauma, sepsis, shock, etc.).

i. Because hypoxemia is by far the most common precipitating event in pediatric arrest, improving oxygenation (*not* administering drugs) is the most important therapeutic intervention.

Definitive therapy of cardiopulmonary arrest in children often depends on correcting the underlying cause of hypoxemia (i.e., sepsis, hypovolemic shock from dehydration or traumatic blood loss, etc.).

iii. Ventricular tachycardia and fibrillation are extremely uncommon terminal events in pediatric arrests. When they do occur, they almost always follow a prolonged period of hypoxemia from a preceding *respiratory* arrest.

iv. Practically speaking, most tachyarrhythmias in children will be *supraventricular.* Despite the fact that heart rates may be extremely rapid (150-200 beats/min, or more), these tachyarrhythmias are often surprisingly well tolerated, especially in older children who are otherwise healthy. Conservative treatment is often best. Rarely is there a need for immediate intervention, and there almost always will be time to consult with an expert (if needed) regarding optimal therapy for the tachyarrhythmia.

BONUS TRACING

Our goal in this chapter has been to emphasize that with cardiac arrhythmias, *children are different.* Lest there be no doubt about this statement, we conclude with this *bonus* (= *stumper*) *tracing.* (At the discretion of your Course Director, *exemption from having to take the arrhythmia quiz portion of the ACLS Course might be granted to anyone able to explain the findings on this tracing.*)

PROBLEM **What is going on in *Figure 17D-10?***

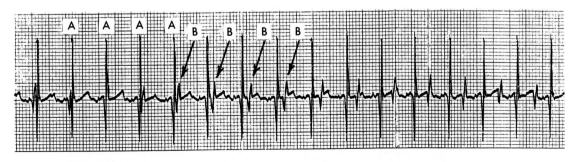

Figure 17D-10. BONUS TRACING: *Can you explain the findings on this tracing?*
(Tracing submitted by Dr. Jim Nimocks—recorded at the Children's Hospital National Medical Center in Washington, DC in 1976.)

ANSWER TO FIGURE 17D-10   At first glance there appears to be one regular complex that occurs throughout the tracing *(Complex A)*. On closer inspection, however, a smaller complex is also seen *(arrows pointing to Complex B)*. Atrial activity is present, although admittedly hard to interpret. Actually, the deflections labeled *A* and *B* are *each* QRS complexes—and the reason they are different and dissociated from each other (as well as each having their own related atrial activity), is that the tracing was taken from *conjoined twins* who were still attached at the time of the recording!

References

American Heart Association Subcommittee on Emergency Cardiac Care: Standards and guidelines for cardiopulmonary resuscitation (CPR) and emergency cardiac care (ECC), *JAMA* 255:2954, 1986.

Brown CG, Kelen GD: High-dose epinephrine in pediatric cardiac arrest, *Ann Emerg Med* 20:104, 1991.

Cavallaro D, Melker R: Comparison of two techniques for determining cardiac activity in infants, *Crit Care Med* 11:189, 1983.

Crespo SG, Schoffstall JM, Fuhs LR, Spivey WH: Comparison of two doses of endotracheal epinephrine in a cardiac arrest model, *Ann Emerg Med* 20:230, 1991.

David R: Closed chest cardiac massage in the newborn infant, *Pediatrics* 81:552, 1988.

Dick M, Campbell RM: Advances in the management of cardiac arrhythmias in children, *Pediatr Clin North Am* 31:1175, 1984.

Eisenberg M, Bergner L, Hallstrom A: Epidemiology of cardiac arrest and resuscitation in children, *Ann Emerg Med* 12:672, 1983.

Fiser DH: Intraosseous infusion, *N Engl J Med* 322:1579, 1990.

Garson A: *The electrocardiogram in infants and children: a systematic approach*, Philadelphia, 1983, Lea & Febiger.

Garson A: Arrhythmias in pediatric patients, *Med Clin North Am* 68:1171, 1984.

Gillette PC, Smith RT, Garson A, Mullins CE, Gutgesell HP, Goh TH, Cooley DA, McNamara DG: Chronic supraventricular tachycardia: a curable cause of congestive cardiomyopathy, *JAMA* 253:391, 1985.

Gillette PC: Advances in treatment of supraventricular tachydysrhythmias in children, *Mod Conc Cardiovasc Dis* 58:37, 1989.

Gillis J, Dickson D, Rieder M, Steward D, Edmonds J: Results of in-patient pediatric resuscitation, *Crit Care Med* 14:469, 1986.

Goetting MG, Paradis NA: High-dose epinephrine improves outcome from pediatric cardiac arrest, *Ann Emerg Med* 20:22, 1991.

Hakim SN: *Cardiac disease in children*. In Rosen P, (ed): *Emergency medicine: concepts and clinical practice*, St Louis, 1988, Mosby–Year Book.

Hoelzer MF: *Recent advances in intravenous therapy*. In Kobernick MS, Burney RE (eds): *Emergency medicine clinics of North America*, Philadelphia, 1986, WB Saunders.

Kanter RK, Zimmerman JJ, Strauss RH, Stoeckel KA: Pediatric emergency intravenous access: evaluation of a protocol, *Am J Dis Child* 140:132, 1986.

Karpawich PP, Gillette PC, Garson AJ, Hesslein PS, Porter CB, McNamara DG: Congenital complete atrioventricular block: clinical and electrophysiologic predictors of need for pacemaker insertion, *Am J Cardiol* 48:1098, 1981.

McGovern B, Garan H, Ruskin JN: Precipitation of cardiac arrest by verapamil in patients with Wolff-Parkinson-White syndrome, *Ann Med Intern* 104:791, 794, 1986.

Medical Letter: H Influenzae vaccine for infants, *Med Letter* 33:5, 1991.

Mehta AV, Casta A, Wolff GS: *Supraventricular tachycardia*. In Roberts NK, Gelband H (eds): *Cardiac arrhythmias in the neonate, infant and child*, Norwalk, Conn, 1983, Appleton-Century-Crofts.

Melker R: *CPR in neonates, infants, and children*. In Auerbach PS, Budassi SA (eds): *Cardiac arrest and CPR*, Rockville, Md, 1983, Aspen.

Orlowski JP: Optimum position for external cardiac compression in infants and young children, *Ann Emerg Med* 15:667, 1986.

Porter C, Garson A, Gillette PC: Verapamil: an effective calcium blocking agent for pediatric patients, *Pediatrics* 71:748, 1983.

Reyes G, Stanton R, Galvis AG: Adenosine in the treatment of paroxysmal supraventricular tachycardia in children, *Ann Emerg Med* 21:1499-1501, 1992.

Roberts NK: *Atrioventricular conduction: disorders of atrioventricular conduction and intraventricular conduction*. In Roberts NK, Gelband H, (eds): *Cardiac arrhythmias in the neonate, infant and child*, Norwalk, Conn, 1983, Appleton-Century-Crofts.

Scott O, Williams GJ, Fiddler GI: Results of 24 hour ambulatory monitoring of electrocardiogram in 131 healthy boys aged 10 to 13 years, *Br Heart J* 44:304, 1980.

Seidel JS, Inkelis SH: *Pediatric resuscitation*. In Harwood AL, (ed): *Cardiopulmonary resuscitation*, Baltimore, 1982, Williams & Wilkins.

Seigler RS, Tecklenburg FW, Shealy R: Prehospital intraosseous infusion by emergency medical services personnel: a prospective study, *Pediatrics* 84:173, 1989.

Shahar E, Barzilay Z, Frand M: Verapamil in the treatment of paroxysmal supraventricular tachycardia in infants and children, *J Pediatr* 98:323, 1981.

Spivey WH, Crespo SG, Fuhs LR, Schoffstall JM: Plasma catecholamine levels after intraosseous epinephrine administration in a cardiac arrest model, *Ann Emerg Med* 21:127, 1992.

Spivey WH, Lathers CM, Malone DR, Unger HD, Bhat S, McNamara RN, Schoffstall J, Tumer N: Comparison of intraosseous, central, and peripheral routes of sodium bicarbonate administration during CPR in pigs, *Ann Emerg Med* 14:1135, 1985.

Vetter VL: Management of arrhythmias in children: unusual features, *Cardiovasc Clin* 16:329, 1985.

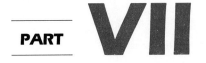

PART **VII**

Medicolegal Aspects

CHAPTER 18

MEDICOLEGAL ASPECTS OF ACLS

Ken Grauer, MD
Arlene Marrin, RN
Marvin Dewar, MD, JD
Ray Moseley, Ph.D.

SECTION A

INTRODUCTION & GENERAL CONCEPTS

Advances in medical care over the past 25 years have complicated and prolonged the dying process. As many as 80% of deaths now occur in hospitals or other long-term health care facilities (President's Commission, 1983). Sophisticated medical technology (ventilators, dialysis machines, organ transplantation, etc.) is often called on to preserve vital function, even for patients whose quality of life is extremely poor. Life support measures may be continued for extended periods of time so that *death is no longer thought of as the final event in the medical process. Instead, death has become a process in itself.* As a result, the focus of much medical decision-making has shifted from whether patients *can* be kept alive to whether they *should* be kept alive. Should patients always receive intensive medical treatment for their primary disease process? Should potentially life-threatening complications be treated if they occur? Should one implement/continue mechanical life support measures? Should CPR be performed? *And how should these decisions be made?*

Two principal factors account for much of the change in our approach to the dying process (Davenport, 1989):

i. *Increased demand by patients and family members for a more active role in making medical care decisions.* Open to question is whether continued intensive medical treatment is really in the best interest of patients who have little or no realistic chance to regain a meaningful quality of life.

ii. *Ever increasing concern about malpractice litigation.* Despite lack of case law to substantiate the common fear of liability for withholding or withdrawing life support measures, many clinicians have become unwilling to proceed with such measures under any circumstances, and especially when disagreement in any form arises between the expressed desires of the patient, the family, and the health care team.

Other issues regarding the principle of self-determination have received increasing attention. Representatives for the incompetent (including deformed newborns and the mentally retarded) want to assure that these individuals are guaranteed rights similar to those of competent individuals. All the while government and the media are demanding cost containment. Because the legal system continues to lag behind medical technology, physicians, nurses, paramedics, and other health care providers often find themselves in a precarious situation. Despite a number of landmark cases, the courts still cannot agree completely on what their role should be in terminating or continuing life support measures. Thus, health care providers face the ethical and legal dilemma of having to make life and death decisions on a daily basis without clearly defined legal standards to support their actions.

An example of how legal changes have not kept up with medical advances is the *double indemnity* clause (Grey, 1986). Life insurance companies sometimes pay double the amount of a policy for accidental death in which the insured party dies within 120 days of the date of the accident. At the time this rule was made, it seemed logical since the victim of a lethal accident could not possibly survive this long. *Times have changed.* With modern advanced life support techniques, some patients have been kept alive for months (and even years) following an accident despite remaining in a vegetative state with little chance for meaningful recovery. Should such irreversibly brain damaged patients be kept alive? Should the family be apprised that if life support measures are not withdrawn, the 120-day clause may expire and significant compensation may be lost? More important, should legal technicalities enter into already difficult ethical questions on what constitutes appropriate medical therapy?

Medicolegal Liability

Let us first examine the concept of medicolegal liability as it applies to health care practitioners. To do this, one should appreciate the meaning and implications of the terms criminal and case law. *Criminal law* is the body of law that prohibits conduct harmful to society as a whole. This includes acts of homicide and suicide (Anderson, 1982). In 1973, the AMA passed a resolution stating that "intentional termination of the life of one human being by another (mercy killing) is contrary to that for which the medical profession stands, and is contrary to the policy of the American Medical Association" (Stevens, 1986). Thus commission of active *euthanasia* by health care professionals is a crime.

Assisting suicide is also considered a homicide crime in many states. In June, 1990, intense controversy and legal inquiry surrounded Dr. Jack Kevorkian and the use of his "suicide machine." Dr. Kevorkian had assisted in the suicide of an Oregon woman, Janet Akins, who had been diagnosed with Alzheimer's disease and wanted to die. With the use of Dr. Kevorkian's device, Mrs. Akins ended her life in the state of Michigan where it is not a crime to commit suicide or assist in this act. Nevertheless, the AMA remained firm in its position that a physician should not intentionally cause death.

While criminal law prohibits conduct harmful to society, *civil law* prohibits conduct harmful to individuals. The broad category of medical malpractice is included in civil law. When a health care professional fails to exercise "reasonable" care and causes an injury, it is said that a *tort* has been committed. In order for **medical negligence** to be successfully prosecuted as an act of **malpractice,** *four* conditions must be satisfied:

   i. A relationship must have been established between the patient and the health care provider.
   ii. Negligence on the part of the health care provider must have occurred.
   iii. The patient must have suffered an injury.
   iv. A *cause-and-effect* relationship between the negligent act and the injury that resulted *must be proved*.

First there must be a duty to care (i.e., establishment of a practitioner-patient relationship). This is usually determined by mutual consent between the parties at the time of first meeting. The courts consider such relationships *contractual* and binding. Equally binding is the practitioner-patient relationship between an unresponsive patient who is brought to an emergency facility and the health care provider. Here the contract is *implied* since the courts assume the patient would request treatment were he/she able to do so. In contrast, if an emergency care provider who is off duty passes the scene of an accident, no medicolegal obligation exists for the practitioner to stop and render assistance. However, a strong moral and ethical obligation to stop and help is still present.

Once a practitioner-physician relationship has been established, it must either be seen through to its conclusion or properly terminated. Failure to do so is considered *abandonment*. For a physician in an ambulatory practice, proper termination of a doctor-patient relationship usually entails informing the patient *in writing* of these intentions, continuing to care for acute needs of the patient for a reasonable period of time, and advising the patient to obtain another source of health care. For the Good Samaritan who decides to help at the scene of an accident, once he/she begins to render care, a medicolegal obligation is formed to continue treatment to the best of one's ability until another capable health care professional arrives on the scene to take over.

A key word in the above description of the ingredients for a malpractice claim is "reasonable." For negligence to be proven, it must be shown that *reasonable* care was not exercised by the health care provider. Reasonable is defined legally as using "ordinary skill and diligence (to) apply the means and methods generally used by (health care providers) of *ordinary* skill and learning in the practice of (their) profession" (Levin and Levin, 1979). For example, the courts do not expect a family physician who stops at the scene of an accident to be able to treat a traumatized victim with the skill of a surgeon. However, if the family physician moonlights in an emergency department, patients treated in that facility should receive the same standard of care from the family physician as from a full-time emergency physician.

Once a duty (contract) to provide care has been established, it must be proved that a *breach* of duty *(negligence)* occurred. Theoretically, with respect to cardiopulmonary resuscitation, a physician might be tried for failure to attempt resuscitation, for improper resuscitation, or for resuscitation against a patient's will—although none of these claims have yet been brought to trial (Hashimoto, 1985).

A case for malpractice cannot be made on the basis of negligence alone. The patient must also suffer some injury, and a *direct causal relationship* must exist between the negligent act and the injury. If all practical precautions were taken, the fact that someone was harmed or injured does not necessarily mean that there was a breach of duty.

The Right to Refuse Treatment

The Bill of Rights adopted by the American Hospital Association recognizes the right of *competent* patients to informed consent. The term *informed consent* is used to convey that a patient has been provided with a reasonable explanation (in language that *they* can understand) of the state of their medical condition. In addition, the patient must be advised of potential diagnostic procedures and treatment alternatives along with the purpose, potential benefits, and risks of each.

The following conditions are viewed by the courts as indicative of sufficient competency to render **informed consent** (Farnsworth, 1989):

   i. The patient should have an adequate understanding of their medical condition.

ii. They should also have an adequate understanding of available therapeutic options, including awareness of the implications and potential consequences from choosing any of these options.

iii. Finally, the patient should be willing and able to make a reasonable choice from the various therapeutic options available.

Clarity is not necessarily needed for competency. Thus a patient could be considered competent enough to refuse a treatment despite some degree of temporal disorientation (i.e., not knowing the day of the week) or not knowing the name of the current president of the United States. Competency is a *dynamic* concept. Patients who lack the capacity to make medical decisions at one point in time may become perfectly capable of directing their care at some later point in time.

Assessment of a patient's competency must also take into account the complexity of the decision to be made. Thus, a patient with marginal mental capability might be able to provide informed consent for antibiotic treatment of pneumonia, but lack the decision-making ability to consent to a complex and potentially dangerous surgical procedure.

Traditionally, the following individuals have been considered legally *incompetent* to provide informed consent on their own: (1) severely retarded persons; (2) unconscious persons; and (3) young children (Drane, 1984). In contrast, acutely ill patients have generally been considered competent to consent to needed treatment even though their mental capabilities may be somewhat impaired by their disease process. Primary care providers should be aware of the fact that **psychiatric consultation is *not* mandatory for determination of medical competency.** Nevertheless, if doubt remains, or if potential conflict exists between the expressed desire of the patient and the family or health care team, psychiatric consultation may prove invaluable in ensuring that the patient's decisions are not unduly influenced by disease processes such as depression or psychosis.

> It should be emphasized that even incompetent patients should be encouraged to participate in their medical care decisions to the fullest extent possible. This is particularly important with decisions about withholding or withdrawing medical treatment.

A corollary of the doctrine of informed consent is that competent patients retain a near absolute right to refuse medical treatment and/or demand that ongoing medical treatment be discontinued (Beauchamp and Childress, 1985). To ensure medicolegal protection of the treating physician in the event of subsequent litigation, complete documentation of a competent patient's informed decision is essential if a medical treatment is withdrawn or withheld.

Advance Directives

One method that allows patients to preserve autonomy and self-determination in health care decision-making in the event of subsequent incompetency is the use of advance directives. There are two types of advance directives: informal and formal (Davidson and Moseley, 1986). *Informal advance directives* often arise when patients communicate their wishes about future medical care to physicians or family members. While these communications are helpful in determining the course of subsequent care, they often fail to completely clarify the patient's wishes in many treatment withdrawal situations.

Formal written advance directives (more commonly known as *"living wills"*) are very helpful to physicians in clarifying treatment wishes of the patient in the event they later become terminally ill and unable to direct their health care. Since their initiation in 1976, more than 40 states have enacted natural death act legislation recognizing the validity of formal advance directives (Cotton, 1989). Although legislation varies to some degree from state to state, most **natural death acts** share a number of common features (Areen, 1987; Marrin et al, 1990):

i. the patient must be competent at the time the living will is executed

ii. the signing of the living will must be witnessed (although notarization of the signing is generally not required)

iii. a properly executed living will becomes part of the medical record, and

iv. physicians making treatment decisions in good faith based on a validly executed living will can expect to receive civil and criminal immunity for their actions.

In many states, the living will becomes applicable only after a patient is diagnosed with a terminal illness and death is imminent. Specific types of medical care that may be withheld or withdrawn differ among the various state statutes. Some statutes allow withholding of "life-prolonging procedures," while others limit withholding to "extraordinary care." Withholding artificial nutrition or hydration is a matter of particular ethical, medical, and legal concern, and many states now specify whether these measures are among the medical treatments that may be forgone. Health care providers may therefore want to consult their hospital attorneys or risk managers for the special provisions of their state's natural death acts.

> Despite the advantages of a living will and the strongly supportive attitude of most physicians toward this document, the living will had only rarely been used in clinical practice—until recently (Emanuel and Emanuel, 1989; Davidson et al, 1989). Many hospitals simply chose not to routinely inquire as to whether patients admitted to their institution had ever made out a living will. Instead, *they required the PATIENT to*

assume responsibility for notifying the hospital if an advance directive had been filled out (McCray and Botkin, 1989). Despite the fact that many (most?) elderly patients have definite preferences regarding the use of life-sustaining treatment, when left to their own, a majority do *not* fill out a living will (Cohen-Mansfield et al, 1991; Gamble et al, 1991). Even when advance directives have been filled out, they all too often do not come to the physician's attention unless specific inquiry is made on the subject (Emanuel and Emanuel, 1989). In clinical practice, most physicians have not been in the habit of routinely recommending advance directives to their patients for a variety of reasons including the time required of them to adequately address the issue, lack of comfort in discussing the process of dying with their patients, and the belief that discussion on the subject should really be patient initiated (Zinberg, 1990; La Puma et al, 1991). Ironically, *it appears that patients and physicians each wait for the other to raise this sensitive issue* (White and Fletcher, 1991).

As recently as 1988, it was estimated that *less* than 20% of adults in this country had completed an advance directive (La Puma et al, 1991). In an attempt to improve on this figure and enhance the ability of the health care team to provide medical care commensurate with patient wishes, Congress passed the **Patient Self-Determination Act** in October of 1990. The Act officially took effect in December, 1991, and requires hospitals, nursing homes, and hospices to advise *all* patients at the time of admission about their *right* to either accept or refuse medical care—and to express their wishes in the form of an advance directive (La Puma et al, 1991). To optimize compliance with the Patient Self-Determination Act, documentation of active discussion on these issues must appear on the medical record of all admitted patients as a condition for approval of Medicare and Medicaid reimbursement—ideally with an indication that such discussion was carried out in a language that the patient could understand.

In addition to the living will, another type of advance directive that may assist the physician with treatment-withholding decisions is the **durable power of attorney (DPA)**. The DPA offers the advantage of greater flexibility than the living will, since the patient need not attempt to anticipate all future treatment dilemmas. Instead, the patient selects a **proxy** *decision-maker* to help with future decisions (in the event they are someday unable to make such decisions themselves). The proxy decision-maker relies on specific instructions from the patient and the general awareness they have of the patient's values and goals to guide future health care decisions.

> All 50 states have statutes recognizing DPAs, and at least eight states have separate statutory authority for durable powers of attorney for health care (Cotton, 1989). In addition, several states have provisions in their natural death acts permitting patients to designate a health care decision-maker in the event they subsequently become incapacitated (Areen, 1987).

Practically speaking, the optimal clinical approach to the use of advance directives is *combination* of the living will *and* DPA. Joint use of these two modalities allows the patient to specify personal treatment goals and instructions in the terms of their living will, thus providing autonomous control over future medical treatment options (such as ventilatory support or artificial nutrition). Extra assurance that their true wishes will be accurately conveyed to the

health care team may then be added by appointing a DPA or proxy designee. In situations specified by the living will, the proxy decision-maker would have clear and convincing evidence of the patient's treatment desires. In situations not specifically covered by the living will, the proxy could rely on other presumptive evidence of the patient's wishes under the circumstances (e.g., prior conversations or awareness of general values or goals).

> The tremendous importance of *written documentation* (IN the medical record) of *ALL discussions* with patients regarding life support measures should be evident from the above (Orentlicher, 1990). Meticulous compliance in this practice may be immensely helpful with legal documentation of a particular patient's preferences for life support (and may prove invaluable at some time in the future if there is no formal advance directive).

At least one court has endorsed the *combined approach* (using the living will *and* DPA) as providing presently competent patients with the optimal opportunity for preserving their decision-making autonomy in the event that they subsequently become incompetent (Browning v Sunset Point Nursing Center, 1989).

> An important additional (and often overlooked) benefit that may result from completion of an advance directive is the positive effect of this action in comforting patients and reducing their anxiety about the process of dying. Knowing that their specific wishes for life support measures have been clearly expressed in a legally recognized form is likely to go a long way toward maximizing the feeling that they retain at least some control of their ultimate fate (La Puma et al, 1991).

> It remains to be seen whether the Patient Self-Determination Act will accomplish its principal objective of improving the clinical utilization of advance directives. Because it eliminates the need for the patient to be the one to initiate discussion of the subject, the Act will certainly increase general awareness of the existence of advance directives, and of the patient's right to exercise autonomy in many of their health care decisions. It should also encourage greater discussion about the process of dying within families—which should ultimately result in improved ability of the proxy to represent the patient's true desires (La Puma et al, 1991).

Recently, several innovations have been suggested in an attempt to improve even more on the clinical utility of the living will (Brett, 1991; Doukas and McCullough, 1991). These include the **"values history"** (in which personal values and attitudes that might influence patient decisions about life support measures are elicited) and the **"Medical Directive."** In this latter document, the person filling out the form is asked to indicate from a checklist those specific diagnostic and therapeutic interventions they would want for a series of hypothetical clinical scenarios if they were the patient involved. The aim of this *detailed intervention-focused advance directive* is to try to anticipate specific clinical situations that might not be covered by the broader terms of a living will. While admittedly still subject to potential misinterpretation (since the *exact* context of any given clinical scenario is not completely predictable), these innovations may help by taking the process of determining patient wishes for life support interventions one step closer to the patient's personal perspectives about life, death, and medical care (Brett, 1991).

Ordinary Versus Extraordinary Means of Prolonging Life Support

As a result of the Cruzan case, *there is no longer any legal distinction between ordinary and extraordinary types of care*. However, because the area has been (and continues to be) a source of great interest and debate, we retrace developments leading up to the Cruzan case (which is further discussed in Section B of this chapter).

In the past, physicians had only been obligated to provide *ordinary* care. They were not bound to provide *extraordinary* care, and could withhold such treatment at any time. The difficulty was in differentiating between these two types of care. Historically, the term extraordinary care had often been used to refer to treatment measures that could not be applied without producing excessive pain, expense, or other inconvenience, and which did not offer much hope of benefit. Other definitions of extraordinary care were broader and included "life-sustaining" and/or other invasive procedures. Ventilators and vasoactive medications were viewed as extraordinary treatments, while oxygen, food, and water tended to be considered as ordinary treatments.

The question of whether artificial feedings should be considered ordinary or extraordinary care has also been greatly debated. **Paul Brophy** was a Massachusetts firefighter who suffered a subarachnoid hemorrhage in March, 1983 as the result of a ruptured cerebral aneurysm. He never regained consciousness after surgery and remained in a persistent vegetative state. Despite numerous verbal advance directives by Brophy to family members before the onset of his coma ("No way do I want to live like that" [Karen Quinlan]), the court initially rejected the family's petition to withdraw nutritional support. Ultimately the case was appealed, and in 1986 the Supreme Court of Massachusetts reversed the trial court decision by finally allowing Mr. Brophy to die. This was the first time a court in the United States directly confronted the issue of withdrawing artificial provision of fluids and nutrition from a patient in a persistent vegetative state. A national precedent was thus set.

Shortly thereafter, the AMA Council on Ethical and Judicial Affairs rendered an opinion consistent with the Brophy decision stating: "Life-prolonging medical treatment includes medication and artificially or technologically supplied respiration, nutrition, or hydration. In treating a terminally ill or irreversible comatose patient, the physician should determine whether the benefits of treatment outweigh its burdens. At all times the dignity of the patient should be maintained" (Rymer, 1989).

Some had argued (as in the Brophy decision), that initial placement of a nasogastric or gastrostomy tube is a medical procedure—but subsequent care of that tube *once it was in place* constituted *ordinary* care. The AMA did not agree with this analysis, and argued that it was not the complexity of an ongoing treatment that defined it as medical, but the fact that the treatment had to first be ordered by the physician, then continually monitored by the physician, and at all times responded to by the physician were any complications to arise.

> Divergence in opinion among physicians has been prevalent as to whether feeding tubes represent ordinary or extraordinary care, and whether their use is principally aimed as a comfort-oriented (prevention of starvation) measure (Quill, 1989). Despite universal acceptance of patient preference as the most important factor in deciding whether to initiate artificial nutrition, permission for insertion of a feeding tube is rarely obtained from the patient (Smith and Wigton, 1987; Paulus, 1986; *Bouvia vs Superior Court*, 1987). This is because the patient most often is (has become) medically incompetent by the time the decision to institute artificial nutrition is made. As a result of the tendency of incompetent patients to pull out nasogastric feeding tubes, restraints are often needed to keep the tube in place (Quill, 1989). Lo and Dornbrand question *how a treatment which requires the patient to be restrained can be viewed as "ordinary" care (or as a "comfort-oriented" measure)*, especially when most such patients are mentally unable to appreciate how the feeding tube will benefit them (1989).

The only case of criminal prosecution that has been brought against physicians for withdrawal of life-sustaining treatment occurred in California in 1982 (Kapp and Lo, 1986). The case involved the legality of withdrawing ventilatory support and intravenous (IV) fluids from a comatose patient. Despite the fact that the decision to withdraw treatment had been made with the family's consent, the district attorney, acting on information provided by a hospital employee, initially ruled that the patient had been "starved to death."

In dismissing the case against the physicians, the California Court of Appeals, in **Barber v Superior Court** (1983) held that there was no legal responsibility to continue treatment that had become medically futile. In addition, the court rejected the contention that IV fluids were ordinary care which must always be provided. Instead, the court adopted the position advocated by the 1983 President's Commission that all medical treatments should be evaluated according to the relative benefits and burdens that they offer the patient.

In Florida, the husband of 75-year-old **Helen Corbett** was able to obtain a court order to discontinue the artificial feeding that was sustaining his wife. In this case, a Court of Appeals reversed a prior decision by a lower court and affirmed that "the right to refuse treatment is protected by both state and federal constitutions, and cannot be abridged by state statute."

In California, alert and competent **Elizabeth Bouvia** was granted the right to refuse nasogastric feeding by the Court of Appeals. "Who shall say what the minimum amount of available life must be? Does it matter if it be 15 to 20 years, 15 to 20 months, or 15 to 20 days, if such life has been physically destroyed and its quality, dignity, and purpose gone?" Thus the court supported the tenet that "the decision must ultimately belong to the one whose life is in issue."

Perhaps the greatest amount of publicity regarding this issue was associated with the **"Baby Doe"** case in Indiana (1982). Baby Doe was a severely defective newborn who died 6 days after birth when the baby's parents requested that physicians withhold IV feeding and forgo corrective surgery. Reaction to the case by the public and the Reagan administration resulted in a clamor that led to the Baby Doe regulations. A warning was issued to health care providers that withholding nutritional sustenance to a deformed infant is unlawful (Waldman, 1985). However, in June 1986 the Supreme Court revoked the Baby Doe regulations and ruled that the federal government cannot force hospitals to treat severely handicapped infants over the objections of their parents.

Among the key points brought out by these illustrative cases is that **withdrawal of *life-prolonging* medical treatment may be sanctioned in cases in which this measure reflects the desires of a competent patient or is in the best interests of an incompetent patient** (as determined by the treating physicians, the next of kin, and/or the patient's legal proxy). The premise for withdrawal of life support in both instances must be either that the underlying disease process is irreversible or that the purpose, dignity, and quality of life have been lost. Physicians are not bound (morally or legally obligated) to provide *futile* treatment in cases where no realistic chance exists to reverse the underlying disease process and achieve meaningful survival. Instead, it should be the physician's objective (and duty) to make the patient as comfortable as possible.

Although still in common use, the terms *ordinary* and *extraordinary* care are vague, ambiguous, and subject to great variation in their interpretation. As a result, it may be best to avoid these terms. Instead, confusion may be minimized by considering the po-

---

tential *burden* of treatment alternatives, and weighing this burden against the potential *benefit* that might result from such treatment. As emphasized, treatment is *not* indicated when the treatment is *futile* (i.e., when it has no potential benefit).

Despite the rulings of these case studies, withholding artificial nutrition from patients unable to feed themselves is still perceived by many health care providers in the emotionally laden terms of "allowing a patient to starve." This may be a misconception. Clearly, nutrition should always be *offered*. However, it is important to emphasize that artificial nutrition will *not* always be beneficial to the patient, and in certain cases it may ultimately add to pain and suffering by prolonging the dying process. *Patients who do not receive artificial nutrition are not necessarily suffering as a consequence of the lack of nutrition.*

> Yarborough stresses the need for us to preserve the right of a patient to refuse our offer of nutrition, especially when artificial feeding goes against that patient's expressed desires (1989). Forced feeding in such cases should no more be enacted than forced breathing. Viewed in this manner, the decision to withhold or withdraw artificial nutrition need not be as emotionally burdensome as many health care providers perceive it to be (Yarborough, 1989).

Brain Death

Brain death was first identified in 1959 when two French physicians described a condition which they termed "coma depassé" (a state beyond coma) (Pallis, 1982). The best known criteria for determining brain death are contained in the report of the Ad Hoc Committee of the Harvard Medical School. The report states that the characteristics of a permanently nonfunctioning brain are:

i. *Unreceptivity and unresponsivity*—"even the most intensely painful stimuli evoke no vocal or other response—not even a groan, withdrawal of a limb, or quickening of respiration." The patient is in an irreversible *coma*.

ii. *No breathing or movements*.

iii. *No reflexes*—absence of reflexes includes corneal and pharyngeal reflexes. There is no ocular movement, blinking, swallowing, yawning, vocalization, or evidence of postural activity. The pupils are fixed and dilated.

iv. *Flat EEG*. (One year after this report, it was decided that an EEG was not essential, although it could provide additional supporting data.)

As brain death criteria became more accepted, criticism was directed at the terminology and testing guidelines used in the above Harvard proposal. Today, 40 states have brain death statutes. Concern for the lack of uniformity in the wording of statutes has led several groups to formulate their own proposals for the legal definition of death and to encourage universal acceptance for their proposals. In 1981 these groups met to form a President's Commission for the Study of Ethical Problems in Medicine and Biomedical and Behavioral Research. The purpose of their meeting was to provide a model wording for a statute defining death. Their proposal, The Uniform Determination Of Death Act, states:

> "An individual who has sustained either of the following is dead:
> 1. Irreversible cessation of circulatory and respiratory functions, or
> 2. Irreversible cessation of all functions of the entire brain, including the brainstem."

Although deceptively simple in its terminology, much of the confusion on the issue might be resolved if this Death Act were to become law in every state (O'Hara, 1983).

Accepted medical standard dictates that when the *possibility* exists that the brain is viable, and there are no compelling medical or legal reasons to act otherwise, resuscitation should be initiated (McIntyre, 1981). Unfortunately in practical terms, it often is impossible for a health care provider to know whether compelling reasons for withholding resuscitation might exist at the time a cardiac arrest is first encountered. How can one determine how long the patient was unconscious before help arrived? Can information obtained from bystanders be considered reliable? Are there potentially extenuating circumstances (for example, drug overdose or hypothermia) that might respond to longer attempts at resuscitation? Is the patient pregnant (and could there be a potentially viable fetus)? Had the patient ever indicated their wishes by an advanced directive? As a result, the emergency care provider will usually be obligated to initiate CPR at the scene of a cardiac arrest. It will then be up to the physician to decide based on cardiovascular responsiveness (or lack thereof), whether or not to continue the resuscitative effort.

> Another reason for the importance of clarifying the definition of brain death resides with the **potential donation of organs** for transplantation from "brain dead" individuals who have no hope of recovery but whose organs remain viable. A recent survey by Youngner et al (1989) revealed that only 63% of responders were aware of the requirement for irreversible loss of *all* brain function before brain death could be declared. Others mistakenly believed that loss of cortical function alone was sufficient to satisfy criteria for brain death. While confusion among clinicians about the definition of brain death in a given case is often understandable (and may well be appropriate), it poses a real concern that potential organ donors may be overlooked because of uncertainty in diagnosis and/or fear of litigation from premature declaration of brain death (Wikler and Weisbard, 1989). Emergency care providers should therefore incorporate consideration of the potential for organ donation in their assessment of nonresponding patients, and seek expeditious specialty consultation as appropriate for making a definitive diagnosis as soon as possible.

Persistent Vegetative State

The clinical state of "brain death" (in which there is total loss of *all* brain function) should be distinguished from the *persistent vegetative state (PVS)*. The American Academy of Neurology (AAN) has recently defined this latter condition in a position statement as "a form of eyes-open permanent unconsciousness in which the patient has periods of wakefulness and physiological sleep/wake cycles, but at no time is the patient aware of him- or herself or the environment" (1989). They add that "neurologically, being awake but unaware is the result of a *functioning brainstem* and the total loss of cerebral cortical functioning."

Patients in a PVS are incapable of any voluntary behavior. Most such individuals retain the capacity to breathe spontaneously (since this is a brainstem function), but normal chewing and swallowing are lost (since these acts are voluntary and require intact cortical functioning). However, reflex withdrawal or posturing, movements in response to noxious stimuli, spontaneous eye opening, and even the utterance of unintelligible, instinctive grunts or screams may all be observed (Council on Scientific, Ethical and Judicial Affairs, 1990). It is important to appreciate that for many cases due to hypoxic ischemic encephalopathy, continued close observation over an extended period of time (of as long as 1-3 months) may be needed before the diagnosis of PVS can be made with a high degree of medical certainty (AAN, 1989).

Perhaps the most difficult aspect for the health care provider (and the family) to accept about PVS is the realization that these patients may survive for months (and even years) if artificial provision of fluids and nutrition is continued. According to the AAN (1989), these patients are therefore *not* "terminally ill."

What is the extent of our medical responsibility toward the patient in a PVS? Need artificial provision of fluids and liquids be continued indefinitely? Or can it be stopped? While still the subject of much controversy, the AAN Position Statement offers helpful guidelines in this regard. We summarize the concepts contained in that Position Statement and in the commentary by Munsat et al as follows:

i. Artificial provision of nutrition and hydration is a form of medical treatment. It is *not* a nursing procedure. As a form of medical treatment, it may be discontinued according to the same principles and practices employed for withholding and/or withdrawing other medical treatments. Such would be the case for a patient in PVS, since by definition there is no hope for recovery and medical treatment will provide no potential benefit for the patient.

ii. Patients in PVS do not have the capacity to experience (consciously perceive) pain or suffering because they do not have cortical function. They will therefore not experience hunger or thirst if fluids and nutrition are withheld, and will not experience dyspnea after removal of a respirator.

iii. Further medical treatment (including artificial provision of fluids and nutrition) may be withdrawn if:
- the diagnosis of PVS is secure
- it is clear that the patient would not want further medical treatment
- the family agrees with the decision to withdraw medical treatment.

iv. No major medical or ethical distinction should be made between the *withholding* and *withdrawal* of medical treatment. It is perfectly appropriate to institute intensive medical treatment during the initial phase of the patient's unresponsiveness before hopelessness of the patient's condition has been confirmed. Such intensive treatment for a period of 1 to 3 months may in fact be required in order to establish the diagnosis of a PVS. *It is equally appropriate to withdraw medical treatment* (including provision of artificial fluids and nutrition) *at a later time after confirmation of PVS has been made* (and after the family has had sufficient time to accept the permanence of the patient's condition).

Although it goes against the intuitive inclination of many health care providers, withdrawal of medical treatment is often a much more logical course of action than withholding the treatment in the first place. *This is because the ONLY way to conclusively demonstrate that medical treatment will be futile is by a trial period of intensive therapy and observation.*

References

American Academy of Neurology: Position on certain aspects of the care and management of the persistent vegetative state patient, *Neurology* 39:125, 1989.

Anderson RD: Legal boundaries of Florida nursing practice, Sacramento, 1982, RD Anderson Publishing Company.

Areen J: The legal status of consent obtained from families of adult patients to withhold or withdraw treatment, *JAMA* 258:229, 1987.

Beauchamp TL, Childress JF: *Principles of biomedical ethics*, New York, 1985, Oxford University Press.

Brett AS: Limitations of listing specific medical interventions in advance directives, *JAMA* 266:825, 1991.

Cohen-Mansfield J, Rabinovich BA, Lipson S, Fein A, Gerber B, Weisman S, Pawlson LG: The decision to execute a durable power of attorney for health care and preferences regarding the utilization of life-sustaining treatments in nursing home residents, *Arch Intern Med* 151:289, 1991.

Cotton P: AMA pushing living wills, guide to life-support use, *Med World News*, p 26, July 24, 1989.

Council on Scientific, Ethical, and Judicial Affairs: Persistent vegetative state and the decision to withdraw or withhold life support, *JAMA* 263:426, 1990.

Davenport J: Common questions about withdrawal of life support, *Am Fam Physician* 39:201, 1989.

Davidson KW, Moseley R: Advance directives in family practice, *J Fam Pract* 22:439, 1986.

Davidson KW, Hackler C, Caradine DR, McCord RS: Physicians' attitudes on advance directives, *JAMA* 262:2415, 1989.

Doukas DJ, McCullough LB: The values history: the evaluation of the patient's values and advance directives, *J Fam Pract* 32:145, 1991.

Drane JF: Competency to give an informed consent: a model for making clinical assessments, *JAMA* 252:925, 1984.

Emanuel LL, Emanuel EJ: The medical directive: a new comprehensive advance care document, *JAMA* 261:3288, 1989.

Farnsworth MG: Evaluation of mental competency, *Am Fam Physician* 39:182, 1989.

Gamble ER, McDonald PJ, Lichstein PR: Knowledge, attitudes, and behavior of elderly persons regarding living wills, *Arch Intern Med* 151:277, 1991.

Grey L: Death and dying: medicine and the law collide, *Generics* 1:19, 1986.

Hashimoto DM: A structural analysis of the physician-patient relationship in no-code decision-making, *Specialty Law Digest: Health Care* 7:7, 1985.

Kapp MB, Lo B: Legal perceptions and medical decision-making, *Milbank Q* 64:163, 1986.

La Puma J, Orentlicher D, Moss RJ: Advance directives on admission: clinical implications and analysis of the patient self-determination act of 1990, *JAMA* 266:402, 1991.

Lo B, Dornbrand L: Understanding the benefits and burdens of tube feedings, *Arch Intern Med* 149:1925, 1989.

Marrin A, Dewar M, Grauer K: Medicolegal aspects of withholding or withdrawing artificial life support, *Fam Pract Recert* 12:88, 1990.

McCray SV, Botkin JR: Hospital policy on advance directives: do institutions ask patients about living wills? *JAMA* 262:2411, 1989.

McIntyre KM: *Medicolegal aspects of CPR and ECC*. In McIntyre KM, Lewis AJ, editors: *Textbook of advanced cardiac life support*, Dallas, 1981, American Heart Association.

O'Hara PJ: Medical-legal agreement on brain death: an assessment of the uniform determination of death act, *Specialty Law Digest: Health Care* 5:7, 1983.

Orentlicher D: The right to die after Cruzan, *JAMA* 264:2444, 1990.

Pallis C: From brain death to brain stem death, *Br Med J* 285:1487, 1982.

Pallis C: Diagnosis of brain stem death, *Br Med J* 285:1558, 1982.

Paulus S: Rasmussen vs Fleming, *Issues Law Med* 2:211, 1986.

President's Commission for the Study of Ethical Problems in Medicine and Biomedical and Behavioral Research: *Deciding to forego life-sustaining treatment decisions: ethical, medical, and legal issues in treatment decisions*, Washington, DC, 1983, Superintendent of Documents, US Government Printing Office.

Quill TE: Utilization of nasogastric feeding tubes in a group of chronically ill elderly patients in a community hospital, *Arch Intern Med* 149:1937, 1989.

Rymer TA: Courts differ on disposition of patient's right to die cases, *The Citation* 58:73, 1989.

Smith DG, Wigton RS: Modeling decisions to use tube feeding in seriously ill patients, *Arch Intern Med* 147:1242, 1987.

Stevens MB: Withholding resuscitation, *Am Fam Physician* 33:207, 1986.

Waldman JS: Termination of life-support for newborns: whose choice is it anyway? *Florida Bar Journal*, October 1985.

White ML, Fletcher JC: The patient self-determination act: on balance, more help than hindrance, *JAMA* 266:410, 1991.

Wikler D, Weisbard AJ: Appropriate confusion over "brain death," *JAMA* 261:2246, 1989.

Yarborough M: Why physicians must not give food and water to every patient, *J Fam Pract* 29:683, 1989.

Zinberg JM: Advance directives: do they provide direction? *JAMA* 263:1764, 1990 (letter).

Court Cases

Barber v Superior Court, 195 Cal Rptr 484, 491, 1983.

Bouvia vs Superior Court, 179 Cal App 3d 1127; 225 Cal Rptr 297 (Apr 1986).

Browning v Sunset Point Nursing Center, 543 SO2d 258 (Fla2d DCA, 1989).

RECENT CASE LAW AND STATUTES

Relying on family members to grant treatment consent for incompetent patients has long been customary medical practice. Interestingly, this practice has not had formal legal support until the last 15 years when a number of courts addressed the issue of withholding treatment from incompetent patients. *Review of these cases suggests* (with a few notable exceptions) *an* **evolving judicial standard** *allowing withholding of treatment from incompetent adult patients under certain circumstances.* Up until recently, all of these cases had been argued at the state court level. With the ruling in the Cruzan decision, the United States Supreme Court has now also become involved in a "right-to-die" issue.

The Case of Karen Quinlan

Very few court cases attracted the media exposure and public attention that the Karen Quinlan case did in 1976. As the result of severe anoxic injury, this 21-year-old woman became comatose and remained in a vegetative state. Purposeful function was nonexistent. However, Karen was not brain dead and continued to exhibit spontaneous, involuntary movements including yawns, facial grimaces, chewing, and eye opening. Karen's father petitioned the courts to terminate life support. After much deliberation, the courts finally consented and allowed the ventilator to be turned off. Ironically, Karen did *not* die. It was not until several years after the ventilator was turned off that she finally passed away.

The importance of the Quinlan case is that the courts sanctioned withdrawal of life support from a patient despite the fact that brain death by the usual criteria was not present. In addition, by granting Karen's family, her treating physician, and a hospital-appointed ethics committee the right to disconnect her ventilator, the court appeared to be defining a legally acceptable medical standard for future decision-making under similar circumstances (Annas, 1982).

The Case of Joseph Saikewicz

This decision-making standard was jeopardized by the ruling in the case of Joseph Saikewicz. Mr. Saikewicz was a 67-year-old mentally incompetent man who had lived most of his life as a ward of the state of Massachusetts. Severely retarded from birth, Mr. Saikewicz never learned to speak, although he was able to communicate through grunts and gestures. In April 1976, he was found to have acute myeloblastic leukemia. The question arose as to whether full treatment with chemotherapy should be given.

Mr. Saikewicz would certainly not have understood the reason or potential benefits to be derived from such therapy. In addition, he would have had to be restrained to receive such treatment and would be subjected to much pain during the course of therapy. Even with maximal treatment, prognosis for his condition would be poor. As a result, the courts allowed chemotherapy to be withheld, and Mr. Saikewicz died quietly of pneumonia shortly thereafter.

Upholding the probate court's decision, the Massachusetts Supreme Court considered the following state (societal) interests that might require that treatment be continued:

   i. the preservation of life
   ii. the protection of innocent third parties
   iii. the prevention of suicide, and
   iv. the maintenance of the ethical integrity of the medical profession.

Finding none of these factors sufficiently compelling to override the right of both competent and incompetent patients to direct the course of their own medical care, the court approved the decision to forgo chemotherapy.

> Saikewicz departed from the Quinlan recommendation that treatment-withholding decisions were best left to the medical profession in consultation with the patient's family. Instead, the probate court was identified as the proper decision-maker, with input from the family, the guardian, and attending physician.

In spite of the medicolegal uncertainty generated by the Saikewicz decision (suggesting the need to seek judicial review of withdrawal decisions), a number of positive outcomes did result. Patients' rights to refuse life-sustaining treatment were strengthened and extended to include *incompetent* patients since "the value of human dignity extends to both (the competent and incompetent)" (Annas, 1982). In addition, the theory of *substituted judgment* was introduced by the Quinlan and Saikewicz cases. According to this theory, a proxy decision-maker could speak for an incompetent patient on the basis of what the proxy feels the incompetent would decide were he or she competent. In the Quinlan case, Karen's father was appointed her legal guardian and allowed to speak for her. The situation was more difficult in the Saikewicz decision because the patient had never been competent. Under these circumstances, the court decided to speak for the patient. It ruled that if Joseph had been competent he would have decided against the painful side effects of chemotherapy which offered little hope for cure or relief from his illness.

DNR Orders: The Case of Shirley Dinnerstein

The Dinnerstein case of 1978 was important in clarifying some of the confusion raised by the Saikewicz decision. Shirley Dinnerstein was a 67-year old woman with Alzheimer's disease who developed a stroke that left her paralyzed on the left side. At the time of the trial, she was bedbound, unable to speak, and being fed by nasogastric tube. Mrs. Dinnerstein's husband and physician both felt she should be conferred DNR status. However, in the wake of the Saikewicz decision (which suggested that *only* the courts could decide if medical care was to be withheld from a patient), the hospital feared legal retribution and refused to allow DNR orders to be written.

The court supported the request of Mrs. Dinnerstein's husband and her physician to write the DNR order. This was the first time such an order had ever been asked for. The court noted that the Saikewicz decision had been . . .

> " . . . (mis)interpreted by some in the medical profession as casting doubt upon the lawfulness of an order (from the physician) not to attempt resuscitation of an incompetent, terminally ill patient . . . and that legally requiring resuscitation of all terminally ill patients, without exercise of medical judgement, is a pointless, even cruel, prolongation of the act of dying."

Thus the court affirmed the legitimacy of physicians withholding resuscitation for certain types of patients without judicial review.

> Withholding resuscitation "presents a question peculiarly within the competence of the medical profession of what measures are appropriate to ease the imminent passing of an irreversibly terminally ill patient in light of the patient's history and condition and the wishes of her family."

As a result of the Dinnerstein decision, physicians were asked to come to court only if they proposed to withhold therapies designed to restore a patient to a normal, cognitive life. The question of chemotherapy in the Saikewicz case is an example of such a therapy. In contrast, performing CPR on Shirley Dinnerstein would do nothing to restore her to a normal existence.

The Case of John Storar

The decision reached in the John Storar case of 1980 contrasted further with the Saikewicz decision. Storar, like Saikewicz, was a lifelong incompetent. At the age of 52, he was diagnosed as having bladder cancer that soon metastasized widely. As a result of extensive bleeding from the urinary tract, blood transfusions were required. However, within several months his mother requested that the transfusions be stopped since her son's condition was terminal and treatment only seemed to prolong his suffering. Because the director of the state facility where John stayed disagreed, the case came to trial. Although the lower court

initially ruled in favor of Mrs. Storar, the New York Court of Appeals reversed this decision. The higher court ruled that *since John was incompetent from birth, there was no way that anyone* (including his mother) *could know for sure what he would have wanted if he were competent.* Legally, therefore, he has to be treated as a child and should be given rights commensurate with his mental age of 18 months. This meant that not even his parents could refuse life-saving therapy for him, especially when such therapy was not unduly burdensome (i.e., there would be minimal pain or discomfort from the blood transfusions that were contemplated).

The Case of Nancy Cruzan

In December 1989, the United States Supreme Court was presented with its first "right-to-die" case. It involved the decision of whether to remove a gastrostomy tube from 32-year-old Nancy Cruzan, who was in a persistent vegetative state. In 1983, Ms. Cruzan sustained severe anoxic brain damage as the sequelae of injuries acquired in an automobile accident. After years of vegetative existence, Ms. Cruzan's parents petitioned the Missouri courts for permission to remove her gastrostomy tube. Although the lower court initially granted permission for this, the Missouri Supreme Court later overruled that decision, affirming the sanctity of life by stating "the state's interest is not in quality of life. . . . Instead, the state's interest is in life; that interest is unqualified" (*Cruzan v Harmon*, 1988). The Missouri constitution did not recognize the right of privacy; it therefore refused to uphold the right of a patient who was not terminal to discontinue life prolonging medical treatment. It also rejected the request by Ms. Cruzan's parents because it felt that they couldn't provide "clear and convincing" evidence of Nancy Cruzan's preferences—despite the statement by her parents that they "knew in their hearts that Nancy would not want to continue to live in her condition" (Lo et al, 1990). Instead, the Missouri Supreme Court placed the state's interest in preservation of life ahead of a patient's liberty right. It avoided ruling on whether use of a gastrostomy tube was a medical treatment, but did state that "common sense tells us that food and water do not treat an illness, they maintain a life."

The United States Supreme Court held that individuals have a constitutionally protected liberty interest in refusing unwanted medical treatment, and that *this right is not lost when patients become incapacitated.* The mechanism and procedures to effectuate this right for incompetent patients, however, was left to the individual states. In this particular case, the major roadblock was the Missouri state court's requirement for "clear and convincing" evidence of the patient's desires—a requirement not in the realm of possibility for many nonautonomous patients to fulfill (Weir and Gostin, 1990; Orentlicher, 1990). As a result, Nancy was to be kept alive *despite* consensus that she would not recover, and at a cost of "immeasurable anguish to her family and $130,000 yearly to the state of Missouri" (Angell, 1990).

> Although this Supreme Court decision disappointed many who were looking for a strong (and unified) national policy, at least it did not alter the situation in most other states where the courts permit (and encourage) surrogates to exercise the right of self-determination to discontinue medical treatment (including nutrition and hydration) when the patient is no longer competent.

Finally in December 1990, it was ruled that the parents of Nancy Cruzan could remove the feeding tube that had kept her alive for the previous seven years. Testimony of three former co-workers of the patient a month earlier that Ms. Cruzan had indicated she would not want to be kept alive in a vegetative state—in addition to prior informal statements made by the patient—led the ruling judge to conclude that there was "no evidence Nancy would continue her present existence, hopeless as it is, and slowly progressively worsening." The feeding tube was removed, and Nancy Cruzan died shortly thereafter.

Summary of Recent Case Law

Additional cases far too numerous to mention (and each with slightly differing circumstances) continually arise in various states across the country. For purposes of space constraints, we attempt to clinically correlate a summary of recent case law decisions as follows:

> *Physicians appear to be on firm ground by agreeing to withhold and/or withdraw life-sustaining treatment or resuscitation from competent, consenting individuals, and from those who have properly executed formal advance directives at a time when they were competent* (Marrin, Dewar, and Grauer, 1990; Orentlicher, 1990). Concerns about legal liability should not deter an otherwise appropriate decision to withdraw life-sustaining treatment. No person has ever been found liable for withdrawing life-support measures without court permission (Orentlicher, 1990).
>
> The Cruzan case notwithstanding, *physicians also seem to be supported by courts in the overwhelming majority of states for agreeing with a proxy to withhold resuscitation and/or withdraw life-sustaining treatment from terminally ill non-lifelong-incompetent patients.* As a result of the Storar case, however, legal recourse may be needed when deciding on these issues for lifelong incompetents. The courts imply that full treatment should be provided in this situation unless a court ruling says otherwise.
>
> In general, decisions regarding withholding or withdrawing of life support measures need not be restricted to cases when death is imminent, but apply

> to all terminally ill patients. *The key is having a clear understanding of the competent patient's true wishes, or of what the incompetent patient would want if they still were competent.*

Regarding the judicial system, *the courts neither require nor desire to be routinely involved in making the decision to withdraw or withhold nutrition and hydration when there is clear and properly executed documentation of a patient's wish for this directive, especially when the family and the health care team are in agreement.* Routinely involving the courts would be expensive, time-consuming, and extraordinarily cumbersome, not to mention that "too many patients have died before their right to reject treatment was vindicated in court" (In re Farrell, 1987; Weir and Gostin, 1990). As a result, most courts seem to have concluded that "judicial intervention is both unnecessary and counterproductive, except to protect the lives of nonautonomous patients who have no surrogate" (Weir and Gostin, 1990).

Regarding medical liability, the following court statement should be comforting to clinicians forced to act (and withhold or withdraw life-sustaining treatment) without prior judicial authorization:

> "Little need be said about criminal liability: there is precious little precedent, and what there is suggests that the doctor will be protected if he (/she) acts on a good faith judgment that is not grievously unreasonable by medical standards."

If anything, the risk of liability is increased if life-sustaining treatment is continued against the wishes of a competent patient or the surrogate of a nonautonomous patient (Weir and Gostin, 1990).

Regarding care of the hopelessly ill, a statement by the Ad Hoc Committee on Medical Ethics is encouraging:

> "The physician has a responsibility to ensure that his (/her) hopelessly ill patient dies with dignity and with as little suffering as possible. The preferences of the patient in regard to use of life-support measures should be given the highest priority. There may be circumstances in which the physician may elect to support the body when clinical death of the brain has occurred, but there is no ethical standard that dictates he (/she) must prolong physical viability in such a patient by unusual or heroic means.
>
> If a physician decides that the disease process or other medical condition that the patient has would not positively be affected by the initiation of resuscitative efforts—in other words, if resuscitative efforts would only prolong the dying process—then a decision to write a DNR order is ethically proper.
>
> When a DNR order has been written, the physician must ensure that the patient is as comfortable as possible. A decision to withhold supportive therapy, while ethically sound, may not be acceptable to some families for religious or other reasons. Their wishes must be considered but not necessarily followed. The physician must be the final arbiter in decisions related to a patient, placing the wishes of the patient above all other considerations."

An editorial by Fox and Lipton (1983) summarizes the factors which enter into the decision-making process:

> "Optimal decisions are made when the prognosis is certain, the patient's premorbid preferences are known, his or her view of the quality of life has been expressed, and the family is in complete agreement. However, the realities of clinical practice are such that this is not always the case. Sometimes the physician believes the treatment is futile, the incompetent patient's previous views are unknown, and family members insist that everything possible be done. Sometimes the treatment is futile, yet the physician, for whatever reason, insists on performing it over the objections of the family and nursing staff."

When conflict arises—assistance in the form of consultation with a medical ethicist, hospital ethics committee or legal recourse may need to be sought. Differences will continue to exist from one state to another. The emergency care provider would therefore do well to become familiar with the standard of practice in the area where he/she resides.

References

Angell M: Prisoners of technology: the case of Nancy Cruzan, *N Engl J Med* 322:1226, 1990.

Annas GJ: *Reconciling Quinlan and Saikewicz: decision-making for the terminally ill incompetent.* In Doudera E, Peters JD, editors: *Legal and ethical aspects of treating critically and terminally ill patients,* Ann Arbor, Mich, 1982, Aupha Press.

Fox M, Lipton HL: The decision to perform cardiopulmonary resuscitation, *N Engl J Med* 309:607, 1983 (editorial).

Lo B, Rouse F, Dornbrand L: Family decision making on trial: who decides for incompetent patients? *N Engl J Med* 322:1228, 1990.

Marrin A, Dewar M, Grauer K: Medicolegal aspects of withholding or withdrawing artificial life support, *Fam Pract Recert* 12:88, 1990.

Orentlicher D: The right to die after Cruzan, *JAMA* 264:2444, 1990.

Weir RF, Gostin L: Decisions to abate life-sustaining treatment for non-autonomous patients: ethical standards and legal liability for physicians after Cruzan, *JAMA* 264:1846, 1990.

Court Cases

In the Matter of Karen Quinlan, 70 NJ 10, 335 A 2d 647, 1976.

Superintendent of Belchertown State School v Saikewicz, 370 NE 2d 417, 1977.

In re Dinnerstein, 380 NE 2d 134, 1978.

In re Spring, 399 NE 2d 493, 1979.

In re Spring, 405 NE 2d 115, 1980.

New York State Court of Appeals Opinions Concerning: In the Matter of John Storar, *New York Law J* 185(63):1, 4-6, 1981.

In re Farrell, 108 NJ 335, 529 A2d 404 (1987).

Cruzan v Harmon, 760 S.W. 2d at 420 (1988).

SECTION C

A SUGGESTED APPROACH FOR DETERMINING CODE STATUS

Determining Code Status *Before* the Arrest

In an attempt to incorporate case law into clinical practice, we suggest the following algorithm for determining patient code status (see **Algorithm #1** shown in *Figure 18C-1*).

1. *IS THERE ANY REASON NOT TO RESUSCITATE?*

CPR is the standard of care for treating victims of cardiopulmonary arrest. Therefore, *unless there are compelling reasons not to initiate CPR, it should always be performed.*

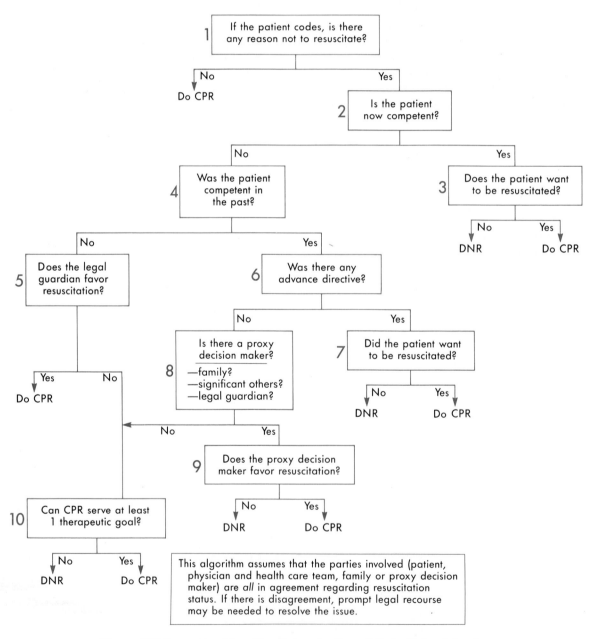

Figure 18C-1.   Algorithm #1—**Determination of Code Status** *before* the arrest.

2. IS THE PATIENT NOW COMPETENT?

If there is reason not to resuscitate, the first question to raise is whether the patient is *now* competent. Does the patient understand the nature of his/her condition? Are potential consequences of refusing resuscitation fully appreciated?

3. DOES THE PATIENT WANT TO BE RESUSCITATED?

If the patient is presently competent and states that he/she does not want CPR performed on them in the event of a cardiac arrest, the medical team is ethically and legally bound to abide by this wish. A **DNR** *("No Code")* **order** should be conspicuously written on the chart, and all members of the health care team informed of this decision. It should be emphasized that *an informed, competent patient has the right to refuse life-sustaining treatment even if the physician and/or family disagree, and even though the patient may not necessarily be in the terminal phase of a terminal illness.*

> The drawback of using terms such as "DNR" or "No Code" is that once they are written, the medical care team may become less diligent in providing other aspects of health care (Lipton, 1986). Stevens (1986) has therefore suggested the term "Care and Comfort Only (CCO)" be used instead, as this would remind all that *caring* for and *comforting* the patient must continue even if resuscitation is no longer indicated.
>
> It is important to remember that other interventions are not necessarily contraindicated simply because a patient is no longer a candidate for resuscitation (Table 18-1). *DNR does not mean do not care!* By the same token, it does not mean do not respond, relieve suffering, and provide symptomatic control (Donnelly, 1987; Fowler, 1989). Dying patients often suffer from nausea, vomiting, diarrhea, anxiety, depression, and skin breakdown, as well as from pain. Relatively simple interventions can often dramatically improve patient comfort while preserving patient dignity and respect without prolonging the dying process. Finally, *DNR does not mean do not re-evaluate* the patient's status. Clinical conditions are subject to change, and a DNR designation at one point may no longer be appropriate at a later point in time. Perhaps instead of DNR, the order should read **"ABC"** (for "**a**ll **b**ut **C**PR") to remind us that an order not to resuscitate has *no* implications for any other treatment decision (Bartholome, 1988).

Table 18-1

The Meaning *(and Non-Meaning)* of DNR
DNR ≠ **DNC** (**D**o **N**ot **C**are)
≠ **DNR**es (**D**o **N**ot **R**espond)
≠ **DNT** (**D**o **N**ot **T**reat, relieve suffering, and provide symptomatic control)
≠ **DNR**eval (**D**o **N**ot **R**eevaluate the patient's status)
DNR = **ABC** (**A**ll **B**ut **C**PR)!!!

An additional caveat to mention regarding DNR status is the lack of justification for performing a *"slow code"*—that is, less than intensive treatment for patients "not deemed worthy of full resuscitation." In such cases, lackadaisical CPR is performed only "for the record" or to reassure the family that "everything was done." Also known as an "intern's code," the "Hollywood code," or a *"light* blue code," this secret designation is circulated only among selected members of the hospital staff. Classification as a "full code" remains on the official hospital record. A double standard results with subpar efforts at resuscitation that are unnecessarily invasive for the patient, expensive for the surviving family, and which undermine morale, promote cynicism and conflict among the staff, and leave the clinician wide open to lawsuit. Improved communication with interactive discussion between the health care team, the family, and patient (if competent) about realistic expectations for survival, the implications of resuscitation attempts, and the maintenance of full supportive care throughout the patient's course comprise a far better approach than the deception inherent in performance of a "slow code" (Lo and Steinbrook, 1983; Perkins, 1986; Neher, 1988).

In contrast, should a competent patient request to be resuscitated in the event of a cardiac arrest, CPR should *almost always* be performed regardless of the patient's age, underlying disease process, or seemingly low quality of life.*

> Ideally the physician will have brought up the possibility of cardiopulmonary resuscitation with the patient *before* the event (and before the patient's illness renders him/her incompetent). Unfortunately this rarely occurs despite common acknowledgment by physicians that patients ought to be involved in the decision to be resuscitated (Davidson and Moseley, 1986; AMA Council on Ethical and Judicial Affairs, 1991). Reasons for avoiding the issue include physician discomfort with the topic, lack of knowledge about the types of advance directives, lack of time, lack of awareness that many patients want to talk about the possibility of resuscitation (and about their preferences for life-sustaining treatment), and the mistaken belief that informing seriously ill patients about their condition is usually harmful (Davidson and Moseley, 1986; Lo et al, 1986).
>
> It is estimated that between 15% to 33% of patients do not want to discuss DNR orders with their physician. This means that *well over two thirds of patients DO want to discuss DNR orders with their physicians* (Lo, 1991; AMA Council on Ethical and Judicial Affairs, 1991). When such discussion is carried out in a caring and compassionate manner, a majority of elderly and/or competent debilitated patients (and/or their families) opt for DNR (Youngner, 1988).
>
> Perkins (1986) has suggested a method for eliciting this sensitive information from the patient in which he proceeds with a line of questioning that begins in a non-threatening manner, gradually leading to more direct inquiry of patient desires.
>
> i. **Assess the patient's grasp of his/her illness:**
>   - What do you think is wrong with you?
>   - Have you ever been seriously ill before?
>   - What bothers you about being sick?
>   - What do you think will happen to you?

---

*The one exception to this generality is when in the judgment of the treating physician CPR would be completely futile. *(See discussion of Step 10, "Can CPR Serve at Least One Therapeutic Goal?")*

ii. **Define therapeutic goals:**
  - What do you like to do at home?
  - What is important in your life?

iii. **Probe for treatment refusals:**
  - Would you refuse any particular treatments in the event of critical illness?
  - Have you signed a Living Will (or other advance directive)?

iv. **Determine patient desires for resuscitation:**
  - Have you thought about whether you would want treatment if your heart suddenly stops beating?
  - How would you want decisions to be made if you became too ill to communicate?

The importance of discussing a patient's desire for resuscitative measures was emphasized in a recent study by Frankl et al (1989) which suggested that patient preference for life support depends closely on *patient perception* of ultimate outcome. Whereas an overwhelming majority of patients believing that life-sustaining measures could restore them to their usual health would elect to have such treatment, *less than 20% would elect treatment if they thought their ultimate chance for recovery was hopeless.* This finding once again underscores how *improved communication with frank discussion of* **realistic expectations** *about outcome (combined with assurance that continued supportive care will be provided) are the key factors in avoiding the need to initiate futile life-support measures.*

> Most older patients have formed definite opinions about the appropriateness of performing CPR for various clinical conditions (Miller et al, 1992). In general, such individuals greatly appreciate being actively involved in the decision-making process—which in itself becomes therapeutic by enhancing their sense of personal control in determining their fate (Kellogg et al, 1992). Given this chance to help with decisions regarding their fate—and given a reasonable chance for survival—older people surprisingly often opt in favor of life. However, older people are also inclined to significantly *overestimate* the chance for survival to actual hospital discharge following in-hospital cardiopulmonary resuscitation (Miller et al, 1992). Awareness of this disturbing tendency may help explain patient preference for performance of advanced life support measures in some seemingly less appropriate cases. It may also assist health care providers in targeting their approach to such patients in the most appropriate manner possible (i.e., assessing the patient's true desires for resuscitation, followed by frank discussion of realistic expectations for outcome).

How the questions are asked is everything!
Imagine yourself as a patient admitted to the hospital with an acute, potentially life-threatening illness. How might you respond to the following questions regarding your code status?

  i. *"Do you want us to do everything possible to save your life if your heart stops beating?"*

  ii. *"If your heart stops beating, you wouldn't want us to pump on your chest and put all those tubes down your throat to breathe for you—would you???"*

Murphy (1988) found the almost uniform (reflexive) response to the first question to be, *"Why of course Doctor, please do everything you can to keep me alive."* It is important to realize that a patient responding in this manner is not necessarily doing so with full understanding of their medical condition, adequate appreciation of what the resuscitation process might entail, and a realistic picture of the chance for ultimate survival.

In contrast, phrasing of the second question is much more likely to elicit a negative response. Of even greater concern is the negative connotation of the wording inherent in this question which may make the patient wonder how much (if at all) the physician really cares. It is easy to imagine how a patient might be made to feel abandoned by this question, and think that they had little to look forward to other than a painful death.

Consider another approach. As a patient, would you feel better if asked about your code status in the following manner?

  iii. "It's our intention to give you the very best care we can to help you recover—as long as recovery will be *meaningful* to you. This includes using the very best technology and medication we have available. If your heart stops beating, we'll try to start it with electricity and medication. If you stop breathing, we'll breathe for you by inserting a tube into your breathing passages and use a breathing machine to move air in and out of your lungs. However, at some time in the future we may reach a point where survival no longer is meaningful to you. Or we may reach a point when it becomes clear to us that even the best of medical technology and medication will not be enough to restore you to a state of health that is meaningful for you. *If ever we reach such a point, I wouldn't want to have to use those machines just to keep you alive. But before we ever get to that stage, I want to know how you feel about the matter. What would you like us to do?"*

Concern for the patient is obvious from this third approach. Additional reassurance can be provided by emphasizing that even if the decision is made not to perform cardiopulmonary resuscitation, every effort will continue to make the patient as comfortable as possible.

Can sedatives and/or analgesics be given to patients in sufficient dose to provide comfort after making the decision to withhold and/or withdraw life support? *Or is this illegal and constitute euthanasia?*

> Considering the dying patient's need for reassurance that pain and suffering will be minimized to the greatest extent possible, the answer to this question takes on paramount importance. Fortunately, the answer is YES! According to the accepted ethical principle of *double effect*, drugs may be given to relieve suffering (the *ethically permissible effect*) as long as the action intended by the health care provider is the ethically permissible one (i.e., relief of pain and suffering)—and that the ethically objectionable effect (i.e., hastening death) is not the intended means for achieving relief of such suffering (Jonsen et al, 1986). Thus, administration of analgesics and/or sedatives in large enough quantity to produce almost certain

death is unethical. However, administration of the same medications in doses primarily intended to prevent or relieve pain, agitation, and/or air hunger is ethical—even if the possibility exists that administration of such medications may inadvertently hasten the patient's demise (Wilson et al, 1992).

Ordering and administering sedatives and analgesics during the process of withholding and withdrawing life support are complex and difficult issues for which guidelines are *not* available (Wilson et al, 1992). It may be helpful for health care providers to realize that it IS ethically acceptable to hold "hastening death" as one goal of such administration as long as *this is not the principal goal*—nor the primary reason for giving such medication. That this situation occurs in practice was shown by Wilson et al (1992) in a study in which physicians were asked to indicate their reasons for ordering sedatives and analgesics for a group of terminally ill patients during the dying process after the decision was made to withhold and/or withdraw life support. Reasons cited for medicating such patients included relief of pain (in 88%), decreasing anxiety (in 85%), reducing air hunger (in 76%), comforting families of the dying patient (in 82%), and "hastening the patient's death" (in 39%). It is comforting to know that *in no case* was hastening death the only reason cited—and that in this small study, death did not appear to be causally hastened in any patient by administration of such medication.

4. WAS THE PATIENT COMPETENT IN THE PAST?

Competent patients enjoy a constitutional right to determine their self-destiny. Is this right lost once the patient becomes incompetent? Obviously not. The question that then arises is once a patient does become incompetent, *who decides?* The family? A legal guardian? The courts? Or the patient by means of an advance directive completed while he/she was still competent? (Marrin et al, 1990).

Thus, the first thing to determine is whether the patient was ever competent (and potentially able to express their wishes for treatment).

5. DOES THE LEGAL GUARDIAN FAVOR RESUSCITATION?

Patients who have never been competent usually have a legal guardian appointed to make decisions in their behalf. If this guardian favors resuscitation in the event of a cardiac arrest, then CPR should be performed.

6. WAS THERE ANY ADVANCE DIRECTIVE?
7. DID THE PATIENT WANT TO BE RESUSCITATED?

If the patient was competent in the past but is not competent now, it is essential to determine if an *advance directive* of the patient's wishes had ever been made in the past. Formal advance directives may be *instructional* or by *proxy*. The former includes the *Living Will*, and instructs the phy-

sician and the family not to use "artificial or heroic measures to prolong the patient's life if he (/she) cannot recover from a physical or mental disability" (Perkins, 1986). Proxy directives involve appointment of a *Durable Power of Attorney (DPA)* to decide about resuscitation status for the patient in the event the patient becomes incompetent. Unfortunately, all too often in clinical practice patients are either not familiar with advance directives, or they fail to make use of them.

Informal advance directives include physician notation of a patient's treatment wishes and family recollection of what the patient had said in the past (i.e., *"Please don't ever let them put me on a respirator"*). Although better than no directive at all, informal directives suffer from lack of proof of informed consent (they are not signed by the patient), and the fact that they are unlikely to be legally binding (Davidson and Moseley, 1986).

If the patient appropriately indicated by advance directive that he/she did not want to be resuscitated, that wish should be honored.

Occasionally, advance directives specify limited treatment such as "chemical code only" or "defibrillate but don't intubate." If properly documented (and written in the orders), such requests by the patient should also be honored.

> The obvious problem with indicating specific treatment measures is the virtual impossibility of foreseeing the multitude of potential developments as the code progresses. For example, should a patient designated for "chemical resuscitation only" be given continued doses of antiarrhythmic agents or a pressor agent for treatment of a ventricular tachycardia associated with significant hypotension? Or can we even say this patient has really "coded" yet, given that they are in a sustained organized arrhythmia (ventricular tachycardia) that *is* associated with a pulse? Cardioversion would be potentially curative in this situation, and one could conceivably justify this measure if one interpreted the sustained ventricular tachycardia as a "pre-code" tachyarrhythmia. On the other hand, if one interpreted the sustained ventricular tachycardia as a "code arrhythmia," the clinician would be bound to "chemical *resuscitation* measures only" and therefore forced to witness the patient's clinical deterioration before being allowed to intervene.
>
> Our feeling is to follow limited treatment directives IF they are appropriately specified and documented by a competent patient whenever this is feasible, realizing the virtual impossibility of foreseeing all circumstances. Clearly, clinical judgment on a case-by-case basis with consideration of the patient's true intent in the context of the clinical situation is needed.

The role of the family in the case where an advance directive has been completed should be to help "interpret" the patient's desires (*"Yes, that's what my father would have done"*), and to see that they are carried out. Even if a family member disagrees with their loved one's decision, the patient's wishes should still be respected.

> Reasons for involving the family in the decision-making process when the patient is no longer competent are that the family usually has the patient's best interests at heart, and that they are frequently in the best position to know what the patient would desire if competent. Because potential conflicts of interest may exist, however (due to feelings of guilt, financial

concerns, or simply becoming tired of caring for the patient), the physician must always assure to the best of his/her ability that the family is truly acting in the patient's behalf.

To repeat, when family is involved in making treatment decisions for an incompetent patient, **decisions must be made on the basis of what the patient would have wanted!** Emphasizing this to family members often goes a long way toward alleviating any feelings of guilt that may have resulted in a request for continuation of care that is futile.

Despite the fact that the family is often in the best *position* to know what the patient would want if he/she was competent, a study by Uhlmann et al (1988) suggests that *family members are all too often wrong in their prediction of patient desires!* In general, patient families and/or surrogate decision makers appear to be much more likely to favor selection of a DNR order than the patient would be (Quill and Bennett, 1992; Torian et al, 1992)—once again highlighting the tremendous importance of advance directives for determining true patient desires. Passage of the Patient Self-Determination Act (which went into effect in December, 1991) will hopefully improve on clinical utilization of advance directives (*see Section A in this chapter*).

8. IS THERE A PROXY DECISION-MAKER?

If the patient did not fill out any advance directive, it is important to determine if there is a *proxy decision-maker*. This may be a family member, a significant other, or a duly appointed legal guardian.

Health care providers often turn to the family for assistance in the decision-making process if there is neither a formal advance directive nor an officially appointed proxy, although there is no basis in common law to support this practice (Areen, 1987). Fortunately, an increasing number of states are accepting the medical custom of obtaining consent from the family to withdraw or withhold treatment for patients unable to speak for themselves (Areen, 1987).

9. DOES THE PROXY DECISION-MAKER FAVOR RESUSCITATION?

If the patient is not now competent and no advance directive was made but the proxy decision-maker favors resuscitation, CPR should be performed.

It should be emphasized that the proxy decision-maker should *never* be asked what he/she personally prefers for the patient. Not only may this question be burdening to the proxy, but it may also produce a conflict of interest. Instead proxy decision-makers *must respond with what they feel the patient would want* were the patient still able to express his/her desires (*substituted judgment*).

The role of the physician in the process is to help the family (or proxy) by defining the standards for making their decision (*"What would your mother want done if she were able to decide?"*).

10. CAN CPR SERVE AT LEAST ONE THERAPEUTIC GOAL?

The question of whether CPR serves at least one therapeutic goal is the *final common pathway* for several points on the algorithm. This entails the reasonable expectations for rehabilitation of the patient in the event that CPR is successful. Even though the patient may have a terminal disease, CPR would still serve a therapeutic purpose if successful resuscitation allows such a patient to return home to spend meaningful time with their family. In general, physicians tend to consider the quality of life of elderly out-patients to be significantly worse than do the patients (Uhlmann and Pearlman, 1991).

" . . . younger family members, nurses and even physicians have difficulty in appreciating the pleasure an elderly incapacitated patient may derive from very simple experiences and just being alive . . . An existence that might be intolerable at age 30 may be pleasurable at age 80" (Charlson et al, 1986).

Time is frequently more precious to elders because it is so limited. Surprisingly, a *majority* of elderly patients are willing to undergo intensive care to achieve as little as one additional month of survival regardless of their age, functional status, perceived quality of life, hypothetical life expectancy, or the nature of previous intensive care experiences (Danis et al, 1988; Torian et al, 1992).

In contrast, a patient with a terminal disease who is bedbound, fed by nasogastric tube, and in constant pain would probably not have any therapeutic goal served by receiving CPR in the event of a cardiac arrest. *CPR in this setting would be "futile," and should not be performed* (Blackhall, 1987).

It is important to try to understand if extenuating circumstances exist that might explain a particular patient's need (desire) to be kept alive for a finite period of time. For example, anticipated arrival of a family member, birth of a grandchild, wedding of a loved one, etc., are all events that might motivate a hopelessly ill patient to remain alive until the event has passed. All out efforts of the health care team to enable the patient to live to see the event would be justified in such cases, regardless of the patient's overall medical condition. It is of interest that terminally ill patients can sometimes delay their death for a short period of time until after an occasion important to them has passed (Smith and Phillips, 1990).

CPR is *not* benign. It should not be routinely performed simply for the reason that there is "nothing to lose." *There may in fact be something to lose*—namely development of a persistent vegetative state, which many believe to be a fate *worse* than death. An even more likely scenario is for the patient to survive initial resuscitation, only to eventually succumb after a prolonged course in the intensive care unit including numerous painful, invasive, and dehumanizing procedures (Blackhall, 1987).

"When an emphysematous nonagenarian lies on the floor, ashen, with a handful of nurses compressing his chest and breathing through his mouth, a sense of *futility* permeates the room . . . . (Is) this effort futile? And if it is, why do we do it?" (Murphy, 1988). That is, why do we "squeeze death out of the chest (eighty) times a minute?" (Konner, 1988).

Not all patients are candidates for CPR! If CPR holds no potential benefit for the patient (i.e., if it is ***futile***), *it does not have to be offered* (Blackhall, 1987; AMA Council on Ethical and Judicial Affairs, 1991). On the other hand, if there is a chance (however small) that CPR may restore the patient to a meaningful level of function, patient autonomy should be preserved (as much as possible) in deciding whether to perform this procedure.

Use of the term "DNR" (i.e., *do not resuscitate*) has probably contributed to the widespread impression that CPR works. As stated by Blackhall (1987), "CPR is a desperate technique that works relatively infrequently (with long-term survival from in-hospital resuscitation being no more than 10-20%), and in many types of patients, virtually never. To solve the ethical problems posed by CPR we must first face that medical fact." A more appropriate term to better reflect the poor success rates of in-hospital resuscitation might therefore be ***DNAR*** or **"D**o **N**ot ***A**ttempt* **R**esuscitation" (Brody, 1989; Hadorn, 1989).

> In general, the courts have indicated that they do not wish to become involved with DNR decisions except under special circumstances. Thus the physician should be on firm ground writing DNR orders for the incompetent patient if CPR will not serve any therapeutic goal and the family, significant others, legal guardian, and medical team all agree that DNR status is in the patient's best interest and is what the patient would have wanted were he/she competent.
>
> Should disagreement exist between any of the involved parties, prompt legal recourse may be helpful in resolving the issue. Physicians may feel more comfortable with *full* code status until either a consensus is reached, or a legal decision is forthcoming. Having stated this, it should be emphasized that no physician has yet been successfully prosecuted for withholding resuscitation deemed to be contraindicated because of "futility"—and that the AMA Council on Ethical and Judicial Affairs supports withholding CPR "when efforts to resuscitate a patient are judged by the treating physician to be futile *even if previously requested by the patient*" (1991).
>
> As previously discussed (the case of John Storar), an exception to this general rule is the procedure for the lifelong incompetent. The difficulty here is the impossibility of knowing what the patient would have wanted, since incompetence has been present since birth. Unless a "reasonable person" standard is invoked by the court ("What would a *hypothetical* reasonable person do under similar circumstances?"), full therapy should be provided for the lifelong incompetent.

The DNR Order

Evans and Brody (1985) have suggested that there are at least two widely understood goals for a hospital policy on resuscitation:

    i. To ensure that physicians decide on the medical and ethical appropriateness of resuscitation attempts *before* they are needed, on the assumption that a better decision will be made if it is made by the physician most familiar with the case, and if it is made without the stress induced by facing a sudden arrest.

    ii. To encourage the physician to discuss the situation with the patient (or the family of an incompetent patient) to determine their wishes concerning further treatment.

All too frequently in the past, both goals fell short. To improve the situation, these same authors have offered a number of suggestions, which we present with a few modifications:*

1. All hospitals with a heavy load of seriously ill patients should develop formal policies for DNR orders.
2. Such policies should insist that competent patients not be bypassed (as they all too frequently are) in decisions to write a DNR order, and that patients and their families (if appropriate) be involved in resuscitation decisions.
3. DNR policies should involve methods to help overcome physician reluctance to discuss these decisions with patients or families. (Consideration should be given to bringing up these issues routinely on admission to the hospital.)
4. The medical and ethical inappropriateness of partial resuscitative efforts should be addressed.
5. The order sheet for each DNR patient must indicate in very concrete terms which medical and supportive efforts will be maintained and which will not. Documentation should also be made in the progress notes of relevant discussions held with the patient and/or family, and of the rationale for such orders.
6. A mechanism must be in place for cooperatively resolving disagreements between housestaff, attending physicians, nursing staff, and families regarding DNR orders.
7. A mechanism should also be in place to assure that decisions regarding the resuscitation of any particular patient are reviewed frequently (ideally on a daily basis, or at least every other day).
8. Finally, *efforts must be taken to ensure that the decision not to resuscitate a patient does not affect other aspects of their care!*

Decision Making *After* an Arrest Is Called

In contrast to the decision-making process for determining code status before an arrest is called, the process becomes much more clearcut *after* the arrest is called. Alternatives of the health care provider are much more

---

*Implementation of these suggestions has been greatly facilitated by passage of the Patient Self-Determination Act (which officially took effect in December, 1992).

limited (as suggested by **Algorithm #2** shown in *Figure 18C-2*).

1. IS THERE A DNR ORDER ON THE CHART?

Practically speaking, about the only reason for not performing CPR once a cardiac arrest is called would be the serendipitous discovery of a heretofore unseen "DNR" order hidden *(written)* in the chart. Verbal recollections of what the patient said (informal directives) are unacceptable in this setting. Thus CPR *must* be initiated and vigorously pursued.

2. IS THE PATIENT RESPONDING TO RESUSCITATION?

If the patient is responding to efforts at resuscitation, CPR should continue.

3. IS THERE A REASON NOT TO CONTINUE?

If the patient does not respond to initial attempts at resuscitation, but no reason exists for stopping CPR, resuscitation should continue until there is firm evidence of cardiovascular unresponsiveness to competently delivered BLS and ACLS.

With respect to when CPR should be terminated in the Emergency Department, Eliastam has suggested a number of guidelines (1979):

   i. Apnea and pulselessness known to have exceeded 10 minutes
   ii. No response after more than 30 minutes of ACLS, including that administered in the pre-hospital setting
   iii. No ventricular ECG activity (asystole) after more than 10 minutes of ACLS
   iv. Preexisting terminal illness.

In contrast, Chipman et al (1981) feel it preferable not to use specific criteria for deciding when to stop CPR because

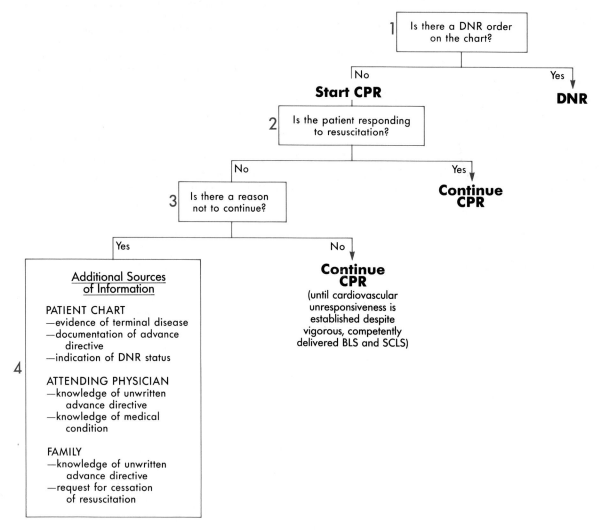

Figure 18C-2. Algorithm #2—**Resuscitation Decision-Making** *after* an arrest is called.

there are "too many uncertainties—clinical, ethical, and emotional—to subject this situation to standardized criteria."

Note should be made of the special situation of *hypothermia*, for which CPR should continue until the patient is "warm and dead" (Chipman et al, 1981). Case reports exist of children who have made full recovery without neurologic deficit following cold water submersion for periods of well beyond 20 minutes. (Other special resuscitation situations are discussed in detail in Chapter 13.)

4. ADDITIONAL SOURCES OF INFORMATION

As noted above, *once a code has started, resuscitation efforts must continue unless compelling reasons exist for stopping.* While in most instances nothing short of cardiovascular unresponsiveness should dissuade the code director from continuing with resuscitation, additional sources of information which come to light as the code is in progress (from the patient's chart and/or discussion with the family or attending physician) may sometimes prove invaluable in helping to make this decision.

References

American Medical Association Council on Ethical and Judicial Affairs: Guidelines for the appropriate use of do-not-resuscitate orders, *JAMA* 265:1868, 1991.

Areen J: The legal status of consent obtained from families of adult patients to withhold or withdraw treatment, *JAMA* 258:229, 1987.

Bartholome WG: "Do not resuscitate" orders: accepting responsibility, *Arch Intern Med* 148:2345, 1988.

Blackhall LJ: Sounding board: must we always use CPR? *N Engl J Med* 317:1281, 1987.

Brody H: Ethics and therapeutic skepticism, *J Fam Pract* 29:611, 1989.

Charlson ME, Sax FL, MacKenzie R, Fields SD, Braham RL, Douglas RG: Resuscitation: how do we decide? a prospective study of physicians' preferences and the clinical course of hospitalized patients, *JAMA* 255:1316, 1986.

Chipman C, Adelman R, Sexton G: Criteria for cessation of CPR in the emergency department, *Ann Emerg Med* 10:11, 1981.

Danis M, Patrick DL, Southerland LI, Green ML: Patients' and families' preferences for medical intensive care, *JAMA* 260:797, 1988.

Davidson KW, Moseley R: Advance directives in family practice, *J Fam Pract* 22:439, 1986.

Donnelly WJ: DNR: the case for early retirement, *Arch Intern Med* 147:37, 1987.

Eliastam M: When to stop cardiopulmonary resuscitation, *Topics in Emergency Medicine* 1:109, 1979.

Evans AL, Brody BA: The do-not-resuscitate order in teaching hospitals, *JAMA* 253:2236, 1985.

Fowler MDM: When did "do not resuscitate" mean do not care? *Heart Lung* 18:424, 1989.

Frankl D, Oye RK, Bellamy PE: Attitudes of hospitalized patients toward life support: a survey of 200 medical inpatients, *Am J Med* 86:645, 1989.

Hadorn DC: DNAR: do not attempt resuscitation, *N Engl J Med* 320:673, 1989.

Jonsen AR, Siegler M, Winslade WJ: *Clinical ethics*, ed 2, New York, 1986, Macmillan.

Kellogg FR, Crain M, Corwin J, Brickner PW: Life-sustaining interventions in frail elderly persons: talking about choices, *Arch Intern Med* 152:2317-2320, 1992.

Konner M: Becoming a doctor: a journey of initiation in medical school, New York, 1988, Penguin.

Lipton HL: Do-not-resuscitate decisions in a community hospital: incidence, implications and outcomes, *JAMA* 256:1164, 1986.

Lo B: Unanswered questions about DNR orders, *JAMA* 265:1874, 1991 (editorial).

Lo B, McLeod GA, Saika G: Patient attitudes to discussing life-sustaining treatment, *Arch Intern Med* 146:1613, 1986.

Lo B, Steinbrook RL: Deciding whether to resuscitate, *Arch Intern Med* 143:1561, 1983.

Marrin A, Dewar M, Grauer K: Medicolegal aspects of withholding or withdrawing artificial life support, *Fam Pract Recert* 12:88, 1990.

Miller DL, Jahnigan DW, Gorbien MJ, Simbartl L: Cardiopulmonary resuscitation: how useful? attitudes and knowledge of an elderly population, *Arch Intern Med* 152:578, 1992.

Murphy DJ: Do-not-resuscitate orders: time for reappraisal in long-term-care institutions, *JAMA* 260:2098, 1988.

Murphy DJ, Matchar DB: Life-sustaining therapy: a model for appropriate use, *JAMA* 264:2103, 1990.

Neher JO: The "slow code": a hidden conflict, *J Fam Pract* 27:429, 1988.

Perkins HS: Ethics at the end of life: practical principles for making resuscitation decisions, *J Gen Intern Med* 1:170, 1986.

Quill TE, Bennett NM: The effects of a hospital policy and state legislation on resuscitation orders for geriatric patients, *Arch Intern Med* 152:569, 1992.

Smith DG, Phillips DP: Postponement of death until symbolically meaningful occasions, *JAMA* 263:1947, 1990.

Stevens MB: Withholding resuscitation, *Am Fam Physician* 33:207, 1986.

Torian LV, Davidson EJ, Fillit HM, Fulop G, Sell LL: Decision for and against resuscitation in an acute geriatric medicine unit serving the frail elderly, *Arch Intern Med* 152:561, 1992.

Uhlman RF, Pearlman RA, Cain KC: Physicians' and spouses' predictions of elderly patients' resuscitation preferences, *J Gerontol* 43:M115, 1988.

Uhlmann RF, Pearlman RA: Perceived quality of life and preferences for life-sustaining treatment in older adults, *Arch Intern Med* 151:495, 1991.

Wilson WC, Smedira NG, Fink C, McDowell JA, Luce JM: Ordering and administration of sedatives and analgesics during the withholding and withdrawal of life support from critically ill patients, *JAMA* 267:949, 1992.

Youngner SJ: Who defines futility? *JAMA* 260:2094, 1988.

MEDICOLEGAL CASE STUDY

We conclude with a hypothetical case study that should "bring home" key concepts discussed in this chapter.

At the Scene

Imagine you are part of the paramedic team dispatched to the scene of a cardiac arrest. On arrival you find CPR being performed by the patient's son. The monitor reveals ventricular fibrillation. There is no spontaneous pulse. The son tells you that it took him "about 5 or 10 minutes" to arrive after his mother called, and that he has been doing CPR ever since. As you prepare to defibrillate the patient, the mother (the patient's wife) grabs your arm and asks you to stop. Her husband has already suffered three myocardial infarctions and "never wanted them to work on me again." *How would you proceed?*

ANSWER: *CPR is the standard of care for treating victims of cardiopulmonary arrest.* As long as there is the slightest possibility that the brain may be viable, resuscitation *must* be started.

With the exception of decapitation or rigor mortis, there is no expedient, reliable method for determining brain death at the scene of a cardiac arrest. The history that it took "about 5 or 10 minutes" before the son was able to start CPR is not extremely helpful since one has no way of knowing what the rhythm was during this period (partially perfusing ventricular tachycardia? or ventricular fibrillation?), and time estimation by the lay public during the stress of an emergency is notoriously inaccurate.

Despite the wife's request and description of an *informal* advance directive (he "never wanted them to work on me again"), EMS was summoned, and there is no evidence of any formal advance directives. The history of three prior infarctions notwithstanding, there is no evidence that the patient's prearrest condition is terminal. Thus there is really no choice for the paramedics other than to initiate and vigorously pursue resuscitative measures.

Currently, a number of states and EMS systems are considering formation of policies and procedures for pre-hospital DNR orders. As effective policies and procedures are developed, pre-hospital DNR orders may soon become an appropriate response for carefully selected patients.

In the Emergency Department

The patient is successfully defibrillated into a supraventricular rhythm with a pulse. He is intubated, an IV line is started, and the appropriate emergency drugs are given. The patient is rushed to the emergency department where the resuscitation effort is continued. Further discussion with the family reveals that the patient's health had deteriorated rapidly since his last admission. The wife states that her husband had told her time and time again how he no longer wished to continue living. She again asks you to stop the resuscitation. Although the son agrees that his father had been depressed of late, he still feels that "everything should be done" at this point. *How would you proceed if you were the physician in charge?*

ANSWER: "Once a physician-patient relationship exists, the physician has an obligation to initiate (continue) CPR when medically indicated and when DNR status is not in force" (JAMA Suppl., 1986). Thus you *must* continue intensive attempts at resuscitation.

Once you have started, the decision to discontinue resuscitation should be based on cardiovascular unresponsiveness (unless an appropriately completed advance directive that states otherwise is produced). In this particular case, the patient has responded to your therapy (Algorithm #2). As a result, resuscitation must continue.

While morally you may feel otherwise, "when the resuscitation decision must be made in an emergency, the decision must be made in favor of life" (Fox and Lipton, 1983). Despite disagreement among the family (and any personal empathy that you may feel for the wife), without a written DNR order, a formal written advance directive, or incontrovertible evidence of a verbal advance directive from the patient indicating otherwise, you are legally bound to treat in the acute setting (Algorithm #1). In this particular case, the conflicting viewpoints of the wife and the son complicate determination of the patient's true desires. It should be emphasized to the son that the decision to continue CPR must be based on what the patient (his father) *would want* were he still able to express his desires—and *not* on what the son wants.

In the Coronary Care Unit the Day After

The patient's vital signs stabilize, but he remains comatose. The wife continues to ask the staff to "let him go." The son remains cautiously optimistic that there may still be hope. A neurologist is consulted on the case. Although the patient is not yet "brain dead," the outlook appears dim. However, because of the conflicting feelings among family members, no DNR order is written.

Imagine yourself as the nurse assigned to the patient's care. As the medical resident in charge leaves, he informs you that the patient is "not a full code." Should he arrest, "we will just go through the motions." Nothing is written regarding this on the chart. Moments after the resident leaves, the patient goes into ventricular fibrillation. *How should you proceed?*

ANSWER: Unless specific interventions to be carried out are clearly spelled out on the order sheet and in the progress notes (that is, "Lidocaine for ventricular tachycardia" or "defibrillate but do not intubate"), no justification exists for performing a *"slow code."* Thus in this case you are once again bound to resuscitate the patient in a vigorous manner *despite* instructions to the contrary from the medical resident.

If a patient suffers irreversible brain damage and shows no sign of recovery, withholding resuscitation and withdrawing life support are reasonable options provided that the family, significant others, and the medical team all agree. Technically, the spouse is the appropriate decision-maker, especially since her wishes (to stop resuscitation) are based on her impression of what the patient (her husband) *would have wanted*. However, because of a conflict in views between mother and son, involving a hospital medical ethics committee (and if necessary, seeking legal council) may prove helpful.

In this particular case, although the overall outlook for the patient is extremely poor, brain death was not present, and adequate time had not yet passed for irreversibility to be diagnosed with certainty. Therefore, in the absence of advance directives indicating otherwise, continued supportive care of the patient was appropriate. In addition, a sympathetic approach toward the family combined with frequent updates on the patient's medical condition and involvement of a hospital social worker and/or psychologist may prove invaluable in helping the family work through their grief. Should significant disagreement between mother and son persist over patient disposition (and uncertainty remain regarding what the pa-tient's true desires for resuscitation would be), legal recourse may be needed to resolve the issue (Marrin et al, 1990).

As a final note, it is important to again emphasize that policies and protocols may differ significantly from state to state (and even from hospital to hospital within the same state). Health care providers are therefore urged to become familiar with the policies in practice within their own institution, and to stay abreast with changes in policy as they occur.

References

American Heart Association Subcommittee on Emergency Cardiac Care: Standards and guidelines for cardiopulmonary resuscitation (CPR) and emergency cardiac care (ECC), VIII, medicolegal considerations and recommendations, *JAMA* 255:2979, 1986.

Fox M, Lipton HL: The decision to perform cardiopulmonary resuscitation, *N Engl J Med* 309:607, 1983 (editorial).

Marrin A, Dewar M, Grauer K: Medicolegal aspects of withholding or withdrawing artificial life support, *Fam Pract Recert* 12:88, 1990.

INDEX

The letter *f* after a page number indicates a figure; *ff* indicates multiple tables; *t* indicates a table.